Metabolic Effects of Gonadal Hormones and Contraceptive Steroids

Edited by
Hilton A. Salhanick

Professor of Obstetrics and Gynecology
Harvard Medical School
Member, Center for Population Studies
Harvard School of Public Health

David M. Kipnis

Professor of Medicine
Washington University School of Medicine

Raymond L. Vande Wiele

Professor of Obstetrics and Gynecology
College of Physicians and Surgeons
Columbia University

METABOLIC EFFECTS OF GONADAL HORMONES AND CONTRACEPTIVE STEROIDS

Based on a Workshop held in
Boston, Massachusetts, December 1-5, 1968

⅌ Plenum Press • New York – London • 1969

First Printing — August 1969
Second Printing — March 1971

Library of Congress Catalog Card Number 71-89792
ISBN-13: 978-1-4684-1784-5   e-ISBN-13: 978-1-4684-1782-1
DOI: 10.1007/978-1-4684-1782-1

The Workshop upon which this volume is based was held in Boston, Massachusetts on December 1-5, 1968 and was sponsored by the National Institute of Child Health and Human Development and the Center for Population Studies of the Harvard University School of Public Health. It was conducted pursuant to Contract No. PH-43-68-1456 with the National Institutes of Health, Department of Health, Education and Welfare. Reproduction in whole or in part is permitted only for purposes of the United States Government.

A division of Plenum Publishing Corporation
227 West 17th Street, New York, N.Y. 10011

United Kingdom edition published by Plenum Press, London
A division of Plenum Publishing Company, Ltd.
Donington House, 30 Norfolk Street, London W.C. 2, England

FOREWORD

The Center for Population Research of the National Institute
of Child Health and Human Development began operations in August
1968 and is engaged in research dealing with health-related population problems. We organize and support projects for the development of new contraceptives and in the broad field of population
research in the social sciences.

The Center also supports a variety of projects dealing with
the mechanism of action and medical effects of contraceptives now
in use, particularly oral contraceptives and intrauterine devices.
These studies were initiated several years ago at the specific
direction of Congress. We were pleased, therefore, with the
opportunity to help organize and support this important and timely
conference on the "Metabolic Effects of Gonadal Hormones and
Contraceptive Steroids," the subject of which forms an integral
part of the Center's research program.

April, 1969   Philip A. Corfman
                                    Director
                                    Center for Population Research
                                    National Institute of Child Health
                                       and Human Development

PREFACE

Progress in science is often associated with either a "sixth sense" or an inevitable timeliness. Both factors, perhaps, led the members of the Endocrinology Study Section of the National Institutes of Health to propose, in 1966, that an expanded view of the effects of gonadal hormones, in general, and the contraceptive steroids, in particular, was needed. There had been ample evaluations of the clinical symptomatology, contraceptive efficacy, and effects on the reproductive system, but there was a dearth of information on their multiple systemic metabolic effects. Since approximately six million women were using the drugs, it was timely and important to examine the biological effects from the point of view of the laboratory and clinical investigator. A subcommittee was established, and for two years, the three members maintained a surveillance of the field. In 1968, they concluded that sufficient information was available to hold a conference on that topic, but it seemed premature to explore the carcinogenic potential of the contraceptive steroids and probably unrewarding to consider again the effects of these substances on the reproductive tract.

Dr. Philip Corfman, Director of the Center for Population Research, NICHD, encouraged us to proceed with the plan to hold a conference on these problems. In June, a contract proposal was funded for such a conference, which was held in Boston, December 1-5, under the auspices of that Center and the Harvard Center for Population Studies. Approximately 55 investigators were invited to present their experience in nine areas; these presentations constitute the contents of this volume.

In general, this volume is an attempt to collate and describe the known metabolic effects as well as to illuminate deficiencies in our knowledge. It emphasizes biological mechanisms and interpretations which supplement information acquired epidemiologically. For the most part, the findings are straightforward and non-controversial. In fact, the most convincing aspect of the reports included in this work is the consistency with which data were replicated in different laboratories.

Certain facts are clear: Not natural substances, contraceptive steroids should not be identified as such. Unique, synthetic compounds of diverse actions whether administered singly or in combinations and regardless of dose, route, or frequency of administration, their effects cannot be equated with phases of the menstrual cycle, pregnancy or pseudopregnancy. In the study of some effects, they yield dose-response curves; in others, they appear to produce quantal responses. Perhaps this is because threshold and maximal doses were not always achievable in these studies. In fact, after more than ten years of use, a dose-response curve for contraceptive action of steroids has not been demonstrated. Thus, in view of the qualitative and quantitative differences between the natural and synthetic steroids, we believe that semantic oversimplification which equates the pharmacological state induced by contraceptive steroids with biological states such as pregnancy should be abandoned.

Contraceptive drugs are not "equal." They are not equal biochemically, physiologically, pharmacologically, or psychologically. Modern chemical ingenuity has synthesized a vast array of steroid molecules and produced a comparatively thorough understanding of their chemical characteristics. Little is known of their metabolic function however. The limited structure-activity data available appear to indicate that it may be possible to separate some of the metabolic effects from the contraceptive effects. Steroids which have metabolic effects and are essentially devoid of contraceptive activity (e.g., cortical hormones), are easily obtainable, but no steroid with contraceptive action has been demonstrated to be without metabolic effects. We see a challenge of the future to free these drugs of unwanted effects and yet retain contraceptive action. Whether it will be possible to develop such a molecule (or combination of molecules) is moot; two of the editors do not believe that it is possible, one of us is more optimistic. Since such disagreements result from lack of knowledge, the acquisition of such information is imperative.

Some of the effects of the steroids appear to be idiosyncratic. Individual patients with such reactions should be identified in order to prevent unnecessary complications as well as to understand the mechanisms of the idiosyncrasy. Unrecognized disease, subclinical disorders, and inborn errors of metabolism are just a few of the conditions which may underlie the idiosyncratic responses.

Many of the metabolic effects are quite commonplace when looked for and the replication of these effects in different laboratories attests to this. There appears to be a consistent pattern: the physiologic reserve is challenged. When ample reserve exists, the effects are less marked; but when the reserve is decreased for any reason, the effects become prominent. It

appears worthwhile therefore to examine the reserve status of
patients' systems prior to prescribing such medications and to
plan re-examinations at measured intervals thereafter.

Throughout this work, the problems of species differences
became apparent because animal data play a prominent role. As
expected, dosages, responses, and even mechanisms of action may be
different in humans from that observed in lower animals. Nevertheless, many experiments cannot be done in humans, and often lack of
knowledge prevents extrapolation from animal models to humans.
On the other hand, animal data are important and except for the
relative sensitivities of human and animal, we are impressed more
with the similarities than the differences.

Until recently, the metabolic effects of the sex steroids have
been inadequately investigated or ignored. These accumulated data
and others suggest that no tissue or organ system is free from a
biological, functional, and/or morphological effect of contraceptive steroids. Many of these changes appear to be reversible after
short periods of treatment, but it is impossible to form judgments
on the reversibility of some of the changes resulting from prolonged administration. This question becomes more important daily
for the many patients who have already had long-term contraceptive
steroid treatment.

The most difficult question to answer relates to the serious-
ness of such changes. Many of the alterations are of small
magnitude and may not be of consequence to most persons under
treatment. In fact, cross-sectional studies may not demonstrate
the effects and longitudinal experiments may be necessary to reveal critical changes. Nevertheless, the consistency of research
reports on such findings rejects the possibility that they are of
no consequence and requires that certain questions be answered. Is
a person liable to the complications of diabetes if the glucose
tolerance curve is abnormal? If certain of the clotting factors
are elevated in the blood, does this imply an increased risk of
thromboembolism? Will alteration of the serum lipid profile
predispose to atherosclerotic cardiovascular disease? These
questions are not raised rhetorically, nor do they deal with the
semantics of words such as the definition of "health" or "death."
The problems are susceptible to scientific analysis by appropriate
long-range research programs and we urge this promulgation.

We are mindful of the tremendous need for new and better
contraceptives and of the impact on our society if the oral contraceptive agents were no longer available. We are also mindful,
however, of the potential hazards if we proceed with inadequate
knowledge. The debate of whether it is wiser to use the contraceptive steroids for "n" years or risk "x" pregnancies is not

relevant for a number of reasons. An intimate relationship
between individuals over a long period of time does not lend itself
to generalizations. Other methods of contraception are available
and are equally effective for many individuals. And, as has been
stated above, one cannot compare the physiologic state induced by
the contraceptive steroids to pregnancy in respect to hazards and
benefits. In the light of such dilemma, better understanding of
current methods of contraception and further development of better
and different ones remain urgent.

That our fund of knowledge is meager is clear from many of
the articles in this volume. More work must be done and new
information gathered even though, at times, it might not always
appear to be "mission-oriented." Nevertheless, we believe that
this collection of information demonstrates that free and independent investigation, performed out of scientific curiosity, has
prompt and significant rewards and is, indeed, relevant to the
problem at hand.

Many persons contributed to the planning and execution of the
meeting. We are especially indebted to the introductory speakers
in each session who played major roles in planning their sessions.
These investigators are: Attallah Kappas, Paul Beck, Edwin Beirman,
Ulysses Seal, Myron Stein, John Laragh, Louis Avioli, Anthony
Fletcher, and Bert Kopell. Chief responsibility for the administration of the conference and this volume rested with Miss Marie
MacDonald. Without her efforts, the meeting might still be in the
planning stages. A number of other persons from the Harvard
Center for Population Studies contributed unstintingly in prepar-
ing bibliographies, monitoring tapes, preparing slides, arranging
for the recording equipment, and in numerous other ways. For this
help, we are indebted to Miss Wilma Winters, Librarian, Dr. Henry
Vaillant, Dr. and Mrs. E. Noel McIntosh, Sister M. Jean Wallace,
C.S.C., and Dr. Clayton L. Thomas. We are especially grateful to
Dean John C. Snyder and Professor Roger Revelle for their support
and the provision of facilities for the preparation of both the
conference and the manuscript.

April, 1969   Hilton A. Salhanick
                                                 David M. Kipnis
                                                 Raymond L. Vande Wiele

CONTENTS

PROTEIN AND AMINO ACID METABOLISM

RESPIRATION

DISCUSSION AND APPENDIX

PARTICIPANTS

Lilla Aftergood, Ph.D.,
Assistant Research Biochemist
School of Public Health,
University of California,
Los Angeles, California.

A. Albert, M.D.
Professor of Physiology
Mayo Graduate School of Medicine,
Rochester, Minnesota.

Irwin M. Arias, M.D.
Associate Professor of Medicine
Albert Einstein College of Medicine,
New York, New York.

Tage Astrup, Ph.D.
Director of Research
Institute for Medical Research,
James F. Mitchell Foundation,
Washington, D.C.

Louis V. Avioli, M.D.
Associate Professor of Medicine
Washington University School of Medicine,
St. Louis, Missouri.

Paul Beck, M.D.
Assistant Professor of Medicine
University of Colorado School of Medicine,
Denver General Hospital,
Denver, Colorado.

Edwin L. Bierman, M.D.
Professor of Medicine
University of Washington School of Medicine,
Seattle, Washington.

Stanley J. Birge, M.D.
Instructor in Medicine
Washington University School of Medicine,
St. Louis, Missouri.

Pieter Brakman, M.D.
Senior Investigator
Institute for Medical Research,
James F. Mitchell Foundation,
Washington, D.C.

Philip A. Corfman, M.D.
Director, Center for Population Research,
National Institute of Child Health and Human Development,
Bethesda, Maryland

Milton G. Crane, M.D.
Research Professor of Medicine
Department of Internal Medicine,
Loma Linda University,
Loma Linda, California.

Julian M. Davidson, Ph.D.
Assistant Professor of Physiology
Stanford University School of Medicine,
Palo Alto, California

John W.H. Doar, M.D.
Lecturer in Human Metabolism
Alexander Simpson Laboratory for Metabolic Research,
St. Mary's Hospital Medical School,
London, W-2, England.

Richard Doll, M.D.
Director, Medical Research Council's Statistical Research Unit,
University College Hospital Medical School,
115 Gower Street,
London, W.C. 1, England.

Eugene Eisenberg, M.D.
Associate Professor of Medicine
University of California School of Medicine,
San Francisco, California

Anthony P. Fletcher, M.D.
Associate Professor of Medicine,
Washington University School of Medicine,
4550 Scott Avenue
St. Louis, Missouri.

Edward H. Frieden, Ph.D.
Professor of Chemistry
Kent State University,
Kent, Ohio.

Robert H. Furman, M.D.
Associate Director of Research, Oklahoma Medical Research
  Foundation;
Professor of Research Medicine,
University of Oklahoma School of Medicine,
Oklahoma City, Oklahoma.

Ernest M. Gold, M.D.
Chief, Endocrinology Section
Veterans Administration Center;
Assistant Professor of Medicine
University of California School of Medicine,
Los Angeles, California.

Robert W. Goy, Ph.D.
Professor of Medical Psychology
University of Oregon Medical School;
Chairman of Department of Reproductive Physiology and Behavior,
Oregon Regional Primate Center;
Beaverton, Oregon

Theodore E. Gram, Ph.D.
Research Associate
Laboratory of Chemical Pharmacology,
National Heart Institute,
National Institutes of Health,
Bethesda, Maryland.

Richard J. Haslam, M.D.
Visiting Assistant Professor
Department of Pathology,
McMaster University School of Medicine,
Hamilton, Ontario.

William R. Hazzard, M.D.
Senior Research Fellow
University of Washington School of Medicine,
Seattle, Washington.

Robert P. Heaney, M.D.
Professor and Chairman,
Department of Medicine,
Creighton University School of Medicine,
Omaha, Nebraska.

Norman B. Javitt, M.D.
Associate Professor of Medicine
The New York Hospital and Cornell University Medical Center
New York, New York.

Albert L. Jones, M.D.
Assistant Professor of Medicine and Anatomy
San Francisco Medical Center,
University of California,
Veterans Administration Hospital,
San Francisco, California.

Ronald K. Kalkhoff, M.D.
Assistant Professor of Medicine
Marquette School of Medicine,
Milwaukee, Wisconsin.

Attallah Kappas, M.D.
Associate Professor and Physician
Rockefeller University Hospital,
Rockefeller University,
New York, New York.

Fred H. Katz, M.D.
Associate Professor of Medicine
Loyola University Stritch School of Medicine,
Hines, Illinois

David M. Kipnis, M.D.
Professor of Medicine
Washington University School of Medicine
St. Louis, Missouri

Charles D. Kochakian, Ph.D.
Professor and Chairman
Department of Experimental Endocrinology
Medical College and School of Dentistry,
University of Alabama in Birmingham,
Birmingham, Alabama.

Bert S. Kopell, M.D.
Assistant Professor of Psychiatry
Stanford University School of Medicine,
Palo Alto, California.

Stephen Krane, M.D.
Associate Professor of Medicine
Harvard Medical School,
Massachusetts General Hospital,
Boston, Massachusetts

Mary J. Kreek, M.D.
Assistant Professor
The Rockefeller University,
New York, New York.

John H. Laragh, M.D.
Professor of Clinical Medicine
Department of Medicine,
Columbia University, College of Physicians and Surgeons,
New York, New York.

John A. Luetscher, M.D.
Professor of Medicine
Stanford University School of Medicine,
Stanford, California.

Harold A. Lyons, M.D.
Professor of Medicine, Downstate Medical Center
State University of New York
Brooklyn, New York.

Richard P. Michael, M.D.
Reader Department of Psychiatry
Institute of Psychiatry,
University of London,
London, England

Rudolph H. Moos, Ph.D.
Associate Professor of Psychiatry
Stanford University School of Medicine,
Palo Alto, California.

Patrick J. Mulrow, M.D.
Associate Professor of Medicine
Yale University School of Medicine,
New Haven, Connecticut.

Bert W. O'Malley, M.D.
Head, Section on Macromolecular Regulation
Endocrinology Branch,
National Cancer Institute,
Bethesda, Maryland 20014.

Robert H. Palmer, M.D.
Assistant Professor of Medicine
University of Chicago,
Chicago, Illinois.

John R.K. Preedy, M.D.
Professor of Medicine
Emory University,
Atlanta, Georgia.

Clayton Rich, M.D.
Professor of Medicine
University of Washington School of Medicine,
Seattle, Washington.

David P. Rose, M.D., Ph.D.
Lecturer in Chemical Pathology
University of Sheffield
Sheffield, England.

Eugenia Rosemberg, M.D.
Research Director
Medical Research Institute of Worcester,
Worcester, Massachusetts

Irving Rothchild, M.D., Ph.D.
Professor of Reproductive Biology
Case Western Reserve University School of Medicine,
Cleveland, Ohio.

Hilton A. Salhanick, M.D., Ph.D.
Professor of Obstetrics and Gynecology
Harvard Medical School;
Member, Center for Population Studies,
Harvard School of Public Health,
Boston, Massachusetts.

Avery A. Sandberg, M.D.
Chief of Medicine C,
Roswell Park Memorial Institute;
Research Professor of Physiology and Associate Research,
Professor of Medicine, University of Buffalo,
Buffalo, New York.

Ulysses S. Seal, Ph.D.
Associate Professor of Biochemistry
University of Minnesota,
Minneapolis, Minnesota.

Daniel G. Seigel, S.D.
Epidemiology & Biometry Branch
National Institute of Child Health and Human Development,
National Institutes of Health
Bethesda, Maryland.

Chull S. Song, M.D., Ph.D.
Assistant Professor
The Rockefeller University,
New York, New York.

William N. Spellacy, M.D.
Associate Professor of Obstetrics and Gynecology
University of Miami School of Medicine
Miami, Florida.

Myron Stein, M.D.
Associate Professor of Medical Sciences
Brown University;
Director, Pulmonary Division,
Rhode Island Hospital,
Providence, Rhode Island.

Alvar Svanborg, M.D.
Head, Clinic II
Chairman, Vasa Hospital
Associate Professor of Medicine
University of Goteborg,
Goteborg, Sweden.

Raymond L. Vande Wiele, M.D.
Professor of Obstetrics and Gynecology
College of Physicians and Surgeons,
Columbia University
New York, New York.

Stanford Wessler, M.D.
Professor of Medicine
Washington University School of Medicine,
St. Louis, Missouri.

James W. Woods, M.D.
Professor of Medicine
University of North Carolina School of Medicine,
Chapel Hill, North Carolina.

Victor Wynn, M.D.
Reader in Human Metabolism
Alexander Simpson Laboratory for Metabolic Research
St. Mary's Hospital Medical School,
London, W-2, England.

OBSERVERS

For the National Institute of Child Health and Human Development:

    Ruth Crozier
    Center for Population Research,
    National Institute of Child Health and Human Development,
    National Institutes of Health,
    Bethesda, Maryland.

    Patricia M. Gabbett
    Information Specialist
    Center for Population Research,
    National Institute of Child Health and Human Development,
    National Institutes of Health,
    Bethesda, Maryland.

    Martin Peller
    Head, Reproduction Information Center,
    National Institute of Child Health and Human Development,
    National Institutes of Health,
    Bethesda, Maryland.

    Allyn Waterman, Ph.D.
    Program Director
    Reproduction and Population Research Branch,
    National Institute of Child Health and Human Development,
    National Institutes of Health,
    Bethesda, Maryland.

For the Endocrinology Study Section:

    H. Leon Bradlow, M.D.
    Institute for Steroid Research,
    Bronx, New York.

Morris Graff
Executive Secretary
Endocrinology Study Section,
National Institutes of Health,
Bethesda, Maryland.

Dr. Mortimer Levitz
Professor of Research Chemistry
Department of Obstetrics and Gynecology,
New York University,
New York, New York.

For the Reproductive Biology Study Section:

J.D. Biggers, D.Sc., Ph.D.
Professor
Johns Hopkins University School of Hygiene,
Baltimore, Maryland.

Kristen B. Eik-Nes, Ph.D.
Professor and Chairman, Division of Endocrinology,
University of California Medical School,
Los Angeles, California.

For the Food and Drug Administration:

Elsie R. Carrington, M.D.
Professor and Chairman
Department of Obstetrics and Gynecology,
Woman's Medical College of Pennsylvania,
Philadelphia, Pennsylvania.

Eleanor Delfs, M.D.
Professor of Gynecology and Obstetrics
Marquette School of Medicine,
Milwaukee, Wisconsin.

John J. Schrogie, M.D.
Division of Research and Liaison,
Bureau of Medicine,
Food and Drug Administration,
Washington, D.C.

Bernard St. Raymond, M.D.
Medical Officer
Bureau of Medicine,
Food and Drug Administration,
Washington, D.C.

Philip G. Walters, M.D.
Medical Officer
Bureau of Medicine,
Food and Drug Administration,
Washington, D.C.

For the Ford Foundation:

Anna L. Southam, M.D.
Program Officer
International Division, Population,
Ford Foundation,
New York, New York.

INTRODUCTORY NOTE

Much hard work by many individuals has gone into the preparation and publication of this volume. The participants, particularly, are to be commended for their willingness to take time from
their research to appraise and evaluate the metabolic effects of
the natural and synthetic steroids. The justification for their
hard work is the knowledge that the conclusions reached will be of
great importance -

to individual women and their families (millions in all);

to scientists seeking an understanding of human reproduction
and the control of fertility (far too few in number);

to industries engaged in producing the several combinations
of contraceptive steroids being used around the world today;

to physicians and other health experts who are seeking to
provide family planning and fertility control services to
people in many countries; and last but by no means least,

to public leaders, whether in or out of government, whether
in or out of religious institutions.

Wisely, the meetings were planned as scientific fact-seeking
sessions, not as public debates. It is also appropriate that this
responsible and dispassionate appraisal be made readily available
for independent consideration by others. My colleagues at the
Harvard School of Public Health and the Harvard Center for Population Studies are keenly concerned with this problem and join me in
support of this endeavor. Where there may be inaccuracies in the
findings, we hope they will be corrected; where there are voids in
our knowledge, we hope they will be filled in the near future. We
are confident that the reasoned approach to both scientific and
social problems is worthwhile.

April, 1969   John C. Snyder, M.D.
                                Henry Pickering Walcott Professor
                                  of Public Health
                                Dean, Harvard School of Public Health

LIVER AND GASTROINTESTINAL TRACT

SEX HORMONES, THE GASTROINTESTINAL TRACT AND THE LIVER :

INTRODUCTORY COMMENTS

Attallah Kappas and Chull S. Song

The Rockefeller University, New York, N.Y.

It is the purpose of this communication to serve as an introduction to the research reports which comprise the program of the
opening session of these meetings. This session is nominally devoted to a general consideration of the ways in which natural and
synthetic sex hormones influence the form or the function of the
gastrointestinal organs. As the subsequent seven papers in this
volume attest, however, the program has been limited to the presentation of studies dealing solely with sex hormone effects on
certain aspects of hepatic physiology and biochemistry, and particularly with those hormone effects on liver function from which inferences relevant to man might be drawn.

This emphasis on the liver reflects several considerations: a
limitation of time with respect to the program; a recent and increasing recognition of the significant alterations in liver function
which are associated with pregnancy or the use of ovulation-suppressing sex hormone mixtures; and the still sparse and anecdotal character of the literature dealing with sex steroid influences on other
organs of the gastrointestinal tract, such as the gall-bladder and
the gut (1-9). Except for the stomach there has in fact been little
interest evinced in systematically studying the possible effects of
sex steroids on the physiology of other gastrointestinal organs; and
what little information is available does not take a form from which
useful generalizations can yet be made. Nevertheless attention may
be called to several comprehensive reviews containing information
somewhat relevant to the nominal topic of the first session's program, i.e. sex hormone effects on the gastrointestinal system. These
reviews collate a large amount of data pertinent to the subjects with
which they deal and carry extensive lists of references to original
reports.

The influence of sex hormones on the metabolism of carbohydrates is considered in detail in the papers presented in a later session of these meetings, but the review by Haist (10) provides useful background information on this topic. Though dealing primarily with corticosteroid effects on pancreatic function and morphology, a good number of the studies quoted point to the existence of interesting related effects of sex steroids as well. These include for example sex hormone influences on the carbohydrate tolerance of man and experimental animals; on the hyperglycemic responses to glucagon; on the insulin content of the pancreas; on islet-cell morphology and histology, etc. No clear pattern emerges but the review is an excellent reference source for a variety of sometimes disparate sex hormone effects on pancreatic function.

The review on nausea and vomiting of pregnancy by Fairweather (11) covers the historical, epidemiological, pathological and etiologic aspects of this and the related clinical problem, hyperemesis gravidarum, the section on endocrine factors being of special interest. Although studies of the effects of sex hormones on esophageal and intestinal secretions, motility, etc., would seem to be a fruitful area of investigation in regard to these problems, little significant work has been done along such lines as is evident from this summation. The reasons for this are not clear, but they may be related in part to the usually inocuous and transient nature of the clinical problem which these symptom complexes present.

The most extensive studies done on the influence of sex hormones on gastrointestinal organs, other than the liver, have been carried out in relation specifically to the stomach, interest in this viscus being largely stimulated presumably by the obvious differences which characterize the course of peptic ulcer disease in men and women. These differences encompass not only the decreased severity and strikingly lower incidence of this disorder in women, but the ameliorative effects which pregnancy and, apparently, estrogens exert on the clinical course of the disease as well. The report by Crean (12) is a thorough, lucidly written review of the relations of endocrine secretions to gastric function, a good deal of the report being devoted specifically to the effects of sex hormones and pregnancy on the physiology of this organ. The mechanism through which a diminution in the severity of peptic ulcer disease is brought about during gestation or estrogen administration remains obscure, the evidence concerning effects on gastric acid secretion, etc. being still contradictory. The material presented in this review is, however, persuasive of the existence of physiologically significant and perhaps clinically meaningful actions of estrogenic hormones on gastric physiology. The paper provides in sum a rich source of literature citations, and constitutes an important reference work for those interested in this aspect of sex hormone pharmacology.

It is the liver which is probably affected in more ways and
with more regularity and intensity by sex hormones than any other
extra-genital organ; these effects encompassing such a spectrum of
sites and types of actions that they raise an important question
concerning the significance of the distinctions made between "primary" target organs of these hormones and those which are presumably
"secondary" in type. A collation of these sex hormone actions, and
the influence of pregnancy as well, on the liver of man and experimental animals has been recently published (13) and these effects
will not be reviewed in detail here. Such actions, however, reach
into nearly every biochemical and physiological system in the liver.
In brief, sex hormones can be shown to significantly influence the
synthesis of hepatic DNA, RNA and total protein including hepatic
cell enzymes, serum enzymes formed in the liver and circulating plasma proteins of various types. Extensive effects on hepatic lipid and
lipoprotein formation, on the intermediary metabolism of carbohydrates and on the activity of certain enzymes relevant to this process have also been demonstrated. These hormones further alter the
rate of chemical transformation and conjugation of drugs and other
substrates; and they have important influences on the formation and
composition of bile and on the transport into the biliary secretion
of numerous endogenous and exogenous substances.

Out of this spectrum of sex hormone actions on hepatic function
two have been chosen for particular examination in the research papers which follow. The first four papers deal essentially with the
excretory activity of the liver (14) and the effects thereon of synthetic and natural sex steroids. Figure 1 shows an electron photomicrograph of a preparation of bile canaliculi from the liver of a rat
obtained by a method we have recently devised (15). These biliary
canaliculi represent the intralobar segments of the biliary tree and
are characterized by a lack of a proper cell wall, their limiting
membrane actually comprising the membranes of adjacent hepatic cells
taking the form of microvillous projections of variable size and
number. These bile canaliculi are the most proximal intrahepatic loci
where various biliary constituents are transported from the parenchymal cells into the bile. Some of these substances, for example
bilirubin and the bile acids, are transported against large concentration gradients, and such active transport of biliary components
for eventual excretion into the intestinal tract constitutes one of
the major functions of liver cells.

It is clear from the material presented in the next four papers
that this transport function of the liver can be regularly and pro-
foundly impaired by a large number of natural estrogens as well as
certain synthetic estrogenic and progestational hormones. The mechanism of this sex hormone action on hepatic excretion is not yet firm-
ly elucidated but the effect undoubtedly finds expression in a substantial number, if not most, women during the course of a normal
gestation or during the prolonged use of synthetic sex hormones for

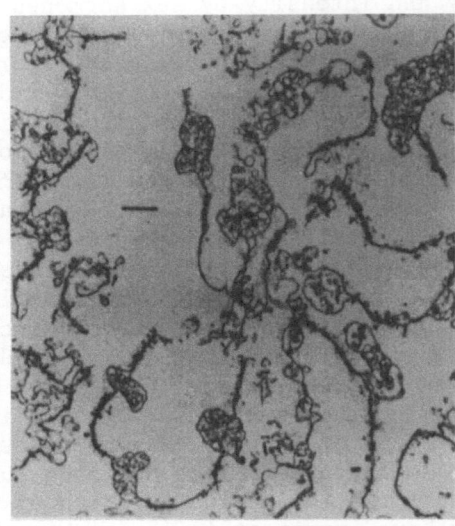

Fig. 1 Electron photomicrograph of a preparation of biliary
canaliculi from rat liver

ovulation-suppression or other purposes. It is not at present
clear whether the impairment in hepatic excretion induced by sex
steroids for dyes, bile acids and certain hormones extends to
other substances which are transported into the bile against large
concentration gradients, although it is reasonable to suggest that
this may well be the case. Such substances include of course a number of drugs in common usage and impaired biliary excretion of such
agents could thus have important pharmacological implications for
drug administration in pregnant women, and related susceptible
groups such as the early neonate (16). There has been to the present
little effort devoted to the study of this problem, but it is not
difficult to conclude, on the basis of the observations presented
in the following papers, that this may be a potentially fruitful
area of clinical and laboratory investigation in endocrine pharmacology.

The last three papers of the opening session's program deal
with certain sex hormone effects on the liver which are perhaps more
directly relevant to its potential capacity for effecting the detoxification of drugs. Figure 2 depicts the pathway by which heme is
synthesized. The rate-limiting step in this pathway is catalyzed by
the mitochondrial enzyme δ-aminolevulinic acid (ALA) synthetase.
This enzyme is usually produced at a low rate in hepatic cells since
the requirements of the liver for heme are normally small. In hereditary hepatic porphyria, however, a genetic defect leads to marked-

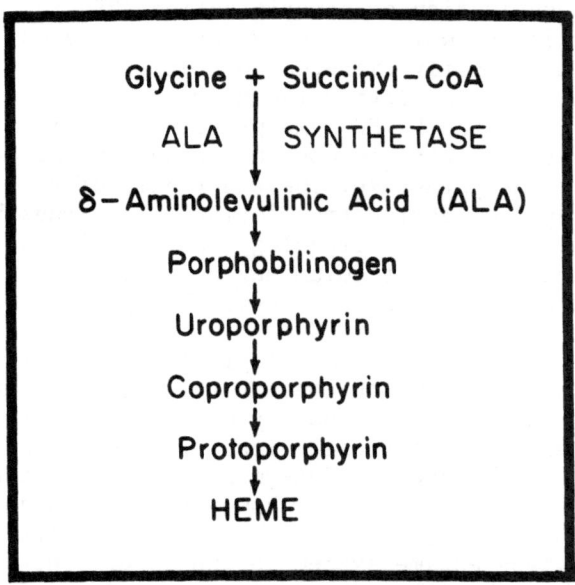

Fig. 2 The biosynthetic pathway for heme

ly enhanced synthesis of the enzyme and heme, as well as all intermediates in the pathway are formed at excessive rates (17, 18). The
enzyme is also inducible in the normal liver, so that enhanced production of ALA-synthetase can be evoked by numerous drugs and foreign chemicals (19). Of particular interest is the fact that such
chemical inducers of ALA-synthetase include not only a variety of
steroids natural to man, but also a majority of the synthetic steroid mixtures widely used for contraceptive purposes (20-22; Song
et al, these proceedings). This newly described enzyme inducing
action of natural and synthetic sex hormones has possible relevance
to the pathogenesis of hereditary hepatic porphyria of man (16). It
may also find expression in the population of apparently normal
women who have been shown to excrete higher than normal amounts of
porphyrins or intermediates in this pathway following the use of
contraceptive steroids (23).

This steroid effect on the liver may have even more important
implications than those related to the genetic disease porphyria.
Heme, the end-product of this pathway, is the prosthetic group of
the P-450 cytochrome, a hemoprotein localized in the endoplasmic
reticulum of the liver cell (24). This cytochrome is the terminal
oxygenase of an NADPH-linked microsomal electron transport system,
the primary function of which appears to be concerned with the oxidative transformation of drugs and certain endogenous substrates.
This oxidative transformation usually, but not always, results in

the biological inactivation or detoxification (25, 26) of the
substrate in question as well as its conversion to a more hydro-
philic and thus more easily excreted derivative. Chemicals which
induce ALA-synthetase can provide the extra heme necessary for
enhanced synthesis of the P-450 heme-protein and this microsomal
cytochrome usually increases in concentration concomitant with
the induction of ALA-synthetase. The end-result of this process is
generally more rapid oxidative transformation of drugs by the liver. Parallel changes in the morphology and certain enzymic activities of the endoplasmic reticulum may be associated with the
induction of the synthetase and the P-450 hemoprotein (25, 26).

Sex hormones which, in pharmacological amounts, induce ALA-
synthetase and the P-450 cytochrome may thus play an important
role in defining the overall capacity of the liver cell to chemically transform and to biologically inactivate drugs and related
substances. This role cannot be determined solely by the enzyme
inducing potency of these steroids, however, since such steroids
are known additionally to serve as substrates for this microsomal drug-metabolizing enzyme system in the liver. They therefore
also compete with such exogenous substances as drugs for oxidative transformation by this enzyme system (25, 26). This dual
role played by sex steroids as both inducers and competing substrates complicates an attempt to predict, without appropriate
study, the capacity of the liver to detoxify specific types or
single examples of drugs although certain data summarized here
(Gram and Gillette, these proceedings, and elsewhere [27]) indicate the occurrence of a net decrease in hepatic drug metabolizing
potential during late pregnancy and in the early neonatal period.
A definitive role for gestational hormones in determining the chemical or physiological background for these altered drug metabolizing activities is not yet established although it seems likely
that such hormones are involved in these changes to some extent.
Perhaps the single most important clinical implication of the material presented in the last three papers thus relates to the possibility that sex hormones and their metabolites can regulate the
responses to certain drugs by effecting changes in the rates at
which they are chemically transformed in the liver. The types and
mechanisms of such hormone-drug interactions in hepatic cells have
not yet been sufficiently explored in man, but it seems reasonable
to predict that the information which such studies will provide may
be of considerable practical as well as theoretical importance to
sex hormone physiology.

Finally, attention may be called to the fact that, with respect
to both of the major hepatic actions of sex hormones which are discussed in the following papers, hormone metabolites are shown to
manifest activities which in potency are equal to or exceeding those
expressed by their chemically unaltered hormone precursors. It is
therefore not inappropriate to again suggest (28,29) that some biolo-

gical actions which we now ascribe to primary hormones may in
fact be mediated, in part, by their chemical transformation products; and that the rates of conversion of primary hormones to
active metabolites and the rates of disposal of these metabolites
by conjugation or other means may be important determinants of
certain types of hormone actions. This idea is well known to pharmacology and may perhaps be of more general relevance to endocrinology than is presently supposed.

REFERENCES

1. Large, A.M., Johnston, C.G., Katsuki, T., and Fachnie, H.L.
    Amer. J. Med. Sci. 239: 713, 1960

2. Imamoglu, K., Wangensteen, S.L., Root, H.D., Salmon, P.A.,
    Griffen, W.O., Jr., and Wangensteen O.H. Surgical Forum 10:
    246, 1959

3. Mann, F.C., and Higgins, G.M. Arch. Surg. 15: 552, 1927

4. Kilpatrick, Z.M., Silverman, J.F., and Betancourt E. New Eng.
    J. Med. 278: 438, 1968

5. Ward, G.W., and Stevensen J.R. New Eng. J. Med. 278: 910, 1968

6. Watson, W.C., and Murray, D. Lancet 1: 65, 1966

7. Editorial, New Eng. J. Med. 278: 452, 1968

8. Mawdesley-Thomas, L.E., and Noel P.R. Vet. Rec. 80: 658, 1967

9. Livrea, G., Longo, G., and Giorgianni, C. Boll. Soc. Ital. Biol.
    Sper. 42 (24): 2053, 1966

10. Haist, R.E. Meth. Hormone Res. 4: 193, 1965

11. Fairweather, D.V.I. Amer. J. Obstet. Gynec. 102: 135, 1968

12. Crean, G.P. Vitamins and Hormones 21: 215, 1963

13. Song, C.S., and Kappas, A. Vitamins and Hormones 26: 147, 1968

14. Bradley, S.E. Harvey Lectures 56: 131, 1959

15. Song, C.S., Rubin, W., Rifkind, A.B., and Kappas, A. J. Cell
    Biol. in press, 1969

16.   Kappas, A. New Eng. J. Med. 278: 378, 1968

17.   Tschudy, D.P., Perlroth, M.G., Marver, H.S., Collins, A.,
      Hunter, G., Jr., and Rechcigl, M., Jr. Proc. Nat. Acad. Sci.
      53: 841, 1965

18.   Nakao, K., Wada, O., Kitamura, T., Uono, K., and Urata, G.
      Nature 210: 838, 1966

19.   Granick, S. J. Biol. Chem. 241: 1359, 1966

20.   Granick, S., and Kappas, A. J. Biol. Chem. 242: 4587, 1967

21.   Kappas, A., and Granick, S. J. Biol. Chem. 243: 346, 1968

22.   Kappas, A., Song, C.S., Sachson, R.A , Levere, R.D., and
      Granick, S. Proc. Nat. Acad. Sci. 61: 509, 1968

23.   Koskelo, P., Eisalo, A., and Toivenen, I. Brit. Med. J. 1:
      652, 1966

24.   Omura, T., and Sato, R. J. Biol. Chem. 239: 2370, 1964

25.   Conney, A.H. Pharmacol. Rev. 19: 317, 1967

26.   Mannering, G.J. In "Selected Pharmacological Testing Methods", 3:
      Burger, A. (Ed.), Marcel Dekker, Inc. New York, 1968, pp. 51-
      119.

27.   Song, C.S., Singer, J.W., Levere, R.D., Harris, D.F., and Kappas,
      A. J. Lab. Clin. Med. 72: 1019, 1968 (Abstract)

28.   Kappas, A., and Palmer, R.H. Pharmacol. Rev. 15: 123, 1963

29.   Kappas, A., and Palmer, R.H. Meth. Hormone Res. 4: 1, 1965

EFFECT OF ETHYNYL ESTRADIOL ON HEPATIC EXCRETORY FUNCTION OF THE RAT

M. Harkavy and N.B. Javitt

Gastroenterology Division, Department of Medicine,
Cornell University Medical College, New York, New York

Current knowledge concerning the effect of natural and synthetic estrogens on hepatic excretory function in man (1,2) and in animals (3) is based for the most part on changes in the rate of disappearance from plasma of compounds that are excreted in high concentration in bile. The increased retention in plasma of phenol-tetrabromphthalein disulfonate (BSP) and phenoldibromphthalein disulfonate (diBSP) (1-3) has been attributed to a decrease in the transport maximum (Tm) of these compounds from the liver cell into the biliary canaliculus. Since Tm was considered to be independent of bile flow, it has been inferred that the hormone interferes with the active transfer process. However, it has been shown by O'Maille, Richards and Short (4) and others (5,6) that the maximum excretion rate of BSP is enhanced more than two-fold by an increase in bile flow rate. Therefore, changes in the hepatic excretion rate of compounds that are present in bile in high concentrations can be attributed to alterations in both bile flow and active transfer. To distinguish between these possibilities, the effect of ethynyl estradiol on bile flow and the concentration of sodium taurocholate and phenoldibromphthalein disulfonate was determined in bile fistula female rats.

METHODS

Female Wistar rats (200-300 g) received a subcutaneous injection of 1.25 mg ethynyl estradiol in propylene glycol (0.25 ml)

Supported by Grant #AM-08043 from the National Institutes of Health.

We wish to thank Dr. Sidney Emerman for his assistance in these studies.

11

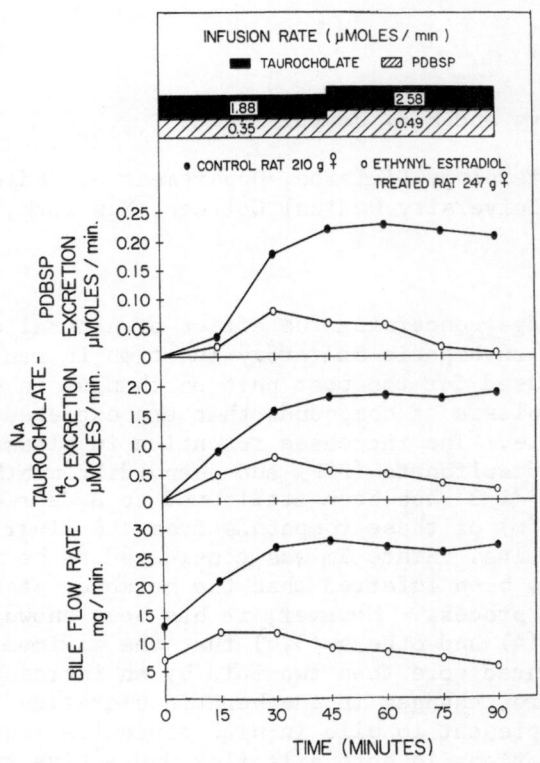

Fig. 1. Maximum bile flow and maximum excretion rates attained during infusion of sodium taurocholate and phenoldibromphthalein disulfonate into control and ethynyl estradiol treated female Wistar rat. The excretion rate of sodium taurocholate is calculated from the specific activity of the infusion rate neglecting the low rate of endogenous bile salt excretion.

24 hours prior to surgery. Control animals received the same volume
of propylene glycol. Surgery was done during intraperitoneal pentobarbital anesthesia. Polyethylene cannulas were inserted in the
common duct, a leg vein and the femoral artery. A second injection
of ethynyl estradiol or polyethylene glycol alone was given. The
animal was placed in a restraining cage and maintained on an infusion of 5% dextrose in 0.45% saline at one ml/hour.

Following overnight collection of bile (18-22 hours) and
collection of control specimens the next morning, each animal received an infusion of sodium taurocholate and diBSP. The infusion
mixture consisted of 45 mM sodium taurocholate (Maybridge Chemical
Co., Tintagel, N. Cornwall, England) 8 mM diBSP (Hynson, Westcott
and Dunning, Baltimore, Md., U.S.A.) and 3% human serum albumin in
5% dextrose and 0.45% saline. The infusion was given for 90 minutes
at rates varying from 0.05 to 0.10 ml/min. No hemolysis was detected in blood samples collected at 15 minute intervals. Bile was
collected into tared tubes and the volume estimated by the change
in weight. To facilitate the estimation of sodium taurocholate,
particularly in serum, a tracer amount of taurocholate-24-^{14}C
(Tracerlab, Waltham, Mass., U.S.A.) was added to the infusion mixture and the specific activity then used to estimate the concentration of sodium taurocholate. Since infusions were given after
depletion of the endogenous bile salt pool, the possible change in
specific activity by endogenous bile salt synthesis was considered
not significant. Confirmation of this assumption was obtained when
it was found that quantitative estimation of the sodium taurocholate
in bile specimens from control and hormone treated animals agreed
within 3% of the value found for total bile salt determined by the
enzymatic method (7,8). Phenoldibromphthalein disulfonate was
quantitatively estimated in plasma and bile by methods described
previously (9).

Polyethylene glycol-^{14}C (S.A. 0.18 µC/mg), molecular weight
8300 (New England Nuclear Corp., Boston, Mass.), was used for
estimation of the porosity of the biliary tree (10). Using liquid
scintillation spectrometry (8), the concentration of polyethylene
glycol in bile and plasma was determined in animals with ligated
renal pedicles two hours following a single intravenous injection
of 5µC.

RESULTS

The results of a typical study are shown in Figure 1. In the
control animal, a maximal bile flow rate and excretion rate of
sodium taurocholate and diBSP is attained within 60 minutes. In
the hormone treated animal, the increase in bile flow and excretion
rate of sodium taurocholate and diBSP is much less and, in some
studied, these rates are not sustained during the entire infusion

period. In all studies, the infusion rate of the compounds exceeded the excretion rate, and a progressive increase in plasma levels of taurocholate and diBSP always occurred. As a consequence of the reduced capacity of the hormone treated animals to excrete the compound, the serum levels of taurocholate and diBSP were greater than in the control group of animals.

The results obtained in five control and 12 ethynyl estradiol treated animals are summarized in Table 1. The most significant difference between the two groups of animals is the maximum bile flow occurring during the infusion. The mean maximum value for the control group was 10.7 mg/min/100 g body weight compared to 5.9 mg/min for the hormone treated group. The bile flow rates in the hormone treated group were also found to be lower than the control group during the overnight and preinfusion periods.

No significant difference was found in the mean value for sodium taurocholate concentration (74mM) between groups. A difference was found for diBSP concentration in bile. Because of the decrease in diBSP concentration and in bile flow in the hormone treated group, the reduction in diBSP Tm is proportionally greater than the reduction in taurocholate excretion rate.

An increase in the bile/plasma concentration ratio for polyethylene glycol 8300 was found in the hormone treated animals. Since the concentration of polyethylene glycol in bile and plasma are at a plateau within two hours following intravenous injection into renal pedicle ligated animals, the concentration ratio represents an equilibrium between the two compartments.

DISCUSSION

The term, Tm, signifying the maximum rate of tubular excretion, was introduced by Smith, Goldring and Chasis (11) to express the concept that the maximum active transport of organic anions such as para-amino hippurate is dependent on renal tubular excretory mass. When the solute load is sufficiently high, the maximum solute excretion rate is considered to be independent of glomerular activity and renal blood flow. When it was found that an organic anion, BSP, is excreted in bile in high concentration at an apparently fixed maximal excretion rate, the analogy to renal tubular transport became apparent and the term, Tm, used to signify the same concept (12).

The decrease in the rate of disappearance of BSP and diBSP from plasma as a consequence of estradiol (1,3) or ethynyl estradiol (2) administration has been attributed to a decrease in Tm. The increased retention of BSP conjugates in plasma and the finding of increased retention of diBSP, a compound that is not

TABLE 1

EFFECT OF ETHYNYL ESTRADIOL[a] ON HEPATIC EXCRETORY
FUNCTION IN FEMALE WISTAR RATS

	CONTROL 5 animals	ETHYNYL ESTRADIOL 12 animals	P VALUE[b]
	MEAN VALUE ± S.D.[c]		
BILE FLOW mg/min/100 g body wt			
Overnight	3.7±0.9	2.6±0.9	<0.05
Preinfusion[d]	4.6±1.6	2.8±1.2	<0.05
Maximum[e] infusion	10.7±1.9	5.9±2.6	<0.005
SODIUM TAUROCHOLATE			
maximum concentration μmole/ml bile	74±9	74±21	n.s.[f]
maximum excretion rate μmole/min/100 g	0.78±0.26	0.40±0.23	<0.02
PHENOLDIBROMPHTHALEIN DISULFONATE			
maximum concentration μmole/ml bile	9.4±4.3	4.3±2.3	<0.05
maximum excretion rate μmole/min/100 g	0.11±0.07	0.026±0.02	<0.02
POLYETHYLENE GLYCOL MOL WT 8300			
concentration ratio bile/plasma[g]	0.06±.03	0.19±.06	<0.05

[a] two subcutaneous injections at 24 hour interval of 1.25 mg ethynyl estradiol in propylene glycol

[b] T test of significance for difference in mean values

[c] standard deviation

[d] flow rate for 15 minutes just prior to start of infusion

[e] maximum value attained during infusion period

[f] not significant

[g] group consisted of four control and three hormone-treated animals

conjugated prior to excretion (9), indicates that the hormone
induced effect is on the excretory process.

In the last few years, it has been shown that the Tm for BSP in
the dog (4), sheep (5) and rat (6) is also dependent on bile flow.
An increase in bile flow as a result of sodium dehydrocholate or
taurocholate administration causes a two- to three-fold increment in
BSP Tm. The relative increase in BSP Tm is greater when control
bile flow is low. At high bile flow rates, little further enhancement in BSP Tm occurs with a further increment in flow (4). Therefore, it seems clear that the Tm concept as applied to hepatic
excretory function is dependent on both an active transport process
and flow rate.

The decrease in maximum diBSP excretion rate induced by
ethynyl estradiol is attributable to a decrease both in maximum
concentration in bile and in maximum bile flow. The reduction in
concentration may reflect a decrease in the active transfer process.
The reduction in the capacity to excrete bile salt accounts for
the reduction in maximum flow rate.

A reduction in bile flow in the hormone treated rats was also
found prior to the infusion of bile salt. It does not seem reasonable to attribute this reduction in flow to a decrease in bile
salt transport since the animal is capable of increasing bile salt
during the infusion period. It is possible that as a result of
hormone treatment, a reduction in bile salt pool and synthesis
occurs thus reducing the endogenous excretion rate. It is also
possible that there is a change in the molecular weight of the
macromolecular complex in bile consisting of cholesterol, lecithin
and bile salt. An increase in the molecular weight of this mixed
micelle or a decrease in the concentration at which mixed micelles
form could cause a reduction in bile flow. The present studies
were not designed to evaluate these possibilities.

Another factor causing a reduction in basal bile flow is a
change in the permeability properties of the biliary tree.
Diffusion of bile salt from the biliary tree would reduce the
osmotic gradient so that there would be a reduction in flow without a change in bile salt concentration. Since diBSP excretion
causes little change in bile flow, diffusion of this compound from
the biliary tree could account, at least in part, for a reduction
in concentration. This speculation is supported by the finding
that the biliary tree of the animal receiving ethynyl estradiol
is relatively more permeable to polyethylene glycol molecular
weight 8300. However, it is difficult to extrapolate from one
molecular weight to another and it is evident that other possibilities have not been excluded. The interpretation however, is
consistent with the known effect of estradiol on rat uterus (13).

SUMMARY

The administration of ethynyl estradiol to female rats causes a reduction in bile flow and the maximum capacity (Tm) to excrete bile salt and phenoldibromphthalein disulfonate. An increase in the relative permeability to polyethylene glycol molecular weight 8300 also occurs. The decrease in phenoldibromphthalein disulfonate Tm is attributable to a reduction in the concentration of the compound in bile and the bile flow rate. The reduction in bile flow may be related to the change in permeability of the biliary tree.

REFERENCES

1. Mueller, M.N. and Kappas, A.: Estrogen pharmacology. I. The influence of estradiol and estriol on hepatic disposal of sulfobromphthalein (BSP) in man. J. Clin. Invest. 43:1905-1914 (1964).

2. Kleiner, G.J., Kresch, L. and Arias, I.M.: Studies of hepatic excretory function. II. The effect of norethynodrel and mestranol on bromsulfalein sodium metabolism in women of childbearing age. New. Eng. J. Med. 273:420-423 (1965).

3. Gallagher, T.F,, Jr., Mueller, M.N. and Kappas, A.: Studies on the mechanism and structural specificity of the estrogen effect on BSP metabolism. Trans. Assoc. Amer. Phys. 78:187-195 (1965).

4. O'Maille, E.R.L., Richards, T.G. and Short, A.H.: Factors determining the maximal rate of organic anion secretion by the liver and further evidence on the hepatic site of action of the hormone secretion. J. of Physiol. 186:424-438 (1966).

5. Gronwall, R. and Cornelius, C.E.: Biliary excretion of sulfobromophthalein in sheep. Fed. Proc. 25:576 (1966).

6. Ritt, D.J., Schenker, S. and Combes, G.: Taurocholic acid stimulation of apparent maximal biliary excretion of sulfobromophthalein sodium. Gastroenterology 52:322 (1967).

7. Iwata, T. and Yamasaki, K.: Enzymatic determination and thin-layer chromatography of bile acids in blood. J. Biochem. 56:424-431 (1964).

8. Javitt, N. and Emerman, S.: Effect of sodium taurolithocholate on bile flow and bile acid excretion. J. Clin. Invest. 47:1002-1014 (1968).

9.   Javitt, N.: Phenoldibromphthalein disulfonate. A new
compound for the study of liver disease. Proc. Soc. Exper. Biol.
Med. 117:254-257 (1964).

10. Javitt, N.: Porosity of the biliary tree to polyethylene
glycols. Gastroenterology 54:157 (1968).

11. Smith, H., Goldring, H. and Chasis, H.: The measurement
of tubular excretory mass, effective blood flow and filtration
rate in the normal human kidney. J. Clin. Invest. 17:263-269
(1938).

12. Wheeler, H.O., Meltzer, J. and Bradley, S.E.: Biliary
transport and hepatic storage of sulfobromophthalein sodium in the
unanesthetized dog, in normal man and in patients with hepatic
disease. J. Clin. Invest. 39:1131-1144 (1960).

13. Spanziani, E. and Gutman, A.: Distribution volumes of
sugars in rat uterus, ileum and skeletal muscle as affected by
estradiol. Endocrinology 76:470-478 (1965).

THE EFFECT OF NATURAL AND SYNTHETIC ESTROGENS ON THE EXCRETION

OF BSP BY THE LIVER

R.H. Palmer, T.F. Gallagher, Jr., M.N. Mueller and
A. Kappas

Department of Medicine and Argonne Cancer Research
Hospital*, The University of Chicago, Chicago, and the
Rockefeller University, New York

There is now general agreement that cholestasis and/or
impairment of certain liver functions can be caused by a wide variety of steroids, including androgens (1), estrogens (1-5), progestins (1,6,7) and bile salts (8,9). (For a recent review and
bibliography, see Song and Kappas (10)). Many of these steroids
are synthetic or unsaturated steroids, often alkylated at the 17
position. This discussion will emphasize the capacity of natural
estrogens to impair hepatic excretion of sulfobromophthalein in
man, and will examine certain structural aspects of this activity
in the rat.

Sulfobromophthalein, or BSP, is rapidly removed from plasma
by the liver following its intravenous injection. As a result of
this characteristic, study of its plasma disappearance rate following injection has come to represent an extremely useful and sensitive indicator of hepatic function in man. There is usually a
rapid early and a slower late plasma disappearance of the dye; the
former has been attributed to uptake of BSP by the liver and the
latter to hepatic processes concerned with excretion of dye into
the bile. Less than six percent of injected dye can be found in
the peripheral circulation 45 minutes after intravenous injection
in subjects with normal liver function.

Initial studies on the effects of natural estrogens on BSP
retention showed that these steroids rapidly and consistently impair the capacity of the liver to dispose of this dye following its
intravenous administration. The striking abnormalities in BSP

---

*Operated by the University of Chicago for the U.S. Atomic
Energy Commission.

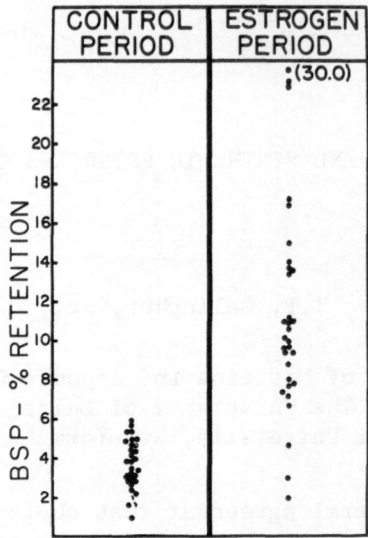

Fig. 1. BSP retention induced by 5 mg/day or more of estradiol or estriol in 31 patients. The duration of therapy varied from 3 to 41 days.

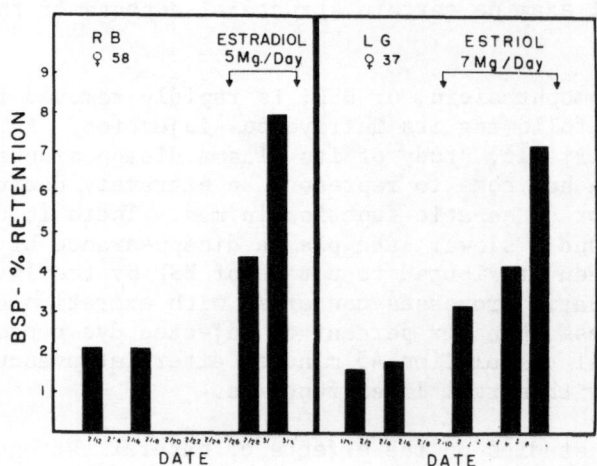

Fig. 2. BSP retention induced by estradiol and estriol in two subjects.

retention produced by the intramuscular injections of varying amounts of estradiol and estriol in 31 subjects are shown in Figure 1. Specific examples of the effects of these natural estrogens in two subjects are shown in Figure 2. The amounts of estrogen used in these studies were higher than those produced during the normal menstrual cycle, but are within the range of total daily estrogen production that characterizes the latter part of pregnancy in humans.

Approximately one half of the patients who received these steroids showed significant elevations in serum alkaline phosphatase as well. Hyperbilirubinemia did not develop in any subject, nor were there alterations in other indices of liver function, such as flocculation tests or appropriate serum enzymes. Furthermore, liver biopsies from patients receiving intensive treatment with estradiol for periods of two to four weeks did not differ by light microscopy from pre-treatment biopsies.

The processes concerned with the uptake of BSP by the liver, its transient storage in liver cells, and its excretion into the bile were assessed by techniques developed by Wheeler and associates (11). The continuous infusion of dye at three different rates, with periodic sampling of its plasma concentration, permits calculation of the relative storage capacity of the liver for dye (S) and the maximum rate at which the liver can secrete the dye into the bile (T_m). The T_m and S for BSP were determined in six subjects before and after treatment with estradiol. The results are shown in Figure 3. Estradiol did not cause any decrease in the storage capacity, but markedly depressed the net capacity of the liver to transfer dye into the bile. The depression, which ranged from 40-95%, reached a level in some subjects within the range characterizing patients with congenital defects of hepatic excretory function. It is not clear whether the variations observed in the responses could be expected in repeated tests in the same individual, or whether they reflect individual inborn or acquired determinants of excretory capacity.

An important element of the hepatic disposal of BSP involves conjugation of the dye with glutathione and its component amino acids. To determine whether impairment of these conjugation processes could account for the effect of estrogens on dye excretion, the amount of conjugated BSP found in plasma was studied in four subjects before and after estrogen treatment. Table 1 shows that there were substantially larger amounts of conjugated dye in the plasma during estradiol administration than during control periods. These data suggest that it it unlikely that estrogens impair hepatic BSP disposal in man by an inhibitory action on dye conjugation.

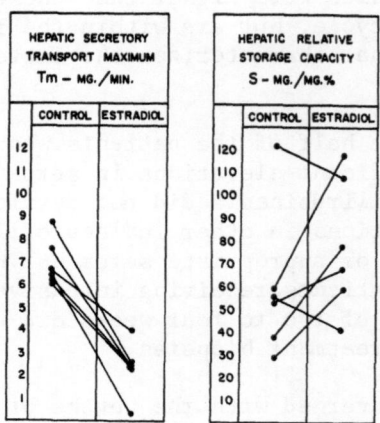

Fig. 3. Effect of estrogens on hepatic T_m and S for BSP.

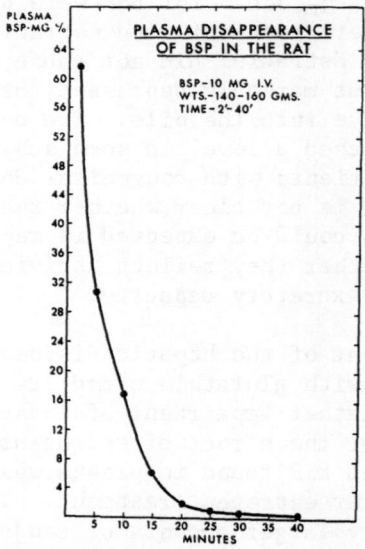

Fig. 4. Plasma disappearance of BSP in the rat.

TABLE 1

Conjugated BSP as a Fraction of Total Plasma BSP

Patient	BSP - % Conjugated	
	Control	Estrogen
CT	6	20
BP	7	50
DH	15	43
CM	15	60

Studies in rats were undertaken to explore the structural basis of this estrogen effect on the liver. The plasma disappearance curve of BSP in the rat resembles that in man, except that rats have a substantially greater capacity for dye excretion (Fig. 4). Estradiol, however, markedly impairs hepatic dye disposal in this species as it does in humans (Fig. 5). Similar results in rats treated with ethinyl estradiol have been reported by Kreek (12) and Javitt (13).

As shown in Figure 6, estrogen impairment of BSP metabolism in the rat, as in man, develops quickly after the hormone is administered and recedes quickly after it is discontinued. Using these and related observations, a test system was developed, in rats treated with steroids, one mg/day for ten days, which permitted an examination of the structural basis for this hormonal effect on the liver.

Table 2 summarizes the activities determined for 42 natural and synthetic steroids. Examination of structure-activity relationships reveals that the presence or absence of functional groups of various types and configurations in the C and D rings of phenolic steroids is not important for activity. The insertion of a double bond between carbons 6 and 7 (XIII, XIV) eliminates activity, but insertion of an additional double bond between carbons 8 and 9 (XII) restores activity. Structural alterations in the phenolic A ring significantly influence the capacity of estrogens to impair liver function. Thus hydroxylation (XXI-XXIII), methylation (XVII,XIX) or methyl ether formation (XXIV,XXV) at carbons 1 or 2 diminishes or abolishes activity; however, additional

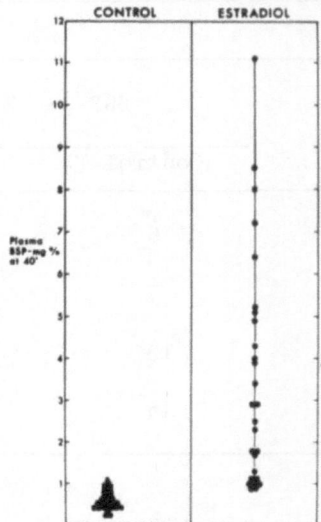

Fig. 5. Plasma BSP concentration forty minutes following dye injection in rats before and after treatment with estradiol, 1.0 mg/day for 10 days.

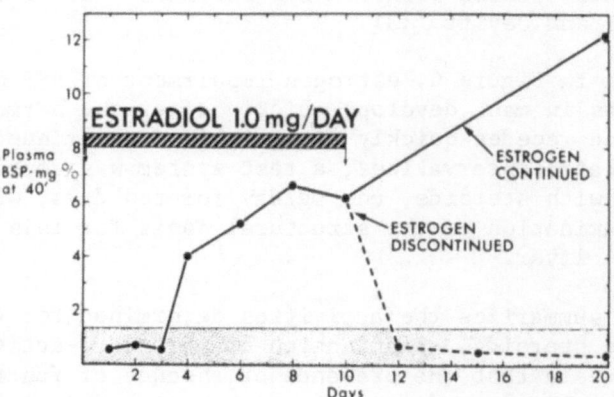

Fig. 6. Onset and recovery from the effects of estrogen on BSP metabolism in the rat. The shaded area represents the normal range for control rats. The points represent mean values from groups of at least six rats.

TABLE 2

EFFECTS OF ESTROGENS AND OTHER STEROIDS
ON BSP METABOLISM IN THE RAT

No.	Compound	Animals tested	Plasma BSP range	Plasma BSP mean	Comment
			mg%	mg%	
I	Estradiol	39	0.6-16.2	5.0	Active
II	Estrone	22	0.7-21.4	10.9	Active
III	α-estradiol	8	0.5- 4.6	1.7	Active
IV	Estriol	26	2.4-22.5	10.5	Active
V	Epi-estriol	8	0.5-10.8	4.0	Active
VI	Estradiol-3-acetate	10	0.8- 8.0	3.4	Active
VII	Estradiol-17-acetate	10	0.7-16.9	6.7	Active
VIII	Estradiol-3-methyl-ether	11	0.8-14.0	4.8	Active
IX	Mestranol	12	0.9- 8.2	2.8	Active
X	11β-hydroxyestrone	5	1.2- 3.9	2.4	Active
XI	16-ketoestrone	6	0.8- 4.6	1.6	Active
XII	Equilenin	10	0.8-20.4	7.9	Active
XIII	6-hydroestrone	26	0.2- 1.0	0.5	Inactive
XIV	6-hydroestradiol	6	0.6- 4.2	1.3	1 value>1.5mg%
XV	17-deoxyestrone	14	1.3-10.4	6.2	Active
XVI	3-deoxyestrone	6	0.5- 0.8	0.7	Inactive
XVII	1-methyl estrone	10	0.3- 1.3	0.7	Inactive
XVIII	1-methyl estrone-3-acetate	8	0.4- 0.8	0.5	Inactive
XIX	2-methyl-estrone	3	0.6- 0.8	0.7	Inactive
XX	2,17α-dimethyl estradiol	5	0.5-13.3	4.7	Active
XXI	2-hydroxyestrone	5	0.4- 5.0	1.5	1 value>1.5 mg%
XXII	2-hydroxyestradiol	4	0.5- 0.9	0.7	Inactive
XXIII	2-hydroxyestriol	6	0.6- 1.9	1.7	4 values>1.5mg%
XXIV	2-methoxyestrone	6	0.5- 1.0	0.8	Inactive
XXV	2-methoxyestradiol	6	0.5- 4.5	1.5	1 value>1.5mg%
XXVI	Diethylstilbestrol	7	2.1- 7.9	5.1	Active
XXVII	Norethynodrel	12	0.6- 1.2	0.7	Inactive
XXVIII	17α-ethinyl-4-estrene-17β-ol,-acetate,3-one	14	0.5- 1.0	0.7	Inactive
XXIX	Norethandrolone	12	0.3- 1.0	0.5	Inactive
XXX	Methyltestosterone	5	0.5- 0.9	0.7	Inactive
XXXI	Testosterone	9	0.4- 0.8	0.6	Inactive
XXXII	Androsterone	8	0.5- 0.7	0.6	Inactive
XXXIII	Etiocholanolone	9	0.4- 0.8	0.5	Inactive
XXXIV	Pregnanediol	9	0.4- 0.7	0.5	Inactive
XXXV	Progesterone	15	0.4- 0.8	0.6	Inactive
XXXVI	Corticosterone	8	0.5- 0.8	0.6	Inactive
XXXVII	Cortisol	7	0.3- 0.6	0.5	Inactive
XXXVIII	Cholic acid	9	0.3- 0.5	0.4	Inactive
XXXIX	Lithocholic acid	8	0.3- 0.7	0.5	Inactive
XL	Taurocholic acid	9	0.3- 0.7	0.5	Inactive
XLI	Taurolithocholic acid	9	0.3- 0.6	0.5	Inactive
XLII	Glycolithocholic acid	8	0.3- 0.8	0.5	Inactive

*The term "active" refers to the ability of the steroid to induce BSP retention in excess of 1.5 mg% 40 minutes after intravenous injection of 10 mg of dye.

methylation at carbon 17 (XX) restores activity. Chemical
substitutions on the C-3 hydroxyl group do not alter activity
(VI, VIII, IX) but an oxygen function at this position does appear
to be essential (XVI). The non-steroid estrogen stilbestrol also
impairs liver function.

A wide variety of other neutral and acidic steroids do not
induce BSP retention in this system. Estrogens, while inducing an
alteration in liver function, do not produce significant morphological changes demonstrable by light or electron microscopy. In
contrast, 17-methyl testosterone (XXX), which did not impair BSP
excretion in the amounts used, did produce marked canalicular di-
latation in the livers of test animals. Forker (14) has also reported recently that rats treated with estrone have impairment of
BSP excretion without morphological cholestasis. These results,
together with the absence of cholestasis by light microscopy in
liver biopsies from our patients, raise the question of whether
morphological cholestasis is a phenomenon separate from functional
impairment and perhaps restricted to unnatural, 17-alkylated steroids, or whether the two are the same process and only differ
quantitatively.

In the rat, as in man, impairment of BSP conjugation does not
appear to be a factor in estrogen-induced BSP retention (5). Substantial amounts of conjugated BSP can be found in rat plasma
during estrogen treatment, and there is no decrease either in the
hepatic content of glutathione or the BSP conjugating activity of
liver homogenates in vitro. Furthermore, the disappearance of
dibromosulfophthalein, which is excreted into the bile without
conjugation, was similarly impaired in estrogen treated rats.

The mechanism by which estrogens impair BSP excretion remains
to be clarified. There is now growing evidence that the T_m of BSP
is dependent on bile salt excretion. Studies by Boyer, Scheig and
Klatskin (15), in the isolated, perfused rat liver, indicate that
the T_m of BSP varies with the excretion of bile salts, which is in
turn related to the total bile flow, so that the concentration of
BSP at its T_m remains practically constant. Estrogens could impair
BSP excretion by interfering with the excretion of bile salts.
This would have its clinical counterpart in the pruritus of pregnancy, now known to be associated with increased plasma levels of
bile salts (16). Javitt (13) has reported recently that ethinyl
estradiol does indeed reduce the maximum excretion of bile salts
by about 50 percent in rats.

In Javitt's work, however, there was an even greater reduction
in the excretion of dibromosulfophthalein, with a decrease in its
concentration relative to bile salt concentration in bile. These
results are compatible with the hypothesis that estrogens facilitate the back-diffusion of substances from bile to plasma. This

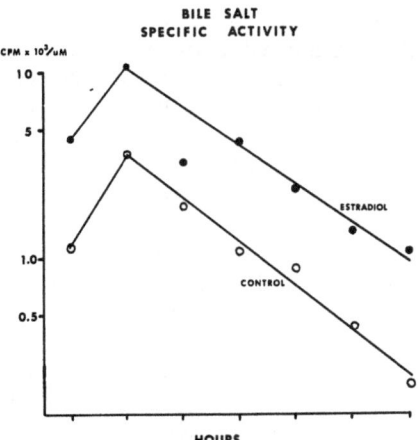

Fig. 7. Decline in specific activity (cpm ^{14}C-taurocholate per μM total bile salts) in estradiol treated (closed circles) and control (open circles) rats. Estradiol, 1 mg/day, was administered subcutaneously for 10 days.

hypothesis would also explain the increased plasma concentration of BSP in our subjects receiving estrogens. Strong support for this hypothesis has come recently form Forker (14), who has shown that estrone increases the permeability of the biliary tree to sucrose and mannitol. Forker also found that estrone was more effective in reducing the plasma clearance of BSP at low plasma concentrations than at transport maximum levels, a finding consistent with the view that estrone enhances back-diffusion of BSP. The normal tubular reabsorption of water has been demonstrated in the rat (17) and the dog (18).

In order to investigate the effect of estrogens on bile acid excretion, we have used rats with externalized bile fistulae. Preliminary results suggest that when the entero-hepatic circulation of these unanesthetized, feeding rats with intact bile salt pools is suddenly interrupted, the initial rate of bile salt excretion in animals pretreated with estradiol is only about one-third that of controls. However, bile flow is decreased even further, so that the concentration of bile salts is actually one-third higher than in control rats. This finding, if confirmed, is consistent with increased fluid reabsorption in estrogen treated animals.

Our data also suggest an effect of bile salt secretion by the hepatocyte. If a tracer dose of ^{14}C-taurocholate is injected intraperitoneally, the label is rapidly taken up by the liver, excreted into the bile, and "washed out" by the secretion of endogenous bile salts. In these preliminary results (Fig. 7), bile from the estrogen treated rat attains a higher specific activity following injection of a standard amount of label than that from the control, as would be expected from the greater excretion of endogenous bile salts in the latter. However, the "wash-out", or decline in specific activity, is essentially similar in the two animals. While other interpretations are possible, this suggests that estrogens do not retard the uptake and excretion of labeled bile salt, nor do they enhance the back diffusion of bile salts, both of which would prolong the wash out, and support the concept that estrogens may also have a direct inhibitory effect on bile salt excretion at the level of the hepatocyte.

In summary, a number of natural and synthetic estrogens impair the biliary excretion of BSP. It is probable that this estrogen action underlies certain functional abnormalities of the liver which characterize the pregnant woman, the neonatal child, and certain women taking synthetic estrogenic compounds. The mechanism of this action has not been established, but there is evidence for both a primary effect on bile salt excretion and for an effect on the back-diffusion of substances from bile to plasma. The clinical importance of this excretory impairment, which presumably affects the disposal of exogenous pharmacological compounds as well as endogenous hormones and their metabolites, remains to be clarified.

REFERENCES

1. Sherlock, S.: Diseases of the Liver and Biliary System. F.A. Davis Company, Philadelphia, Penna., 1963. p. 309.

2. Mueller, M.N. and Kappas, A.: Impairment of hepatic excretion of sulfobromophthalein (BSP) by natural estrogens. Trans. Assoc. Am. Phys. 77:248-258 (1964).

3. Mueller, M.N. and Kappas, A.: Estrogen pharmacology. I. The influence of estradiol and estriol on the hepatic disposal of sulfobromophthalein (BSP) in man. J. Clin. Invest. 43:1905-1914 (1964).

4. Kottra, L.L. and Kappas, A.: Estrogen pharmacology. III. Effect of estradiol on plasma disappearance rate of sulfobromophthalein in man. Arch. Intern. Med. 117:373-376 (1966).

5. Gallagher, T.F., Jr., Mueller, M.N. and Kappas, A.: Estrogen pharmacology. IV. Studies on the structural basis for estrogen-induced impairment of liver function. Medicine 45:471-479 (1966).

6. Tyler, E.T. and Olson, H.J.: Fertility promoting and inhibitory effects of new steroid hormonal substances. J.A.M.A. 169:1843-1854 (1959).

7. Perez-Mera, R.A. and Shields, C.E.: Jaundice associated with norethindrone acetate therapy. New Eng. J. Med. 267:1137-1138 (1962).

8. Javitt, N.B.: Cholestasis in rats induced by taurolithocholate. Nature 210:1262 (1966).

9. Javitt, N.B. and Emerman, S.: Effect of sodium taurolithocholate on bile flow and bile acid excretion. J. Clin. Invest. 47:1002-1014 (1968).

10. Song, C.S. and Kappas, A.: The influence of estrogens, progestins and pregnancy on the liver. Vitamins and Hormones 26:147-195 (1968).

11. Wheeler, H.O., Meltzer, J.I. and Bradley, S.E.: Biliary transport and hepatic storage of sulfobromophthalein sodium in the unanesthetized dog, in normal man, and in patients with hepatic disease. J. Clin. Invest. 39:1131-1144 (1960).

12. Kreek, M.J., Peterson, R.E., Sleisinger, M.H. and Jeffries, G.H.: Influence of ethinyl estradiol-induced cholestasis on bile flow and biliary excretion of estradiol and bromosulfophthalein by the rat. Abstract. J. Clin. Invest. 46:1080 (1967).

13. Javitt, N.B. and Harkavy, M.: Ethinyl estradiol induced cholestasis in female Wistar rats. Abstract. Gastroenterology. (In press).

14. Forker, E.L.: Increased permeability of the rat biliary tree induced by estrone. Abstract. Gastroenterology. (In press).

15. Boyer, J.L., Scheig, R. and Klatskin, G.: The effect of bile salts on the hepatic metabolism of BSP. Abstract. Gastroenterology (In press).

16. Sjövall, K. and Sjövall, J.: Serum bile acid levels in pregnancy with pruritus. Bile acids and steroids 158. Biochim. Biophys. Acta 13:207-211 (1967).

17. Schanker, L.S. and Hogben, C.A.M.: Biliary excretion of inulin, sucrose and mannitol: analysis of bile formation. Am. J. Physiol. 200:1087-1090 (1961).

18. Wheeler, H.O., Ross, E.D. and Bradley, S.E.: Canalicular bile production in dogs. Am. J. Physiol. 214:866-874 (1968).

SOME EFFECTS OF CONTRACEPTIVE STEROIDS ON HEPATIC FUNCTION IN
NORMAL WOMEN AND IN PATIENTS WITH ACQUIRED AND INHERITABLE DEFECTS
IN HEPATIC EXCRETORY FUNCTION

Irwin M. Arias

Department of Medicine, Albert Einstein College of
Medicine and Bronx Municipal Hospital Center, New York,
New York

Although the development of oral contraceptive pills represents
a major advance in population control, the use of these agents has
introduced several problems relating to jaundice. Table 1 classi-
fies three types of hepatic effects of oral contraceptive steroids.
Decreased hepatic excretion of sulfobromophthalein (BSP), regularly
seen in women taking oral contraceptives, is not associated with
hyperbilirubinemia, and mimics that seen in the last trimester of
pregnancy (1) or following administration of estrogens (2) or C-17
alkylated anabolic steroids (3). Jaundice occurring during administration of oral contraceptives may be classified on the basis of
whether or not the patient was previously anicteric. The disorders
listed in Group 2 are characterized by bile secretory failure mani-
fested by accumulation in serum of conjugated bilirubin, bile salts
and cholesterol, increased serum alkaline phosphatase and 5'-
nucleotidase activities, and a relatively characteristic lesion of
bile canaliculi and lysosomes which is best seen by enzyme histochemical and electron microscopic examinations (4). Occasionally,
patients receiving oral contraceptives manifest non-dosage related
bile secretory failure and are presumed to be sensitive to the drug
although the mechanism is unknown (5). Other patients develop bile
secretory failure in association with pregnancy (6) or without obvious precipitating cause (7) and manifest recrudescence of the
syndrome following administration of oral contraceptive drugs. A
similar syndrome occurs in patients with chronic liver disease such
as cirrhosis or hepatitis. Group 3 consists mainly of patients with
chronic, subclinical hyperbilirubinemia due to the Dubin-Johnson

The studies performed in the author's laboratory were supported
by research grants from the USPHS (AM-02019), the New York Heart
Association and Heart Fund, Inc. and the G.D. Searle Co.

syndrome (8,9) who become clinically jaundiced during administration of oral contraceptive steroids.

In truth, oral contraceptive agents have resulted in a small epidemic of jaundice which is restricted to the disease categories indicated in Table 1. The patients listed in Table 1 were studied within the past eleven months. Patients in Group 3 and many in Group 2 would probably not have come to medical attention had it not been for the oral contraceptive agent. The patients with the Dubin-Johnson syndrome and those with recurrent cholestasis of pregnancy represent more than a three-fold increase in the number of similar cases seen in the previous two years. This presentation will concern several aspects of the pathogenesis of these alterations in hepatic function.

TABLE 1

CLASSIFICATION OF HEPATIC EFFECTS OF ORAL CONTRACEPTIVE STEROIDS

		Patients*
1.	Reduced hepatic excretory function	every patient studied
2.	Jaundice in previously anicteric patients	
	A. Drug "sensitivity"	2
	B. Benign familial recurrent cholestasis	2
	C. Recurrent cholestasis of pregnancy	12
	D. Chronic liver disease (cirrhosis or hepatitis)	3
3.	Accentuated pre-existing hyper-bilirubinemia	
	A. Dubin-Johnson syndrome	19
	B. Chronic liver disease (cirrhosis or hepatitis)	2

*The number of patients refers to new cases studied during the previous 11 months.

TABLE 2

EFFECT OF NORETHYNODREL AND MESTRANOL AND ESTRADIOL ON BROMSULFALEIN
SODIUM METABOLISM IN WOMEN OF CHILDBEARING AGE

Subject	S(mg stored/mg dye/100 ml in plasma)			Tm(mg excreted/min)		
	Before Rx*	During Rx	After Rx	Before Rx	During Rx	After Rx
Cyclic treatment of 5 mg norethynodrel and 0.075 mg mestranol:						
D.T.	51	48	59	7.9	4.8	8.2
C.W.		89			4.9	
M.C.		48			5.2	
E.S.		39			4.2	
H.M.		54			5.1	
Mean		56 ± 17			4.8 ± 0.3	
Continuous daily treatment of 9.85 mg norethynodrel and 0.15 mg mestranol:						
F.W.	46	61	52	8.4	2.8	7.3
W.O.		67			2.1	
M.L.		58			2.2	
F.W.		62			2.4	
Mean		64 ± 3			2.4 ± 0.8	
Continuous daily treatment of 2.5 mg estradiol:						
A.B.	72	88	75	7.9	7.2	7.0
D.B.	56	49	50	8.1	6.8	6.6
M.K.		51			8.5	
C.H.		62			7.4	
Mean		62 ± 16			7.5 ± 0.5	

*Rx has been substituted for the word treatment or administration.
(From: Kleiner, G.J., Kresch, L. and Arias, I.M.: New Eng. J. Med. 273:421-423 (1965))

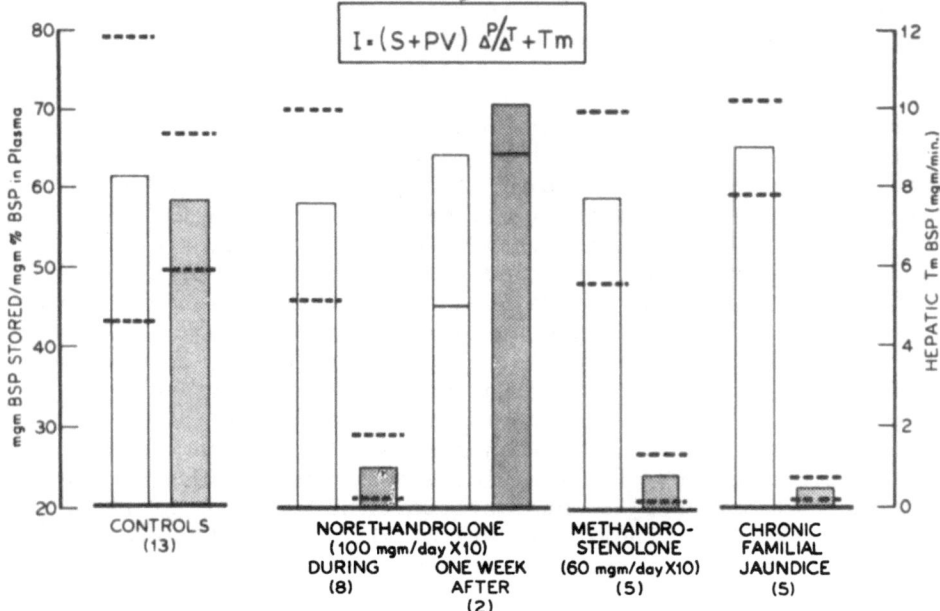

Fig. 1. Estimates of the relative hepatic storage (S) and hepatic transport maximum (T_m) for BSP in normal subjects, in patients receiving norethandrolone or methandrostenolone, and in patients with chronic familial jaundice (Dubin-Johnson syndrome). (From Arias, I.M., <u>Protein Metabolism, an International Symposium</u>, Springer-Verlag, Berlin, 434-444, 1962.)

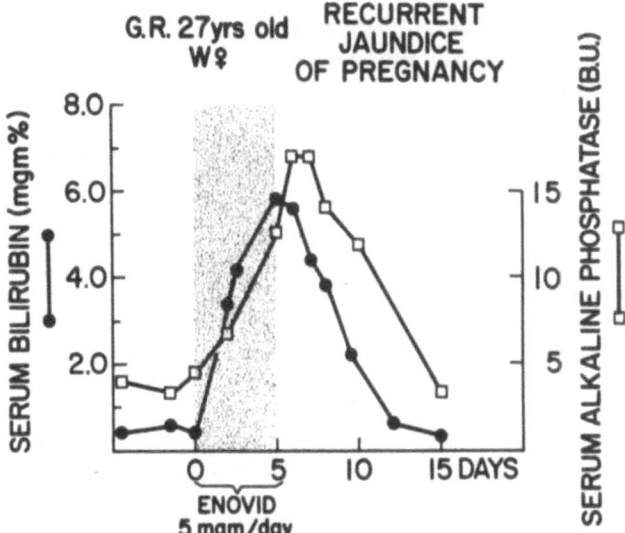

Fig. 2. Effect of Enovid administration on serum bilirubin concentration and alkaline phosphatase activity in a patient with recurrent jaundice (cholestasis) of pregnancy.

In 1965, the effect of Enovid on the hepatic metabolism of BSP was studied in normal women in the childbearing age (10) using the intravenous infusion technique of Wheeler et al (11) which permits quantitative estimation of the relative hepatic storage of BSP (S, expressed as mgm of dye stored per mgm% dye in plasma) and the biliary transport maximum for BSP (Tm_{BSP}, expressed as mgm dye excreted per minute). In all forms of acquired liver disease, both storage and Tm_{BSP} are reduced (11); however, as shown in Table 2, there is selective reduction in Tm_{BSP} after cyclic or continuous administration of Enovid but not after parenteral administration of 2.5 mgm estradiol for ten days. Following cessation of Enovid administration, Tm_{BSP} returned to normal within 48 hours. Similar results were observed previously in normal subjects receiving C-17 alkylated anabolic steroids and the effect was also rapidly reversed following cessation of steroid administration (3 and Fig. 1). In each of these studies, BSP conjugation with glutathione was unimpaired and light and electron microscopic examinations of liver did not reveal morphologic abnormalities (3,10). None of the patients who received Enovid or C-17 alkylated anabolic steroids became jaundiced. The hepatic excretory reserve for bilirubin has not been quantitated in man but has been estimated to be approximately ten-fold and must be substantially reduced before hyperbilirubinemia occurs (12). Based upon these considerations, it was suggested that jaundice may follow administration of oral contraceptive agents to patients with inheritable or acquired reduction in hepatic excretory function. Subsequent clinical experience has supported this postulate and several examples will be considered:

1. Thirteen families have been described in which affected individuals of either sex develop many episodes of bile secretory failure ("intrahepatic cholestasis") with the biochemical and morphologic features previously mentioned. The entity is called benign familial recurrent cholestasis (7). No precipitating cause for the exacerbations is known; the episodes usually last for two to ten weeks and normal functional and morphologic results are obtained during remission (13). In three women with this disorder, we have observed recrudescence of bile secretory failure following administration of Enovid for five to fourteen days. Pruritis and jaundice disappeared within ten days after cessation of drug administration and conventional liver function tests gave normal results by twenty days. None of these women had ever been pregnant.

2. Some women manifest bile secretory failure in late pregnancy with complete amelioration following delivery (6). Often, there is more than one woman affected in a family although no detailed genetic studies have been performed. Nonpregnant women who experience this disorder during pregnancy have a recrudescence of the syndrome following administration of oral contraceptive agents

as illustrated in Figure 2. Hyperbilirubinemia and increased serum
alkaline phosphatase activity and bile acid concentrations occur
within ten days after the onset of oral contraceptive administration and all biochemical parameters return to normal within 14 days
after cessation of drug administration.

3. Occasionally, women with chronic liver disease (cirrhosis
or hepatitis) continue to menstruate and take ovulation-suppressing
drugs as oral contraceptives. In five icteric women with post-
necrotic cirrhosis, Enovid administration was followed within three
weeks by increased hyperbilirubinemia and serum alkaline phosphatase activity which abated within two weeks following cessation of
drug administration. Two women complained of pruritus.

Different manifestations were seen following administration of
oral contraceptives to patients with chronic familial jaundice
(Dubin-Johnson syndrome) (8,9). This syndrome is clinically characterized by mild, perhaps lifelong, and often intermittent jaundice of mild to moderate severity with predominantly conjugated
bilirubin in the plasma. There is retention of BSP in serum 45
minutes after the intravenous administration of 5 mgm of dye per
kg body weight and the gall bladder usually fails to visualize
radiographically after ingestion of appropriate contrast media.
Clinical jaundice becomes apparent during the last trimester of
pregnancy and occasionally in association with menstruation. The
disorder occurs in both sexes and in more than one generation.
The mode of inheritance is unknown and there is no satisfactory
test for detecting heterozygotes. Using the continuous BSP infusion technique, hepatic Tm_{BSP} is virtually zero and relative hepatic storage of BSP is normal (9,11) (Fig. 1). Direct analysis of
BSP in bile in a patient with the Dubin-Johnson syndrome and a
biliary fistula confirmed the defect in BSP excretion in this disorder (14). In this patient, biliary excretion of iopanoic acid
was reduced and administration of sodium dehydrocholate increased
bile flow but did not increase Tm_{BSP}. Plasma bile acid concentrations are normal in the Dubin-Johnson syndrome and pathologically
there is no cholestasis although parenchymal cells contain large
amounts of a poorly defined brown-black pigment. With Dr. Charles
Cornelius, we described mutant Corriedale sheep with a defect appearing morphologically and functionally identical to the Dubin-
Johnson syndrome in man (15). The biliary excretion of various
organic anions and an organic cation has been studied in normal and
mutant sheep. The maximal biliary excretion of BSP in mutant
Corriedale sheep was less than 7% of that observed in normal sheep
whereas maximal biliary excretion of taurocholate, the major organic anion in sheep bile, was not different in normal and mutant
sheep (16). Taurocholate infusion enhanced maximal hepatic excretion of of BSP in normal but not in mutant sheep. In addition,
biliary excretion of the following organic anions was greatly

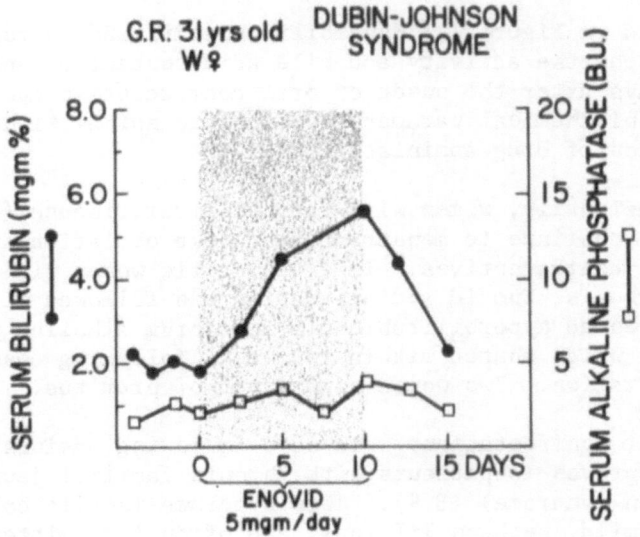

Fig. 3. Effect of Enovid administration on serum bilirubin
concentration and alkaline phosphatase activity in a patient with
chronic familial jaundice (Dubin-Johnson syndrome).

reduced in mutants: iopanoic acid (used for radiologic visualiza-
tion of the gall bladder), metanephrine (which is related to the
hepatic pigmentation), phylloerythrin (a porphyrin derived from
chlorophyll in ruminants and quantitatively excreted unchanged in
the bile) and conjugated bilirubin. The organic cation, procaine
amide ethobromide, was excreted normally in the bile. These
studies, in an inheritable disorder, demonstrate that bile salt excretion which is not required by other organic anions such as bile
pigments, porphyrins, drugs and dyes. The effect of Enovid administration in the Dubin-Johnson syndrome in man is illustrated in
Figure 3. Conjugated hyperbilirubinemia was accentuated without
change in the serum alkaline phosphatase activity. Plasma bile
acid and cholesterol concentrations remained normal and there was
no cholestasis seen on light and electron microscopic study of
liver biopsies. Following cessation of Enovid administration,
there was prompt return of the serum bilirubin concentration to
pre-treatment levels. A comparable effect has been observed during
the first or second cycle of administration of different oral contraceptives in nine women with the Dubin-Johnson syndrome. Because
this syndrome is associated with mild hyperbilirubinemia, patients
are often unaware of its presence unless a coexistent event occurs.
Administration of oral contraceptives converts mild chemical hyperbilirubinemia into overt clinical jaundice and, therefore, serves
to bring such patients to medical attention.

SUMMARY

These observations indicate that oral contraceptives normally reduce hepatic excretion of organic anions, at least for BSP and probably for bilirubin and bile salts at higher dosage as has been shown in animals. In the Dubin-Johnson syndrome, there is a selective defect in hepatic excretory function which is accentuated by oral contraceptives although if drug administration were continued, it is possible that bile secretory failure (i.e., involvement of the bile salt excretory mechanism) would occur. In recurrent cholestasis with or without pregnancy, an initial effect of oral contraceptives on BSP excretion may occur, but this has not been specifically studied. In the latter disorders, a non-dose related response to oral contraceptives affects the bile salt excretory mechanism producing bile secretory failure and cholestasis. In patients with post-necrotic cirrhosis, oral contraceptives result in bile secretory failure probably because hepatic excretory function is greatly reduced in this disease. The major determinant for the effect of oral contraceptive agents in these various diseases appears to be the nature of the underlying disorder. This is consistent with a general effect of these steroids on the bile canaliculi and/or its presumed carrier molecules.

Oral contraceptive steroids also affect the entry of bilirubin into liver cells as well as its subsequent conjugation with glucuronic acid; however, the foregoing discussion concerns those aspects most relevant to clinical jaundice seen with these drugs.

REFERENCES

1. Combes, B., Sjibato, H., Adams, R., Mitchell, B. and Trammell, V.: Alterations in sulfobromophthalein sodium removal mechanisms from blood during normal pregnancy. J. Clin. Invest. 42:1431-1442 (1963).

2. Mueller, M.N. and Kappas, A.: Estrogen pharmacology. I. The influence of estradiol and estriol on hepatic disposal of sulfobromophthalein (BSP) in man. J. Clin. Invest. 43:1905-1914 (1964).

3. Scherb, J., Kirschner, M. and Arias, I.M.: Studies of hepatic excretory function. The effect of 17-ethyl-19-nortestosterone on sulfobromophthalein sodium (BSP) metabolism in man. J. Clin. Invest. 42:404-408 (1963).

4.   Goldfischer, S., Arias, I.M., Essner, E. and Novikoff, A.B.: Cytochemical and electron microscopic studies of rat liver with reduced capacity to transport conjugated bilirubin. J. Exp. Med. 115:467-474 (1962).

5.   Urban, E., Frank, B.W. and Kern, F.: Liver dysfunction with mestranol but not with norethynodrel in a patient with Enovid-induced jaundice. Ann. Int. Med. 68:598-602 (1968).

6.   Haemmerli, U.P.: Jaundice during pregnancy: with special emphasis on recurrent jaundice during pregnancy and its differential diagnosis. Acta. Med. Scand. 179: (supp. 444): 1, (1966).

7.   Summerskill, W.H.J.: The syndrome of benign recurrent cholestasis. Amer. J. Med. 38:298-305 (1965).

8.   Dubin, I.N.: Chronic idiopathic jaundice. Am. J. Med. 24:268-279 (1958).

9.   Arias, I.M.: Studies of chronic familial non-hemolytic jaundice with conjugated bilirubin in serum with and without an unidentified pigment in the liver cells. Am. J. Med. 31:510-514 (1961).

10. Kleiner, G., Kresch, L. and Arias, I.M.: Studies of hepatic excretory function. II. The effect of norethynodrel and mestranol on bromsulfalein sodium metabolism in women of child-bearing age. New Eng. J. Med. 273:420-423 (1965).

11. Wheeler, H.O., Meltzer, J. and Bradley, S.E.: Biliary transport and hepatic storage of sulfobromophthalein sodium in the unanesthetized dog, in normal man and in patients with hepatic disease. J. Clin. Invest. 39:1131-1144 (1960).

12. Arias, I.M.: Effects of a plant acid (icterogenin) and certain anabolic steroids on the hepatic metabolism of bilirubin and sulfobromophthalein (BSP). Ann. N.Y. Acad. Sci. 104:1014-1025 (1963).

13. Biempica, L. and Arias, I.M.: Biochemical, histochemical and ultrastructural studies of the liver in familial recurrent cholestasis. Gastroenterology 52:521-535 (1967).

14. Gutstein, S., Alpert, S. and Arias, I.M.: Biliary excretion of sulfobromophthalein sodium (BSP) in a patient with the Dubin-Johnson syndrome and a biliary fistula. Israel J. Med. 4:36-41 (1968).

15.   Cornelius, C., Arias, I.M. and Osburn, B.I.:   Hepatic pigmentation with photosensitivity: a syndrome in Corriedale sheep resembling Dubin-Johnson syndrome in man.   J. Amer. Veter. Med. Assoc.   146:709-713 (1965).

16.   Alpert, S., Mosher, M., Shanske, A. and Arias, I.M.: Multiplicity of hepatic excretory mechanisms for organic anions. J. Gen. Physiol.   (In press).

CHOLESTASIS OF PREGNANCY AND DURING ETHINYL ESTRADIOL ADMINISTRATION IN THE HUMAN AND RAT

Mary Jeanne Kreek

The Rockefeller University, New York, N.Y.

Cholestasis of pregnancy may be subdivided into two syndromes, pruritus gravidarum and the idiopathic cholestatic jaundice of pregnancy, which represent varying degrees of severity of a common disorder. These syndromes were first differentiated from other causes of itching and jaundice during pregnancy by Svanborg, Thorling, Arfwedson and others (1-5). These syndromes tend to occur in the third trimester of pregnancy. Pruritus gravidarum and the idiopathic cholestatic jaundice of pregnancy tend to occur in the third trimester of pregnancy, although symptoms may appear as early as the first trimester, and are usually characterized by symptoms of generalized pruritus, mild anorexia, nausea and occasional vomiting. In the more severe form, jaundice then appears. The liver may become slightly enlarged and tender, and liver function tests reflect cholestasis, with elevated levels of serum alkaline phosphatase, 5'-nucleotidase, conjugated bilirubin and bromsulphthalein retention, with minimal evidence of hepatocellular necrosis. The major pathological lesion, as seen in the liver biopsy, is intrahepatic cholestasis with centrilobular bile staining of liver cells and canalicular bile plugs, possibly accompanied by minimal parenchymal cell necrosis in areas of bile stasis, but without inflammatory cells or proliferation of mesenchymal cells (see Figure 1).

Complete remission of clinical biochemical and histologic abnormalities promptly follows delivery, but the syndromes tend to recur in subsequent pregnancies. It is of particular interest that the syndromes tend to recur when the patients receive oral contraceptive agents. Conversely, in approximately fifty percent of all reported cases of jaundice occurring during oral contraceptive usage, a history of cholestasis during pregnancy was elicited (6-8).

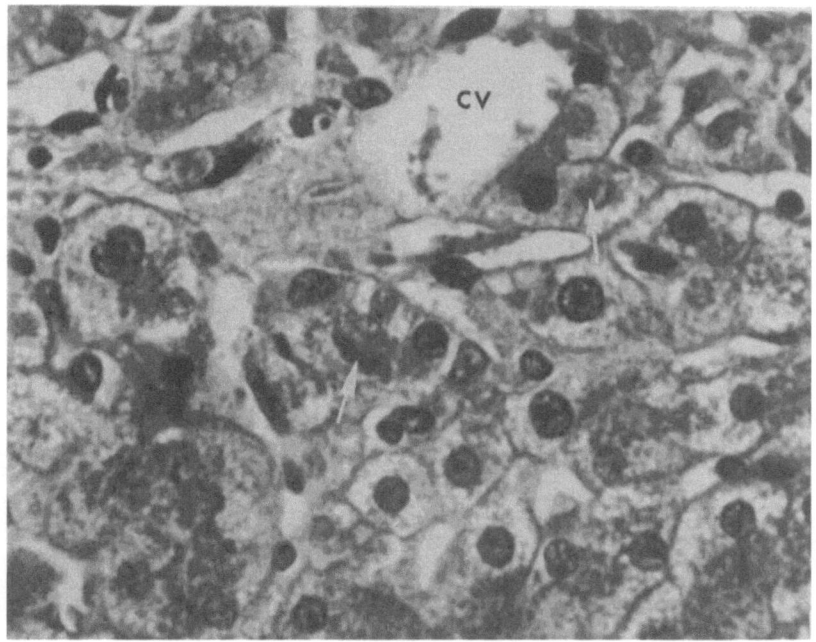

Figure 1. Liver biopsy specimen obtained from a patient with
recurrent cholestatic jaundice of pregnancy. Centrilobular area
showing bile stasis and bile plugs in bile canaliculi. C.V. =
central vein. (From Kreek, Sleisenger and Jeffries, Am. J. Med.
1964)

The following studies were carried out to determine what degree
of subclinical cholestasis occurs during normal pregnancy when endogenous estrogen and progesterone levels are high, and whether estrogen may play an etiologic role in the syndromes of cholestasis of
pregnancy and during oral contraceptive usage in sensitive individuals. Further studies were carried out in the rat to determine the
effects of estrogen therapy on bile flow and estrogen metabolism.

LIVER FUNCTION DURING NORMAL PREGNANCY AND PUERPERIUM

Liver function tests performed during normal pregnancy frequently
have been shown to deviate from those performed in the normal, non-
pregnant state. These deviations have been reviewed in many of the
monographs concerning jaundice during pregnancy (2,4,5). Most of
the studies of liver function tests during pregnancy have been
conducted either on a retrospective basis or by determining function
at one point in time during pregnancy, thus using different patients
to establish each set of values. It was considered of interest to
follow prospectively a group of women throughout pregnancy, labor

TABLE I

LIVER FUNCTION TESTS - LATE PREGNANCY

Test	Week of Pregnancy		Labor	Normal Level
	37-38	39-40		
Alkaline Phosphotase				
Mean	5.7	6.2	5.1	
Range	1.9-14.9	3.3-14.6	0.6-11.6	<5.0 Bodansky Units
# of Cases	50	49	81	
5'-Nucleotidase				
Mean	1.8	2.1	2.0	
Range	0.5-6.7	1.0-11.0	0.3-9.3	<1.7 Bodansky Units
# of Cases	50	50	71	
Leucine Aminopeptidase				
Mean	594	650	780	
Range	145-2050	230-1525	400-1240	85-210 Units
# of Cases	93	72	98	

and the post-partum period, so that the changes in liver function tests of each individual could be determined during these times, and so that concomitant changes in symptoms and physical findings could be observed. In this recent prospective study, 200 unselected women, admitted consecutively to an ante-partum clinic, were followed throughout pregnancy and an additional 100 unselected women, admitted during active labor, were followed through the post-partum period (9). It was further documented that during the third trimester of normal pregnancy, the serum activity of certain enzymes, including non-specific alkaline phosphatase, 5'-nucleotidase and leucine aminopeptidase may exceed the serum levels in non-pregnant women (see Table 1). It has been well documented that the placenta produces a heat-stable alkaline phosphatase which contributes to the circulating level of maternal non-specific alkaline phosphatase in late pregnancy (10-12). Similarily, it has been clearly demonstrated that the substrate used in the routine determination of leucine aminopeptidase, L-leucine-β-naphthylamide, is also readily split by oxytocinase, an oxytocin inactivating enzyme of placental origin which is present in increasing amounts during late pregnancy (13). Therefore, although these changes in alkaline phosphatase and leucine aminopeptidase levels are in part due to the release of enzymes from the placenta, the elevation of 5'-nucleotidase and the wide variation of all enzyme levels in women with functioning placentae suggest that the elevations may in part be due to a variable increase in enzyme production at the hepatobiliary level and decrease in maternal hepatic excretory function, also reflected by a reduced clearance of bromsulphthalein at this time (14).

In this study it was also shown that serum glutamic-pyruvic transaminase and bilirubin levels do not become elevated in late pregnancy or in labor (see Table 2).

TABLE 2

LIVER FUNCTION TESTS - LATE PREGNANCY

Test	Week of Pregnancy 37 40 + Labor	Normal Level
Bilirubin, Total		
Mean	0.3	
Range	0.1-1.2	<0.8mg/100ml.
# of Cases	297	
Serum Glutamic-Pyruvic Transaminase		
Mean	11	
Range	2-52	<40 units
# of Cases	299	

As over 70% of this patient population received ethinyl estradiol 1.0mg per day in the post-partum period to suppress lactation, it was possible to study the effects of this synthetic estrogen on liver function immediately following the endogenous production of high levels of hormones. It was noted that the regression of liver function test values towards normal in the post-partum period was similar in the treated and untreated groups (see Table 3).

TABLE 3

LIVER FUNCTION TESTS POST - PARTUM

EFFECT OF ETHINYL ESTRADIOL THERAPY (E)

	39 Wk. Labor	2-4d. Post-Partum No E	E
5'-Nucleotidase			
Mean	2.0	1.4	1.7
# of Cases	(121)	(22)	(87)
Alkaline Phosphotase			
Mean	5.8	4.9	5.0
# of Cases	(130)	(22)	(94)
Leucine Aminopeptidase			
Mean	740	550	554
# of Cases	(170)	(44)	(167)

However, bromsulphthalein retention at 45 minutes, which was mildly elevated to a mean value of 5% in the untreated patients two to four days post-partum was strikingly more elevated to 10.3% retention at the same time in the estrogen treated group (see Table 4).

TABLE 4

BROMSULPHTHALEIN RETENTION 2 TO 6 DAYS
POST-PARTUM IN "NORMAL" FEMALES

Effect of Ethinyl Estradiol Therapy

No Ethinyl Estradiol	43 patients	mean	5%
		range	1-22%
Ethinyl Estradiol	129 patients	mean	10.3%
		range	1-32%

Normal Value - <4% retention at 45 minutes after BSP, 5mg/kilo body weight, administered intravenously.

CHOLESTASIS OF PREGNANCY

The incidence of cholestasis during pregnancy is unknown.
During the years 1956-1968, thirty cases have been identified at
the New York Hospital on basis of referral within the hospital.
Twenty-eight of these were found from 1963-1968 when these studies
were being conducted and two of these patients were discovered
within the 300 patient prospective study described above. The
classification of each case into the various syndromes of cholestasis
of pregnancy and the number of pregnancies thus complicated in each
sub-group are shown in Table 5. Included in this group are five
patients with known pre-existing liver disease who in the setting
of late pregnancy developed superimposed cholestasis with pruritus
and jaundice. These patients were not considered to have "idiopathic cholestasis of pregnancy" and were not used in any of the
subsequent estrogen or progesterone challenge studies. Similarly
Shelton and Sherlock have recently described the effects of
pregnancy on liver function in thirteen women with chronic active
hepatitis or biliary cirrhosis with increased jaundice during that
time, presumably due to "the additive effects of endogenous sex-
hormones" (15). It is of interest that of ten patients we have
observed with signs and symptoms of cholestasis while taking oral
contraceptive agents, five had a past history of cholestasis of

TABLE 5

CHOLESTASIS OF PREGNANCY - N.Y.H.
1957-1968 (30 Cases)
12 cases - 1963-66
16 cases - 1967-68

Classification	# Women	# Pregnancies with Symptoms / Total # Pregnancies
Recurrent Jaundice & Pruritus	4	11/11
Recurrent Jaundice alone	1	8/8
Recurrent Pruritus	3	6/8
Jaundice & Pruritus	12	12/17
Jaundice alone	1	1/6
Pruritus	4	4/10
Jaundice & Pruritus with Preexistent Liver Disease	5	5/5

pregnancy with otherwise normal hepatobiliary function and the other five had co-existent underlying liver disease documented before or after discontinuing the medication.

In our patients with the so-called idiopathic cholestasis of pregnancy, many diverse ethnic and racial groups were represented and no familial incidence of this order was documented, although one patient suggested that a sibling, unavailable for study, might be affected.

Although no real "treatment" or measures to prevent the development of cholestasis have been described, it has been suggested that cholestyramine, an anion exchange resin which binds bile salts in the gastrointestinal tract, may abolish the annoying symptom of pruritus (5). This agent was used in five of our patients with only partial response in two, and no subjective response in the other three patients. Since it has been recently shown that phenobarbital may enhance the clearance of bromsulphthalein as well as lower serum bilirubin levels in human beings with adult congenital non-hemolytic unconjugated hyperbilirubinemia and also enhances bile flow, excretion of an exogenous bilirubin load, and biliary transport maximum for bromsulphthalein in the rat, the possibility of using barbiturates to attempt to reverse the decreased hepatic excretory function in the cholestasis of pregnancy has been considered (16-18). Although no formal studies have been conducted at this time, two patients have been observed during late pregnancy complicated by cholestasis who received moderate doses of barbiturate (200mg pentobarbital per day) for sedation to relieve the insomnia resulting from pruritus. In these two women no subjective decrease in symptoms and no apparent improvement in liver function studies resulted.

ESTROGEN AND PROGESTERONE CHALLENGE STUDIES

Fourteen of these patients, seven "normal" women previously studied throughout pregnancy, demonstrating a typical wide variation in liver function at that time, and including one patient with documented unconjugated hyperbilirubinemia, and seven "abnormal" women with cholestasis of pregnancy, three with a history of pruritus gravidarum and four with a history of cholestatic jaundice of pregnancy, underwent estrogen challenge studies (see Table 6) (8).

These three groups were shown to differ significantly from each other on basis of liver function tests performed during the early post-partum period (see Table 7). Those who had suffered jaundice in pregnancy differed from the normal group with respect to bromsulphthalein retention and serum levels of alkaline phosphatase, 5'-nucleotidase and bilirubin, and those patients who had

TABLE 6

PATIENTS CHALLENGED POST-PARTUM WITH ETHINYL ESTRADIOL

7 "Normal" Females

Previously studied during pregnancy - typical liver function
abnormalities; mean post-partum BSP retention - 9.6%
(One patient with idiopathic unconjugated
hyperbilirubinemia.)

7 "Abnormal" Females

2 - Pruritus during pregnancy
1 - Recurrent pruritus of pregnancy
2 - Pruritus and jaundice of pregnancy
1 - Recurrent pruritus and jaundice
1 - Recurrent jaundice (X8)

suffered from pruritus gravidarum differed significantly from the
normals with respect to serum alkaline phosphatase levels. All of
these patients were receiving ethinyl estradiol for lactation
suppression at the time these studies were performed.

The challenge studies were carried out several months to several
years post-partum. After history, physical examination and liver
function tests were performed, each patient was placed on ethinyl
estradiol, 1.0 or 0.5mg per day p.o. Liver function tests in all
groups were essentially normal prior to the estrogen challenge
(see Table 8). After one week of therapy, the patients with a
past history of jaundice of pregnancy differed significantly from
the normal group with respect to bromsulphthalein retention and
serum levels of leucine aminopeptidase. Mean serum levels of
5'-nucleotidase and bilirubin were also elevated. Although the
liver function tests of patients with a history of pruritus
gravidarum did not differ significantly from the normal group,
mean levels of bromsulphthalein retention and serum 5'-nucleotidase
were elevated (see Table 9).

Similarly the three groups could be separated on basis of
clinical findings during the challenge studies. Women who had
been free of symptoms during pregnancy had only mild early morning
nausea during the first two days of hormone administration or remained free of symptoms. Those with a past history of pruritus
gravidarum developed generalized pruritus within 24 hours after
the first dose of ethinyl estradiol. The pruritus persisted 1-2
days and then subsided, despite continued hormone usage. Two of
these patients suffered from persistent nausea for two days. Two

TABLE 7

POST-PARTUM LIVER FUNCTION TESTS IN NORMALS AND PATIENTS WITH INTRAHEPATIC
CHOLESTASIS OF PREGNANCY*

	Patients with Jaundice		Normals	Patients with Pruritus	
	Mean	P	Mean	P	Mean
BSP Retention	41.5	$0.001 < t$	9.6	n.s.	12.0
Alkaline Phos.	7.5	$0.01 < t < 0.001$	4.7	$0.05 < t < 0.02$	7.8
5'-Nucleotidase	3.30	$0.01 < t < 0.001$	0.81	n.s.	1.73
Total Bilirubin	2.0	$0.001 < t$	0.30	n.s.	0.4
S.G.P.T.	61	n.s.	11	n.s.	7

*For normal values, see Table 1,2,4

TABLE 8

LIVER FUNCTION TESTS PRIOR TO CHALLENGE WITH ETHINYL ESTRADIOL*

	Patients with Jaundice		Normals	Patients with Pruritus	
	Mean	P	Mean	P	Mean
BSP Retention	2.5	n.s.	3.3	n.s.	3.0
Alkaline Phos.	3.5	n.s.	2.5	n.s.	3.6
5'-Nucleotidase	1.37	n.s.	1.11	n.s.	1.18
Total Bilirubin	0.6	n.s.	0.4**	n.s.	0.3
S.G.P.T.	7	n.s.	14	n.s.	11
Leucine-aminopeptidase	206	n.s.	148	n.s.	168

*For normal values, see Tables 1,2,4.

**Mean serum bilirubin excluding value from patient with unconjugated hyperbilirubinemia

TABLE 9

LIVER FUNCTION TESTS AFTER ONE WEEK OF CHALLENGE WITH ETHINYL ESTRADIOL*

	Patients with Jaundice		Normals	Patients with Pruritus	
	Mean	P	Mean	P	Mean
BSP Retention	26.0	0.05<t<0.02	5.7	n.s.	13.0
Alkaline Phos.	4.0	n.s.	2.6	n.s.	2.4
5'-Nucleotidase	2.48	n.s.	1.44	n.s.	2.39
Total Bilirubin	1.3	n.s.	0.4	n.s.	0.2
S.G.P.T.	22	n.s.	19	n.s.	20
Leucine-aminopeptidase	330	0.05<t<0.02	185	n.s.	213

*For Normal values, see Table 1,2,4

TABLE 10

LIVER FUNCTION TESTS AFTER ONE WEEK OF CHALLENGE WITH MEDROXYPROGESTERONE ACETATE

TWO PATIENTS WITH CHOLESTASIS OF PREGNANCY AND WITH POSITIVE
ETHINYL ESTRADIOL CHALLENGE STUDIES

	Prior to Challenge	After One Week Challenge	Normal
BSP Retention	0.6	0.3	0.8mg/100ml
Alkaline Phos.	1.5	1.5	5.0 B.U.
Total Bilirubin	0.3	1.1	4%-45 min.
S.G.P.T.	6	7	30 units
S.G.O.T.	7	5	30 units

*Average value of two cases

patients had enlarged, tender livers after one week. Of the women
who had a past history of cholestatic jaundice of pregnancy, three
developed persistent nausea, throughout the duration of hormone
administration, one developed generalized pruritus within one day
lasting for one week. Two women suffered from right upper quadrant
pain and were found to have enlarged, tender livers at the end of
one week of hormone usage. One patient who had suffered from
jaundice without pruritus during each of eight pregnancies noted
dark urine on the second day of challenge and became jaundiced on
the fifth day, at which time estrogen challenge was terminated.
Therefore, ethinyl estradiol administration precipitated, in a
mild degree, the same symptoms and liver function test abnormalities
which had been noted during pregnancy in the three groups.

Subsequently, two further patients with a past history of
cholestasis of pregnancy and with positive estrogen challenge
studies when not pregnant, have been similarly challenged with
the synthetic progesterone, medroxyprogesterone acetate, 20mg per
day p.o. No symptoms and no alterations in liver function tests
occurred during this challenge (see Table 10).

These studies suggest that estrogens may be of importance in
the pathogenesis of the syndromes of cholestasis of pregnancy and
may also be responsible in part for the alterations in liver
function observed during normal pregnancy. Evidence now available
would suggest that an increased sensitivity of the hepatic excretory
mechanisms to endogenous or exogenous estrogen is the primary defect
in those patients who have had cholestasis of pregnancy and are
abnormally responsive to challenge. However, qualitative or
quantitative differences in estrogen metabolism may also play a
role. The exact nature of this demonstrated estrogen sensitivity
remains undefined. However, the estrogen sensitive individual may
be expected to develop liver function impairment during usage of
oral contraceptive agents containing estrogen.

EFFECTS OF ESTROGEN TREATMENT ON BILE FLOW AND BILIARY EXCRETION OF ESTROGENS IN THE RAT

Gallagher, Mueller and Kappas have shown that the treatment of
rats with a large variety of estrogen compounds will cause a
diminished clearance of bromsulphthalein, whereas progesterone
compounds do not have a similar effect (19). To further elucidate
the effects of estrogen administration on hepatobiliary function,
the following studies were carried out (20,21).

Sprague-Dawley female rats weighing 150-180 grams were fed
ethinyl estradiol 0.5mg per day p.o. for nine days. At the end of
that time liver function tests revealed elevated levels of serum

5'-nucleotidase and alkaline phosphatase, reflecting cholestasis
(21). Litter mate control animals were sham fed. Liver function
tests were normal at the end of the feeding period in these animals.
On the tenth day, common duct cannulation and femoral vein cathe-
terization were performed under light ether anesthesia. The animals
were maintained on intravenous hydration under constant room temperature conditions in modified restraining cages. Eighteen to twenty
hours after surgery, thus 40-48 hours after last estrogen dosage,
the following studies were carried out: Ten milligrams of BSP and
a tracer dose of tritiated estradiol were administered intravenously.
Bile was collected in fractions over a nine hour period, and volume
and radioactivity of bile were measured.

Bile flow in the estrogen treated rats was significantly decreased to as low as 43% of the flow in control rats from the time
of surgery throughout the control and study period (see Figure 2).

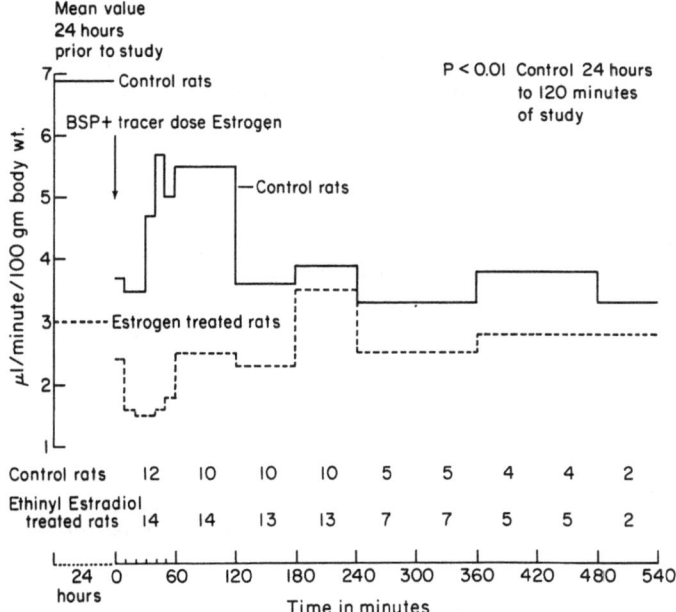

Figure 2. Bile flow, expressed in μl per minute per 100 grams
body weight, in control and ethinyl estradiol treated rats. Mean
value for 24 hours following bile duct cannulation and values for
each bile fraction taken during excretion studies are charted.
(From Kreek, Peterson, Sleisenger, Jeffries, 1969.)(21).

Delayed appearance of bromsulphthalein in the bile occurred in
the estrogen treated rats, within 20 to 30 minutes after adminis-

tration as compared with 0-10 minutes in control animals. The
appearance of estradiol in the bile was also delayed in the estrogen
treated animals, appearing at 30-40 minutes as opposed to within
10 minutes in the controls. Lower radioactivity per unit volume
of bile and per unit time was present in the early bile fractions
of the estrogen treated animals. There was a decreased biliary
excretion of estradiol during the nine hour study period in the
estrogen treated animals (see Figure 3). Thirty-two percent of
the total administered dose of labeled estradiol was excreted
during the study period in the treated animals as compared with
52% of the administered dose in the control group. The recovery
of 52% of the radioactivity from the administered dose of estradiol,
which has been reported to be essentially completely converted to
estrone in the rat, compares well with the biliary recovery of 58%
of radioactivity from an administered dose of estrone in the rat
recently reported by Sandberg and associates (22).

Similarly, despite an overall increased biliary excretion in
both groups, there was a significantly diminished biliary excretion
of radioactivity from an administered dose of estradiol glucuronide
in the estrogen treated animals, 40% of the administered dose as
compared with 81% in the control animals (see Figure 4). This

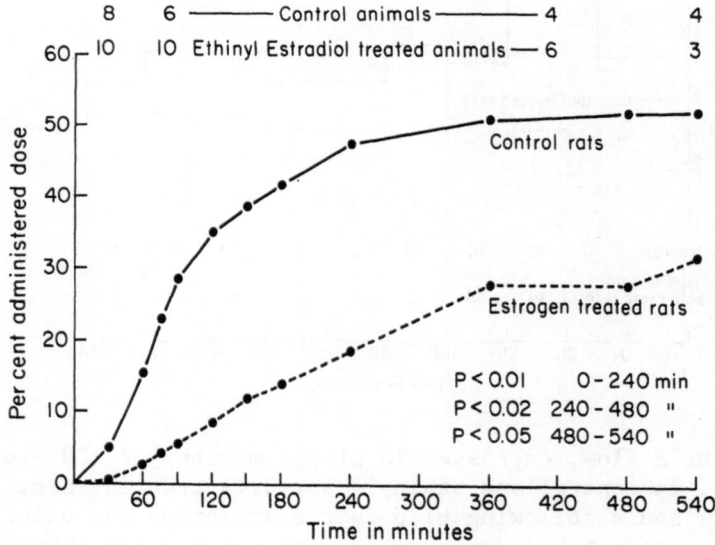

Figure 3. Biliary excretion of estradiol-17 -6,7-H^3 in control
and ethinyl estradiol treated rats during nine hours following
intravenous administration of tracer doses of estrogen and 10mg
bromsulphthalein (From Kreek, Peterson, Sleisenger, Jeffries,
1969) (21).

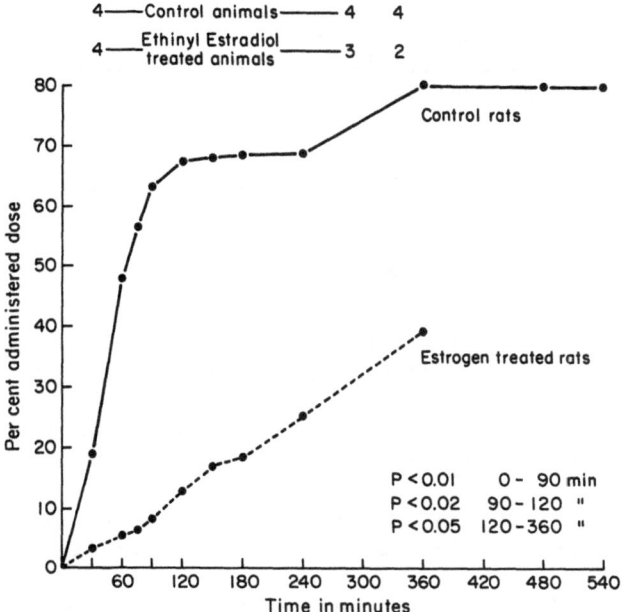

Figure 4. Biliary excretion of estradiol 6,7-H^3-17 -D-glucuronide
in control and ethinyl estradiol treated rats during nine hours
following the intravenous administration of tracer doses of estrogen
and 10mg bromsulphthalein (From Kreek, Peterson, Sleisenger,
Jeffries, 1969) (21).

suggested that glucuronide or other polar conjugate formation was
not the limiting step in biliary excretion of estrogen in the
treated animals and suggested that the major defect caused by
estrogen treatment probably was an impairment of the hepatocellular
excretory mechanisms or of the biliary conduct system.

These studies demonstrating the effects of estrogen therapy
resulting in a reduction of bile flow and a diminution of biliary
excretion of estrogen, a major pathway of estrogen metabolism in
man, suggest a possible role of estrogens in the pathogenesis of
biliary tract disease in pregnancy and also suggest that in the
setting of endogenous or exogenous estrogen-induced cholestasis,
a resultant alteration of estrogen metabolism may occur, possibly
leading to an accumulation of normal or abnormal metabolites which
in turn might intensify cholestasis by the initial yet undefined
mechanism of action.

ACKNOWLEDGMENT

The author would like to acknowledge the contributions made to these studies by several collaborators and assistants, and to especially acknowledge the valued association and close collaboration with Dr. Marvin H. Sleisenger and Dr. Graham H. Jeffries in most of the clinical studies. She would also like to thank Miss Irmgard Olbert for her expert assistance in the preparation of this manuscript.

REFERENCES

1. Svanborg, A.: A study of recurrent jaundice in pregnancy. Acta Obst. et Gynec. Scandinav. 33:434-444 (1954).

2. Thorling, L.: Jaundice in pregnancy. A clinical study. Acta Med. Scand. Suppl. 302:1-123 (1955).

3. Arfwedson, H.: General pruritus in pregnancy. Symptom of liver dysfunction. Obstet. Gynec. 7:274-276 (1956).

4. Ikonen, E.: Jaundice in late pregnancy. Acta Obstet. Gynec. Scand. 43:Suppl. 5, 1-130 (1964).

5. Haemmerli, U.P.: Jaundice during pregnancy: with special emphasis on recurrent jaundice during pregnancy and its differential diagnosis. Acta Med. Scand. 179:Suppl. 444, 1-111 (1966).

6. Kreek, M.J., Sleisenger, M.H., and Jeffries, G.H.: Recurrent cholestatic jaundice of pregnancy with demonstrated estrogen sensitivity. Am. J. Med. 43:795-803 (1967).

7. Orellana-Alcade, J.M. and Dominquez, J.P.: Jaundice and oral contraceptive drugs. Lancet 2:1278-1280 (1966).

8. Kreek, M.J., Weser, E., Sleisenger, M.H., and Jeffries, G.H.: Idiopathic cholestasis of pregnancy: the response to challenge with the synthetic estrogen, ethinyl estradiol. New Eng. J. Med. 277:1391-1395 (1967).

9. Kreek, M.J., Raziano, J., Weser, E., Sleisenger, M.H., Fuchs, F., and Jeffries, G.H.: Liver function in pregnancy (In Preparation).

10. Boyer, S.H.: Alkaline phosphatase in human sera and placentae. Science 134:1002-1004 (1961).

11. McMaster, Y., Tennant, R., Clubb, J.S., Neale, F.C., and
    Pasen, S.: The mechanism of the elevation of serum alkaline
    phosphatase in pregnancy. J. Obst. Gynec. Brit. Cwlth., 71:
    735-739 (1964).

12. Kitchener, P.N., Neale, F.C., Pasen, S., and Brudenell-Woods,
    J.: Alkaline phosphatase in maternal and fetal sera at term
    and during the puerperium. Am. J. Clin. Path. 44:654-661
    (1965).

13. Tuppy, H.: Biochemical studies of oxytocinase. In:
    Proceedings of an International Symposium on Oxytocin held
    in Montevideo, 1959, p. 315. Edited by Caldeyro-Barcia, R.
    and Heller, H. New York, 1961. Pergamon Press, Inc.

14. Combes, B., Shibata, H., Adams, R., Mitchell, B., and
    Trammell, N.: Alterations in sulfabromophthalein sodium
    removal mechanisms from blood during normal pregnancy. J.
    Clin. Invest. 42:1431-1442 (1963).

15. Whelton, M.J. and Sherlock, S.: Pregnancy in patients with
    hepatic cirrhosis: management and outcome. Lancet 2:995-999
    (1968).

16. Kreek, M.J. and Sleisenger, M.H.: Reduction of serum-
    unconjugated bilirubin with phenobarbitone in adult congenital
    non-hemolytic unconjugated hyperbilirubinemia. Lancet 2:73-
    78 (1968).

17. Roberts, R.J. and Plaa, G.L.: Effect of phenobarbital on the
    excretion of an exogenous bilirubin load. Biochem. Pharm.
    16:827-835 (1967).

18. Klaassen, C.D. and Plaa, G.L.: Studies on the mechanism of
    phenobarbital-enhanced sulfobromophthalein disappearance.
    J. Pharm. Expt. Ther. 161:361-366 (1968).

19. Gallagher, T.F. Jr., Mueller, M.N., and Kappas, A.: Studies
    on the mechanism and structural specificity of the estrogen
    effect on BSP metabolism. Tr. A. Am. Physicians 78:187-195
    (1965).

20. Kreek, M.J., Peterson, R.E., Sleisenger, M.H., and Jeffries,
    G.H.: Influence of ethinyl estradiol-induced cholestasis on
    bile flow and biliary excretion of estradiol and bromsulfo-
    phthalein by the rat. (Abstract) J. Clin. Invest. 46:1080
    (1967).

21. Kreek, M.J., Peterson, R.E., Sleisenger, M.H., and Jeffries, G.H.: Effects of ethinyl estradiol-induced cholestasis on bile flow and biliary excretion of estradiol and estradiol glucuronide by the rat. (In Preparation).

22. Sandberg, A.A., Kirdani, R.Y., Back, N., Weyman, P., and Slaunwhite, W.R. Jr.: Biliary excretion and enterohepatic circulation of estrone and estriol in rodents. Am. J. Physiol. 213:1138-1142 (1967).

δ-AMINOLEVULINATE SYNTHETASE OF THE CHICK EMBRYO LIVER : THE EFFECT OF NATURAL AND SYNTHETIC SEX STEROIDS ON ITS ACTIVITY

Chull S. Song, Arleen B. Rifkind, Richard D. Levere,
Peter N. Gillette, Genevieve S. Incefy, and Attallah Kappas

The Rockefeller University, New York, N.Y.

δ-Aminolevulinate (ALA) synthetase is the initial enzyme in the porphyrin and heme biosynthetic pathway and catalyzes the formation of ALA from glycine and succinyl coenzyme A. The production of ALA is the rate-limiting step in the hepatic formation of porphyrins and heme (1, 2). The activity of ALA synthetase, as measured by the rate of production of ALA by hepatic mitochondria (1) or homogenate (3) can be markedly enhanced by administration of a large number of chemicals and drugs that induce experimental porphyria in animals (4). In hereditary porphyria of acute intermittent type in man, the activity of this enzyme is also greatly increased (5, 6), which explains, at least in part, the augmented urinary excretion of porphyrins and their precursors, ALA and porphobilinogen, characterizing this disease.

Previous studies in our laboratory demonstrated that certain natural steroids of the 5β-H configuration (Fig. 1) markedly enhanced the production of porphyrins by chick embryo liver cells growing in primary culture (7, 8) and the activity of ALA synthetase in the livers of whole chick embryos (9). In view of the possible relevance of this new biological activity of steroids to the relationship between sex hormones and the clinical expression of hereditary porphyria of man, and the implications of steroid control of heme synthesis in relation to hemoprotein formation in the liver, we have examined the effect of a number of natural and synthetic sex steroids and their metabolites on the ALA synthetase activity of the chick embryo liver.

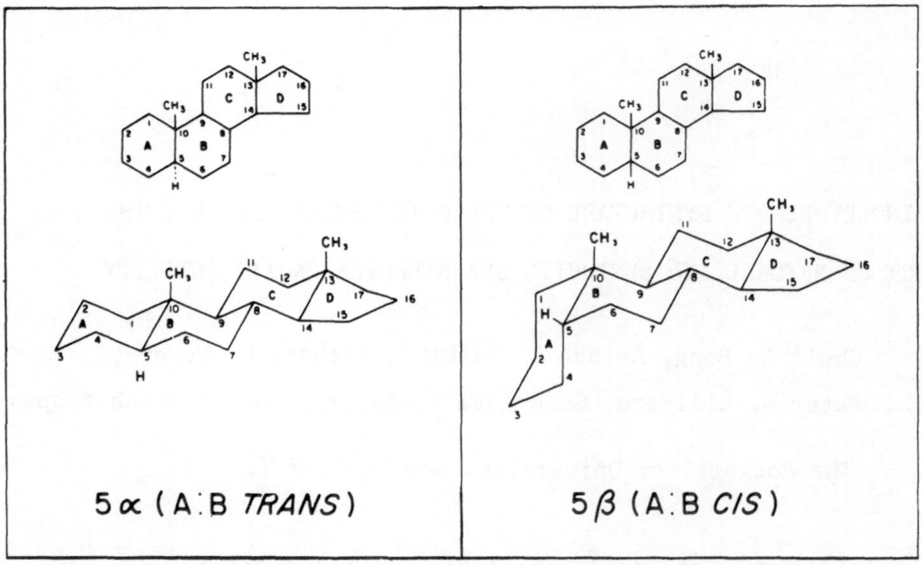

Fig. 1 Stereoisomerism of the steroid ring nucleus. 5α isomer, in which the A:B ring junction is planar, carries the C-10 methyl group and C-5 hydrogen atom in a <u>trans</u> configuration. 5β isomer, in which the A:B ring junction is highly angulated, carries the C-10 methyl group and C-5 hydrogen atom in a <u>cis</u> configuration.

Experimental Methods and Results

The steroid hormones and metabolites were dissolved in propylene glycol containing 10% N,N'-dimethylacetamide and sterilized by passage through Millipore filters. The steroids were injected into the extraembryonic sac of 16-day old chick embryos through a small hole drilled into the blunt end of the egg where the air cavity can usually be located by means of transillumination. Eggs were incubated at 37 degrees for various lengths of time. Embryos were then removed from the shells and their livers quickly excised. Two to three livers were pooled, homogenized, and ALA synthetase activity determined according to the method of Marver et al. (3). The applicability of this method to determination of ALA-synthetase activity in chick embryo liver has previously been established (9).

Table I summarizes mean activities of ALA synthetase in chick embryo livers 8 hours after the administration of various natural sex steroids and their metabolites. At 5 mg per egg, a number of steroid metabolites of the 5β-H configuration such as pregnane-3α,

Table I. Effect of sex steroids and their metabolites on ALA
synthetase activity of the chick embryo liver. 5 mg of each of the
steroids were injected into 16-day old chick embryos and the hepatic activities of ALA synthetase were determined 8 hours later.
The unit of enzyme activity is expressed as mμmoles of ALA formed
per gram wet weight of the liver per hour. Figures in parentheses
indicate the number of experiments.

Steroids	ALA synthetase
	mμmole ALA/g/hour
Control	27 (41)
Etiocholanolone [a]	450 (7)
Etiocholanedione [b]	359 (2)
11-Ketopregnanolone [c]	385 (5)
17α-OH-11-ketopregnanolone [d]	525 (29)
Pregnanedione [e]	522 (5)
Progesterone	93 (6)
Estradiol	46 (14)
Estriol	30 (9)
Testosterone	56 (7)

a   5β-Androstane-3α-ol-17-one
b   5β-Androstane-3,17-dione
c   5β-Pregnane-3α-ol-11,20-dione
d   5β-Pregnane-3α,17α-diol-11,20-dione
e   5β-Pregnane-3,20-dione

17α-diol-11,20-dione, etiocholanolone, etiocholanedione, pregnane-
dione, and 11-ketopregnanolone greatly stimulated the hepatic activity for ALA synthetase. These steroids are not primary endocrine
secretions but are the products of hepatic biotransformation of primary sex hormones such as progesterone and testosterone or intermediates in the steroid biosynthetic scheme. They had previously been
shown to strongly induce the synthesis of porphyrins in chick embryo
liver cells growing in primary culture (7, 8). The magnitude of enhancement of hepatic ALA synthetase activity in the chick embryo liver (Table I) by these 5β-H steroids was comparable to that induced

by the same amount of allylisopropylacetamide, a potent porphyrinogenic chemical (4).

The responses of the chick embryo liver to 5β-H steroids and
to allylisopropylacetamide were somewhat variable and the variability was in part seasonal in nature; but the increase in ALA synthetase activity by these agents was nearly always greater than 5-
10 times the activity noted in control animals. In the case of 5β-
pregnane-3α,17α-diol-11,20-dione, for example, the mean value of
ALA-synthetase activity from 29 experiments was 525 mμmoles of ALA
produced per hour per gram liver, which represents an increment exceeding 19-fold over the mean value of 27 mμmoles ALA produced per
hour per gram of control livers.

The effect of primary sex steroids such as progesterone, estradiol, and testosterone on ALA synthetase activity of the chick embryo liver is also presented in Table I. It is of interest that the
stimulation of the enzyme activity by these sex steroids was considerably less than that produced by their metabolites; such stimulation was of statistically significant magnitude, however, for progesterone and testosterone. Only a small increment was noted for estradiol; and none for estriol.

Fig. 2 depicts the time course of stimulation of ALA synthe-

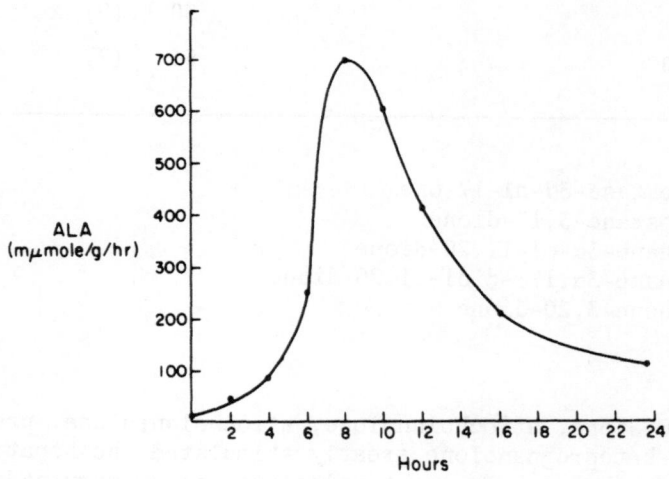

Fig. 2.   Time course of enhancement of ALA synthetase activity of the
chick embryo liver by 5β-pregnane-3α,17α-diol-11,20-dione. 5 mg of
the steroid metabolite were injected into 16-day old chick embryos at
zero time and ALA synthetase activities of the livers were measured
at intervals up to 24 hours. Each point represents the mean value obtained from 4 embryos. The unit of enzyme activity is expressed as
mμmoles of ALA formed per gram wet weight of the liver per hour.

tase activity by the 5β-H metabolite 5β-pregnane-3α,17α-diol-11,20-
dione. Following the administration of 5 mg of the steroid, detectable but slight elevation of the enzyme activity was noted by 2
hours. The activity increased rapidly thereafter and reached a maximum level by 8 hours, following which a quick decline was noted.
It is of note that the maximum level of ALA synthetase subsequent
to treatment with the steroid metabolite preceded by a few hours
the maximum porphyrin accumulation within the embryonic liver cells
as noted by porphyrin fluorescence (2).

    The enhancement of ALA synthetase activity was essentially pro-
portional to the amount of the steroid metabolite injected into the
egg (Fig. 3). With larger doses of the steroid, the response diminished, in a manner similar to those observed with cultured liver
cells (7). The reason for this phenomenon is not clear at this time,
but may be related in part to the toxicity of a large amount of the
steroid metabolite. Many nonsteroid porphyrinogens show a similar
dose-response relationship in chick embryo liver. We have not detected evidence of formation of an inhibitor substance in liver
homogenates to account for the decline of enzyme activity after the
peak level is reached.

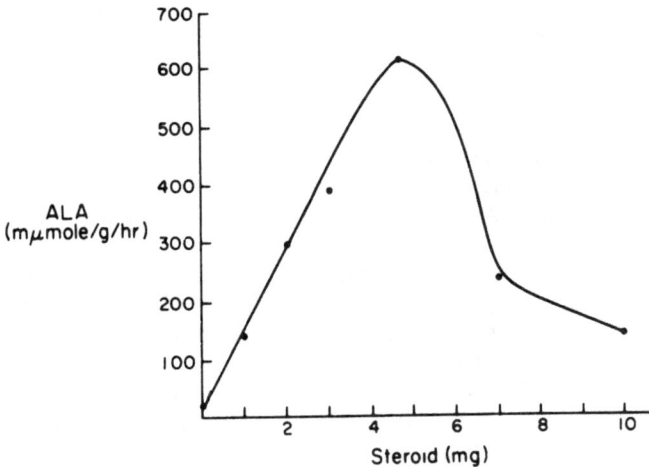

Fig. 3. Relationship between the amount of steroid administered
and the enhancement of ALA synthetase activity in the chick embryo
liver. The steroid metabolite, 5β-pregnane-3α,17α-diol-11,20-dione,
was injected into chick embryos in amounts ranging from 2 mg to
10 mg per embryo. The activity of ALA synthetase was measured 8 hours
later. The enzyme activity is expressed as mμmoles of ALA formed per
gram wet weight of the liver per hour.

The effects of actinomycin D and cycloheximide administered to the chick embryo together with the maximum inducing dose of 5β-pregnane-3α,17α-diol-11,20-dione have also been studied. The inhibitory effects of these substances on the steroid-induced enhancement of ALA synthetase activity became evident as early as 2 hours after treatment. By 8 hours, the inhibitions by actinomycin D (250 µg/embryo) and cycloheximide (5 µg/embryo) were 80% and 96%, respectively. The cultured liver cells display an extreme sensitivity to the inhibitory effect of actinomycin D (8); and the relatively large amount of the antibiotic required to produce a substantial inhibitory effect on the steroid-induced increase in ALA synthetase activity in the whole embryo liver may reflect its insolubility in the egg and difficulty in crossing the extraembryonic membranes into the fetus. This was evidenced by the precipitation of much of the administered antibiotic on the extraembryonic membranes in many of our experiments. Glucose (20-100mg/embryo), when administered with the steroid metabolite, reduced the inducing effect by approximately 50%.

In addition to the natural sex steroids and their metabolites, we have also examined various synthetic estrogens and progestins, singly and in combination, for their effect on ALA synthetase activity of the chick embryo liver. These steroids include the synthetic estrogens such as ethinylestradiol and its 3-methoxy derivative (mestranol) and synthetic progestins such as norethindrone, ethynodiol diacetate, norethynodrel, chlormadinone acetate, norethindrone acetate, medroxyprogesterone acetate, and dimethisterone. These hormones are constituents of oral contraceptive preparations that are currently in common use.

The synthetic estrogens, when administered in amounts ranging from 0.33 mg to 9 mg per embryo and examined 8 hours later, had little or no effect on the ALA synthetase activity of the liver.

On the other hand, all the synthetic progestins were inducers of ALA synthetase activity, with the exception of chlormadinone acetate which showed little or no effect. At 3 mg per embryo, the synthetic progestins enhanced the activity of this enzyme to a magnitude comparable to that brought about by the 5β-H metabolites. Addition of synthetic estrogens to the progestins in proportions found in commercial preparations of oral contraceptives (estrogen:progestin ration ranging from 1:10 to 1:250 in weight) did not alter the response of the embryo liver to the progestins.

Discussion

The chick embyro liver preparation used in the present investigation represents a simple and sensitive technique for the initial studies of a large number of drugs and chemicals for their porphyrino-

genic properties. Our studies demonstrate that 5β-H metabolites of
sex steroids are potent inducers of ALA production by the liver
cells of chick embryos. Such increased rate of synthesis of ALA is
followed in a few hours by a maximum accumulation of porphyrins in
the liver cell, consistent with the currently accepted view that ALA
synthetase is the rate-limiting enzyme in porphyrin and heme biosynthesis in the liver.

Because of the natural occurrence in various species of animals
of steroids structurally resembling, or identical with, the 5β-H metabolites that are strong porphyrinogens, the suggestions have been
made (7, 8) that these steroids may represent one category of physiological agents which control, by increasing the formation of ALA synthetase, the rate of porphyrin and heme biosynthesis in the liver.
Derangement in such a control mechanism, e.g. by defective disposal
of the steroid metabolites, may be related to the clinical expression
of the genetic disease, acute intermittent porphyria, although this
possibility remains speculative at present.

The results of our studies, though consistent with the de novo
formation of ALA synthetase by the steroid metabolites, are not final
proofs for such a mode of action of the steroids. Rigorous proof for
de novo formation of ALA synthetase must await the successful solubi-
lization of this enzyme from cell membranes and a means of measuring
its amount independent of its catalytic activity.

There have been various, and at time conflicting, reports that
estrogens, progestins and oral contraceptive agents (10, 11, 12, 13,
14) precipitate acute exacerbations of clinical symptoms associated
with acute intermittent porphyria or increased urinary outputs of porphyrins and precursors (15, 16). There are reports, on the other hand,
in which oral contraceptive agents were shown to ameliorate the clinical symptoms of women with cyclic exacerbations of porphyria in relation to menstrual periods (17). The biochemical basis for these findings remains presently uncertain. The explanation may lie in part in
the effect of exogenous steroids on the production of certain potent
endogenous inducers of porphyrin synthesis in such individuals. Our
observations suggest that it may in particular be the progestational
components of the oral contraceptive preparations which produce clinical exacerbations of acute intermittent porphyria or the increased
urinary excretion of porphyrins and their precursors.

In view of the wide variations of drug effects that can be observed among different species (18), our studies obviously must be extended to other animals including man before a firm clinical implication of the porphyrinogenic effect of the sex steroids can be drawn.
Such studies involving various mammalian experimental animals and men
are currently in progress in our laboratory. One area in which this
steroid effect may find physiological expression relates to the hepa-

tic capacity to effect drug detoxification by oxidative metabolism catalyzed by a heme-containing oxygenase, cytochrome P-450. The rate of oxidation of various drugs and the concentration of microsomal cytochrome P-450 in the rat have been shown to vary greatly in relation to the sex and gestational status (Gram and Gillette, these proceedings). The effect of sex steroids on the rate of porphyrin and heme production may therefore find physiological expression in the activity of certain hepatic enzymes in which heme serves as a prosthetic group.

REFERENCES

1. Granick, S., and Urata, G. J. Biol. Chem. 238: 821, 1963

2. Granick, S., J. Biol. Chem. 241: 1359, 1966

3. Marver, H.S., Tschudy, D.P., Perlroth, M.G., and Collins, A. J. Biol. Chem. 241: 2803, 1966

4. De Matteis, F. Pharmacol. Rev. 19: 523, 1967

5. Tschudy, D.P., Perlroth, M.G., Marver, H.S., Collins, A., Hunter, G., Jr., and Rechcigl, M., Jr. Proc. Nat. Acad. Sci. 53: 841, 1965

6. Nakao, K., Wada, O., Kitamura, T., Uono, K., and Urata, G. Nature 210: 838, 1966

7. Granick, S., and Kappas, A. J. Biol. Chem. 242: 4587, 1967

8. Kappas, A., and Granick, S. J. Biol. Chem. 243: 346, 1968

9. Kappas, A., Song, C.S., Levere, R.D., Sachson, R.A., and Granick, S. Proc. Nat. Acad. Sci. 61: 509, 1968

10. Welland, F., Hellman, E.S., Collins, A., Hunter, G., Jr., and Tschudy, D.P. Metab. Clin. Exptl. 13: 251, 1964

11. Wetterberg, L. Lancet II, 1178, 1964

12. Burton, J.L., London, N.B., and Wilson, A.T. Lancet II, 1326, 1967

13. Levere, R.D. Blood 28: 569, 1966

14. Levit, E.J., Nodine, J.H., and Perloff, W.H. Amer. J. Med. 22: 831, 1957

15. Koskelo, P., Eisalo, A., and Toivonen, I. Brit. Med. J. 1: 652,
     1966

16. Redeker, A.G., South Afr. J. Lab. Clin. Med. 9: 302,
     1963

17. Perlroth, M.G., Marver, H.S., and Tschudy, D.P. J. Amer. Med.
     Assoc. 194: 1037, 1965

18. Conney, A.H., and Burns, J.J. Adv. in Pharmacol. 1: 31, 1962

THE EFFECTS OF PROGESTERONE ADMINISTRATION ON HEPATIC ENDOPLASMIC RETICULUM: AN ELECTRON MICROSCOPIC AND BIOCHEMICAL STUDY

A.L. Jones and J.B. Emans

Departments of Medicine and Anatomy, University of
California, San Francisco, and Department of Anatomy,
Harvard Medical School, Boston, Massachusetts

It is now well known that there are tiny membrane-limited channels ramifying throughout the cytoplasm of most cells. Porter (24) was the first to describe this lace-like reticulum of membranes with the electron microscope. Because of its association with the endoplasmic portion of the cell rather than the ectoplasm, it was referred to as the "endoplasmic reticulum" (25,26). In 1955, Fawcett (7) noted that two forms of the endoplasmic reticulum existed in the hepatic parenchymal cell. One form consisted of a system of membranes studded with ribosomes (rough-surfaced endoplasmic reticulum) and the other consisted of only a membranous network (smooth-surfaced endoplasmic reticulum).

In the liver parenchymal cell, the rough-surfaced reticulum characteristically is arranged in parallel profiles of flattened cisternae while the smooth-surfaced endoplasmic reticulum is usually visualized as anastomosing interwoven tubules scattered in small patches throughout the cytoplasm (8,14) and (Fig. 1). Areas of direct continuity between these two categories of intracytoplasmic membranes are occasionally encountered. Besides differing in basic structure and distribution, the agranular (smooth) and granular (rough) reticulum also differ with respect to their association with glycogen. When present, glycogen almost invariably is closely

The authors gratefully acknowledge the assistance of Dr. Harvey Marver, Department of Medicine, University of California Medical Center, San Francisco, in determining the δ ALA synthetase and P-450 values and in the preparation of this manuscript. The authors are also indebted to the technical assistance of Mr. Edward Miller and Miss Gabrielle Rouiller. Supported in part by V.A.G.I. TR-48.

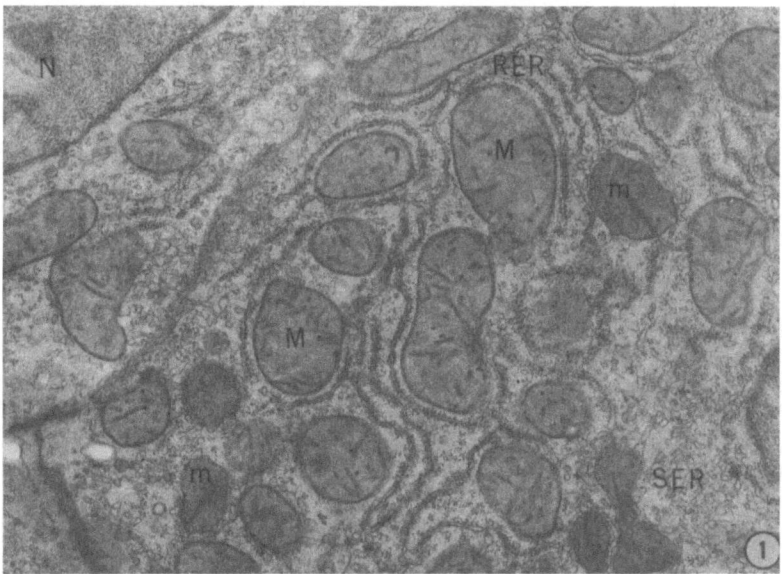

Fig. 1.   An electron micrograph of a portion of liver from
a control hamster. Note the long flattened cisternal profiles
of the rough surfaced endoplasmic reticulum (RER) and the tubular
smooth surfaced reticulum (SER) scattered in small patches throughout the cytoplasm. Nucleus (N), mitochondria (M) and microbodies
(m) are also observed.(x 27,000, reduced 30% for reproduction.)

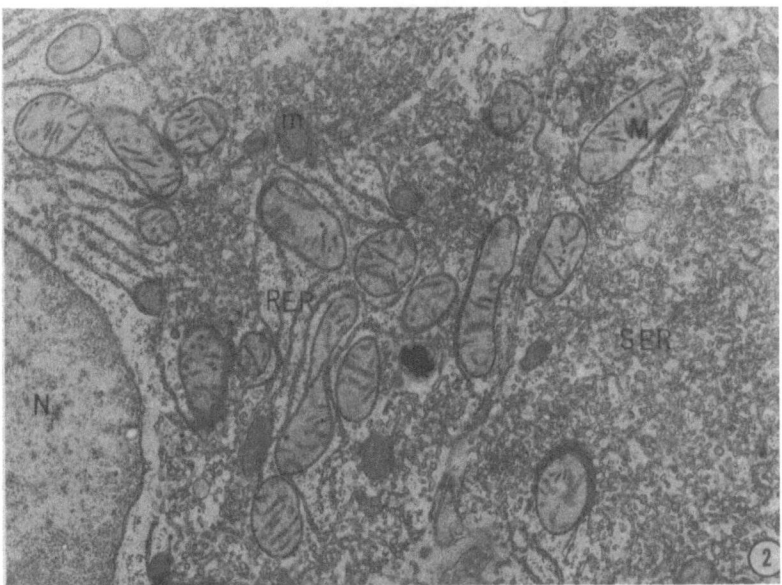

Fig. 2.   Portions of two liver cells from an animal treated
with phenobarbital. A striking hypertrophy of the smooth reticulum
(SER) is in evidence. (x 22,000, reduced 30% for reproduction.)

associated with the smooth reticulum and not the rough surfaced variety (14). The close spatial association between glycogen and the smooth endoplasmic reticulum provided the first evidence that the two forms of endoplasmic reticulum were perhaps functionally as well as structurally (14) and, as shown later, chemically different (4,9). Subsequently, many studies have led us to believe that the rough reticulum plays a principal role in protein synthesis (4) while the smooth reticulum has been implicated in glycogen (14), cholesterol (13), lipoprotein (15) and, of importance to this paper, drug and steroid-metabolism (5,14).

Two important recent discoveries have provided much of our insight into the possible functions of both categories of endoplasmic reticulum. These are the development of methods capable of subfractionating microsomes into a rough and smooth variety (6,14), and the discovery that certain lipid soluble drugs such as phenobarbital promote a selective increase in the hepatic smooth-surfaced reticulum (14) (Figs. 2,4).

Previous work by Fouts (6) indicated that the majority of drug metabolizing enzyme activity resided in the smooth-surfaced microsomal fraction and that this activity increased mainly in the smooth-surfaced fraction following administration of phenobarbital. In addition to this increase in drug metabolizing enzymes, it is now well established that phenobarbital promotes a striking increase in the quantity of smooth reticulum seen with the electron microscope (14). These findings have led to the understandable conclusion that the smooth reticulum plays a significant role in the metabolism of many drugs.

The ability of the liver to increase its smooth-surfaced reticulum and certain enzymes in response to drugs probably represents an adaption to alterations in environment rather than a manifestation of toxicity. The value of such a response in the detoxification of drugs, carcinogens and insecticides is apparent since it allows the liver to metabolize the inducing substance more readily.

If what is known about membrane turnover is correct (28), induction of membranes and enzymes probably occur continuously in the normal cell and is, in all likelihood, influenced by naturally occurring endogenous compounds rather than controlled by exogenous chemicals. The phenobarbital effect is probably an exaggeration of a normal process in which enzyme synthesis is regulated to meet the metabolic needs of the organism. Several pieces of information led us to a consideration of the possible influence of the sex steroids on the induction process:
    1. All of the some 200 known exogenous compounds considered inducers are lipid soluble (2).

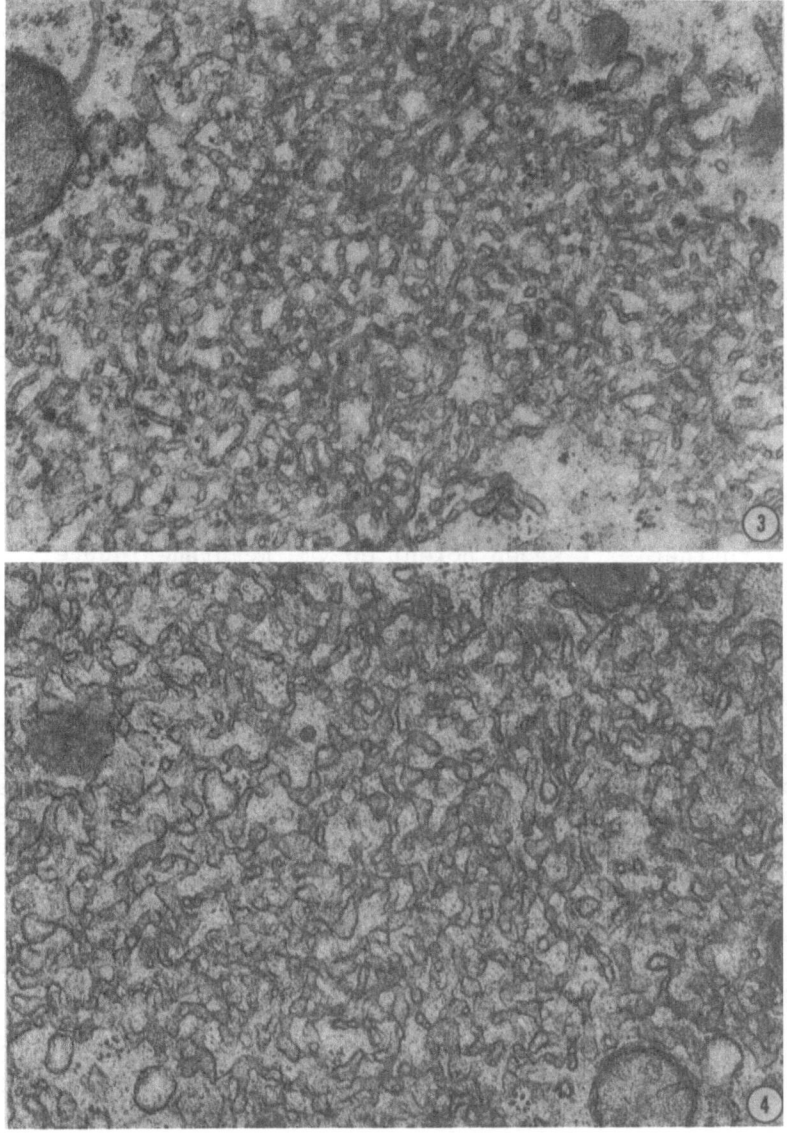

Figs. 3 and 4. Smooth reticulum rich areas from experimentally
treated liver cells. Figure 3 is from a male hamster given 10 mg
of progesterone/day and Figure 4 is from a phenobarbital treated
animal. In both micrographs the tubular form of the smooth reticulum from progesterone treated animals (Fig. 3) are often smaller
and more tightly packed than those of the phenobarbital treated
group (Fig. 4). The significance of this observation, if any, is
not known. (x 47,000, reduced 30% for reproduction.)

2.   There is a striking similarity between certain steroid hydroxylases and drug metabolizing enzymes (3).

3.   Steroids, according to the data of Kuntzman (17), are metabolized more efficiently by liver microsomes, than are drugs, suggesting that steroid metabolism is a normal function of these mocrosomal enzymes.

4.   Evidence has been reported indicating that progesterone administration to hamsters promoted an increase in hepatic smooth reticulum (5,14).

5.   Granick's list of substances which induce the formation of enzymes involved in porphyrin(or heme) metabolism includes the sex steroids (10).

The approach taken in this and in our previous paper (5) has been to compare the effects of progesterone administration in the hamster with that of a known potent enzyme membrane inducer, phenobarbital.

MATERIALS AND METHODS

The details of the materials and methods are described elsewhere (5) and will not be reiterated here. In summary, male golden hamsters (110-120 gm) were given either 10, 30, or 60 mg of progesterone in oil intraperitoneally each day in divided dosages for four days, and, after 24 hours, were sacrificed on the fifth day. Another group of male animals were given 10 mg of phenobarbital and one ml oil intraperitoneally each day for four days and again sacrificed on the fifth day following an overnight fast. Livers from all animals were removed and weighed, and one portion was processed for electron microscopy and another portion was used for total microsomal phospholipid determination.

In subsequent experiments, four female golden hamsters, 110 gm, were placed on either the 10 mg or 30 mg progesterone regimen and the effects on the liver endoplasmic reticulum analyzed by electron microscopy. In addition, nine males were divided into three groups and were given either 10 mg phenobarbital, 30 mg of progesterone/day or the oil vehicle alone for four days and, after a 24 hour fast, a portion of their livers were again evaluated by electron microscopy and another portion removed and processed for δ ALA synthetase activity by the method of Marver et al (18) and for the microsomal heme protein P-450, according to the method of Omura and Sato (21). The extinction coefficient employed was 91mM-1 cm-1.

TABLE 1

EFFECT OF PROGESTERONE ON LIVER WEIGHT

Liver
(% of Body Weight)

	Mean	S.D.	P
Control (10)	2.91	± .36	
10 mg Prog/day (4)	3.68	± .33	.01
30 mg Prog/day (9)	3.89	± .44	< .001
Phenobarbital (9)	3.60	± .42	< .001

100-120 gm male hamsters were injected as described in Materials and Methods for 4 days and sacrificed on the fifth day. Liver weights are expressed as % of total body weight occupied by the liver. P is calculated from the "t" distribution and expresses the probability that the difference in mean % body weight observed between treated and control groups is not statistically significant. Each experimental group was compared independently with the control group in these calculations. Numbers in parentheses indicate the number of animals in each group.

(From Emans, J. B. and Jones, A. L. J. Histochem. Cytochem. 16: 561: (1968)).

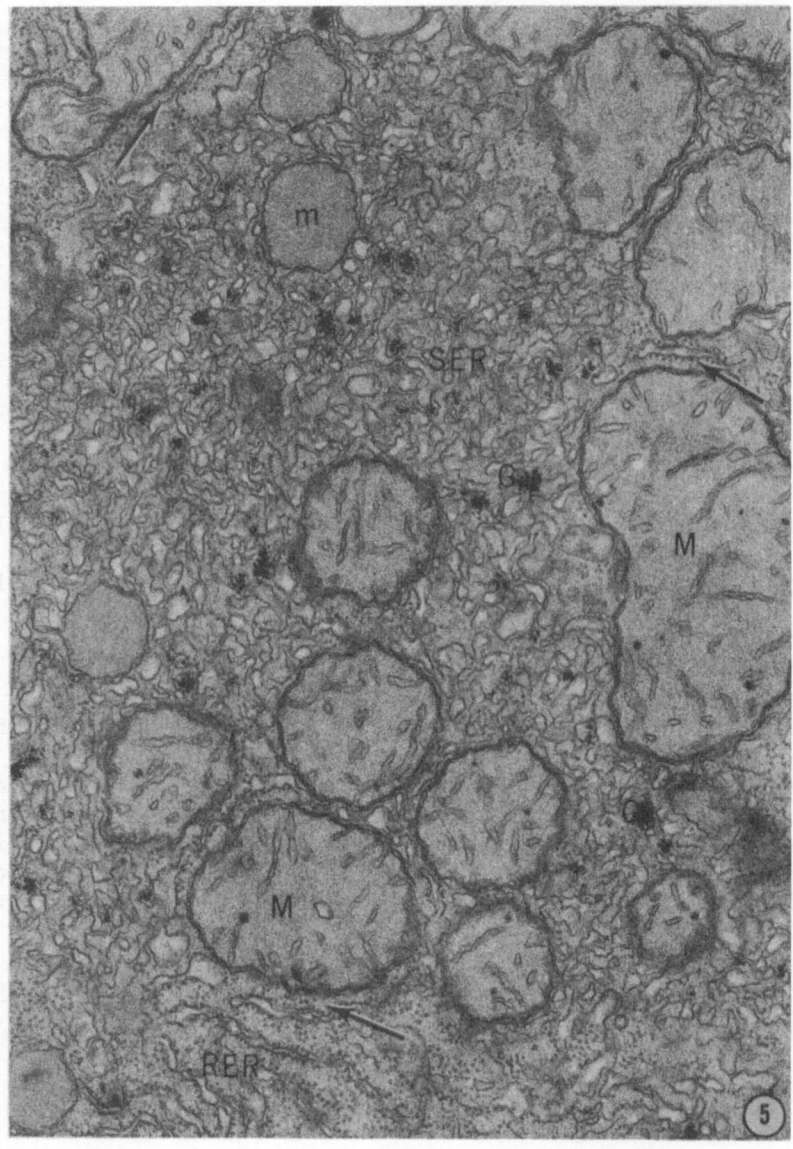

Fig. 5. An electron micrograph of a portion of liver from
a female hamster given 30 mg of progesterone daily for four days.
In the female as well as the male, progesterone administration promotes hypertrophy of the hepatic smooth endoplasmic reticulum. An
association between the rough-surfaced reticulum and the mitochondria are observed at the arrows. A few electron opaque glycogen
rosettes (G) are noted in the smooth reticulum rich areas. Rough
reticulum (RER), nucleus (N), Golgi (G) and mitochondria (M).
(x 31,000, reduced 20% for reproduction.)

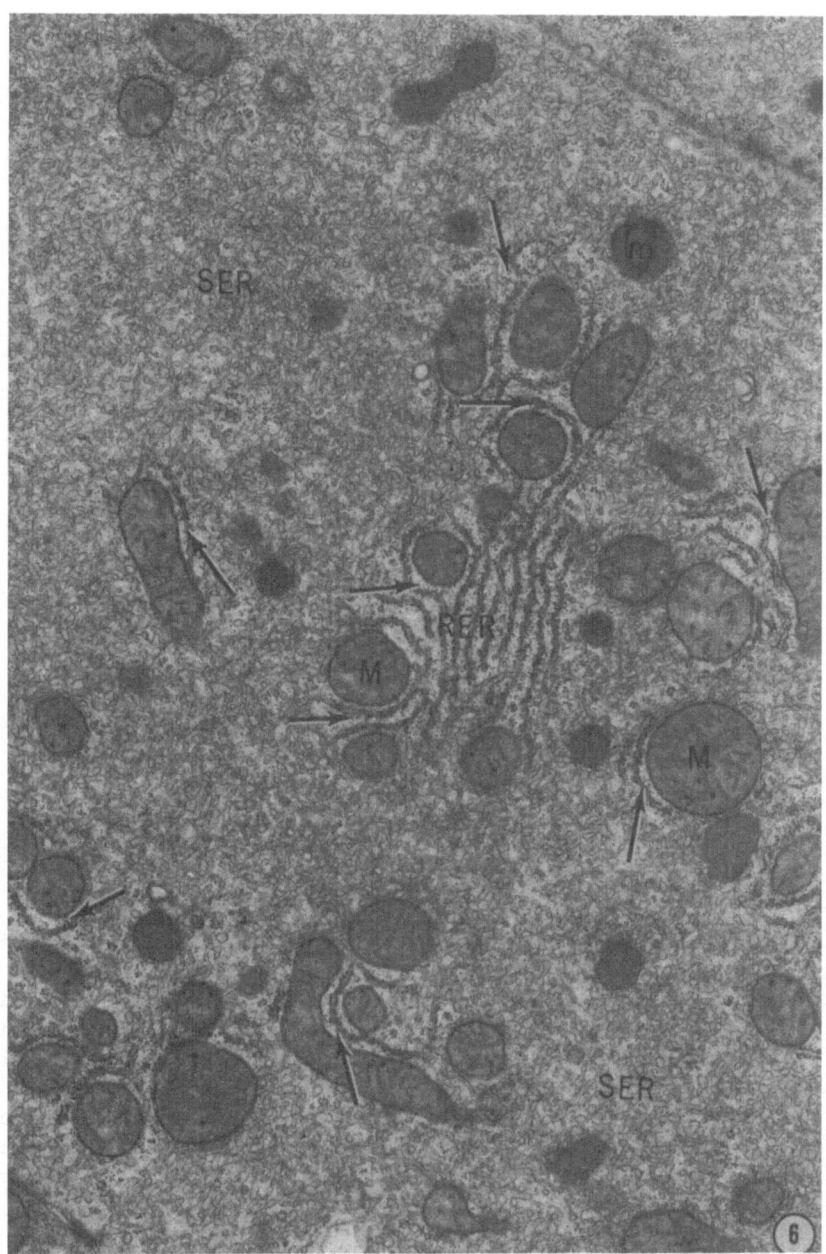

Fig. 6. After administration of 30 mg of progesterone per day to male hamsters, there is a spectacular increase in liver cell smooth reticulum. Many areas of continuity between the rough and smooth surfaced membranes are observed. Note the close association between the mitochondria (M) and the rough reticulum (RER) at the arrows. (x 25,000, reduced 20% for reproduction.) (From Emans, J.B. and Jones, A.L.: J. Histochem. Cytochem. 16:561, 1968.)

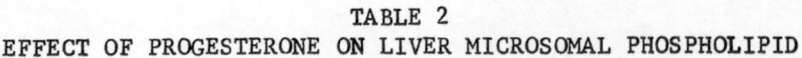

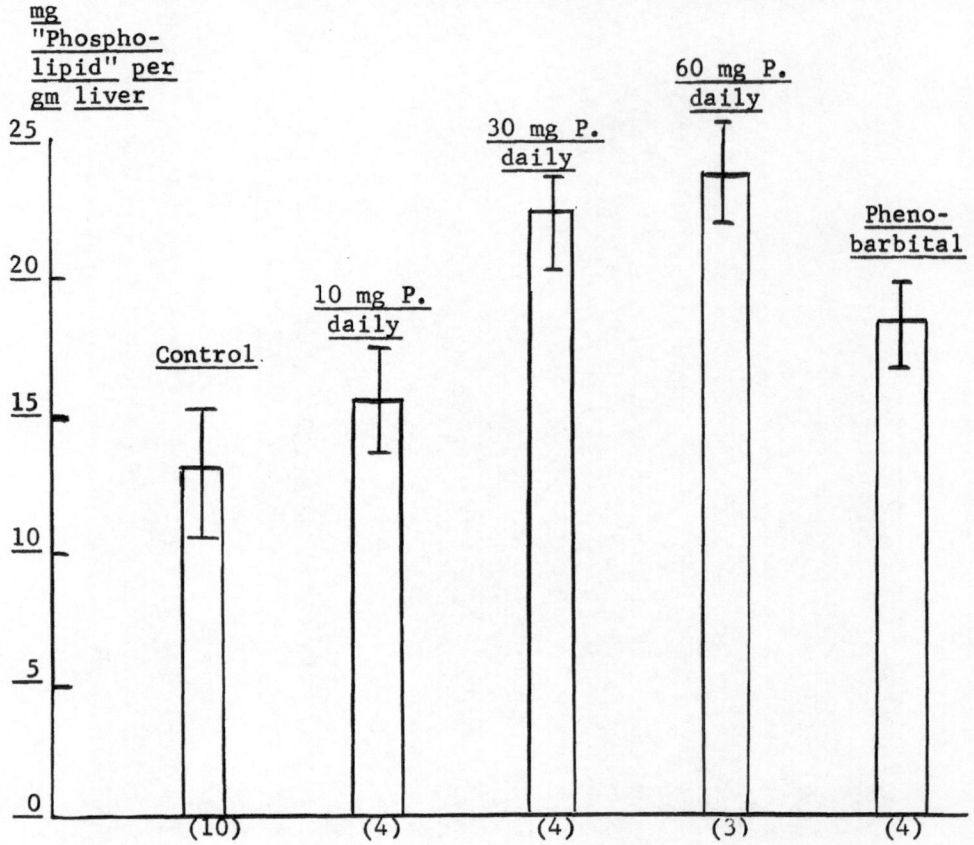

TABLE 2
EFFECT OF PROGESTERONE ON LIVER MICROSOMAL PHOSPHOLIPID

Animals were treated as described in Materials and Methods. As an indication of the quantity of microsomal membrane present in the liver, total phosphorus in the phospholipid fraction of micro-somes from each liver was determined, and a factor of 25 used to convert phosphorus to "phospholipid." The graph indicates the means and range of values obtained in each group and the number of animals in each group is indicated in parenthesis. (P refers to progesterone.)

(From Emans, J. R. and A. L. Jones. J. Histochem. Cytochem. 16: 561 (1968)).

RESULTS

Morphology

Both progesterone and phenobarbital-treated animals showed a prominent increase in liver size (Table 1). With the electron microscope, a spectacular selective increase in the quantity of smooth-surfaced endoplasmic reticulum was seen in both male (Figs. 2-4,6) and female (Fig. 5) (14) hamsters given either progesterone (Figs. 3,5,6) or phenobarbital (Fig. 2). In animals receiving the higher dosages of progesterone (Figs. 5,6), this apparent increase in new membrane appeared even more striking than in the phenobarbital-treated animals (Fig. 2). Hypertrophy of the smooth endoplasmic reticulum in both progesterone and phenobarbital-treated animals was apparently not at the expense of the rough reticulum; rather, it represented an absolute increase in the smooth form unaccompanied by changes in the rough category. Other organelles, including the nucleus and mitochondria did not appear altered by phenobarbitol or progesterone treatment. A preferential association between the long slender segments of the rough reticulum and the mitochondria was seen in all groups including controls (Fig. 1) but was particularly noteworthy in the progesterone-treated group (Fig. 6).

Biochemistry

Levels of microsomal phospholipid per gram of liver increased two-fold in the 30 and 60 mg progesterone-treated livers and somewhat less in the phenobarbital and 10 mg progesterone group (Table 2). The apparent discrepancy between the modest increase noted in the microsomal phospholipid levels and the many-fold increase in smooth endoplasmic reticulum seen by the electron microscopy relates to the fact that total microsomal phospholipid measures the sum of rough and smooth-surfaced microsomal fractions. If only the smooth membranes increase as we believe, and the normal ratio of rough to smooth reticulum in the intact cell is approximately 3/2, then the smooth reticulum would have to increase $3\frac{1}{2}$ fold in order to realize a two-fold increase in microsomal phospholipid. Thus, a relatively small increase in total microsomal phospholipid is consistent with the larger increase in the smooth endoplasmic reticulum seen with the electron microscope.

Cytochrome P-450 (21), a carbon monoxide binding microsomal heme-protein necessary for certain steps in hydroxylation reactions, was found to increase per mg microsomal protein in both the phenobarbital and progesterone-treated groups (Table 3). Since the quantity of microsomes/gm liver also increased in both cases (5), this represents a several-fold increase in P-450/gm liver. The rise in cytochrome P-450 was somewhat greater in the phenobarbital

TABLE 3

COMPARISON OF THE ENZYMATIC EFFECTS OF PHENOBARBITAL AND
PROGESTERONE

	δ ALA Synthetase mμ Moles ALA/gm Liver/ 1/2 hr	P-450 mμ Moles/mg Protein
Control	23.1	1.17
Phenobarbital	38.1	2.6
Progesterone	68.5	1.94

100-120 gm male hamsters were given either 10 mg/day
phenobarbital or 30 mg/day progesterone for four days as decribed
in Materials and Methods. Three animals were used in each group
and their livers pooled. δ ALA Synthetase was measured by the
method of Omura and Sato (21).

as compared to the progesterone-treated group but the rise in δ-aminolevulinic acid synthetase activity was approximately three-fold in the progesterone-treated group and less than two-fold in the phenobarbital group. Although there are some quantitative differences in enzyme induction, the data clearly indicates that qualitatively phenobarbital and progesterone have similar inductive effects on the proteins and enzymes studied.

DISCUSSION

Classification of Inducers

It is now recognized that there are two principal classes of microsomal enzyme inducers (2). One class is represented by such compounds as phenobarbital and many insecticides, and another by certain carcinogenic compounds such as methycholanthrene and 3'4' benzopyrene. Inducers in the first group promote a marked hypertrophy of the liver smooth endoplasmic reticulum as well as a generalized increase in activity of many microsomal enzymes with the possible exception of glucose-6-phosphatase (23). Inducers in the second group promote a more subdued proliferation of the smooth endoplasmic reticulum and induce only a few rather specific enzymes. It is also reported that under special circumstances, hypertrophic hypoactive smooth endoplasmic reticulum can exist but this is probably a manifestation of hepato-toxicity (11). The finding of smooth membrane hypertrophy, an elevation in cytochrome P-450, and increases in mitochondrial δ ALA synthetase, do not allow the firm assignment of progesterone to either of these categories of inducers, but progesterone's biochemical and morphological inductive properties do appear more in keeping with the phenobarbital group. The normal existence of progesterone in the body and the above data raise the possibility that progesterone or its metabolites may be natural inducers of smooth endoplasmic reticulum and by virtue of this inductive capacity, it may participate in the maintenance of normal levels of the smooth reticulum and associated enzymes.

Steps in Enzyme Induction

Granick's model for the induction of microsomal heme-containing cytochromes suggests that the intranuclear concentration of heme regulates the production of heme and microsomal cytochromes (10). In this model, heme, which may be derived from the turnover of liver cytochromes, combines with an intranuclear aporepressor to form a repressor which inhibits an operator gene. When the operator gene is rendered inactive, no mRNA is synthesized and the microsomal cytochrome production is diminished. If heme is not available to bind the aporepressor then there is an increase in endoplasmic reticulum (microsomes) with its associated enzymes. Inducing substances presumably act by competing with heme for

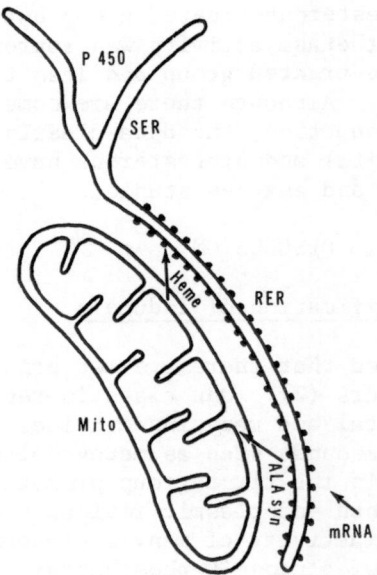

Fig. 7. The close association of the rough-surfaced reticulum with the mitochondria seen in the electron micrographs is diagrammatically represented here. This kind of a relationship may represent a unit necessary for the production of smooth reticulum and heme containing cytochromes. Under the influence of mRNA the rough-surfaced endoplasmic reticulum (RER) synthesizes the enzyme δ ALA synthetase which is transferred to the inner membrane of the mitochondria. This results in an increased production of heme of which a part is transferred back to the endoplasmic reticulum and utilized for the production of the microsomal heme protein P-450.

binding to the aporepressor, and once bound to the aporepressor render it inactive and unable to inhibit the operon.

Evidence suggesting nuclear control is also derived from the observation that livers from animals pretreated with Actinomycin D showed a marked reduction in ability to induce microsomal enzymes, membrane formation (22) and δ ALA synthetase (19). Steroid molecules entering the liver cell normally may be sequestered in the lipid portion of the smooth reticulum where they would come to be in juxtaposition to the metabolizing enzymes presumably located in the protein moiety of the same membrane. Excess steroids not bound by the endoplasmic reticulum would contribute to the intracellular concentration of the same steroid which may then influence through the nucleus the production of mRNA necessary for the synthesis of new endoplasmic reticulum and its associated hydroxylases. We proposed in a previous paper (5) that exogenous lipid soluble compounds such as phenobarbital may only indirectly induce membrane and enzyme synthesis by taking up binding sites on the endoplasmic reticulum normally reserved for steroids, thereby increasing the cytoplasmic and nuclear concentration of the steroid. Elevated concentrations of free hormone might then result in greater inhibition of the aporepressor, less repression of the operon and increased production of specific mRNA, enzymes and microsomal protein. A hypothesis of this nature might easily be evaluated by investigating the ability of exogenous inducers to induce membrane and enzyme synthesis in castrated animals or in animals with other endocrinologic manipulation. Cardell (1) has noted a decrease in hepatic smooth endoplasmic reticulum following hypophysectomy in rats. This observation would support our hypothesis of an endocrine control mechanism, possibly mediated through the sex hormones, for the maintenance of normal levels of endoplasmic reticulum. However, the fact that porphyrin synthesis can be induced in steroid-free chick embryo liver cultures (10) by exogenous compounds argues against this proposal.

One point which has puzzled morphologists is that most of the inducing substances promote an increase in δ ALA synthetase, a mitochondrial enzyme, yet very little if any alteration in mitochondrial morphology is noted in the electron micrographs. Even after the potent stimulator of δ ALA synthetase, allylisopropylacetamide, was administered to rats, no mitochondrial alterations were noted. Nevertheless, as elegantly demonstrated by Posalaki and Barka (27), this compound promotes a marked increase in liver smooth endoplasmic reticulum. Since heme production is carried on in the liver almost exclusively by the mitochondria, it appears likely that the increased mitochondrial heme production may precede the increased synthesis of microsomal heme containing enzymes. Although the precise location of δ ALA synthetase production is not known, from a consideration of the work of Marver et al (19) on the inhibitory effect of puromycin on the synthesis of δ ALA synthetase, and from what we know about the ability of the endoplasmic reticulum to synthesize and transfer certain enzyme proteins to the mitochondria (16), the rough-surfaced reticulum seems the most likely site of synthesis of δ ALA synthetase. In our micrographs, particularly of the progesterone-treated animals, there was an apparent preferential association of rough-surfaced reticulum with the mitochondria. It may well be that this represents a spatial association enabling the newly synthesized δ ALA synthetase to be transferred efficiently from the rough-surfaced reticulum to its functional location on the inner membrane of the mitochondria (20), and the newly formed heme necessary for the final synthesis of heme containing enzymes to be transferred back to the rough endoplasmic reticulum where the protein components of the new smooth membrane and enzymes are being synthesized. If this is true, then the formation of the heme cytochrome rich new smooth membrane may require both the rough-surfaced endoplasmic reticulum

and mitochondria working as a unit. Although the association observed between mitochondria and rough-surfaced endoplasmic reticulum was more apparent in the progesterone-treated livers, it was
also observed in the controls. This is not surprising considering
the rather short half-life of the endoplasmic reticulum (two to
three days) (28) and δ ALA synthetase (67-72 minutes) (19) which
necessitate continuous synthesis of new membrane and enzyme.

We have inferred throughout the discussion that hypertrophy
of the smooth reticulum is a result of increased synthesis and
the establishment of a new steady state rather than a lack of
breakdown or prolonged turnover. This area remains unsettled and
arguments for increased synthesis (22,28) as well as for decreased
breakdown (12,27,29) exist. Our observations do not lend support
to either theory, but we are inclined to favor the data of
Schimke et al (28) which indicates that increased synthesis
account for most of the net increase in membrane.

CONCLUDING REMARKS

In the present paper, we have tried to point out that there
are two categories of endoplasmic reticulum in the liver cell
which are distinctly different morphologically and probably functionally. The rough reticulum undoubtedly plays the principal
role in the synthesis of protein including enzyme protein while
the smooth reticulum plays an important role in drug and steroid-
metabolism. The results indicate that, in the hamster, progesterone is an inducer of the smooth reticulum, the microsomal
heme-protein P-450, and δ ALA synthetase, and raise several
questions about the normal interrelationship between sex steroids
and the smooth endoplasmic reticulum. Are the sex steroids or
their metabolites natural inducers of hepatic enzymes, and to what
extent do they influence the normal quantity of endoplasmic
reticulum and associated enzymes when present in the circulation
in physiologic levels? Does the administration of sex hormones
affect hepatic drug metabolizing enzymes so that certain drug
therapy may be significantly altered and results may be unpre-
dictable? To what extent, if any, is there potentiation in the
enzyme and membrane-inductive effects when exogenous inducers
such as phenobarbital are given with the sex steroids? And,
lastly, the more basic question, what initiates the hepatic
events which result in increased membrane synthesis in response
to either exogenous or endogenous compounds? It is hoped that
in the future the answers to these important questions will be
forthcoming.

SUMMARY

The liver cell smooth endoplasmic reticulum has been implicated in a number of hepatic metabolic processes including drug and steroid metabolism. Evidence for its role in drug metabolism has been derived from the observation that phenobarbital or certain other lipid soluble compounds promote an increase in this organelle and many of its associated enzymes. This effect is considered an adaptive response enabling the liver to metabolize the inducing substance more rapidly and may be an exaggeration of a normal and continuous inductive process necessary for the maintenance of smooth endoplasmic reticulum. The present paper demonstrates that repeated administration of a naturally occurring endogenous compound, progesterone, produces hepatocellular events similar to those produced by exogenous compounds; namely, an increase in liver weight, hypertrophy of the smooth endoplasmic reticulum and elevated levels of the heme-protein P-450 and δ ALA synthetase. The data indicate that progesterone may be a natural inducer of hepatic endoplasmic reticulum and certain associated enzymes and that this steroid may normally influence the quantity of these liver cell components.

REFERENCES

1. Cardell, R.R. Subcellular alterations in rat liver following hypophysectory. Biochem. Biophys. Acta 148:539 (1967).

2. Conney, A.H. Pharmacological implications of microsomal enzyme induction. Pharm. Rev. 19:317 (1967).

3. Conney, A.H., Schneidman, K., Jacobson, M., and Kuntzman, R. Drug induced changes in steroid metabolism. Am. N.Y. Acad. Sci. 123:(Art. 1) 98 (1965).

4. Dallner, D., and Ernster, L. Subfractionation and composition of microsomal membranes: A review. J. Histochem. Cytochem. 16:611 (1968).

5. Emans, J.B., and Jones, A.L. Hypertrophy of liver cell smooth surfaced reticulum following progesterone administration. J. Histochem. Cytochem. 16:561 (1968).

6. Fouts, J.R., Rogers, L.A., and Gram, T.E. The metabolism of drugs by hepatic microsomal enzymes. Studies on intramicrosomal distribution of enzymes and relationships between enzyme activity and structure of the hepatic endoplasmic reticulum. Exp. Molec. Path. 5:475 (1966).

7. Fawcett, D.W. Observations on the cytology and electron microscopy of hepatic cells. J. Nat. Cancer Inst. 15:1475 (1955).

8. Fawcett, D.W. Structural and functional variations in the membranes of the cytoplasm. In Intracellular Membraneous Structure, p. 15. Japan Society for Cell Biology, Okayama (1965).

9. Glaumann, H., and Dallner, G. Lipid composition and turnover of rough and smooth microsomal membranes in rat liver. J. Lipid Res. 9:720 (1968).

10. Granick, S. The induction in vitro of the synthesis of δ aminolevulinic acid synthetase in chemical porphyria: a response to certain drugs, sex hormones, and foreign chemicals. J. Biol. Chem. 241:1359 (1966).

11. Hutterer, F., Schaffner, F., Klion, F.M., and Popper, H. Hypertrophic, hypoactive smooth endoplasmic reticulum: a sensitive indicator of hepatotoxicity exemplified by Dieldrin. Science 161:1017 (1968).

12. Jick, H., and Shuster, L. The turnover of microsomal reduced nicotinamide adenine dinucleotide phosphate-cytochrome reductase in the livers of mice treated with phenobarbital. J. Biol. Chem. 241:5366 (1966).

13. Jones, A.L., and Armstrong, D.T. Increased cholesterol biosynthesis following phenobarbital induced hypertrophy of agranular reticulum in liver. Proc. Soc. Exp. Biol. Med. 119:1136 (1965).

14. Jones, A.L., and Fawcett, D.W. Hypertrophy of the agranular endoplasmic reticulum in hamster liver induced by phenobarbital (with a review on the function of this organelle in liver). J. Histochem. Cytochem. 14:215 (1966).

15. Jones, A.L., Ruderman, N.B., and Herrera, M.G. Electron microscopic and biochemical study of lipoprotein synthesis in the isolated perfused rat liver. J. Lipid Research 8:429 (1967).

16. Kadenback, B. Synthesis of mitochondrial proteins: demonstration of a transfer of proteins from microsomes into mitochondria. Biochem. Biophys. Acta 134:430 (1966).

17. Kuntzman, R., Lawrence, D., and Conney, A.H. Michaelis constants for the hydroxylation of steroid hormones and drugs by rat liver microsomes. Molec. Pharmacol. 1:163 (1965).

18. Marver, H.S., Tschudy, D.P., Perlroth, M.G., and Collins, A. δ aminolevulinic acid synthetase: I. Studies in liver homogenates. J. Biol. Chem. 241:2803 (1966).

19. Marver, H.S., Tschudy, D.P., Perlroth, M.G., and Collins, A. δ aminolevulinic acid synthetase: II. Induction in rat liver. J. Biol. Chem. 241:4323 (1966).

20. McKay, R., Druyan, R., and Rabinowity, M. Intramito-chondrial loci for δ aminoleuvulinic acid synthetase and ferroche-latase. Fed. Proceed. 27:774 (1968).

21. Omura, T., and Sato, R. The carbon monoxide binding pigment of liver microsomes. J. Biol. Chem. 239:2370 (1964).

22. Orrenius, S., and Ericsson, J.L.E. Enzyme-membrane re-lationship in phenobarbital induction of synthesis of drug-metabolizing enzyme system and proliferation of endoplasmic reticulum. J. Cell Biol. 28:181 (1966).

23. Orrenius S., and Ericsson, J.L.E. On the relationship of liver glucose-6-phosphatase to the proliferation of endoplasmic reticulum in phenobarbital induction. J. Cell Biol. 31:243 (1966).

24. Porter, K.R., Clause, A., and Fullam, E.F. A study tissue of culture cells by electron microscopy. J. Exp. Med. 81:233 (1945).

25. Porter, K.R., and Thompson, H.P. A particulate body associated with epithelial cells cultured from mammary carcinomas of mice of a milk-factor strain. J. Exp. Med. 88:15 (1948).

26. Porter, K.R. Observations on a submicroscopic basophilic component of cytoplasm. J. Exp. Med. 97:727 (1953).

27. Posalaki, Z., and Barka, T. Alterations of hepatic endoplasmic reticulum in porphyric rats. J. Histochem. Cytochem. 16:337 (1968).

28. Schimke, R.T., Ganschow, R., Doyle, D., and Arias, I.M. Regulation of protein turnover in mammalian tissues. Fed. Proceed. 27:1223 (1968).

29. Shuster, L., and Jick, H. The turnover of microsomal protein in the livers of phenobarbital-treated mice. J. Biol. Chem. 241:5361 (1966).

THE ROLE OF SEX HORMONES IN THE METABOLISM OF DRUGS AND OTHER

FOREIGN COMPOUNDS BY HEPATIC MICROSOMAL ENZYMES

T. E. Gram and J. R. Gillette

Laboratory of Chemical Pharmacology, National Heart
Institute, National Institutes of Health, Bethesda, Md.

It has long been recognized that there is a sex difference in
the duration of action of many drugs administered to intact animals.
For example, after the administration of certain barbiturates to
male and female rats, females sleep considerably longer than do
males (1,2,3). A sex difference in the duration of hypnosis (sleeping time) has also been reported for certain strains of mice but,
in contrast to rats, males sleep longer than do females (4,5). Examples of such sex differences in other animal species are rare.

In 1958, Quinn, Axelrod and Brodie (6) showed sex differences
in the rate of metabolism of drugs by hepatic microsomes and demonstrated an inverse relationship between the sex difference in hexobarbital metabolism and the sex difference in hexobarbital sleeping
times,i.e., males had short sleeping times and high microsomal enzyme activity, whereas females had prolonged sleeping times and low
enzyme activity. Furthermore, the differences in microsomal enzyme
activity were under the control of gonadal hormones, for they were
not present in sexually immature animals (6,7,18), and could be
reversed by administration of the antagonistic gonadal hormones. Thus,
chronic administration of estradiol-17β to male rats caused a prolongation of sleeping time and reduction in microsomal enzyme activity, whereas chronic testosterone treatment of female rats shortened
the sleeping time and markedly enhanced enzyme activity (6). Moreover, it has been shown that castration of adult male rats reduced
microsomal enzyme activity, whereas castration of females had no
significant effect (6,10). Thus, androgen seems to play an active
role in the control of microsomal enzyme activity, whereas that of
estrogen appears to be passive. Indeed, development of the sex
difference in drug metabolism at puberty appears to be the result
of a rapid increase in enzyme activity in males at a time when
activity in females does not change appreciably (8).

I.   EFFECT OF ANABOLIC STEROIDS ON DRUG METABOLISM

The effect of testosterone on microsomal drug metabolism is apparently more closely related to its androgenic than to its anabolic effects. Booth and Gillette (9) showed that testosterone and 19-nortestosterone administered to castrated male rats increased the rate of microsomal drug metabolism and the levator ani muscle weight (anabolic effect) to about the same extent, whereas testosterone produced a considerably greater increase in seminal vesicle weight (androgenic effect) than did 19-nortestosterone. Moreover, Kato et al (10) showed that 4-chlorotestosterone, a steroid which has little androgenic action, markedly enhanced the activity of the drug metabolizing enzymes.

II.   THE ROLE OF SUBSTRATE SPECIFICITY IN DETERMINING SEX DIFFER- IN DRUG METABOLISM

The magnitude of the sex difference in drug metabolism by liver microsomes depends upon the drug substrate investigated (11). Aminopyrine, hexobarbital and pentobarbital are metabolized about three to five times more rapidly by microsomes from male rats than by those from females. Cocaine and p-nitroanisole are demethylated about twice as rapidly by liver microsomes from male animals as those from females, but little or no sex difference was noted for the hydroxylation of aniline or zoxazolamine by rat liver microsomes (11). None of the 15 microsomal enzymes examined was more active in female rats than in males. It is noteworthy that a variety of treatments and alterations in physiological status of the animals resulted in diminution in the magnitude of the sex difference in microsomal drug metabolism (12). Examples of these conditions in which the sex difference declined or disappeared are starvation (72 hours), adrenalectomy, hypoxia, and the administration of ACTH, epinephrine, thyroxine or alloxan.

III. SIMILARITIES BETWEEN OXIDATIVE DRUG METABOLIZING ENZYMES AND STEROID HYDROXYLASES IN HEPATIC MICROSOMES

Conney, Kuntzman and their coworkers (13,14) observed that factors which stimulated the metabolism of drugs also enhanced the activity of certain steroid hydroxylases, whereas factors which impaired drug metabolism also decreased steroid hydroxylation. Moreover, both steroid hydroxylation and drug metabolism are catalyzed by enzyme systems that are localized in liver microsomes, require NADPH and O_2 and are inhibited by carbon monoxide (Table I). These findings suggested that steroid hormones and drugs are metabolized through a common microsomal electron transport pathway. Accordingly, as shown in Table II, certain steroid hormones competitively inhibit drug metabolism (15, 16, 17). The current view of the mechanism of these enzymes is illustrated in Fig. 1.

TABLE I

Similarities between Hepatic Steroid Hydroxylases
and Drug-Metabolizing Enzymes[1]

---

1. Localized in microsomal fraction and require NADPH, oxygen and cytochrome P-450 for activity.
2. Higher activity in adult male rats than in adult females.
3. Activity higher in adult male rats than in immature rats.
4. Inhibited in vitro by SKF 525-A.
5. Activity is increased after treatment of rats with phenobarbital or chlordane.
6. Activity is not increased after treatment of rats with 3-methyl-cholanthrene.

---

[1] Data taken from Kuntzman et al (13).

TABLE II

Inhibition of Microsomal Drug Metabolism by Steroid
Hormones in vitro

Substrate	Inhibitor	Inhibition
Ethylmorphine or hexobarbital[1]	Estradiol-17β	Competitive
	testosterone	"
	androsterone	"
	progesterone	"
	cortisol	"
Hexobarbital	Progesterone	Competitive
zoxazolamine	or	--
aniline	ethynodrel	--
3,4-benzpyrene[2]		--
Aniline	Prednisolone	Competitive
aminopyrine[3]	cortisol	"

[1] Data taken from Tephly and Mannering (15).

[2] Data taken from Juchau and Fouts (16).

[3] Data taken from Wada et al (17).

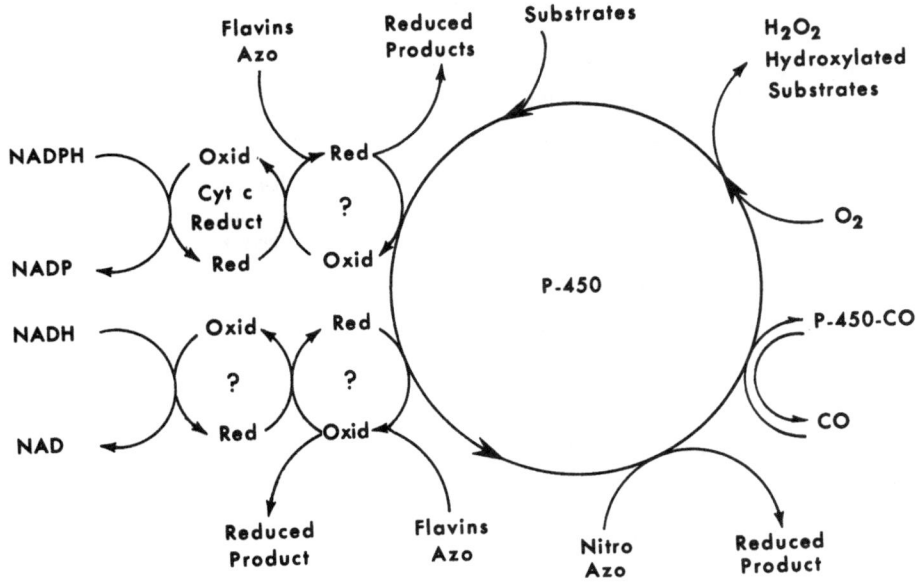

Fig. 1. Electron Transport in Liver Microsomes

IV. KINETIC ASPECTS OF THE SEX DIFFERENCE IN MICROSOMAL DRUG META-BOLISM

With few exceptions, investigators have been unsuccessful in obtaining soluble preparations from mammalian liver microsomes which are active in metabolizing drugs. Accordingly, purification of microsomal enzymes has not yet been achieved and thus explicit kinetic analysis has not been possible. However, in lieu of a solubilized and purified system, several groups have undertaken kinetic analyses of crude microsomal preparations in an effort to account for the sex difference in drug metabolism. Davies et al (18) studied the N-demethylation of ethylmorphine by liver microsomes from adult male and female rats and observed that the activity (Vmax) was 3-4 times as great in males as in females (Table III). The apparent affinity constant (Km) in males was 0.26 mM in males and 0.66 mM in females. That these latter differences were sex-related was shown in experiments employing immature (21-day-old) rats of both sexes in which no sex difference in Km was observed (Table III).

In another study of sex differences in microsomal drug metabolism, Schenkman et al (19) reported good correlation between differences in enzyme activity measured with aminopyrine or hexobarbital as substrates and differences in substrate "binding" (i.e., the magnitude of the spectral change associated with the addition of substrate to microsomes in the absence of NADPH. However, in

TABLE III

Sex Differences in the N-demethylation of Ethylmorphine
by Rat Liver Microsomes[1]

	Km (mM)	Vmax (nmoles HCHO/mg protein per min)
Adult male	0.26	11.6
female	0.66	3.2
Immature male	0.51	---
female	0.52	---

[1]Data taken from Davies et al (18).

other studies, Davies and collaborators (20), employing ethylmorphine as a substrate for microsomal enzymes, reported that the nearly
three-fold sex difference in demethylation could not be accounted
for by corresponding differences in cytochrome P-450 content, cytochrome c or cytochrome P-450 reductase activity, or substrate "binding" (Fig. 1). Thus, although the sex difference in the metabolism
of some substrates may be well correlated with their binding, this
explanation is apparently not universally applicable, and we are
left without a unified kinetic explanation for the sex difference
in microsomal drug metabolism. Recent findings (21), however, indicate that ethylmorphine causes a much greater enhancement of cytochrome P-450 reductase activity in microsomes from male rats than
in those from females. Inasmuch as P-450 reductase may be the rate-
limiting step in microsomal drug metabolism (20), the differential
effect of ethylmorphine on P-450 reduction may account for the sex
difference at least for ethylmorphine metabolism.

V.   DRUG METABOLISM DURING CONTRACEPTION AND PREGNANCY

A. Exogenous steroids. The literature dealing directly with
steroid effects on drug metabolism in vivo is inconsistent and difficult to interpret. Reports of diminished bromsulfalein (BSP) clearance following steroid administration (22) are more likely to reflect changes in biliary transport of the dye than changes in metabolic disposition (23). In contrast, the in vitro addition of progesterone or norethynodrel significantly inhibits the metabolism
of hexobarbital, zoxazolamine, aniline and 3,4-benzpyrene by rat

liver microsomes, but the injection of either steroid into rats influences the metabolism of only two of the nine substrates examined
(16). Norethynodrel, administered either acutely (4 hr before sacrifice) or chronically (once daily for 3 weeks) stimulates the metabolism of hexobarbital and zoxazolamine. Progesterone administration
appears to cause a transitory inhibitory effect on drug metabolism
and subsequently enhanced drug metabolism. Oral administration to
rats of the commercial mixture "Enovid" either acutely (4 hr before
sacrifice) or chronically (for 3 weeks) inhibits hexobarbital metabolism by approximately 50%. In contrast, either acute or chronic
oral administration of "Enovid" to mice (24) significantly reduces
hexobarbital sleeping times, which suggests enhanced metabolism.
Whether this represents a species difference or not is unclear.

B. **Pregnancy**. During the past five years, there has been a
tremendous upsurgence of interest in the fields of teratology and
perinatal pharmacology, i.e. in drug action in the fetus and newborn.
A thorough perusal of the literature, however, reveals that very
little information has accrued, either in animals or in humans, concerning drug metabolism during pregnancy.

The inhibitory effect of steroids on microsomal glucuronyl
transferase (25) and reduced glucuronidation of both endogenous and
exogenous substrates during pregnancy (26) are well-known and will
not be discussed here.

Employing pentobarbital-induced sleeping time as a measure
of drug-metabolizing activity, King and Becker (3) reported that
pregnant rats studied one day prior to expected delivery, had markedly prolonged sleeping times as compared with non-pregnant controls.
At a time following drug administration, when about 65% of the control animals had regained their righting reflexes, only about 5% of
the pregnant rats had recovered, thus suggesting impaired drug metabolizing capacity in the latter group. Parallel studies (27) comparing pregnant rats with controls which were in either the estrus
or diestrus phase of the sexual cycle again revealed prolonged sleeping time in pregnant animals, but no significant differences between
estrus and diestrus. This finding was construed to indicate that
sex hormones **per se** play a minor role in the sleeping time prolongation associated with pregnancy. In collaboration with Drs. Guarino
and Schroeder, we found no differences in microsomal aniline hydroxylase or ethylmorphine N-demethylase activity between female rats
sacrificed during estrus and anestrus (unpublished results). In
mice, a difference in hexobarbital sleeping time has been reported
(28) between estrus and diestrus.

Indirect studies in humans suggest that the metabolism of at
least some drugs is impaired during gestation. Four groups of hospitalized female patients were injected with meperidine (50 mg, i.v.)
and urines were collected and examined for unchanged meperidine and

its N-demethylated product normeperidine, a major metabolite (29,30).
"Non-obstetric" and post-menopausal controls excreted about twice
as much normeperidine as unchanged drug over a 48-hr period. By
contrast, women receiving various oral contraceptives excreted markedly diminished amounts of normeperidine and proportionally greater
amounts of meperidine. Full-term pregnant females excreted even
less metabolite and more of the unchanged drug, thus suggesting impaired capacity for N-demethylation under these conditions (29).

    Studies on the metabolism of drugs by microsomal preparations
from pregnant animals indicate that inhibition occurs at least during the late stages of gestation. Guarino et al (31) examined the
hydroxylation of aniline and the N-demethylation of ethylmorphine
by liver microsomes from rats at early, middle and late times during gestation and found no significant alterations in activity during early (day 6) or middle (day 14) periods. Similarly, no changes
in microsomal cytochrome P-450 content were noted at these times.
However, microsomal preparations from pregnant rats sacrificed 1-2
days prior to term (day 20) exhibited significantly reduced (40%)
aniline hydroxylase activity and N-demethylase (30%) activity; cytochrome P-450 levels were also significantly reduced (~30%). The
apparent Km for ethylmorphine and aniline metabolism was the same
in microsomes from control and pregnant animals, which would rule
out a competitive type of inhibition. Interestingly, the enzyme
activities and cytochrome P-450 content returned to control levels
in rats sacrificed one day post-partum. In similar work, Creaven
and Parke (32) reported inhibition of borneol glucuronidation in
pregnant rats and inhibition of the hydroxylation of coumarin and
biphenyl by hepatic microsomes from pregnant rats and rabbits. Thus
data derived from direct measurements of microsomal enzyme activity,
as well as indirect appraisals based on the pattern of urinary metabolites or changes in gross parameters such as sleeping time, suggest
that the metabolism of many drugs by hepatic microsomes is reduced
during pregnancy. The effects of pregnancy on drug metabolism and
on therapeutic effects in man is not clear at present. In this context, it is important to bear in mind that the duration of action of
many drugs is not regulated solely by their rate of metabolism, but
may be determined by other factors such as tissue binding, distribution or excretion by the kidney, liver or lung. In such instances,
moderate changes in hepatic microsomal drug metabolism would not be
expected to be accompanied by gross changes in the duration of drug
action. Moreover, recent work has indicated enormous individual
differences in drug metabolism by humans (33) and this would also
tend to obscure the clinical significance of changes in the rate of
drug metabolism. Finally, from a standpoint of clinical toxicology,
changes in drug metabolism are probably of greatest importance only
for those agents whose therapeutic index (toxic dose/therapeutic
dose) is low.

SUMMARY

In rats, a sex difference exists in the metabolism of xeno-
biotics by hepatic microsomal enzymes. Hepatic microsomes from male
rats metabolize many drugs 3-4 times as rapidly as microsomes from
females; these differences are inversely correlated with differences in the duration of action of drugs such as hexobarbital in
intact animals. The sex difference in microsomal drug metabolism
in rats is dependent on gonadal hormones for it is absent in immature animals and is influenced by castration or by injection of
the antagonistic steroid. The stimulatory effect of testosterone
on drug metabolism has been shown to be more closely related to its
anabolic activity than to its androgenic action. Sex differences
in drug metabolism are a function of the substrate investigated;
for some substrates the male:female activity ratio ranges between
3 and 4, whereas for other substrates the sex difference is small
or virtually non-existent. The magnitude of the sex difference is
diminished by starvation, hypoxia, or by the administration of epinephrine, thyroxine, or alloxan.

Many similarities between microsomal drug metabolism and microsomal steroid hydroxylation have lead to the suggestion that drugs
and steroids are substrates for the same microsomal enzymes.
Accordingly, steroids competitively inhibit microsomal drug metabolism in vitro. Kinetic analysis of drug metabolism by microsomal enzymes has demonstrated that the sex difference is accompanied
by differences both in enzyme activity (Vmax) and in apparent
affinity constant (Km). Only slight and insignificant sex differences occur in microsomal cytochrome P-450 content. Moreover, the
sex difference in drug metabolism cannot be accounted for on the
basis of differences in cytochrome P-450 reductase or cytochrome
c reductase activities.

During treatment with contraceptives or during the late
phase of gestation, microsomal drug metabolism appears to be diminished both in animals and in humans. This does not appear to be
the result of a competitive mechanism. The significance of these
findings in relation to human therapeutics is discussed.

REFERENCES

1. Nichols, J. S. and D. H. Barron, J. Pharmacol. 46: 125, 1932.
2. Holck, G. O., M. A. Kanan, L. M. Mills and E. L. Smith, J.
   Pharmacol. 60: 323, 1937.
3. King, J. E. and R. F. Becker, Am. J. Obstet. Gynecol. 86: 856,
   1963.
4. Jay, G. E., Proc. Soc. Exp. Biol. Med. 90: 378, 1955.
5. Vesell, E. S., Pharmacology 1: 7, 1968.

6. Quinn, G. P., J. Axelrod and B. B. Brodie, Biochem. Pharmacol. 1: 152, 1958.
7. Streicher, E. and J. Garbus, J. Gerontol. 10: 441, 1955.
8. Bresnick, E. and J. G. Stevenson, Biochem. Pharmacol. 17: 1815, 1968.
9. Booth, J. and J. R. Gillette, J. Pharmacol. 137: 374, 1962.
10. Kato, R., E. Chiesara and G. Frontino, Biochem. Pharmacol. 11: 221, 1962.
11. Kato, R. and J. R. Gillette, J. Pharmacol. 150: 279, 1965.
12. Kato, R. and J. R. Gillette, J. Pharmacol. 150: 285, 1965.
13. Kuntzman, R., M. Jacobson, K. Schneidman and A. H. Conney, J. Pharmacol. 146: 280, 1964.
14. Kuntzman, R., R. Welch and A. H. Conney, Advances in Enzyme Regulation 4: 149, 1966.
15. Tephly, T. R. and G. J. Mannering, Mol. Pharmacol. 4: 10, 1968.
16. Juchau, M. R. and J. R. Fouts, Biochem. Pharmacol. 15: 891, 1968.
17. Wada, F., H. Shimakaga, M. Takasugi, T. Kotake and Y. Sakamoto, J. Biochem. (Tokyo) 64: 109, 1968.
18. Davies, D. S., P. L. Gigon and J. R. Gillette, Biochem. Pharmacol. 17: 1865, 1968.
19. Schenkman, J. B., I. Frey, H. Remmer and R. W. Estabrook, Mol. Pharmacol. 3: 516, 1967.
20. Davies, D. S., P. L. Gigon and J. R. Gillette, Life Sciences (in press) 1969.
21. Gigon, P. L., T. E. Gram and J. R. Gillette, Biochem. Biophys. Res. Comm. 31: 558, 1968.
22. Kottra, L. L. and A. Kappas, Arch. Int. Med. 117: 373, 1966.
23. Kottra, J. and A. Kappas, Ann. Rev. Med. 18: 325, 1967.
24. Roberts, R. J. and G. L. Plaa, Biochem. Pharmacol. 15: 333, 1966.
25. Hsia, D. Y. Y., S. Riabov and R. M. Dowben, Arch. Biochem. Biophys. 103: 181, 1963.
26. Dutton, G. J., ed. "Glucuronic Acid, Free and Combined", Academic Press, New York, 1968.
27. King, J. E. and R. F. Becker, Am. J. Obst. Gynecol. 86: 865, 1963.
28. Catz, C. and S. J. Yaffe, J. Pharmacol. 155: 152, 1967.
29. Crawford, J. S. and S. Rudofsky, Brit. J. Anesthes. 38: 446, 1966.
30. Burns, J. J., B. L. Berger, P. A. Lief, A. Wollach, E. M. Papper and B. B. Brodie, J. Pharmacol. 114: 289, 1955.
31. Guarino, A. M., D. S. Schroeder, J. B. Call and T. E. Gram, Fed. Proc. (in press) 1969.
32. Creaven, P. J. and D. V. Parke, Abstracts, Federated European Biochemistry Societies, second meeting, 1965, p. 88.
33. Kalow, W., in "Pharmacogenetics", W. B. Saunders Co., Philadelphia, 1962.

CARBOHYDRATE METABOLISM

EFFECTS OF GONADAL HORMONES AND CONTRACEPTIVE STEROIDS ON GLUCOSE AND INSULIN METABOLISM

Paul Beck

Endocrinology Division, Department of Medicine,
University of Colorado, School of Medicine,
Denver, Colorado

Considerable data have been accumulated regarding the effect of naturally-occurring and synthetic sex steroids on glucose and insulin metabolism. The studies have been performed largely to elucidate the mechanisms responsible for changes in carbohydrate metabolism during pregnancy. Initially, studying glucose tolerance in women treated with contraceptive steroids seemed to be a logical way to dissociate the effects of gonadal steroids from the metabolic effects of human placental lactogen during gestation. However, such studies have been confusing and often apparently contradictory. Yet, if the structural characteristics of the steroid compounds tested are considered, these results are basically in agreement with, rather than contradictory to, data obtained earlier in laboratory animals. If one correlates the changes in glucose or insulin metabolism with the chemical structure of the estrogen or progestin tested, it is possible to show that there are clear structure-activity relationships between the compounds tested and the results observed, which appear to be modified by the functional state of the pancreatic islet cells in the subjects tested.

It is the purpose of this paper: 1) to review studies of carbohydrate tolerance in laboratory animals treated with gonadal steroids; 2) to postulate structure-activity relationships of gonadal and contraceptive steroids in Rhesus monkeys with regards to glucose and insulin metabolism; 3) to correlate changes in glucose and insulin metabolism observed in experimental animals treated

Supported by USPHS research grant HD-02455 and by a grant-in-aid from Syntex Research.

TABLE I. EFFECT OF DIFFERENT SUBSTANCES INJECTED DAILY DURING 6 MONTHS ON THE INCIDENCE OF DIABETES IN MALE AND FEMALE CASTRATED RATS, AFTER REMOVAL OF 95% OF THE PANCREAS

(Lewis, Foglia and Rodriguez, 1950)

Substance injected	Daily dose per rat μg.	Castrated females				Castrated males	
		exp. A-D		exp. B-C			
		Dia-betics	Per-centage	Dia-betics	Per-centage	Dia-betics	Per-centage
Lactose	25 (mg.)	12/23	52	26/35	74	16/18	89
Cholesterol	500	4/15	27	5/9	55		
Oestrone	15	3/10	30				
Oestrone	50	0/8	0				
Diethylstilboestrol	15	3/10	30				
Diethylstilboestrol	50			1/8	12	3/6	50
Phenocycline	15	0/9	0				
Phenocycline	50	1/11	9				
Dieneoestrol				1/15	6		
Ethinyl-oestradiol	50			4/16	25		
Ethinyl-testosterone	500			4/9	44		
Equilenine	50	6/8	75				
Progesterone	500			6/9	66		
Desoxycorticosterone	100			8/12	66		
Testosterone	50	11/15	73				
Testosterone	500	8/8	100	9/11	83	13/14	92
Methyltestosterone	500						
17β-ethyldihydro-testosterone	500			8/11	72		

Rodriquez, "On the Nature and Treatment of Diabetes", 1965

with gonadal and contraceptive steroids with the changes in carbohydrate tolerance observed in human subjects treated with birth
control pills; 4) to contrast these results with those obtained in
pregnant human subjects; and 5) to demonstrate the special sensitivity of individuals with subclinical diabetes to the hyperglycemic effects of some contraceptive steroids.

HISTORICAL BACKGROUND

In general, previous experimental studies have indicated that
most estrogenic substances ameliorate rather than aggravate diabetes. These tendencies vary, however, with the severity of the
diabetes, with the estrogen preparation tested, and with the duration of exposure to estrogens. Androgens, on the other hand,
generally produce a deterioration of carbohydrate tolerance in
mammals. The effect of progesterone and its derivatives are variable and depend on the species tested and on the type of progestin
administered. The diabetic state of the subject appears to influence his response to progestin treatment. In none of the early
studies were there any measurements of peripheral plasma insulin
concentrations to corroborate these findings. Moreover, except
for the recent studies in women taking oral contraceptive agents,
there are no data concerning the combined effects of estrogens with
progestins on glucose and insulin metabolism. These conclusions
are discussed in detail in the remainder of this section.

The work of Houssay and co-workers clearly delineated the
effect of estrogenic substances on carbohydrate tolerance (1).
When rats were subjected to a subtotal (95%) pancreatectomy and
treated with a variety of estrogenic substances, a diaphasic
effect was observed (2). During the first month of estrogen
treatment, the severity of diabetes was greater in the estrogen-
treated than in the control animals. This diabetogenic effect was
most pronounced in force-fed animals. Subsequently, the hyperglycemia and glycosuria were attenuated or suppressed completely in the
estrogen-treated animals. As shown in Table 1, the beneficial
effect of the estrogen depended on the preparation used. For
example, dienestrol and diethylstilbesterol were more beneficial
than estrone or ethinyl estradiol. By contrast, no benefit was
seen following treatment with equilenin. Mestranol, the 3-methyl-
ether of ethinyl estradiol, was not tested. Houssay and his associates attributed the beneficial effects of the estrogens to the
induction of islet cell hyperplasia (1). However, it should be
pointed out that no measurements of peripheral insulin levels were
made in these studies. An additional possible reason for the improvement in glucose tolerance may be the enhancement of peripheral
glucose utilization by some estrogens (notably estradiol dipropionate). Talaat and co-workers have reported that estradiol dipropionate administration results in an increase in arterio-venus

glucose differences and in increased sensitivity to exogenous insulin both in rabbits (3) and in non-diabetic women (4).

Nevertheless, treatment with estrogens has not always resulted in improvement in glucose metabolism. In some depancreatized diabetic animals, estrogens either have been without effect (5,6) or have increased the severity of diabetes (7). When administered concomitantly with glucocorticoids in rats, stilbesterol induced glycosuria whereas treatment with neither hormone alone produced these effects (8). Nelson has also reported that ethinyl estradiol enhanced the glycosuric effect of hydrocortisone in diabetic human subjects (9).

Androgens generally produce a deterioration of carbohydrate tolerance in mammals. Foglia and co-workers observed that following subtotal pancreatectomy, the deterioration of carbohydrate tolerance was greater in male than in female rats (10). Diabetes in these animals was aggravated by testosterone administration (Table 1), and the incidence of diabetes was reduced in comparable animals by castration prior to pancreatectomy (10). Moreover, the incidence of diabetes in the subtotal pancreatectomized female rats who had been subjected to castration was identical to that of the castrated male rats. Recently, Landon and associates reported that the administration of 1-dehydro-17-α-methyltestosterone (Dianabol, methandienone) produced impairment of glucose tolerance in man (11). Nevertheless, not all androgens will produce deterioration of carbohydrate tolerance. In the experiments of Foglia and co-workers, ethinyl testosterone administration reduced the frequency and severity of diabetes in rats although there was no change after the administration of methyltestosterone or dihydrotestosterone. These findings imply that chemical modification of the basic testosterone nucleus may affect it diabetogenicity.

Much less information is available from the literature about the effects of progesterone and its derivatives on carbohydrate metabolism. The data indicate that these compounds may produce variable effects on carbohydrate metabolism. Although Lewis, Foglia and Rodriguez (2) were unable to observe any change in glucose metabolism in rats subjected to subtotal pancreatectomy, Ingle (12) observed an increase in glycosuria in partially pancreatectomized rats who were force-fed during treatment with 50-100 mg of progesterone daily. Recently, Benjamin and Casper reported that the carbohydrate tolerance improved in women with endometrial hyperplasia or carcinoma after treatment with 17-α-hydroxyprogesterone caproate (13). By contrast, Schreibman has recently reported that glucose tolerance deteriorated in several diabetic subjects treated with the same compound (14).

It is difficult to relate these findings to the changes in

glucose and insulin metabolism observed during human gestation (30).
First, there have been no studies in human subjects treated with
unesterified naturally-occurring estrogens and/or progesterone in
quantities sufficient to reproduce the hormonal milieu of pregnancy.
Second, such changes must be related to the well-documented effects
of human placental lactogen (29,32,52) on carbohydrate metabolism.
Much remains to be learned about the interactions of these steroid
and peptide hormones.

COMPARATIVE STUDIES IN RHESUS MONKEYS

Because of the relatively sparse amount of information about
progesterone in the literature, a series of studies were undertaken to ascertain the effect of progesterone (15) and its synthetic analogues on glucose and insulin metabolism. Intravenous
glucose tolerance tests were performed following an overnight fast
in female Rhesus monkeys anesthetized with phencyclidine hydrochloride and atropine. Glucose (1 g/kg) was administered via the
femoral vein and blood samples were collected from the contralat-
eral femoral vein by percutaneous puncture for glucose and insulin
determinations. Prior to testing, a progestin dissolved in olive
oil was administered subcutaneously for three weeks; the hormone
was not given on the day of the test. The progestins tested were:
progesterone, 20 mg daily; ethynodiol diacetate, 1 mg daily; norethindrone, 2.5 mg daily; norethynodrel, 5 mg daily; and chlormadinone acetate, 0.75 mg daily. The progesterone dosage was selected in an attempt to reproduce effective plasma progestin levels
comparable to those observed for progesterone during pregnancy.
The daily doses for the synthetic progestins are equivalent to the
amounts contained in most commercially available oral contraceptive
pills, but are approximately 15 times greater than the latter on a
body weight basis. Intravenous glucose tolerance tests were also
performed in these animals following administration of the vehicle
alone for three weeks and following provocation with hydrocortisone,
5 mg, administered intramuscularly two and twelve hours before the
administration of glucose.

Three weeks of treatment with pure progesterone produced no
consistent changes in either the mean fasting serum glucose or
insulin concentrations even though the mean serum progesterone level
(17 mμg/ml) 16 hours after the last progesterone injection was 12
times greater than the control value and four times higher than reported by Neill, Johannson and Knobil (16) in pregnant Rhesus
monkeys.

Figure 1 shows the serum glucose and insulin responses to
intravenous glucose in a typical monkey before and after hydrocortisone or progesterone treatment. Natural progesterone produced

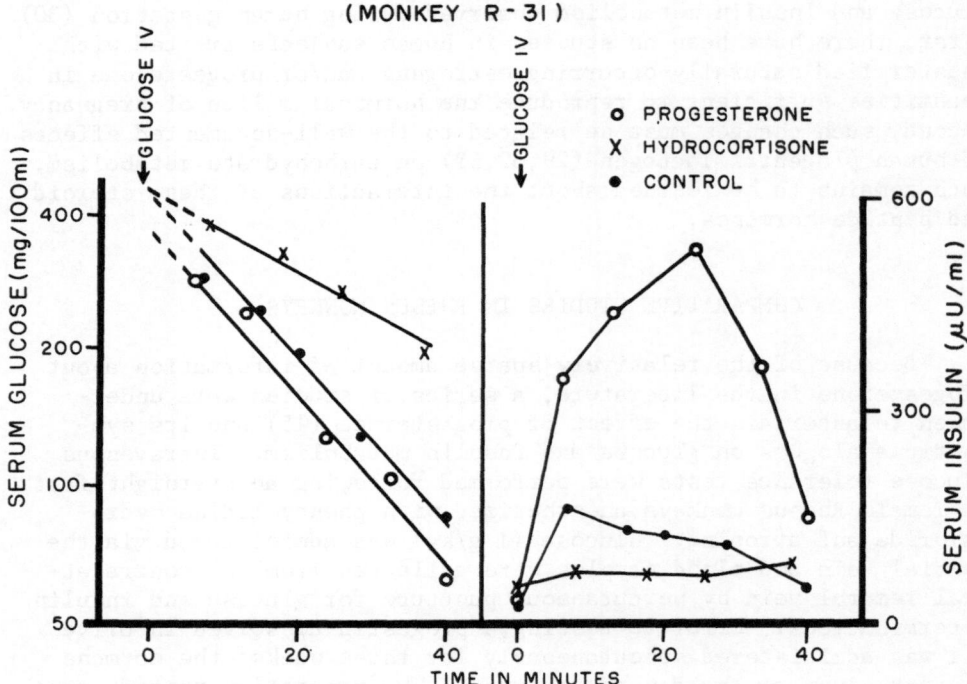

Fig. 1. Serum glucose and insulin responses to intravenous glucose after progesterone or hydrocortisone treatment. (Beck (15))

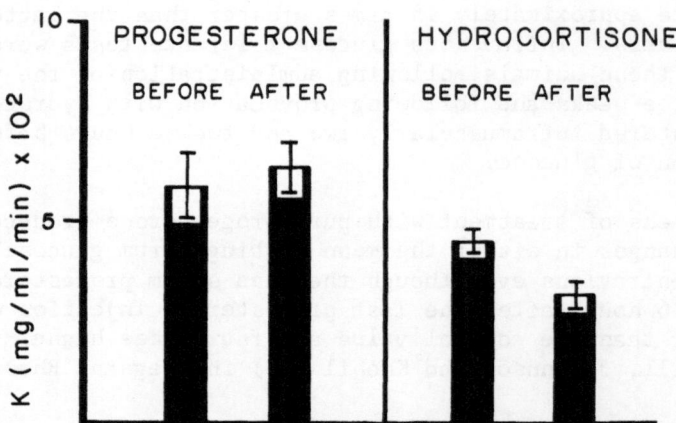

Fig. 2. Mean (± S.E.M.) serum glucose disappearance rates (K) after progesterone or hydrocortisone treatment in Rhesus monkeys. (Beck (15))

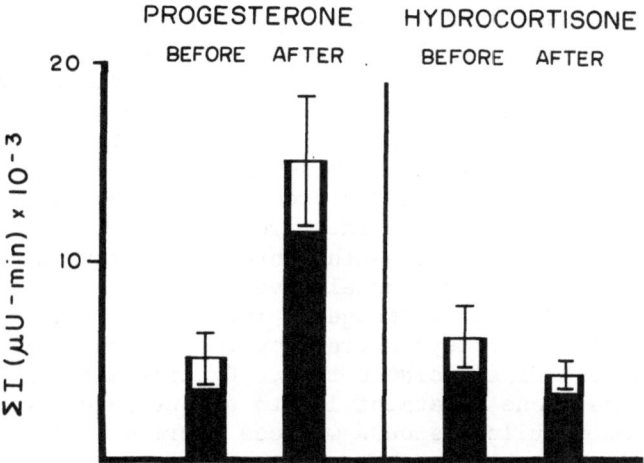

Fig. 3. Mean (± S.E.M.) integrated serum insulin responses (ΣI) after progesterone or hydrocortisone treatment in Rhesus monkeys. (Beck (15))

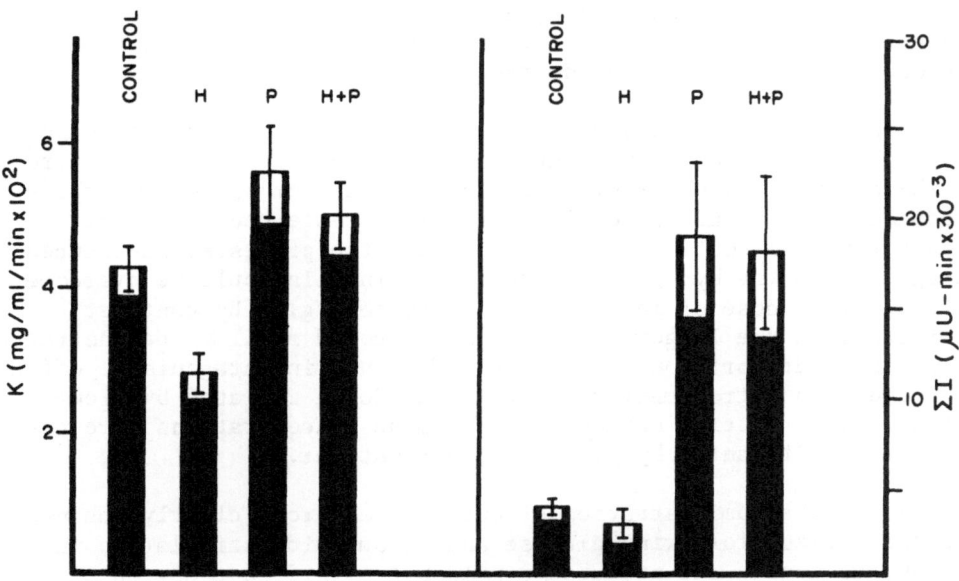

Fig. 4. Reversal of the diabetogenic effect of hydrocortisone in Rhesus monkeys by pre-treatment with progesterone for 3 weeks. (Beck (15))

no change in the rate of glucose disappearance whereas glucose
tolerance deteriorated markedly after hydrocortisone treatment.
Much to our surprise, however, progesterone treatment produced
a marked increase in the plasma insulin response to intravenous
glucose. This increased insulin response was not seen after hydrocortisone administration. These observations have been confirmed
in nine monkeys, and the data are presented in the next two figures
with the glucose disappearance rates recorded as the rate constant,
K, and the insulin responses as the integrated areas under each
insulin response curve above basal levels (ΣI). As shown in Figure
2, there was no significant change in the mean K $\pm$ S.E.M. in the
progesterone-treated monkeys whereas hydrocortisone uniformly
slowed the glucose disappearance rate. By contrast, as shown in
Figure 3, progesterone treatment led to a four-fold increase in
the mean plasma insulin response whereas there was no change after
hydrocortisone treatment. Enhancement of the mean plasma insulin
response without significant alterations in the glucose disappearance rates were also seen in the same progesterone-treated monkeys
following intravenous tolbutamide administration.

To ascertain whether the extra insulin found in peripheral
plasma following progesterone treatment was metabolically active,
hydrocortisone provocative tests were repeated in five progesterone-
treated monkeys. As seen in Figure 4, progesterone treatment prevented the deterioration of glucose tolerance observed following
hydrocortisone treatment alone, and the hydrocortisone treatment
did not alter the magnitude of the plasma insulin response to
glucose following progesterone treatment.

Progesterone treatment also reduced the sensitivity of these
animals to the hypoglycemic action of insulin. As shown in Figure
5, the administration of 0.5 units of insulin per kg body weight
produced hypoglycemia more slowly after progesterone treatment
than during the control period. However, the progesterone-induced
antagonism to the hypoglycemic action of insulin could be overcome
with a larger dose of insulin (0.1 units per kg). By contrast,
resistance to the larger dose of insulin could still be demonstrated
following hydrocortisone treatment. The insulin antagonistic effect
of progesterone treatment did not appear to be mediated by growth
hormone since fasting serum growth hormone concentrations were not
altered significantly by progesterone treatment.

Thus, the administration of pure progesterone clearly enhanced
insulin release following glucose and tolbutamide stimulation in
the Rhesus monkey and produced a mild but significant degree of
peripheral resistance to the hypoglycemic action of insulin.

What effect did the synthetic progestins have on glucose and
insulin metabolism in these same monkeys? An increase in the mean

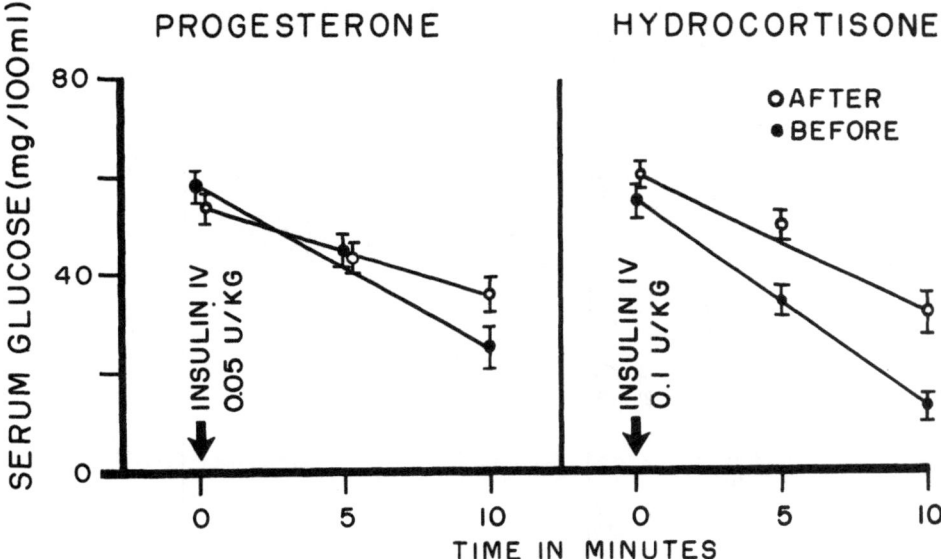

Fig. 5. Mean serum glucose responses to exogenous insulin in Rhesus monkeys after progesterone or hydrocortisone treatment. (Beck (15))

Table 2

PROGESTIN-INDUCED ALTERATIONS IN THE MEAN ($\pm$ S.E.M.)
INTEGRATED INSULIN RESPONSES (ΣI) AND GLUCOSE DISAPPEARANCE RATES
(K) FOLLOWING INTRAVENOUS GLUCOSE, AND IN MEAN GLUCOSE DISAPPEARANCE
(Δ G) 10 MIN. AFTER INTRAVENOUS INSULIN ADMINISTRATION.

Hormone[†]	No. Animals	Dosage (mg)	$\Sigma I_{40'}$ (μU- min)	K (mg%/min)	ΔG (mg%)
Progesterone	9	20	15,433*** (937)	6.35 (0.58)	18.4* (2.8)
Norethynodrel	6	5	9,828* (1,078)	4.91 (0.52)	14.0* (1.9)
Norethindrone	4	2.5	15,561 (2,237)	5.77 (0.46)	–
Ethynodiol diacetate	5	1	6,013 (808)	6.34 (0.83)	–
Chlormadinone acetate	10	0.75	11,128*** (613)	7.27* (0.71)	–
Olive oil	13	–	5,349 (1,049)	6.16 (0.57)	26.9 (2.6)

[†]Injected daily for three weeks. Compared with paired olive oil control,
*p <0.05, **p< 0.01, ***p< 0.005.

Table 3

ESTROGEN-INDUCED ALTERATIONS IN THE MEAN ($\pm$ S.E.M.) INTEGRATED RESPONSES (Σ I) AND GLUCOSE DISAPPEARANCE RATES (K) FOLLOWING INTRAVENOUS GLUCOSE, AND IN MEAN GLUCOSE DISAPPEARANCE (Δ G) 10 MIN. AFTER INTRAVENOUS INSULIN ADMINISTRATION.

Hormone[†]	No. Animals	Dosage (mg)	Σ I$_{40}$' (μU-min)	K (mg%/min)	Δ G (mg%)
Estradiol	9	2	5,350 (1,101)	5.80 (0.51)	–
Estriol	6	0.5	4,296 (538)	5.37 (0.72)	17.1* (2.5)
Ethinyl estradiol	6	1	5,021 (240)	6.65 (0.76)	16.6 (5.2)
Mestranol	9	2	7,779* (937)	6.72 (0.77)	16.4* (0.9)
Olive oil	13	–	5,349 (1,049)	6.16 (0.57)	26.9 (2.6)

[†]Injected daily for two weeks. *p<0.05, **p<0.01, ***p<0.005.

plasma insulin response to glucose was seen following treatment
with chlormadinone, norethynodrel, norethindrone, but not after
ethynodiol diacetate (Table 2). Likewise, there was no change
in the fasting serum glucose or insulin concentration or in the
glucose disappearance rate following treatment with the nortestosterone derivatives (norethynodrel, norethindrone and ethynodiol
diacetate). However, treatment with chlormadinone acetate produced
a significant increase in both the fasting serum insulin level and
in the glucose disappearance rate without change in the fasting
serum glucose concentration. Thus, these data suggest that some,
but not all, synthetic progestins increase the sensitivity of the
pancreatic islet cell to the stimulus of hyperglycemia resulting
in an increase in the magnitude of the circulating plasma insulin
response to glucose. However, only one of the progestins, chlormadinone, produced any significant change in glucose metabolism
or in basal insulin levels. These differences in response could
not be attributed solely to the amounts of hormone administered,
since the daily dose for chlormadinone (0.75 mg) was significantly
smaller than for the other progestins.

In agreement with earlier studies (1), the administration of
pure estradiol, estriol and ethinyl estradiol (1,0.5, and 2 mg
respectively) daily for two weeks produced no significant change
in the serum glucose disappearance rate or the plasma insulin
response following intravenous glucose administration, although
there was a significant decrease in the sensitivity of these animals to the hypoglycemic action of exogenous insulin following the
administration of estriol and ethinyl estradiol (Table 3). By contrast, the administration of mestranol produced a significant increase in the plasma insulin response to glucose and resistance to
the hypoglycemic action of exogenous insulin, even though there was
no significant alteration in the rate of disposal of glucose.
Hence, it appears that mestranol behaves in a significantly different way with respect to carbohydrate metabolism than do the
other estrogens.

Unfortunately, these studies leave several questions unanswered. 1) Is the insulin secreted by the progesterone-treated
animals an abnormal insulin such as proinsulin? 2) Do mestranol
and the synthetic progestins alter the nature of the insulin secreted by the islets or are these changes in insulin secretion due
to alterations in the rate of insulin degradation? 3) Are the
diabetogenic effects of mestranol and the synthetic progestins
synergistic or additive?

STRUCTURE - ACTIVITY RELATIONSHIPS

On the basis of these data, it is possible to postulate some
preliminary structure-activity relationships for pregnene and

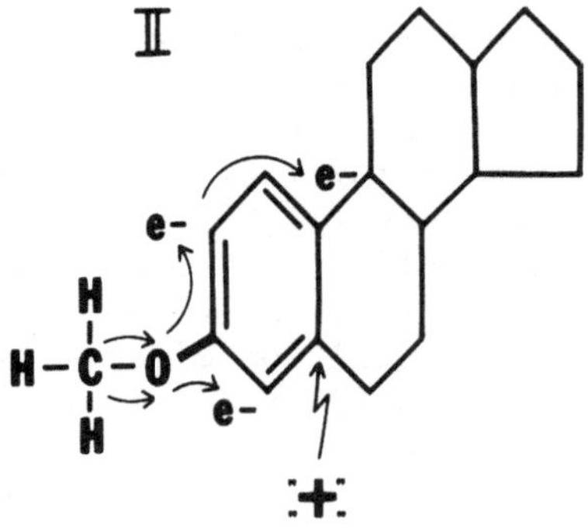

Fig. 6. Structural features of pregnene or nortestosterone (I) and estrogen (II) steroids which are essential for insulinogenic activity. + denotes a partial positive charge; e⁻, electrons. Progesterone, and norethindrone are 4-dehydro-, 3-keto-pregnene steroids; norethynodrel is a 5(10) dehydro-, 3-keto-steroid; chlormadinone, 4-dehydro-, 6 dehydro-, 6 chloro-, 3-keto-steroid. Mestranol is a 3-methyl-ether estrogen.

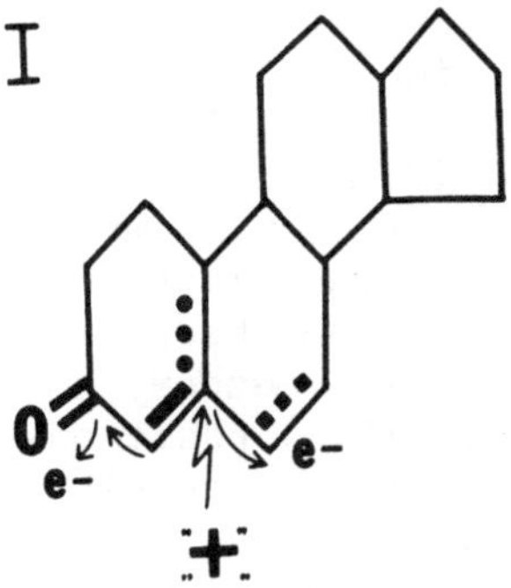

estrogen derivatives with regard to glucose and insulin metabolism.
This is done with full recognition that future studies may modify
this hypothesis. The presence or absence of the C_{19}-methyl group
or of hydroxyl, ethinyl, acetyl, or acetoxy substitution at the
C_{17} position do not appear to alter glucose or insulin metabolism.
On the other hand (Fig. 6), the presence of a partial positive
charge at the C_5 carbon is common to mestranol and all of the
pregnene and nortestosterone derivatives which are associated with
increased insulin production following glucose stimulation. With
progesterone,norethynodrel, norethindrone and chlormadinone, the
requisite charge results from the presence of a single unsaturated
bond at the C_4 or $C_{5(10)}$ position in association with a ketone
group at C_3 which tends to draw electrons away from C_5. With
mestranol, the partial positive charge at C_5 may be achieved by
donation of electrons from the methoxy substituent at C_3 to the
ortho (C_2 and C_4) and para (C_{10}) positions on the A ring. Under
these conditions, the C_5 position should be positively charged
relative its adjacent carbon atoms. That these particular molecules do not produce dramatic changes in blood glucose concentrations would be predicted from past experience with desoxy analogues
of cortisol since they lack hydroxyl groups at the C_{21} and C_{11}
positions (17,18). That chlormadinone improves peripheral glucose
utilization (Table 2) is in agreement with previous studies with
cortisol in which it has been demonstrated that introduction of
unsaturation at the C_6 position leads to a significant reduction
in the gluconeogenic effect of cortisol (19). Although 6α-chloro
(20) and 6α-methyl substitutions (21,22) increase the anti-inflammatory effects of cortisol, (effects generally associated with
changes in glucose metabolism (23) and although 6α-methyl groups
increase the liver glycogen-deposition effects of prednisolone
(1-dehydro-cortisol) and its 9α-fluoro derivative (22), it is
possible that the gluconeogenic effects of 6α-chloro and 6α-methyl
substitutions may be counteracted by other chemical alterations of
the cortisol nucleus (21), including C_6 unsaturation.

Introduction of a double bond at the C_6 position also appears
to be. a convenient way of separating the gluconeogenic or hyperglycemic effects of the steroid nucleus from its ability to stimulate the islet cells of the pancreas or sensitize them to glucose
stimulation. Whereas in the monkey the contra-insulin effect of
progesterone on peripheral target organs appears to counter-
balance the increase in insulin production following glucose stimulation, the acceleration of the glucose disappearance rate following chlormadinone administration suggests that the islet cell
stimulatory effect predominates (Table 2). Hence, one might predict
that the 6α-methyl, 6 dehydro-derivative of 17α-hydroxy-progesterone
acetate might be insulinogenic and non-diabetic in man, a prediction
to be reviewed in more detail later in this discussion.

Thus, in monkeys, steroid compounds with a relatively positive

Table 4

SUMMARY OF INSULINOGENIC AND INSULIN-ANTAGONISTIC
PROPERTIES OF GONADAL AND CONTRACEPTIVE STEROIDS
IN RHESUS MONKEYS.

	Insulin Response	Resistance To Insulin	Δ Glucose Tolerance
Insulinogenic, non-antagonistic			
Pregnene derivative			
Chlormadinone	↑	—	↑
Insulinogenic, insulin-antagonistic			
Pregnene derivatives			
Progesterone	↑	↑	0
Nortestosterone derivatives			
Norethynodrel	↑	↑	0
Norethindrone	↑	—	0
Estrogen derivative			
Mestranol	↑	↑	0
Non-insulinogenic			
Nortestosterone derivative			
Ethynodiol diacetate	0	—	0
Estrogens			
Estradiol	0	—	0
Estriol	0	↑	0
Ethinyl estradiol	0	↑	0

↑ = increased or improved
↓ = decreased or worse
0 = no change
— = not measured

charge at C_5 (Table 4) possess insulinogenic as well as insulin-
resistance activities which generally neutralize each other when
measured in terms of the disposal of intravenously administered
glucose. These two activities may be separable by the introduction of unsaturation at the C_6 position of the B ring.

With these structure-activity relationships in monkeys in
mind, it becomes possible to interpret the many reports of carbohydrate tolerance tests in women receiving oral contraceptive
agents more easily. It should be kept in mind that amounts of
contraceptive steroids usually administered to human subjects are
approximately 1/15 the amount employed in the monkey studies and
that the hormones are typically administered orally rather than
subcutaneously. Nevertheless, there is considerable parallelism
between the human studies and the monkey studies.

COMPARATIVE STUDIES IN MAN

On the basis of the studies performed on experimental animals
with estrogen and progestins, one might predict that normal human
subjects treated with contraceptive steroids would show no change
in glucose tolerance but would have an increase in the plasma
insulin response to glucose in the presence of normal pancreatic
function. By contrast, individuals with compromised pancreatic
islet insulin reserve might show deterioration of glucose tolerance because, unlike their non-diabetic counterparts, they would
be unable to produce the extra insulin required to overcome the
peripheral resistance to insulin produced by these agents. Moreover, because of the tendency of human placental lactogen to retard
insulin release in subclinical diabetic subjects (29), glucose
tolerance might deteriorate more during pregnancy than during contraceptive steroid treatment. Of course, if a test population were
a mixture of non-diabetic and subclinical diabetic individuals,
mixed results would be obtained. Furthermore, one might predict
that oral contraceptives containing mestranol would be more diabetogenic than those containing ethinyl estradiol, and that those
containing mestranol plus norethynodrel or norethindrone might cause
more deterioration of glucose tolerance than following treatment
with mestranol alone or when given in combination with ethynodiol
diacetate. Finally, one might predict that 6-dehydro-progestins
could actually improve carbohydrate tolerance. The clinical data
thus far published support these hypotheses.

Estrogens

Mestranol: Responses of subclinical diabetic vs. non-diabetic
individuals.

Gershberg and associates were probably first to show that

glucose tolerance might deteriorate in human subjects treated with
mestranol alone (24) as well as with mestranol in combination with
norethynodrel (25). In their studies, there was a greater tendency
for glucose tolerance to deteriorate in individuals who had a family
or obstetrical history of diabetes than in those who did not. However, it·was not determined whether those individuals in whom glucose tolerance deteriorated while taking mestranol were actually
subclinical diabetics. Recent studies by Beck and Wells (26) have
affirmed the fact that the state of insulin metabolism in patients
receiving an oral contraceptive containing mestranol distinctly
affects their glucose and insulin responses to a carbohydrate
challenge. In this study, individuals were classified as gestational (subclinical) diabetic or non-diabetic on the basis of oral
glucose tolerance tests administered during the third trimester of
pregnancy. It is significant that of the 12 individuals in this
group who were classified as gestational diabetic subjects, 11
also had abnormal prednisolone provocation tests six weeks post-
partum by the criteria of Fajans and Conn (27). All of the subjects, both gestational diabetic and non-diabetic, had normal
glucose tolerance tests five weeks post-partum. Subsequently, the
subjects were placed on either a combination contraceptive containing mestranol and ethynodiol diacetate, or on a sequential
agent containing mestranol for the first 15 days of the cycle and
mestranol supplemented by chlormadinone during the last five days
of the cycle. Oral glucose tolerance tests were performed in each
subject two weeks, ten weeks, and six months after starting these
contraceptive agents. These time intervals were selected so that
the tests would be performed during the portion of the sequential
agent cycle in which no progestin was administered.

Two weeks of treatment with these contraceptive agents produced no change in the mean fasting or post-prandial plasma glucose concentration in either group. There was no significant difference in the plasma glucose responses of the individuals taking
mestranol alone, as compared to those taking mestranol with
ethynodiol diacetate. Nevertheless, as shown in Table 5, when
the plasma glucose responses of the gestational diabetic subjects
were examined more carefully, it was evident that three of the 12
subjects developed clearly abnormal glucose tolerance tests after
two weeks of mestranol treatment, and an additional five showed a
clear cut deterioration of glucose tolerance as compared with their
post-partum control tests. Glucose tolerance tests were considered
to be deteriorated if at least two of the post-prandial plasma glucose concentrations, after mestranol treatment, were at least 30 mg%
higher than the corresponding values in the post-partum control
tests. These results are in clear contrast to those observed during
the third trimester or following prednisolone provocation in these
same subjects at which time virtually all of the glucose tolerance
tests were abnormal. Although deterioration of glucose tolerance

Table 5

FREQUENCY OF ABNORMAL OR DETERIORATED ORAL
GLUCOSE TOLERANCE TESTS IN 12 SUBCLINICAL
DIABETIC WOMEN DURING TREATMENT WITH
MESTRANOL-CONTAINING ORAL CONTRACEPTIVE
AGENTS. (Beck and Wells(26))

	Abnormal	Deteriorated
3rd Trimester	12	0
Post-partum (5 weeks)	0	0
Prednisolone	11	1
Oral contraceptive (2 weeks)	3	5

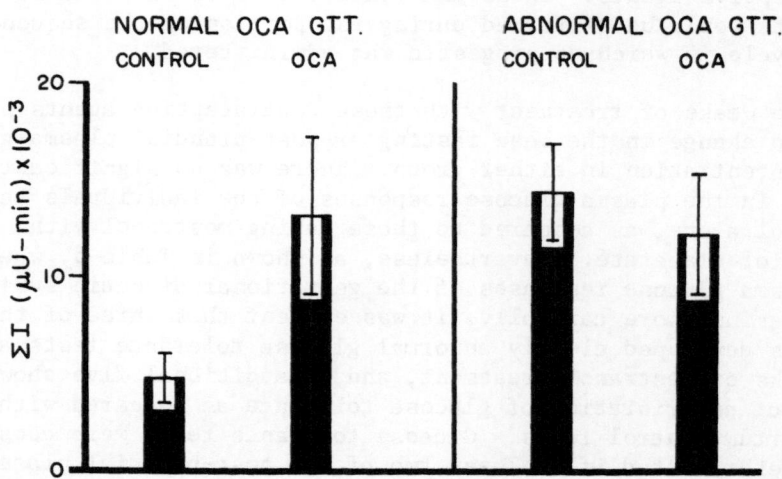

Fig. 7. Mean (±S.E.M.) plasma insulin responses to oral
glucose in non-diabetic and subclinical diabetic subjects treated
for 2 weeks with mestranol or mestranol and ethynodiol diacetate.
(Beck and Wells (26))

was observed in four of the non-diabetic subjects after two
weeks of contraceptive treatment, none of their third trimester,
glucocorticoid provocative, or contraceptive steroid glucose
tolerance tests were abnormal. No further increase in the incidence of abnormal or deteriorated glucose tolerance tests were
observed for either group of subjects after 2½ or 5½ months of
treatment with either agent.

In agreement with previous studies in man (28-30), the mean
integrated plasma insulin responses (ΣI) to oral glucose following
prednisolone provocation and during pregnancy were greater in the
non-diabetic subjects and following prednisolone provocation in
the gestational diabetics than during the post-partum control tests.
As might have been predicted from the monkey studies (Fig. 7), two
weeks of mestranol treatment produced a significant increase in the
mean ± S.E.M. ΣI of the non-diabetic subjects, but there was virtually no change in the plasma insulin responses of the gestational
diabetics. This increased ΣI was maintained throughout the next
three to six months of oral contraceptive treatment in the non-
diabetic subjects. Moreover, when the plasma insulin responses of
the gestational diabetics were compared to their plasma glucose
responses (Fig. 8), the three subjects who showed clear-cut abnormalities of glucose tolerance after two weeks of mestranol were
unable to produce any change in their plasma insulin response to
glucose whereas the individuals with normal glucose tolerance were
able to produce a distinct increase in peripheral insulin levels.

As in monkeys, the human findings suggest that mestranol not
only antagonized the peripheral hypoglycemic action of insulin, but
also enhanced the plasma insulin response to a glucose stimulus in
the non-diabetic individuals. Furthermore, inasmuch as there were
no significant differences in the responses of the women tested
while receiving mestranol alone and in those treated with ethynodiol diacetate plus mestranol, it would appear that the ethynodiol
diacetate played no role in the changes in glucose and insulin
metabolism, a finding which is also in consonance with the monkey
studies.

The results of this study also indicate that subclinical diabetic individuals are much more subject to deterioration of glucose
tolerance than non-diabetic individuals following exposure to
mestranol. On the other hand, mestranol in the dose employed is
not nearly so diabetogenic as prednisolone or pregnancy (Table 5).
This difference appears to be primarily due to the fact that
plasma insulin response to an acute elevation of the blood sugar
concentration is delayed more in the subclinical diabetic individual
during pregnancy or following prednisolone provocation than during
treatment with mestranol. Kalkhoff and associates have also reported a similar sluggishness of the initial plasma insulin response

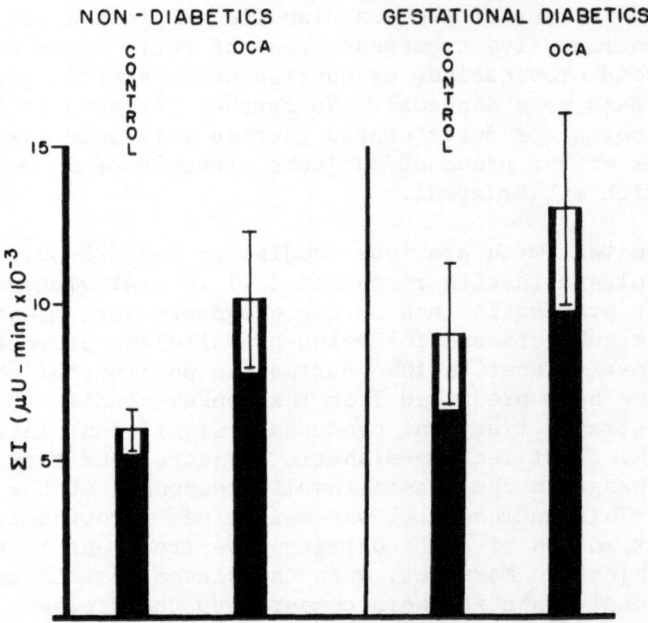

Fig. 8. Comparison of integrated plasma insulin responses
in the gestational diabetic subjects with and without normal glucose tolerance test responses after 2 weeks of oral contraceptive
treatment. (Beck and Wells (26))

Table 6

MEAN (± S.E.M.) INTEGRATED PLASMA INSULIN
RESPONSES TO GLUCOSE (Σ I) AFTER CHLORMADINONE
ACETATE TREATMENT (0.5 MG DAILY) FOR TEN WEEKS
(Beck, Ohaver, Bestley (47))

		Before	After
Non-diabetics	(7)	7,688 ± 2,050	17,294* ± 7,924
Diabetics	(10)	11,090 ± 1,784	12,732 ± 2,213

*P<0.01

to glucose in subclinical diabetic subjects following prednisolone
provocation and after treatment with human placental lactogen (29).
These changes in insulin secretion undoubtedly supplement the
peripheral resistance to the hypoglycemic action of insulin reported
during pregnancy by Burt (31) and observed in the laboratory after
administration of human placental lactogen (32). This inhibition
or retardation of insulin secretion may contribute significantly to
the development of gestational diabetes and to the deterioration of
glucose tolerance after glucocorticoid exposure. Mestranol, however, appears to produce deterioration of glucose tolerance only
if the increased peripheral resistance to the hypoglycemic action
of insulin is not compensated by an additional elaboration of
insulin. Consequently, only those subjects with borderline or
limited pancreatic islet insulin reserve will show a deterioration
of carbohydrate tolerance following exposure to mestranol. The
fact that subclinical diabetic individuals are more subject to
deterioration of glucose tolerance following exposure to oral contraceptive agents than non-diabetic individuals undoubtedly accounts
for some of the variation in the incidence of deterioration of
carbohydrate tolerance in women taking oral contraceptive agents
which have been reported in the literature.

Ethinyl estradiol does not appear to produce hyperglycemia as
readily in man as its 3-methyl ether, mestranol. DiPaola and
associates (33) have reported that prednisolone provocative glucose
tolerance tests are much more frequently abnormal in women treated
with mestranol combined with norethisterone (17α-ethinyl testosterone) (66.7%) than in women treated with ethinyl estradiol
combined with norethisterone (11.1%). Moreover, Yen and Vela (34)
observed no change in glucose tolerance (either intravenous or
oral) in 11 non-diabetic non-obese subjects tested on the 10th and
15th day of the third cycle of therapy with ethinyl estradiol plus
dimethisterone (6α-,21-dimethyl, 17α-ethinyl-testosterone). An
increase in the plasma insulin response to both intravenous and
oral glucose was observed together with an increase in the mean
fasting serum insulin levels. It should be pointed out that Yen
and Vela could not differentiate the magnitude of the plasma insulin
responses in the subjects treated with sequential ethinyl estra-
diol-dimethisterone therapy from those treated with combination
mestranol-ethynodiol diacetate therapy, thereby suggesting either
that ethinyl estradiol may be insulinogenic in man or that there
some carry-over effect from prior exposure to dimethisterone.
Finally, Pyorala and Lampinen (35) have reported a significant
slowing of glucose disappearance rates in 5 subjects treated for
20 days with ethinyl estradiol, thereby indicating that this
estrogen may be an insulin antagonist in man as well as monkey
(Table 3).

Progestins

Human studies now provide good evidence that the progestin components of at least some oral contraceptive agents may alter the glycometabolic effect of synthetic estrogens. In a preliminary communication (36), Spellacy reported that the incidence of abnormal and borderline abnormal glucose tolerance tests were greater in women taking combination-type (12% and 39% respectively) than in those treated with sequential-type (3% and 23%) birth control pills. Nevertheless, analysis of the data for individual birth control pills shows that not all contraceptive progestins affect carbohydrate tolerance adversely, and suggests that demonstration of an effect may depend on the quantity and chemical structure of the progestin administered and the type of glucose tolerance test employed.

Norethynodrel - mestranol. Carbohydrate and insulin metabolism has been studied more frequently in women taking norethynodrel with mestranol (Enovid) than any other oral contraceptive agent, yet there is far from uniform agreement as to the incidence of altered glucose tolerance or insulin metabolism. For example, the data of Javier, Gershberg and Hulse (24) indicate that 53% of women treated with five mg norethynodrel with mestranol developed abnormal or borderline carbohydrate tolerance. On this same dosage of norethynodrel and mestranol, one may see a significant increase in the mean plasma insulin response to glucose (37). Peterson, Steel and Coyne (38) reported a high incidence of borderline or abnormal glucose tolerance tests in women who received ten mg of norethynodrel with mestranol. On the other hand, Pi-Sunyer and Oster (39) observed no significant change in the mean serum glucose or insulin responses to glucose in 20 women treated with a smaller amount of norethynodrel (2.5 mg) with mestranol. Likewise, Posner and co-workers (40,41) found that there was a significant decrease in the mean glucose disappearance rate during intravenous glucose tolerance tests in women treated with five mg of norethynodrel plus mestranol after two or three months of treatment, but that this effect was reversed after four to six months of treatment with this agent. They attributed the improvement in carbohydrate tolerance following long-term treatment to unspecified compensatory changes in metabolism. The fact that intravenous glucose tolerance was normal in Posner's study whereas a significant number of women had abnormal oral glucose tolerance after a comparable period of treatment with the same amount of norethynodrel in other studies (24,37) suggests that the intravenous and oral glucose tolerance tests are not measuring identical phenomena. A similar lack of correlation between intravenous and oral glucose tolerance tests in women during gestation has been reported previously by Benjamin and Casper (42). Moreover, the work of McIntyre (43) and of Unger (44) clearly demonstrates that oral glucose

administration results in a release of intestinal factors which
may play a part in regulating the rate of insulin secretion. In
none of these studies was it clearly established whether or not
the subjects tested had any tendency towards diabetes other than
a suggestive family or obstetrical history before the institution
of oral contraceptive treatment. As has been demonstrated by many
investigators (27,42), the correlation between family or obstetrical history of diabetes and actual subclinical diabetes as demonstrated during pregnancy or during prednisolone provocation is far
from complete. Other data with regard to the effect of norethynodrel on glucose tolerance in normal subjects are difficult to interpret because of the absence of appropriate pre-treatment tests
or lack of appropriate control of the amount or duration of
therapy (45).

6-dehydro - progesterone derivatives. At least two studies
in the literature suggest that the progestin contained in certain
oral contraceptives may actually improve carbohydrate tolerance by
counteracting the diabetogenic effect of the estrogen contained in
the same preparation. Pyorala (35) reported that one mg of megesterol acetate (6-methyl-6-dehydro-17α-acetoxy-progesterone) administered daily for five days reversed the deterioration of
glucose tolerance observed in the same subjects following the administration of ethinyl estradiol alone for the preceding 20
days. Likewise, in 27 normal women, Starup, Date and Deckert (46)
observed no change in the fasting blood glucose or serum insulin
concentrations, in glucose disappearance rates, or in the plasma
insulin responses to intravenous glucose after 12 months of cyclic
combination megesterol acetate (five mg) mestranol treatment. Nevertheless, in one diabetic subject glucose tolerance deteriorated
and there was an increase in the fasting blood glucose level.

There is further evidence that the 6-dehydro derivatives of
progesterone may be free of diabetogenic activity in man. In
preliminary studies by Beck, O'Haver and Bestley (47), neither
subclinical nor non-diabetic individuals showed consistent changes
in oral glucose tolerance over a 2½ month period of treatment with
0.5 mg chlormadinone (6α-chloro, 6-dehydro, 17α-acetoxyprogesterone)
daily. However, the mean integrated plasma insulin response to
glucose was elevated in the non-diabetic subjects, but not in the
diabetic subjects, after 2½ months of treatment (Table 6). These
data would indicate that this 6-dehydro-progestin produces no
significant alteration in glucose tolerance in the dosage employed
but does not rule out the possibility that if larger doses were
employed, deterioration of glucose tolerance might be seen in susceptible individuals. Furthermore, one must ask whether the increase in immunoreactive insulin observed in the non-diabetic individuals after chlormadinone treatment represents a metabolically
inactive form of insulin.

Ethynodiol diacetate. Not all data in the literature coincide
with the thesis outline above. Goldman, Ovadia and Eckerling (48)
observed no change in intravenous glucose tolerance in women
treated with 100 mg pure progesterone daily for five days or with
medroxyprogesterone acetate (6α-methyl, 17α-acetoxy-progesterone)
15 mg every seventh day for three weeks. The amount of progesterone administered was approximately 1/20th the amount administered to the monkeys and does not necessarily preclude glycometabolic effects. Also, no measurement of serum insulin concentrations was made in this study. Halling,Michals and Paulsen (49)
have reported that glucose tolerance was abnormal in six of 15
patients treated with cyclic ethynodiol diacetate-mestranol therapy
for a period of three to 48 months. Their data suggests that ethynodiol diacetate with mestranol produced a greater deterioration of
glucose tolerance than did mestranol treatment alone, although
their data on this point are scanty. One may ask whether these
subjects were entirely normal since they attended an Endocrine
Clinic, and the possibility that they had endocrine abnormalities
which might affect their carbohydrate metabolism must be considered. Wynn and Doar (50), in their now classic study of carbohydrate tolerance in women taking oral contraceptives, reported that
18% of the women had abnormal oral glucose tolerance tests after
three or more months of treatment, a much higher incidence than
one would expect from mestranol alone (24). Inasmuch as 75% of
these women received ethynodiol diacetate plus mestranol, it would
seem likely that the ethynodiol was enhancing the diabetogenic
effect of the mestranol. The possibility exists that the 18 women
who received norethynodrel or norethisterone as part of their combination contraceptive agent may have been those subjects with
the greater proclivity for abnormal carbohydrate tolerance. Jackson
and Clarke (51) reported no alterations in the fasting circulating
glucose or in the daily requirement of antihyperglycemic agents in
six diabetic subjects treated for three months or longer with
Ortho-Novum,(norethindrone and mestranol). No measurements of
plasma insulin or glucose responses following glucose administration
were made in their subjects.

SUMMARY AND CONCLUSIONS

It is clear that gonadal and contraceptive steroids may significantly affect glucose and insulin metabolism in man and experimental animals. Whether any particular steroid has glycometabolic
effects appears to depend on its chemical structure, the amount
administered, and sensitivity of the individual tested to these
metabolic effects. Mestranol, by virtue of its methoxyl group at
the C_3 position, possesses insulinogenic and insulin-antagonistic
activities in monkey and in man which are apparently not present in
the parent estrogen compound. Women with compromised pancreatic

insulin reserve are most likely to develop carbohydrate intolerance while under treatment with contraceptive agents containing mestranol. That the basic pregnene and nortestosterone nuclei also possess insulinogenic and insulin-antagonistic activities is clearly obvious from the results of comparative studies in Rhesus monkeys. Progesterone and several nortestosterone derivatives enhance the stimulatory effect of glucose on plasma immunoreactive insulin production in the monkey without significantly altering the rate of peripheral glucose utilization. Interestingly, the introduction of unsaturation into the B ring of the steroid nucleus at the C_6 position (as in chlormadinone) appears to reduce the insulin-resistance activity of progesterone while preserving or increasing its beta cell stimulatory activity. From the limited number of human studies, it is evident that synthetic progestins often modify the glycometabolic effect of the estrogenic component of oral contraceptive agents in man. Present evidence indicates that oral contraceptive agents are not as diabetogenic in man as pregnancy. Future evaluations of gonadal and contraceptive hormones in man must take into account the structure-activity relationships of these compounds as well as the underlying tendency of the tested subjects to develop diabetes.

REFERENCES

1. Houssay, B.A., Foglia, V.G., and Rodriguez, R.R.: Production or prevention of some types of experimental diabetes by estrogens or corticosteroids. Acta. Endoc. 17:146-164 (1954).

2. Lewis, J.T., Foglia, V.G., Rodriguez, R.R.: The effects of steroids on the incidence of diabetes in rats after subtotal pancreatectomy. Endocrinology 46:111 (1950).

3. Talaat, M., Habib, Y.A., Abdel Naby, S., Hambi, H., Malek, A.Y., Ibrahim, Z.A., and Saad, A.F.: Effects of oestradiol dipropionate on the glucose tolerance and insulin sensitivity curves in normal and ovarectomized female rabbits. Arch. Int. Pharmacodyn. 2:153 (1965).

4. Talaat, M., Habib, Y.A., Higazy, A.M., Abdel Naby, S., Malek, A.Y., and Ibrahim, Z.A.: Effect of sex hormones on the carbohydrate metabolism in normal and diabetic women. Arch. Int. Pharmacodyn. 2:154 (1965).

5. Barnes, B.O., Regan, J.F., and Nelson, W.O.: Improvement in experimental diabetes following the administration of amniotin. J. Am. Med. Ass. 101:926 (1933).

6. Nelson, W.O., and Overholser, M.D.: The effect of oestrogenic hormone on experimental pancreatic diabetes in the monkey. Endocrinology 20:473 (1936).

7. Dalin, G., Joseph, S., and Gaunt, R.: Effect of steroid and pituitary hormones on experimental diabetes mellitus of ferrets. Endocrinology 28:840 (1941).

8. Ingle, D.J.: The relationship of the diabetogenic effect of diethylstilbesterol to the adrenal cortex in the rat. Am. J. of Physiol. 138:577 (1943).

9. Nelson, D.H., Tanney, H., Mestman, G., Geishen, V.W., and Wilson, L.D.: Potentiation of the biologic effect of administered cortisol by estrogen treatment. J. Clin. Endoc. 23:261-265 (1963).

10. Foglia, V.G., Schuster, N., and Rodriguez, R.R.: Sex and diabetes. Endocrinology 41:428 (1947).

11. Landon, J., Wynn, V., Cooke, J.N.C., and Kennedy, A.: Effects of anabolic steroid methandienone on carbohydrate metabolism in man. Metabolism 11:501-512 (1962).

12. Ingle, D.J., Beary, D.F., and Purmalis, A.: Comparison of effect of progesterone and 11-ketoprogesterone upon glycosuria of partially depancreatized rat. Proc. Soc. E.B. Med. 82:416-419 (1953).

13. Benjamin, F., and Casper, D.J.: Alterations in carbohydrate metabolism induced by progesterone in cases of endometrial carcinoma and hyperplasia. Am. J. Ob. Gyn. 94:991-996 (1966).

14. Schreibeman, P.H.: Alterations in carbohydrate and lipid metabolism by a progestin. Diabetes 17:341 (1968).

15. Beck, P.: Progestin enhancement of the plasma insulin response to glucose in Rhesus monkeys. Diabetes (In Press)

16. Neill, J.D., Johansson, E.D.B., and Knobil, E.: Patterns of circulating progesterone concentrations during the fertile menstrual cycle and the remainder of gestation in the Rhesus monkey. Proc. 3rd Int. Congress of Endocrinology 157-158 (1968).

17. Kendall, J.W., Jr., Liddle, G.W., Federspiehl, C.F., and Cornfield, J.: Dissociation of corticotropin - suppressing activity from the eosinpenic and hyperglycemia activities of corticosteroid analogues. J. Clin. Invest. 42:396-403 (1963).

18. Fajans, S.S., Louis, L.H., and Conn, J.W.: Metabolic effects of compound S (11-desoxy-17-hydroxy-corticosterone) in man. J. Lab. Clin. Med. 38:911-915 (1951).

19. Fried, J., Florey, K., Sales, E.F., Herz, J.E., Restivo, A.R., Borman, A., and Singer, F.M.: Synthesis and biological activity of 1- and 6-dehydro-9α-halo corticoids. J. Am. Chem. Soc. 77:4181-4182 (1955).

20. Ringold, H.J., Mancera, O., Djerassi, C., Bowers, A., Batres, E., Martinez, H., Neceoches, E., Edwards, J., Velasco, M., Casa Cámpillo, C., and Dorfman, R.I.: A new class of potent cortical hormones. 6α-chlorocorticoids. J. Am. Chem. Soc. 80: 6464-6465 (1958).

21. Liddle, G.W.: Studies of structure-function relationships of steroids. II. The 6α-methylcorticosteroids. Metabolism 7:405-415 (1958).

22. Dulin, W.E., Barnes, L.E., Glenn, E.M. Lyster, S.C., and Collins, E.J.: Biologic activities of some C_{21} steroids and 6α-methyl C_{21} steroids. Metabolism 7:398-404 (1958).

23. Liddle, G.W., and Fox, M.: Structure-function relationships of anti-inflammatory steroids. In Inflammation and Diseases of Connective Tissue, Mills, L.C., and Moyer, J.H. (Eds.) (Philadelphia:Saunders, 1961), 302-309.

24. Javier, Z., Gershberg, H., and Hulse, M.: Ovulating suppressants, estrogens and carbohydrate metabolism. Metabolism 17: 443-456 (1968).

25. Gershberg, H., Javier, Z., and Hulse, M.: Glucose tolerance in women receiving an ovulatory suppressant. Diabetes 13: 378-382 (1964).

26. Beck, P., and Wells, S.A.: Plasma insulin responses to glucose in nondiabetic and subclinical diabetic women treated with oral contraceptive agents containing mestranol. (Submitted to New Eng. J. Med.)

27. Fajans, S.S., and Conn, J.W.: The early recognition of diabetes mellitus. Annals N.Y. Acad. Sc. 82:208-218 (1959).

28. Kalhoff, R.K., Richardson, B.L., and Stoddard, F.J.: Defective plasma insulin response during prednisolone glucose tolerance tests in subclinical diabetic mothers of heavy infants. Diabetes 17:37-47 (1968).

29. Kalkhoff, R.K., Richardson, B.L., and Beck, P.: Relative effects of pregnancy human placental lactogen and prednisolone on carbohydrate tolerance in normal and subclinical diabetic subjects. Diabetes (In Press)

30. Kalkhoff, R.K., Schalch, D.S., Walker, J.L., Beck, P., Kipnis, D.M., and Daughaday, W.H.: Diabetogenic factors associated with pregnancy. Trans. Asso. Am. Physicians 77:270-278 (1964).

31. Burt, R.L.: Peripheral utilization of glucose in pregnancy. III. Insulin tolerance. Ob. & Gyn. 7:658-664 (1956).

32. Josimovich, J.B.: Potentiation of somatotrophic and diabetogenic effects of growth hormone by human placental lactogen (HPL). Endocrinology 78:707-714 (1966).

33. di Paola, G., Pucholo, F., Robin, M., Nicholson, R., and Marti, M.: Oral contraceptives and carbohydrate metabolism. Am. J. Ob. Gyn. 101:206-216 (1968).

34. Yen, S.S.C., and Vela, D.: The effects of contraceptive steroids on carbohydrate metabolism. J. Clin. Endoc. (In Press)

35. Pyorala, K., Pyorala, T., and Lempinen, V.: Sequential oral contraceptive treatment and intravenous glucose tolerance. The Lancet ii:776-777 (1967).

36. Spellacy, W.N., Buhi, W.C., Moses, L.C., and Goldzieher, J.W.: Carbohydrate studies in long-term users of oral contraceptives. Diabetes 17:(Supp. 1):344-345 (1968).

37. Spellacy, W.N., Carlson, K.L., Birk, S.A., and Schade, S.L.: Glucose and insulin alterations after one year of combination-type oral contraceptive treatment. Metabolism 17:496-501 (1968).

38. Peterson, W.F., Steel, M.W., and Coyne, R.V.: Analysis of the effect of ovulatory suppressants on glucose tolerance. Am. J. Ob. Gyn. 96:484-488 (1966).

39. Pi-Sunyer, F.X., and Oster, S.: Effect of an ovulatory suppressant on glucose tolerance and insulin secretion. Ob. & Gyn. 31:482-484 (1968).

40. Posner, N.A., Silverstone, F.A., Pomerance, W., Baumgold, D.: Oral contraceptives and intravenous glucose tolerance. I. Data noted early in treatment. Ob. & Gyn. 29:79-86 (1967).

41. Posner, N.A., Silverstone, F.A., Pomerance, W., and Singer, N.: Oral contraceptives and intravenous glucose tolerance. II. Long term effect. Ob. & Gyn. 29:87-92 (1967).

42. Benjamin, F., and Casper, D.J.: Comparative validity of oral and intravenous glucose tolerance tests in pregnancy: A study of 144 patients tested both during pregnancy and in the non-pregnant state. Am. J. Ob. Gyn. 97:488-492 (1967).

43. McIntyre, N., Holdsworth, C.D., and Turner, D.S.: Intestinal factors in the control of insulin secretion. J. Clin. Endoc. 25:1317-1324 (1965).

44. Unger, R.H., Ohneda, A., Valverde, I., Eisenstraut, A.M., and Exton, J.: Characterization of the responses of circulating glucagon-like immunoreactivity to intraduodenal and intravenous administration of glucose. J. Clin. Invest. 47:48-65 (1968).

45. Danowski, T.S., Sabeh, G., Alley, R.A., Robbins, T.J., Tsai, C.T., and Sekaran, K.: Glucose tolerance prior to and during therapy with contraceptive steroids. Clin. Pharm. & Therap. 9:223-227 (1968).

46. Starup, J., Date, J., and Deckert, T.: Serum insulin and intravenous glucose tolerance in oral contraception. Acta. Endoc. 58:537-544 (1968).

47. Goldman, J.A., Ovadia, J.L., and Eckerling, B.: Effect of progesterone on glucose tolerance in women. Israel J. Med. Sci. 4:878-882 (1968).

48. Beck, P., Ohaver, S.R., and Bestley, K.J.: Unpublished results.

49. Halling, G.R., Michals, E.L., and Paulsen, C.A.: Glucose intolerance during ethynodiol diacetate-mestranol therapy. Metabolism 16:465-468 (1967).

50. Wynn, V., Doar, J.W.H., and Mills, G.L.: Some effects of oral contraceptives on serum-lipid and lipoprotein levels. The Lancet, II:720-723 (1966).

51. Jackson, L.A., and Clark, J.F.J.: The effect of steroids on the glucose metabolism of non-pregnant diabetics. J. Nat. Med. Assoc. 58:105-106 (1966).

52. Beck, P., and Daughaday, W.H.: Human placental lactogen: Studies of its acute metabolic effects and disposition in normal man. J. Clin. Invest. 46:103-110 (1967).

THE EFFECT OF OVARIAN STEROIDS ON GLUCOSE, INSULIN, AND GROWTH HORMONE

W.N. Spellacy

Department of Obstetrics and Gynecology, University of
Miami School of Medicine, Miami, Florida

As the popularity of the oral method for fertility control
increased, so did the recognition of potentially serious complications. One area which has been extensively investigated is the
effect of these medications on carbohydrate metabolism. Our
investigations involve five areas of study:

1) prospective studies of blood glucose and insulin
    levels in women using several types of oral con-
    traceptives;

2) cross-sectional studies of blood glucose and insulin

The author wishes to express his appreciation to the many
individuals who have assisted on these projects, namely Dr. R.P.
Bendel, Mr. W.C. Buhi, Miss S.A. Birk, Mrs. K.L. Carlson, Mrs. S.L.
Schade, Mrs. K. Noer, Miss M. McShan, and Mrs. C.E. Spellacy. He
also wishes to thank Mr. H. Gravem, Dr. J.R. Boen, and Mrs. J.
Cassady for their help in the statistical analysis of these data.
Finally, he would like to acknowledge and thank Dr. J.W. Goldzieher
and Dr. L.E. Moses of the Southwest Foundation for Research and
Education in San Antonio, Texas and Dr. E.R. Zartman of Planned
Parenthood of Columbus, Ohio, for allowing him to study their
patients who were taking these drugs.
These studies have been supported by funds from the Population
Council of New York Grant No. M65.030, M65.111, M67.144; The Food
and Drug Administration Contract No. 67.34 and 68-48; The National
Institute of Child Health and Human Development Grant No. HD 01463;
and grant-in-aid from the Eli Lilly Company of Indianapolis,
Indiana, and the G.D. Searle and Co. of Chicago, Illinois.

126

levels in women who have used various types of oral
contraceptives for prolonged periods of time;

3) investigations of the individual components (estrogens
   and progestins) of the oral contraceptive drugs;

4) studies of the characteristics of women developing
   the most marked alterations in order to determine a
   profile for the high risk group;

5) studies of human growth hormone (HGH) levels in women
   using oral contraceptives thus seeking to determine
   a mechanism involved in these alterations.

These studies are all still in progress. It is the purpose
of this report to review the status of these five areas of study.

METHODOLOGY

The subjects tested were all volunteers and were not selected
for any chracteristic. In order to have control conditions prior
to beginning these studies the subjects had to be at least six
weeks postpartum or three months without steroid hormone usage.
All subjects were instructed to eat a high carbohydrate (300 gram)
diet for at least three days prior to testing. They were all
brought into the laboratory between 0700 and 0900 after fasting
overnight so as to control any circadian rhythms in hormone secretion. Prior to any test, a detailed history was obtained and
height and weight were recorded. During the testing procedure
physical activity was restricted to sitting for the insulin tests
or lying for the HGH tests.

A. Tests

1. Intravenous Glucose Tolerance Test. In this test, a
fasting venous blood sample was drawn and the subject was given
an intravenous injection of twenty-five grams of glucose as a
50% solution over a two minute period. Repeat blood samples were
then drawn at 0.25, 0.5, 1 and 2 hours after the injection.

2. Oral Glucose Tolerance Test. After a venous blood sample
was drawn, the subjects were asked to drink a solution containing
100 grams of glucose. Repeat blood samples were drawn at 0.5,
1, 2, and 3 hours.

3. Growth Hormone (HGH) Hypoglycemic Test. The subjects for
this test were placed at complete bed rest and a venous catheter
was placed in the antecubital fossa to limit the stress of the test

procedure. The subjects rested for 15 minutes and then a blood
sample was drawn. They were then given a rapid injection of regular insulin (0.1 unit/kilogram body weight) dissolved in 2 milli-
liters of water. Repeat blood samples were drawn from the catheter at 0.25, 0.5, 1, 1.5, 2 and 3 hours after the injection. The
catheter was filled with saline when not in use. This insulin
dose resulted in a blood glucose fall to less than 50% of the
fasting level in all instances. This has been shown to be a maximal stimulus to HGH release (1).

B. Assays

    1. Glucose. The blood for glucose determination was placed
in tubes containing fluoride to inhibit glycolysis and potassium
oxalate as an anticoagulant. These were mixed well and then
frozen at -20° C. Later the glucose content was measured in
duplicate by the method of Nelson and Somogyi (2,3).

    2. Insulin. The blood for insulin determination was placed
in tubes containing heparin. These were immediately mixed, centrifuged at 2000 r.p.m. and the plasma was separated and frozen
at -20° C. For all of the hormone tests, all of the plasma
samples (control and drug) from a given subject were assayed in
duplicate in the same assay determination. The insulin content
was measured by a radioimmunoassay procedure of Goetz and
Herbert (4,5).

    3. Growth Hormone. The plasma for HGH determination was
handled in the same manner as that for insulin. The concentration of heparin used has been tested in both hormone studies and
it has been shown to not cause any modification in the results.
The HGH content was determined in duplicate by a double antibody
radioimmunoassay technique (6).

C. Characterizing Data

    The subjects were all interviewed at each testing and
a record was made of the age, parity, infant birth weights, drugs
used, family history of diabetes mellitus in parents, siblings, or
grandparents, incidence of anomalous or stillborn children, and
previous glucose abnormalities. All of these facts, along with
the physical and laboratory data were punched on computer cards
for later analysis.

D. Data Analysis

    Since the subjects were all tested prior to receiving the
drugs and then serially thereafter (except for the cross-sectional
studies) the subjects served as their own controls. The analysis

involved correlated pairs and by using a computer, calculations
were made of the means, standard deviations, standard errors,
differences, means of the differences, standard errors of these
means and Student's t scores. The probability of occurrence for
each t was taken from two tail tables. Two hundred and twenty-
five correlation coefficients were also determined at each testing
between differences produced in the physical and laboratory data
and the characterizing historical data on each subject.

RESULTS

The results from each of the five study areas will be considered separately. All drugs were administered in the routine
cyclic manner.

A. Prospective Studies

These original studies were conducted at the University
of Minnesota and involved subjects taking either a combination
type (a) or a sequential type (b) oral contraceptive.

1. Menstrual Cycle. One group of women were studied to see
if the natural ovarian hormones produced any alterations in glucose or insulin levels (7). These women had ovulatory menstrual
cycles on the basis of both basal body temperature records and a
secretory endometrial histologic pattern in biopsy specimens.
There were 19 women tested with the intravenous glucose tolerance
test measuring both blood glcose and plasma insulin levels. Each
subject was tested on day 5 and day 25 of the cycle. The statistical results of these tests are shown in Tables 1 and 2. It
can be seen that at the proliferative and secretory phases of the
cycles that were tested, there was no significant difference in
the results. This also allowed the control test to be performed
at any phase of the menstrual cycle.

2. Combination Agent (Enovid-5). Originally 130 subjects were
started in this phase of the study and they are currently in their
third year of testing. After the control intravenous glucose tolerance tests the subjects were started on the drug. Both blood
glucose and plasma insulin were measured. Selected subjects were
brought back for repeat testing at 1, 6, 12, 24, and 36 months,
and an attempt was made to schedule the test on the nineteenth day
of the cycle. There were 25 subjects tested at 1 month (8), 32
subjects tested at 6 months (9), 93 subjects tested at 12 months
(10), 49 subjects were tested at 24 months, and 8 subjects were
tested at 36 months. The statistical studies of these test results
are shown in Tables 1 and 2. The total glucose (Σg) and insulin
(Σi) values during the test for the mean curves and also the ratio

Table 1

BLOOD GLUCOSE LEVELS IN MGM/100 ML MEASURED DURING AN INTRAVENOUS GLUCOSE TOLERANCE
TEST IN SUBJECTS DURING THE MENSTRUAL CYCLE AND IN ORAL CONTRACEPTIVE CYCLES

TIME IN HOURS		FASTING	0.25	0.5	1	2	FASTING	0.25	0.5	1	2
				DAY 5					DAY 25		
				CONTROL					DRUG		
Menstrual Cycle (N=19)	Mean	85.0	230.9	158.7	85.3	73.5	83.8	222.9	146.7	85.6	75.6
	SEM	1.3	8.5	6.4	4.8	2.3	2.1	5.8	7.9	6.4	2.2
Combination Agent											
Enovid 1 mo. (N=25)	Mean	79.4	196.4	124.9	75.9	74.6	81.0	214.6*	146.9*	92.7**	75.8
	SD	8	33	38	23	8	7	40	42	28	8
Enovid 6 mo. (N=32)	Mean	81.8	228.4	159.8	91.2	72.8	81.6	225.5	157.8	93.1	75.7
	SEM	1.5	9.4	6.3	5.3	1.4	1.3	4.7	5.8	4.6	1.8
Enovid 12 mo. (N=93)	Mean	81.5	216.4	146.0	83.1	73.3	81.8	219.0	167.0**	96.1**	76.3**
	SEM	0.8	3.8	4.1	2.9	7.8	0.7	4.7	7.0	2.9	0.8
Enovid 24 mo. (N=49)	Mean	82.8	218.8	150.2	84.8	73.8	82.0	213.6	153.7	97.9*	76.7
	SEM	1.0	5.3	5.3	3.9	1.2	1.2	3.9	4.4	4.1	1.4
Enovid 36 mo. (N=8)	Mean	83.8	209.6	138.1	87.5	72.5	80.0	209.8	149.0	104.3	81.0
	SEM	1.7	12.2	15.7	12.3	2.8	3.5	14.7	14.1	12.3	6.3
Sequential Agent											
C-Quens 6 mo. (N=35)	Mean	83.0	225.1	148.7	82.3	74.3	77.9**	201.7**	126.9**	73.6	70.8
	SEM	1.1	6.5	5.8	3.6	1.4	1.2	4.7	5.5	3.0	1.3
C-Quens 12 mo. (N=28)	Mean	83.5	223.2	146.6	82.2	74.7	82.8	204.0	140.9	85.0	78.4
	SEM	1.2	7.8	6.6	4.3	1.7	1.0	6.2	7.1	4.5	1.4

*p<0.05; **p<0.01; ***p<0.001

Table 2

PLASMA INSULIN LEVELS IN μ UNITS/ML MEASURED DURING AN INTRAVENOUS GLUCOSE TOLERANCE
TEST IN SUBJECTS DURING THE MENSTRUAL CYCLE AND IN ORAL CONTRACEPTIVE CYCLES

TIME IN HOURS		DAY 5 (CONTROL)					DAY 25 (DRUG)				
		FASTING	0.25	0.5	1	2	FASTING	0.25	0.5	1	2
Menstrual Cycle											
(N=19)	Mean	18	66	50	26	15	16	77	52	28	17
	SD	2	8	6	2	1	1	11	6	3	1
Combination Agent											
Enovid 1 mo.	Mean	18	52	39	25	16	25	76*	52	29	23*
(N=25)	SD	11	32	35	23	8	21	46	43	16	17
Enovid 6 mo.	Mean	18	73	47	29	19	26**	106**	80**	41**	22**
(N=32)	SEM	2	8	3	4	2	3	15	12	3	2
Enovid 12 mo.	Mean	11	59	40	19	11	15**	73	56**	30**	15**
(N=93)	SEM	0.8	4.9	2.7	1.9	0.7	1.2	5.8	4.8	1.9	0.9
Enovid 24 mo.	Mean	10	45	29	13	9	9	46	36	22***	11
(N=49)	SEM	1.1	5.0	2.6	1.4	0.9	1.2	3.8	3.4	2.3	1.8
Enovid 36 mo.	Mean	17	58	29	21	14	14	61	37	24	14
(N=8)	SEM	5.8	13.0	6.2	5.1	3.7	2.9	21.2	8.7	4.8	2.7
Sequential Agent											
C-Quens 6 mo.	Mean	12	60	43	22	14	19**	91**	65*	30*	19
(N=35)	SEM	1.1	5.5	3.0	2.4	1.9	1.7	9.0	8.8	3.0	1.6
C-Quens 12 mo.	Mean	8	38	24	11	17	6	39	23	12	7
(N=28)	SEM	1.6	4.9	1.9	1.1	10.1	0.6	4.4	2.1	1.4	0.9

*p<0.05; **p<0.01; ***p<0.001

Table 3

SUMMARY OF TOTAL GLUCOSE (Σg) AND TOTAL INSULIN
(Σi) DURING INTRAVENOUS GLUCOSE TOLERANCE TESTS

	Σg	Σi	$\Sigma i/\Sigma g$	Σg	Σi	$\Sigma i/\Sigma g$	Change in $\Sigma i/\Sigma g$
Control		Day 5			Day 25		
Menstrual Cycle	633.4	175	0.276	614.6	190	0.309	0.033
		Control			Drug		
Combination Oral Agent							
Enovid 1 mo.	551.1	150	0.272	611.0	205	0.336	0.064
Enovid 6 mo.	634.0	186	0.293	633.7	275	0.434	0.141
Enovid 12 mo.	600.3	140	0.233	640.2	189	0.295	0.062
Enovid 24 mo.	610.4	106	0.174	623.9	125	0.200	0.026
Enovid 36 mo.	591.4	139	0.235	624.0	150	0.241	0.006
Sequential Oral Agent							
C-Quens 6 mo.	613.4	151	0.246	550.9	224	0.407	0.161
C-Quens 12 mo.	610.2	98	0.161	591.1	87	0.147	-0.014

Table 4

CRITERION USED IN INTERPRETATION OF THE
ORAL GLUCOSE TOLERANCE TEST RESULTS

Classification	Blood Glucose mgm/100 ml			
	Fasting	Peak	2 hour	3 hour
Normal	<110	<160	<120	<110
Borderline Abnormal	111–119 or	>160	>120	>110
Abnormal	>120 or	>160	and	>120

($\Sigma i/\Sigma g$) are shown in Table 3. It can be seen that both the group
glucose and insulin levels are elevated after taking the drugs.
This is seen during the first month of treatment. After six months
of treatment the glucose values decrease whereas the insulin levels
remain elevated. After 12 months of treatment glucose is again
elevated as is insulin. There were no abnormal glucose curves in
these studies. At the two year test the group glucose and insulin
curves are similar to the control curves except for the one hour
values which are significantly elevated in the drug group. There
are also two abnormal glucose curves (4%) in the drug group where
the 2 hour glucose is greater than 100 mgm% and the K is less than
1. There are data on only eight subjects at a three year test and
the group results are not significantly different. There is one
abnormal glucose curve in this group also (12.5%). Thus the ratio
$\Sigma i/\Sigma g$ is elevated at all tests with peak difference occurring at
6 months. The decrease in the ratio which occurred in subsequent
tests can be due to an elevation of some of the subjects glucose
levels.

   3. Sequential Agent (C-Quens). The original group having a
control test and being started on this type of oral contraceptive
treatment consisted of 43 subjects. Here too the intravenous glucose tolerance test was employed and both blood glucose and plasma
insulin were measured. After 6 months of treatment 35 subjects
were tested (11), and after 12 months of treatment 28 subjects were
tested (12). The statistical data from these studies are shown in
Tables 1 and 2. The Σg and Σi for the group data and also the ratio
$\Sigma i/\Sigma g$ are shown in Table 3. Both the glucose and insulin values
are elevated after 6 months of treatment but they have returned to
normal at the 12 months test. This is in contradistinction to the
results described for the combination type drug group.

   B. Cross-Sectional Studies

      In order to obtain an estimate of the effect of long-term
usage of oral contraceptives on carbohydrate metabolism, several
cross-sectional studies were undertaken fully realizing the limitation of interpretation of these results. In the first study, subjects who had never been tested, and who had been continuously
taking one type of oral contraceptive for long periods of time
were studied with an oral glucose tolerance test (13,14). In this
study, 31 subjects who had been taking Orthonovum - 2 mgm - were
tested. The criterion for interpretation of the glucose results is
shown in Table 4. The results of these tests are shown in Table 5.
The average duration of usage of this drug was 114.6 cycles with all
of the subjects taking the drug for more than 100 cycles (over 8.3
years). Another population of 31 women in the same area were
similarly studied after they had been using a sequential type
drug (C-Quens) for more than 72 cycles (6 years) or averaging 78.2

Table 5

RESULTS OF GLUCOSE TOLERANCE TESTS IN CROSS SECTIONAL STUDIES

Drug Study	Mean Treatment Cycle	Number of Subjects	Results		
			"Normal"	"Borderline"	"Abnormal"
Sequential Agent (C-Quens) San Antonio, Texas	78	31	23(74.2%)	7(22.6%)	1(3.2%)
Combination Agent (Ortho-Novum) San Antonio, Texas	114	31	7(22.6%)	12(38.7%)	12(38.7%)
Sequential Agent (C-Quens) Columbus, Ohio	85	45	34(75.5%)	11(24.5%)	0
Combination Agent (Ovulen) Columbus, Ohio	78	19	12(63.2%)	5(26.3%)	2(10.5%)

cycles. The same criterior of interpretation was applied to these data and the results of the tests are shown in Table 5. Although the incidence of abnormality is significantly different between these two groups, so is the duration of treatment. As the blood glucose results became more abnormal, the plasma insulin patterns showed two changes; first, the levels reached were higher and secondly, the time period to that peak level was more prolonged.

Another population of long-term drug users were studied in Columbus, Ohio. One group of 45 subjects had used the sequential agent C-Quens for more than 65 cycles or an average of 85 cycles. The results of these tests are shown in Table 5. In the same area, another group of 19 women who had used a combination agent (Ovulen) (R) for more than 72 cycles or an average of 78 cycles were tested and these results are also shown in Table 5. Again there appears to be a difference between these agents despite a reversal in the length of treatment. Similar patterns were seen in the insulin levels.

C.   Component Parts: Estrogen (Mestranol)

An additional set of experiments has been started in humans and animals investigating the effects of various estrogens and pro-gestins, the oral contraceptive component parts, upon carbohydrate metabolism. One such preliminary study involved the oral glucose tolerance testing of women after hysterectomy. They were then given mestranol 80 micrograms per day for 21 days each month. A repeat test was performed after six months. The blood glucose and plasma insulin results are shown in Tables 6 and 7 respectively. It can be seen that there are only minor changes after this estrogen is used. This is true if the whole group is reviewed or if it is divided on the basis of the interpretation of the original glucose results. The group did significantly gain weight during the six months (156.2 to 164.3 pounds with $t = 4.7682$ and $p < 0.001$).

D.   Characteristics of High Risk Groups

Many historical variables were studied as to their pre-dictive value in deciding who would manifest the greatest change in insulin or glucose while using these drugs. None of these factors were significantly correlated with the cross-sectional study results. In the prospective study with the combination type drug no significant correlations were demonstrated until after one year of use. At that time, those subjects who had delivered in-fants weighing more than 9 pounds, who were of older age, and who gained excessive weight while taking the drugs had the most marked alterations. In the sequential type drug group there were no sig-nificant correlations until after one year of use and then those subjects who had a positive family history of diabetes mellitus

Table 6

STATISTICAL STUDIES OF BLOOD GLUCOSE (mgm/100 ml) BEFORE
AND AFTER SIX MONTHS OF MESTRANOL (80 μgm) TREATMENT

Time in Hours	CONTROL					DRUG				
	Fasting	0.5	1	2	3	Fasting	0.5	1	2	3
Total Group (N=18)										
Mean	88.7	132.6	146.1	124.8	102.1	86.6	138.9	145.0	126.7	110.8
SD	18.5	41.9	55.7	64.2	62.6	21.8	38.9	58.4	71.9	67.9
-SEM	4.5	10.5	13.5	15.6	15.2	5.3	9.5	14.2	17.5	16.5
T	0.6155	1.0769	0.1716	0.2137	0.9519					
P	NS	NS	NS	NS	NS					
Sub-group With Normal Control Test (N=11)										
Mean	81.1	109.3	118.2	93.0	71.5	81.2	120.7	119.2	93.6	79.0
SD	8.9	13.3	16.9	22.3	21.4	7.9	19.7	33.6	22.3	22.6
SEM	2.7	4.2	5.1	6.7	6.4	2.4	5.9	10.1	6.7	6.8
T	0.3720	0.1653	0.1388	0.1286	0.1916					
P	NS	NS	NS	NS	NS					
Sub-group With Abnormal Control Test (N=7)										
Mean	102.7	171.5	197.2	183.2	158.3	96.5	172.2	192.3	187.3	169.0
SD	24.0	45.2	67.1	76.7	75.8	34.8	45.1	67.0	93.6	86.3
SEM	9.8	18.4	27.4	31.3	30.9	14.2	18.4	27.4	38.2	35.2
T	0.6879	0.0444	0.3943	0.1684	0.4061					
P	NS	NS	NS	NS	NS					

NS = Not significant.

Table 7

STATISTICAL STUDIES OF PLASMA INSULIN (μ Units/ml) BEFORE
AND AFTER SIX MONTHS OF MESTRANOL (80 μgm) TREATMENT

Time in Hours	CONTROL					DRUG				
	Fasting	0.5	1	2	3	Fasting	0.5	1	2	3
Total Group (N=18)										
Mean	18	111	144	143	73	13	108	126	115	71
SD	9.7	81.1	105.7	120.5	71.0	8.8	76.4	103.7	104.6	83.2
SEM	2.4	20.3	25.6	29.2	17.2	2.1	18.5	25.1	25.4	20.2
T	3.5674	0.2471	2.2716	1.5815	0.0877					
P	<0.01	NS	<0.05	NS	NS					
Sub-group With Normal Control Test (N=11)										
Mean	19	106	143	121	42	14	134	128	105	62
SD	9.4	64.1	102.2	112.3	29.3	8.6	81.4	96.5	85.4	91.7
SEM	2.8	20.3	30.8	33.8	8.8	2.6	24.5	29.1	25.7	27.7
T	2.9067	1.0425	1.5969	0.6885	0.8428					
P	<0.05	NS	NS	NS	NS					
Sub-group With Abnormal Control Test (N=7)										
Mean	16	120	145	182	130	12	60	122	136	87
SD	10.9	110.4	121.8	135.6	91.4	9.7	33.6	125.4	140.4	69.6
SEM	4.4	45.1	49.7	55.3	37.3	3.9	13.7	51.2	57.3	28.4
T	1.8878	1.5698	1.5324	2.2864	1.1209					
P	NS	NS	NS	NS	NS					

NS = Not significant.

Table 8

HUMAN GROWTH HORMONE STUDIES DURING MENSTRUAL
AND CONTRACEPTIVE CYCLES (μgm / ml PLASMA)

Time in Hours		Day 5 (CONTROL)							Day 25 (DRUG)						
		Fasting	0.25	0.5	1	1.5	2	3	Fasting	0.25	0.5	1	1.5	2	3
Menstrual Cycle (N=19)	Mean	8.8	11.6	17.8	48.6	56.9	38.3	12.8	7.2	5.7	9.1	45.1	57.2	60.7	23.4
	SEM	1.3	2.3	4.3	7.2	11.9	8.6	2.9	1.2	0.9	1.7	5.1	9.7	15.1	7.2
Combination Agent Enovid 3 mo. (N=26)	Mean	8	8	11	55		48	18	28**	24**	48**	71	–	74	30
	SEM	1.5	1.4	2.5	7.3		7.9	3.6	5.1	3.7	10.4	7.6	–	14.1	5.2
Enovid 12 mo. (N=16)	Mean	10.1	5.9	7.6	35.8	40.0	24.6	9.2	22.1	15.6	17.4	62.4	83.1	54.1*	30.1***
	SEM	4.0	1.9	3.0	11.0	–	3.6	1.4	5.9	4.7	5.8	14.4	19.1	11.2	7.1
Sequential Agent C-Quens 3 mo. (N=25)	Mean	5.2	5.4	7.2	37.0	55.5	45.8	14.9	13.6***	12.8*	22.3*	53.5	75.0	70.6	26.3
	SEM	0.7	1.1	1.9	5.3	8.1	8.4	3.0	2.5	3.1	6.3	6.9	11.2	11.9	5.1

*p<0.05; **p<0.01; ***p<0.001

(parents, grandparents, or siblings) experienced the greatest glucose and insulin change. At the two and three year test with the
combination agent there is significant elevation of glucose and
insulin in those subjects who are of older age, high parity, have
delivered excessively large infants, or who have gained excessive
weight while taking these drugs.

E. Growth Hormone Studies

Previous studies by Young have demonstrated that GH is
diabetogenic (15). Recent data by Frantz and Rabkin showed that
estrogens could elevate GH levels (16). Because of these results
it was decided to investigate plasma HGH levels in women taking
oral contraceptives. The HGH was measured both in a fasting
resting state and also serially in response to a hypoglycemic
stimulus.

The first studies were done in order to establish the
effect of the normal ovarian cycle on HGH levels (17). Nineteen
subjects with ovulatory cycles on the basis of basal body temperature records and endometrial biopsy patterns were tested on the
5th and 25th days of the cycle. The statistical results of those
tests are shown in Table 6 and it is seen that no significant
difference was noted.

Additional studies were done in subjects taking the combination type drug Enovid 5 mgm. There were 36 subjects initially
tested and 26 were retested after 3 months of drug use (18), and 16
were retested after 12 months of drug use (19). The results of
these studies are seen in Table 6 and it is noted that the drug
usage was associated with an elevation of HGH levels in both test
periods.

The sequential type drug C-Quens was given to another group
of 39 subjects and 25 of these were retested after 3 months of drug
use (20). These results are shown in Table 8 and again as was noted
with the combination agent, the HGH levels are significantly elevated.

In order to ascertain whether the glucose HGH feed-back
mechanism stayed intact in long-term drug users, HGH was measured
during the oral glucose tolerance tests in the cross-sectional
study patients. In all cases while the fasting resting level of
HGH was elevated, these levels suppressed normally as the blood
glucose concentration rose (14).

DISCUSSION

Because of the greatly expanded use of ovarian steroid hormone therapy in medicine, and the general concern as to any detrimental consequences resulting from this form of therapy, an expanded research program has developed. The results presented here
from both prospective and cross-sectional research studies seems
to clearly show that some of the carbohydrate metabolic parameters can be altered by these steroids. The prospective studies
suggest that both blood glucose and insulin levels are elevated
soon after these steroids are used. It would appear that the
insulin levels become high enough so that the glucose levels return to their pre-treatment range after several months of use.
With prolonged usage the glucose levels in some subjects will again
rise. The incidence of decompensation with the resultant abnormal
glucose tolerance curves appears to increase with the duration of
treatment. The cross-sectional studies suggest that long periods of
time may be required to elevate many of the glucose levels. From
these studies it is suggested that the insulin levels have remained
elevated, but an alteration has occurred in the secretion mechanism,
thus delaying the insulin release and perhaps even altering the
type of insulin that is released (Proinsulin) (21).

It would also appear that the extent of these alterations may be
partially determined by the characteristics of the individuals
taking the hormones. The "high risk" group seems to be the women
of older age, high parity, those with a positive family history of
diabetes mellitus, those who have delivered large infants, and
those who gain excessive weight while taking these drugs. The
type of hormone preparation used, the dosage, the duration of
treatment, and the way it is administered may also be important.

Although several possible mechanisms for these alterations
have been suggested, such as the production of liver or adrenal
dysfunction, the change in growth hormone secretion must also be
considered. Perhaps not one, but a combination of mechanisms
are involved in producing the carbohydrate alterations.

Additional studies are being conducted with different drugs
and different steroids. Perhaps an effective drug for fertility
control can be found which will not produce significant metabolic
alterations.

SUMMARY

Blood glucose and plasma insulin levels were measured during
an intravenous or an oral glucose tolerance test in subjects taking
oral contraceptives. In a prospective study design both glucose

and insulin levels were elevated and remained elevated for 24 months
when a combination type oral contraceptive was taken. These returned to normal between 24 and 36 months for the group. The glucose and insulin levels were also elevated after six months of use
of a sequential type drug but not after 12 months. In cross-
sectional studies there was a high incidence of altered glucose
and insulin responses. It appears that individuals who are older,
of high parity, who have delivered large infants, or who have a
positive family history for diabetes mellitus, are the ones most
likely to demonstrate changes in the glucose or insulin levels.
Fasting growth hormone levels are elevated in women taking these
drugs as is the amount of HGH released during a stimulatory test.
These elevated HGH levels are suppressible with glucose. The
possible role of HGH in changing the glucose or insulin levels is
still unknown.

ACKNOWLEDGMENT

The authors also wish to thank the publishers of the various
journals listed in the text and bibliography for allowing the data
listed in the tables to be published.

REFERENCES

1. Greenwood, F.C., Landon, J., and Stamp, T.C.B.: The
plasma sugar, free fatty acid, cortisol, and growth hormone
response to insulin I in control subjects. J. Clin. Invest.
45: 429-436 (1966).

2. Nelson, N.: A photometric adaptation of the Somogyi
method for the determination of glucose. J. Biol. Chem.
153:375-380 (1944).

3. Somogyi, M.: Determination of blood sugar. J. Biol. Chm.
160:69-73 (1945).

4. Goetz, F.C., Greenberg, B.Z., Ells, J., and Meinert, C.:
A simple immunoassay for insulin: application to human and dog
plasma. J. Clin. Endocr. 23:1237-1246 (1963).

5. Herbert, V., Lau, K., Gottlieb, C.W., and Bleicher, S.J.:
Coated charcoal immunoassay of insulin. J. Clin. Endocr. 25:1375-
1384 (1965).

6. Spellacy, W.N., Carlson, K.L., and Schade, S.L.: Human
growth hormone studies in patients with galactorrhea (Ahumada del
Castillo Syndrome). Am. J. Obst. & Gynec. 100:84-89 (1968).

7. Spellacy, W.N., Carlson, K.L., and Schade, S.L.: Menstrual cycle carbohydrate metabolism. Am. J. Obst. & Gynec. 99:382-386 (1967).

8. Spellacy, W.N., and Carlson, K.L.: Plasma insulin and blood glucose levels in patients taking oral contraceptives. Am. J. Obst. & Gynec. 95:474-478 (1966).

9. Spellacy, W.N., Carlson, K.L., and Birk, S.A.: Carbohydrate metabolic studies after six cycles of combined type oral contraceptive tablets. Measurement of plasma insulin and blood glucose levels. Diabetes 16:590-594 (1967).

10. Spellacy, W.N., Carlson, K.L., Birk, S.A., and Schade, S.L.: Glucose and insulin alterations after one year of combination-type oral contraceptive treatment. Metabolism 17:496-501 (1968).

11. Spellacy, W.N., Carlson, K.L., and Schade, S.L.: Effect of a sequential oral contraceptive on plasma insulin and blood glucose levels after six months treatment. Am. J. Obst. & Gynec. 101:672-676 (1968).

12. Spellacy, W.N., Buhi, W.C., and Bendel, R.P.: Insulin and glucose studies after one year of treatment with a sequential type oral contraceptive. Obst. & Gynec. In Press.

13. Spellacy, W.N., Buhi, W.C., Spellacy, C.E., Moses, L.E., and Goldzieher, J.W.: Carbohydrate studies in long-term users of oral contraceptives. Diabetes 17:(Supp. 1)344 (1968).

14. Spellacy, W.N., Buhi, W.C., Spellacy, C.E., and Moses, L.E., and Goldzieher, J.W.: Glucose, insulin, and growth hormone studies in long-term users of oral contraceptives. Am. J. Obst. & Gynec. In Press.

15. Young. F.G.: Permanent experimental diabetes produced by pituitary (anterior lobe) injections. Lancet ii:372-374 (1937).

16. Frantz, A.G., and Rabkin, M.T.: Effects of estrogen and sex difference on secretion of human growth hormone. J. Clin. Endocr. 25:1470-1480 (1965).

17. Spellacy, W.N., Buhi, W.C., and Bendel, R.P.: Human growth hormone levels during the menstrual cycle. Am. J. Obst. & Gynec. In Press.

18. Spellacy, W.N., Carlson, K.L., and Schade, S.L.: Human growth hormone levels in normal subjects receiving an oral contraceptive. J.A.M.A. 202:451-454 (1967).

19. Spellacy, W.N., Buhi, W.C., and Bendel, R.P.: Growth hormone and glucose levels after one year of combination type oral contraceptive treatment. Int. J. Fert. In Press.

20. Spellacy, W.N., Buhi, W.C., and Bendel, R.P.: Growth hormone alterations by a sequential type oral contraceptive. Obst. & Gynec. In Press.

21. Steiner, D.F., Cunningham, D., Spigelman, L., and Aten, B.: Insulin biosynthesis: evidence for a precursor. Science 157:697-700 (1967).

INSULIN PRODUCTION IN OVERT (MATURITY-ONSET) DIABETES: ABSENCE OF
HYPERINSULINEMIA DESPITE HYPERGLYCEMIA INDUCED BY CONTRACEPTIVE
STEROIDS

E.M. Gold, J. Carvajal, P.A. Rudnick and K.E. Gerszi

Department of Medicine, Veterans Administration Center
and UCLA Center for the Health Sciences, Los Angeles,
California

During the course of recent studies with glyhexamide, a new
cyclic sulfonylurea, it was found that while this agent was an
effective hypoglycemic agent in adult diabetics (1), this activity
was unaccompanied by increases in serum (immunoreactive) insulin
concentrations (2). These studies fully confirmed reports by other
workers with chlorpropamide (3), tolbutamide (4), and acetohexamide
(5). The failure of sulfonylureas to raise serum insulin not only
leaves uncertain the mode of sulfonylurea action during prolonged
treatment but, in addition, invites questions regarding the insulin
response of untreated diabetics to hyperglycemia. Thus, while
glyhexamide failed to elevate circulating insulin, it was equally
apparent from our data that, unlike normals (6) and untreated maturity-onset diabetics (7), restoration of hyperglycemia following
treatment was also an ineffective stimulus to insulin secretion.

Supported in part by grants from G.D. Searle & Co., Chicago,
Illinois, E.R. Squibb & Co., New Brunswick, N.J. and the Diabetes
Association of Southern California.

Glyhexamide as Subose, and Placebo (lactose) tablets, simulating Subose, were supplied by Squibb. The average amount of
Subose prescribed in this study was two grams daily in divided
doses. Ovulen and tablets simulating Ovulen, but without mestranol,
were supplied by Searle. The assistance of Mr. C. Demos (Squibb)
and Dr. W. Stewart (Searle) in supplying these preparations is
gratefully acknowledged.

The authors wish to acknowledge the technical assistance of
Miss Anita Sarner, Mrs. Daisie Johnson, and Mrs. Judith Nikazy and
the secretarial assistance of Mrs. Elizabeth Ash in the completion
of this work.

The present report describes the failure of patients with overt diabetes to raise plasma insulin despite further blood glucose elevation induced during treatment with a hyperglycemic agent, namely the ovulatory suppressant combination of ethynodiol with mestranol.

MATERIALS AND METHODS

The present data were obtained from 18 patients with overt diabetes of the maturity-onset type. More precisely, all cases had fasting blood glucose levels in excess of 100 mg/100 ml without ketosis. In addition, all were males with an average age of 63 years and with diabetes of less than five years' duration. All of the group had been seen once monthly in a special out-patient clinic for as long as one to four years prior to inception of the present studies.

Throughout this period all patients received continuous treatment with glyhexamide, except for interposed study periods described below.

Glucose tolerance was evaluated during four treatment periods as follows:

1) Glyhexamide: 18 patients were tested after continuous treatment for at least one year.

2) Glyhexamide placebo: 17 patients from the first group were tested after placebo treatment for one month.

3) Ethynodiol diacetate: 12 patients from the second group were tested after one month of treatment with ethynodiol in doses of 1.0 mg daily; no glyhexamide was taken during this period.

4) Ethynodiol - mestranol: 10 patients from the third group received Ovulen for one month, again off glyhexamide therapy.

The treatment periods were non-concurrent. Since glyhexamide was omitted during steroid contraceptive treatment, the experimental design allowed the independent effects of each treatment to be assessed directly.

Patients were admitted to the hospital during study periods and placed on a 300 gram carbohydrate diet for three days prior to study. Oral glucose (OGT) loads were estimated on the basis of 1.75 grams/kg (ideal) body weight and intravenous glucose (IGT) was given as 0.5 gram/kg (actual) body weight. Insulin tolerance tests (ITT) were performed in ten patients given glyhexamide and

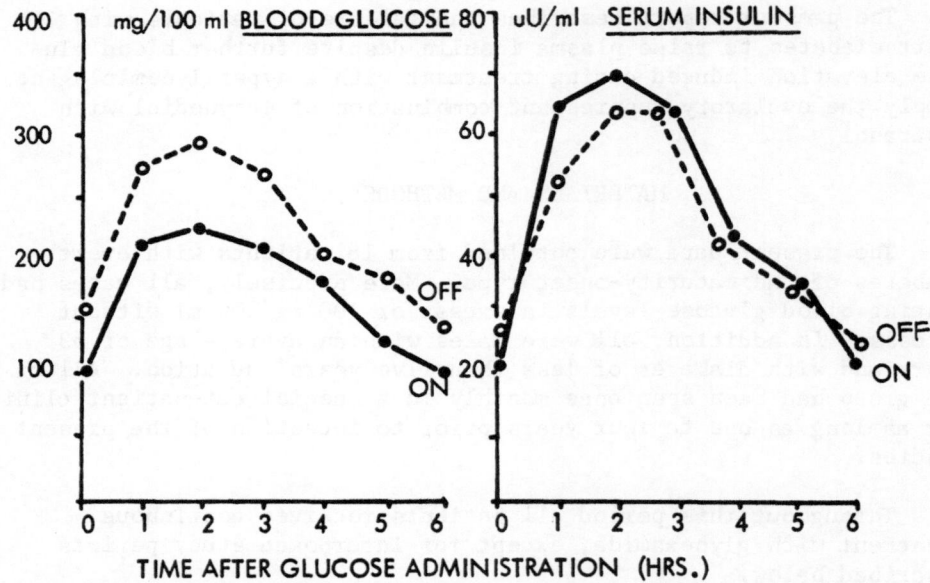

Fig. 1. Oral Glucose Tolerance: Glucose removal and serum insulin concentrations during glyhexamide (on) and placebo treatment (off).

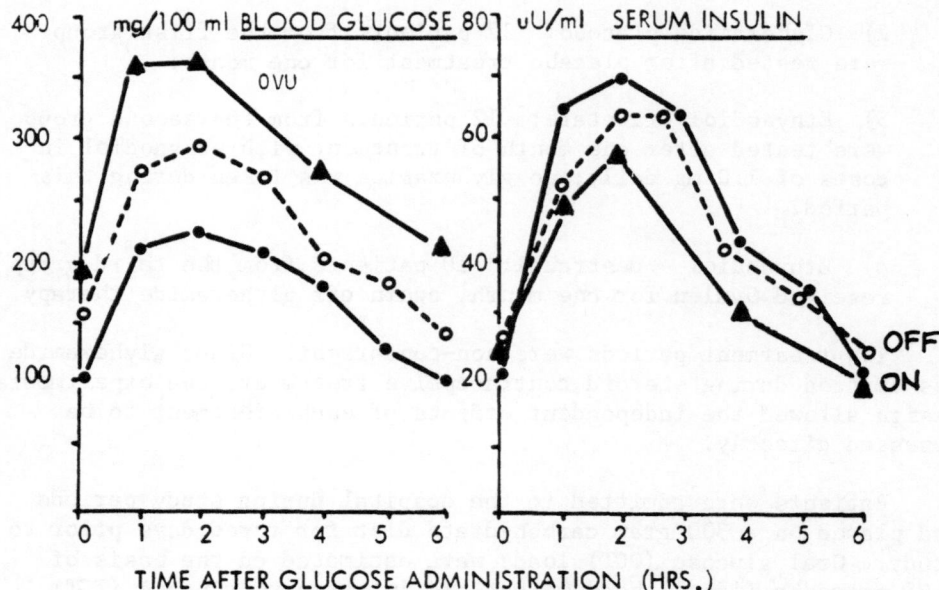

Fig. 2. Oral Glucose Tolerance: Glucose removal and serum insulin concentrations during Ovulen (OVU) treatment.

again after Ovulen treatment; the intravenous insulin dose given
was 0.3 units/kg (actual) body weight. No significant change in
weight was noted after any of the treatment periods.

Samples of venous blood were obtained at 15 time intervals
during six-hour oral tests, at 12 points during four-hour intravenous tests, and at ten points during two-hour insulin tests.
Each sample was assayed for blood glucose (8), serum immunoreactive
insulin (9), and growth hormone (10), the latter two measurements
employing the paper chromatoelectrophoresis techniques of Berson,
Yalow, and their associates. The present report deals principally
with the measurements of insulin in almost 2,000 samples. The data
presented are mean values for each group. Statistical analyses,
including "T-test" comparisons of matched group means, employed
standard techniques (11).

RESULTS

Oral Glucose Tolerance

Measurements of blood glucose during glyhexamide treatment
(on) demonstrated a significant rise in both fasting and post-
glucose values as compared to when placebo (off) treatment was substituted. However, no change in serum insulin concentrations was
observed (Fig. 1).

Following one month of Ovulen treatment, mean blood glucose
values rose even higher to average fasting values of 185 mg/100 ml
with peak levels of 377 mg/100 ml 90 minutes after glucose (Fig. 2).
However, serum insulin concentrations, both basal and post-glucose,
remained unchanged despite the broad range of glucose concentrations
represented.

Ethynodiol alone induced a modest increase in mean blood glucose values (Fig. 3). While, as with Ovulen, this rise was significant with respect to glyhexamide, only in the case of Ovulen
was a significant increase above placebo values obtained. Some
increase in average serum insulin was seen with ethynodiol, but
except for one point, the changes seen were not significant.

Intravenous Glucose Tolerance

During placebo treatment higher blood glucose values were also
observed following intravenous loads as compared to those during
glyhexamide (Fig. 4). However, glucose removal rates, as determined
by "K", the percent change per minute, were essentially identical.
Increases in serum insulin amounted to only about 60% of those obtained following oral glucose, and again, no significant differences
between placebo and glyhexamide treatment were noted.

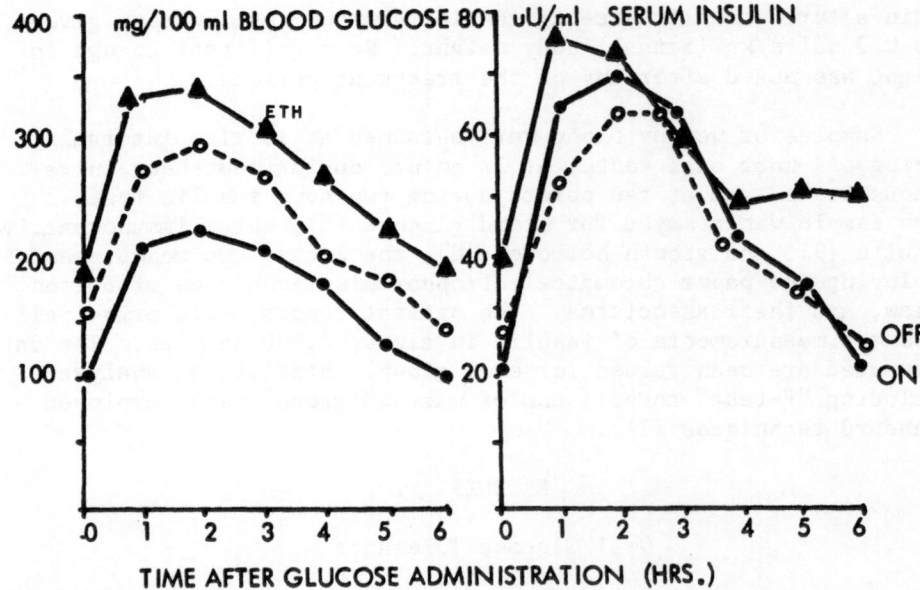

Fig. 3. Oral Glucose Tolerance: Glucose removal and serum insulin during ethynodiol (ETH) treatment.

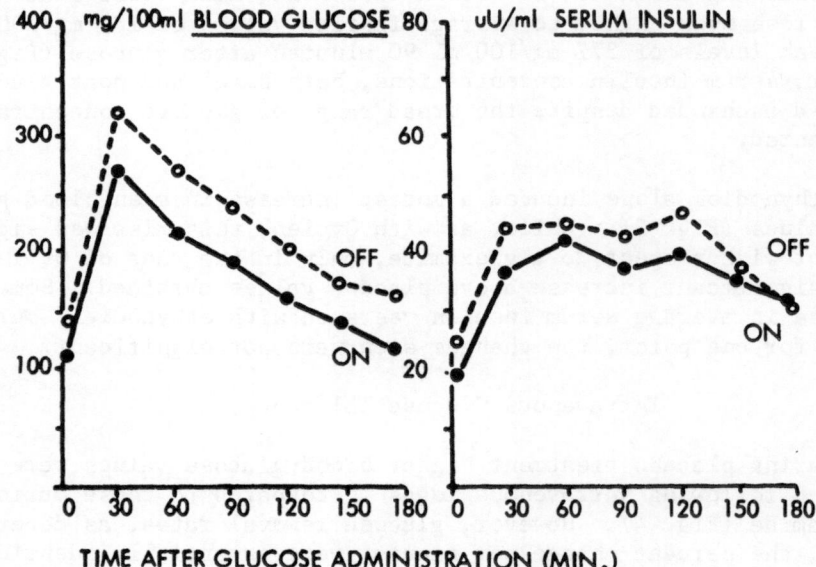

Fig. 4. Intravenous Glucose Tolerance: Glucose removal and serum insulin concentrations during glyhexamide (on) and placebo (off).

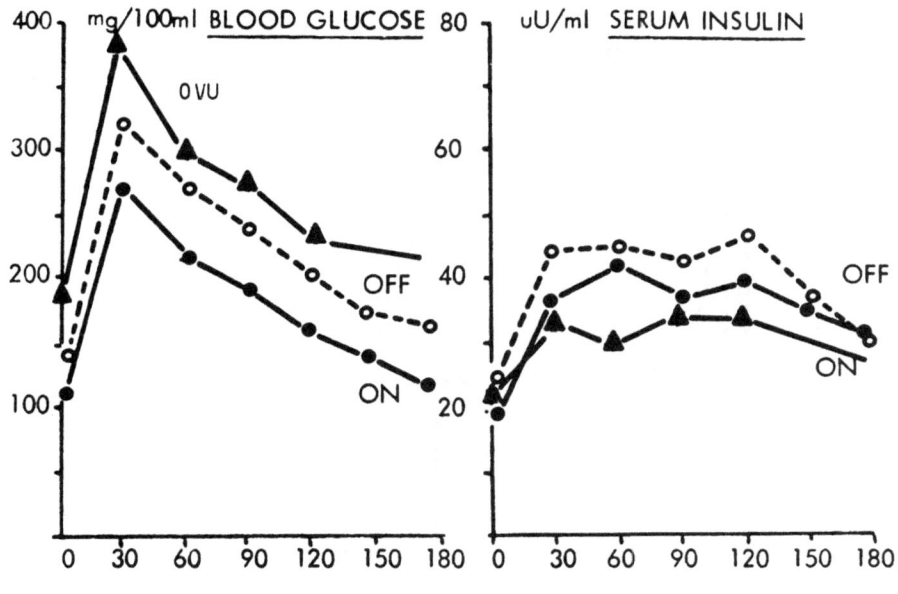

Fig. 5.   Intravenous Glucose Tolerance: Glucose removal and
serum insulin concentrations during Ovulen (OVU) treatment.

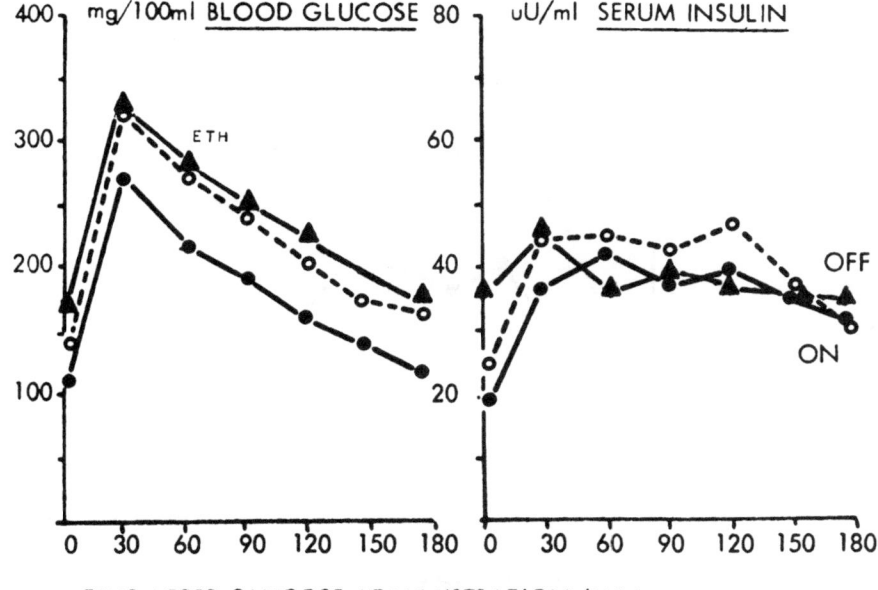

Fig. 6.   Intravenous Glucose Tolerance: Glucose removal and
serum insulin concentrations during ethynodiol (ETH) treatment.

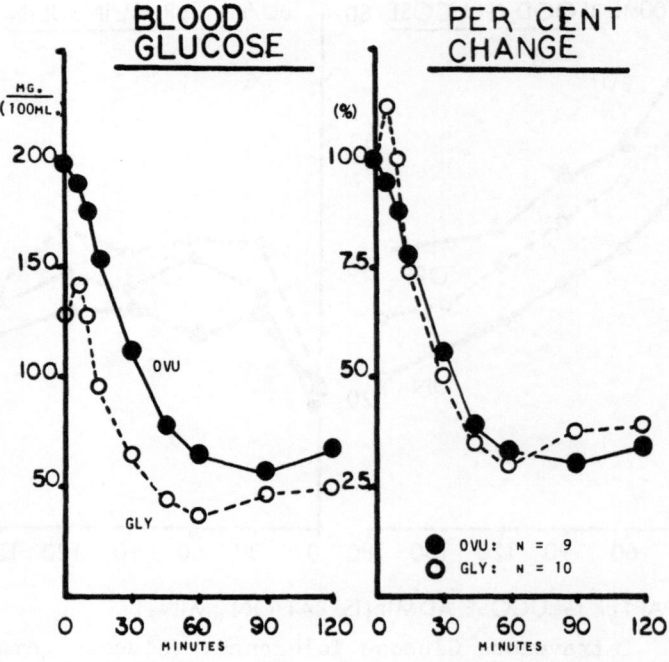

Fig. 7. Insulin Tolerance: Glucose removal during glyhexamide (GLY) versus Ovulen (OVU) treatment.

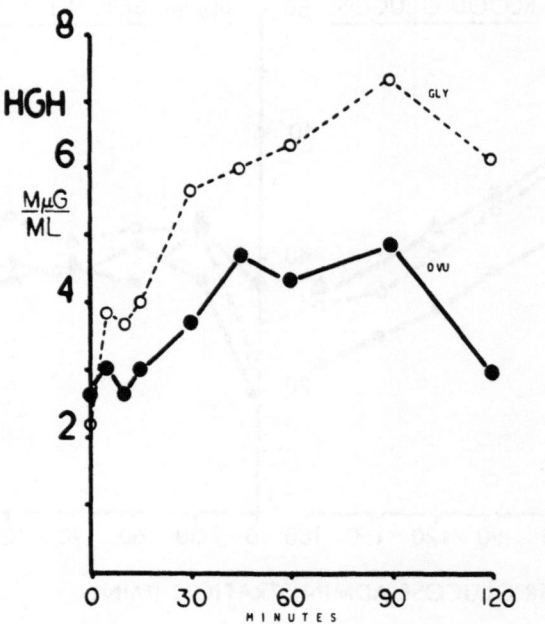

Fig. 8. Insulin Tolerance: HGH response during hypoglycemia.

Blood glucose was further increased by Ovulen, particularly
during the initial 30 minutes following intravenous glucose
(Fig. 5). However, no significant rise in serum insulin beyond
that observed during glyhexamide and placebo treatment occurred.

Following ethynodiol treatment, blood glucose levels and removal rates following intravenous glucose loads again were identical
to those obtained with placebo administration (Fig. 6). Serum
insulin concentrations also remained unchanged.

Insulin Tolerance Test

As indicated from studies thus far, the insulin response of
diabetics remained essentially indifferent to progressive hyperglycemia ranging from that seen with glyhexamide to post-glucose
levels almost 150 mg/100 ml, higher associated with Ovulen treatment. The possibility that increasing peripheral resistance to
these comparable levels of insulin might account for the hyperglycemia observed was explored by measurements of glucose following
identical intravenous doses of insulin during glyhexamide and
Ovulen treatment. Despite higher initial values, no difference in
the proportional decrease of blood glucose was found to support
the possibility that hyperglycemia with Ovulen was the result of
resistance to the peripheral action of insulin (Fig. 7).

Moreover, during both treatment periods, hypoglycemia with
exogenous insulin was accompanied by a significant rise in serum
growth hormone (HGH), although the rise obtained with Ovulen was
somewhat blunted (Fig. 8). Thus, no excessive responsiveness of
HGH was demonstrable in association with the elevated blood glucose levels associated with Ovulen.

The possibility that Ovulen-induced hyperglycemia resulted
from delayed insulin release during the early periods following
glucose loading was examined for both oral and intravenous glucose
loads. Multiple samplings during the initial 90 minutes of both
tests demonstrated significant increases above fasting serum insulin concentrations within the first 30 minutes following oral loads.
However, the absolute levels attained with each treatment were not
statistically different despite some decrease in mean values observed with Ovulen. Serum insulin concentrations after intravenous
loads were uniformly lower and also did not differ significantly
among the treatment groups (Fig. 9).

DISCUSSION

In summary the present study demonstrates that:

1) Blood glucose rises significantly in overt diabetics

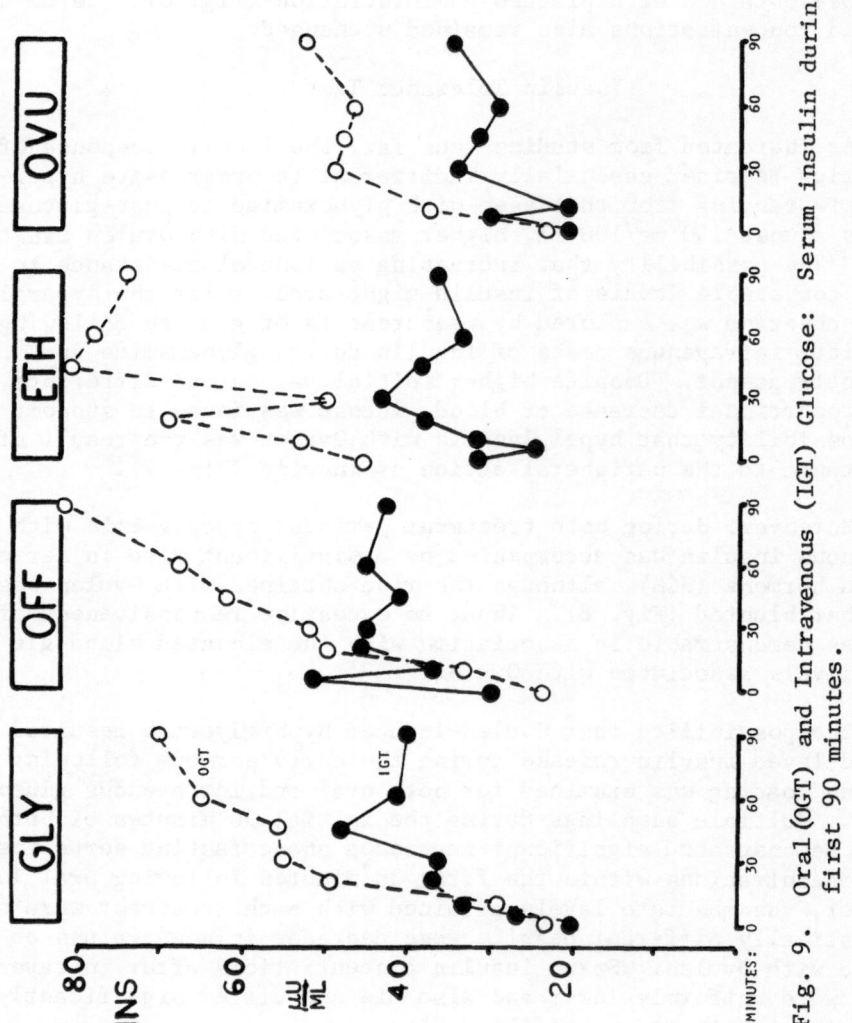

Fig. 9. Oral (OGT) and Intravenous (IGT) Glucose: Serum insulin during first 90 minutes.

treated with Ovulen for one month. While ethynodiol diacetate alone also tends to increase glucose concentrations, the levels attained were not significantly greater than those observed with placebo treatment.

2) Ovulen-induced hyperglycemia, demonstrable both during fasting and following glucose loads, was not accompanied by:

A) Increased concentrations of endogenous (plasma) insulin.
B) Increase resistance to administered insulin.

These findings in patients with established diabetes emphasize the hyperglycemic potency of steroid contraceptives even more strikingly than noted in earlier studies with non-diabetics. Thus, the deterioration in glucose tolerance found by Spellacy and Carlson (12) with Enovid was not associated with the significant elevation in fasting blood sugar found above, and, while Wynn and Doar (13) reported glucose tolerance impairment in 17% of their patients given Ovulen, this was observed in all ten diabetics similarly treated in the present study. Moreover, unlike these previous reports, no increase in serum insulin accompanied the significant hyperglycemia induced in overt diabetes by Ovulen.

The steroid component chiefly responsible for the hyperglycemic action of Ovulen appears to be the estrogen analogue, mestranol. This finding concurs with conclusions reported earlier by others (14) employing this agent. However, the rise in mean blood glucose found during ethynodiol diacetate treatment (above), albeit insufficient to attain statistical significance, nonetheless suggests that mestranol may not be the sole contributor to hyperglycemia associated with Ovulen.

The present study also bears upon the role of glucose in stimulating insulin production in patients with overt diabetes. In particular, the fixed insulin concentrations in the fasted state, despite a mean glucose rise of 70 mg/100 ml (glyhexamide vs. Ovulen) suggests that the pancreatic β-cell of the diabetic is either indifferent or incapable of responding to ambient hyperglycemia. The latter alternative seems less likely inasmuch as oral glucose loads regularly stimulated a prompt two- to three-fold increase in plasma insulin, inconsistent with either an "exhausted insulinogenic reserve" (15) or a constant compensatory attempt to restore blood glucose to levels found in non-diabetic normal subjects (16). An interpretation more in keeping with the present data is a loss of β-cell sensitivity or "indifference" to fasting hyperglycemia while still retaining the capacity to respond to acute increments in blood glucose. Moreover it would appear that in the diabetics presently studied, the insulin secretory response, once initiated, assumes a fixed, somewhat autonomous pattern no longer related either to the

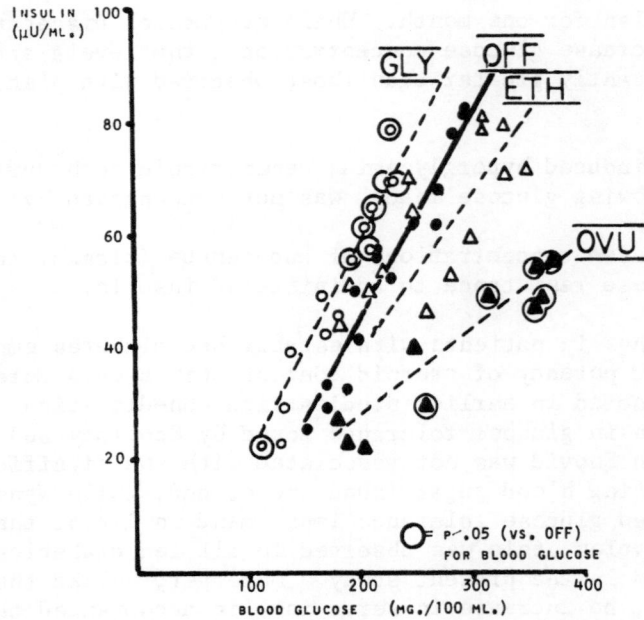

Fig. 10. Oral Glucose: Serum insulin versus blood glucose regression for all four treatment groups.

magnitude or the duration of the hyperglycemic stimulus. These considerations are not incompatible with those advanced by Seltzer (6), Kipnis (17) and others (16), namely that insulin production in maturity-onset diabetics, while maintained and, in some cases, at secretory rates even greater than normal, is nonetheless inappropriate or impaired relative to blood glucose concentrations. Indeed, such a situation offers one explanation for the glucose tolerance improvement noted with glyhexamide, since insulin concentrations while on the sulfonylurea, although similar to those off the drug, were nonetheless greater relative to simultaneous blood glucose levels (Fig. 10). However, the present study with oral contraceptives emphasizes two features of the failing but responsive β-cell which are difficult to interpret solely on the basis of glucose concentrations or an arbitrary response threshold which attempts to maintain glucose levels similar to those in non-diabetics, i.e., below 100 mg/100 ml. The possibility presently advanced is that under the special circumstances studied, insulin secretion may be dissociable from and no longer proportional to sustained (fasting) hyperglycemia but instead is characterized by a fixed, repetitive response to glucose increments irrespective of initial or final concentrations of blood glucose. Further studies are required to establish whether these characteristics are part of the natural history of diabetes mellitus.

REFERENCES

1. Gold, E.M., Carvajal, J., Rudnick, P. and Stein, R.B.: Prolonged use of glyhexamide, a new oral hypoglycemic agent. Third International Congress of Endocrinology, Mexico City, D.F., June 30-July 5, 1968. Excerpta Medica Fon. ICS #157, 1968 (Abstr).

2. Gold, E.M., Carvajal, J., Rudnick, P., Gerszi, K. and Seltzer, H.: Insulin production in overt (maturity-onset) diabetes: Hypoglycemia without changes in serum insulin during prolonged sulfonylurea therapy. (In preparation).

3. Reaven, G. and Dray, J.: Effect of chlorpropamide on serum glucose and immunoreactive insulin concentrations in patients with maturity-onset diabetes mellitus. Diabetes 16:487 (1967).

4. Fox, O.J., McAdam, G.L. and Boshell, B.R.: Effect of sulfonylureas on insulin secretion and reserve. Clin. Res. 15:42 (1967).

5. Sheldon, J., Taylor, K.W. and Anderson, J.: The effects of long-term acetohexamide treatment on pancreatic islet cell function in maturity-onset diabetes. Metabolism 15:874 (1966).

6. Seltzer, H.S., Allen, E.W., Herron, A.L., Jr. and Brennan, M.T.: Insulin secretion in response to glycemic stimulus: Relation of delayed initial release to carbohydrate intolerance in mild Diabetes Mellitus. J. Clin. Invest. 46:323 (1967).

7. Yalow, R.S. and Berson, S.A.: Plasma insulin concentrations in non-diabetic and early diabetic subjects. Determinations by a new sensitive immuno-assay technic. Diabetes 9:254 (1960).

8. Nelson, N.A.: A photometric adaption of the Somogyi method for the determination of glucose. J. Biol. Chem. 153:375 (1944).

9. Yalow, R.S. and Berson, S.A.: Immunoassay of endogenous plasma insulin in man. J. Clin. Invest. 39:1157 (1960).

10. Glick, S.M., Roth, J., Yalow, R.S. and Berson, S.A.: Immunoassay of human growth hormone in plasma. Nature, London 199:784 (1963).

11. Snedecor, G.W.: Statistical Methods: Applied to Experiments in Agriculture and Biology. Fifth edition. Iowa State University Press, 1956.

12. Spellacy, W.N. and Carlson, K.L.: Plasma Insulin and blood glucose levels in patients taking oral contraceptives. Amer. J. Obst. & Gynec. 95:474 (1966).

13. Wynn, V. and Doar, J.W.H.: Some effects of oral contraceptives on carbohydrate metabolism. Lancet ii:715 (1965).

14. Pyorala, K., Pyorala, T. and Lampinen, V.: Sequential oral contraceptive treatment and intravenous glucose tolerance. Lancet ii:776 (1967).

15. Seltzer, H.S. and Harris, V.L.: Exhaustion of insulinogenic reserve in maturity-onset diabetic patients during prolonged and continuous hyperglycemic stress. Diabetes 13:6 (1964).

16. Cerasi, E. and Luft, R.: Plasma insulin responses to glucose infusions in healthy subjects and in diabetes mellitus. Acta Endocr. (Kobenhavn) 55:278 (1967).

17. Kipnis, D.M.: Insulin secretion in diabetes mellitus. Ann. Int. Med. 69:891-901 (1968).

LONGITUDINAL STUDIES OF THE EFFECTS OF ORAL CONTRACEPTIVE THERAPY
ON PLASMA GLUCOSE, NON-ESTERIFIED FATTY ACID, INSULIN AND BLOOD
PYRUVATE LEVELS DURING ORAL AND INTRAVENOUS GLUCOSE TOLERANCE TESTS

V. Wynn and J. W. H. Doar

Alexander Simpson Laboratory for Metabolic Research
St. Mary's Hospital Medical School, London

Relative impairment of oral and intravenous glucose tolerance
has been found in certain women receiving oestrogen-progestagen
combinations (1-6). In a cross-sectional study of 105 women taking
oral contraceptives we found 18% of oral and 15% of intravenous
glucose tolerance tests to be abnormal (2). Changes of circulating
levels of other compounds related to glucose tolerance, including
insulin (5-7), non-esterified fatty acid (NEFA) (2) and pyruvate
(2) have also been noted by various investigators.

In view of the known association of asymptomatic chemical
diabetes mellitus with clinical manifestations of atherosclerosis
(8) these findings are important. It is unknown whether these
changes occur with all oestrogen-progestagen combinations, whether
they occur in all women, whether they regress after therapy is
stopped, whether they become progressively more marked with
prolongation of therapy and whether they are due to the oestrogen
and/or progestagen.

The present longitudinal study of plasma glucose, NEFA and
insulin and blood pyruvate levels in groups of women off and during
oral contraceptive therapy attempts to answer some of these questions.

Supported by NIH Contract No. PH-43-67-1344. We gratefully
acknowledge the assistance of Miss G. Robertson, Mr. D. G. Cramp
and Mr. T. K. Audhya in carrying out the analyses and of Dr. R.
Sharp, Mr. P. Samuel and Mr. G. Randall of Hatfield College of
Technology for computing aid.

SUBJECTS

Two groups of women were studied. Sixty-seven women in Group A were tested before and again while receiving oral contraceptive therapy. Twenty-four women in Group B were initially tested during therapy and again after this had been discontinued. Known diabetics were excluded, and no subject was taking any drug known to affect carbohydrate or intermediary metabolism (excepting oral contraceptives). Details of the two groups of subjects are shown in Table 1. The nature of the oestrogen-progestagen combinations used by the groups is shown in Table 2. No attempt was made to perform tests at the same time of the menstrual cycle. All women were advised to consume at least 200 g carbohydrate for three days before their tests. Any subject with a diabetic sibling, parent, grandparent, uncle or aunt was regarded as having a family history of diabetes.

Table 1

DETAILS OF GROUPS A AND B SUBJECTS

	Group A	Group B
No. of women	67	24
Mean age (years)	26 (17-46)*	32 (23-50)
Mean body weight as % 'ideal body weight'	100 (63-159)	118 (83-196)
Obese women (%)	7	46
Mean parity	1 (0-5)	2 (0-7)
Positive family history of diabetes mellitus (%)	48	46
Mean time (months) on (Group A) and off (Group B) OC therapy	6.2 (3-23)	4.6 (2-15)
Mean duration (months) of OC therapy in Group B subjects	--	23.3 (3-48)

*Range

Table 2

DRUG THERAPY OF GROUP A AND B SUBJECTS

	Group A	Group B
Ovulen	28	12
'Step-Up'*	13	--
Orthonovim	1	1
Norinyl	8	--
Lyndiol	5	3
Gynovlar/Anovlar	9	3
Volidan	2	3
C-Quens	1	1
Enovid/Enovid E	--	1

*'Step-Up' (0.1 mg mestranol + 0.1 mg ethynodiol diacetate for 16 days, 0.1 mg mestranol + 0.5 mg ethynodiol diacetate for 7 days).

PROCEDURES AND METHODS

Oral (OGTT) and intravenous glucose tolerance tests (IVGTT) were carried out by methods previously described (2) using glucose loads of 1.0 g and 0.5 g/kg body weight respectively. The interval between the two tests varied from one to seven days. Plasma glucose was measured by an automated glucose oxidase method (9), pyruvate by an automated enzymatic fluorimetric method (11) and plasma insulin by a double antibody radio-immunoassay technique (12). Plasma samples from paired tests off and on oral contraceptive therapy were always assayed for insulin on the same experimental run.

INTERPRETATION OF TESTS AND ANALYSIS OF RESULTS

Plasma glucose, NEFA, insulin and blood pyruvate levels following oral/intravenous glucose in the two groups were assessed as the mean levels at each time interval. IVGTT 'K' values were calculated from the logarithms of the 30-60 minute plasma glucose levels using the method of least squares. A value of 0.95 is conventionally regarded as the lower limit of normal (13). Individual curves were also assessed as the total area between the curve and

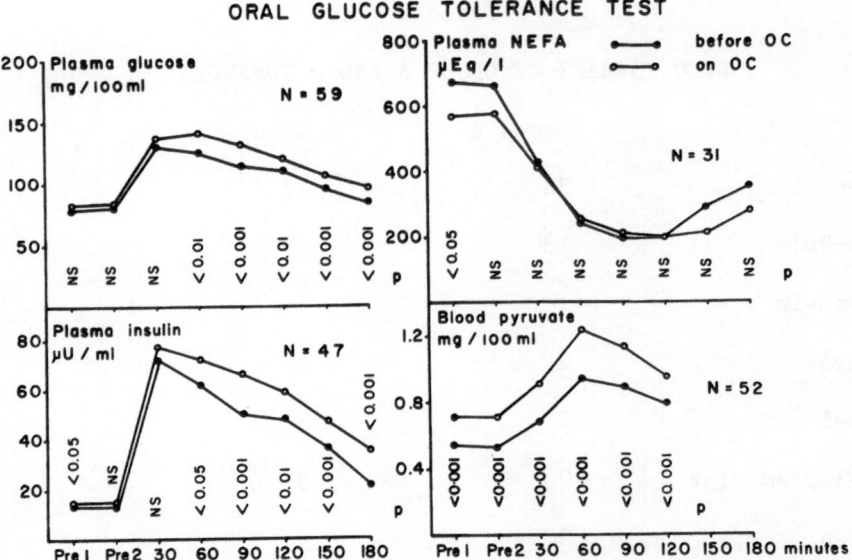

Fig. 1. OGTT mean plasma glucose, NEFA, insulin and blood pyruvate levels in Group A subjects before and during therapy. In this and subsequent figures, 'N' refers to the number of subjects studied and P to the significance of the mean difference.

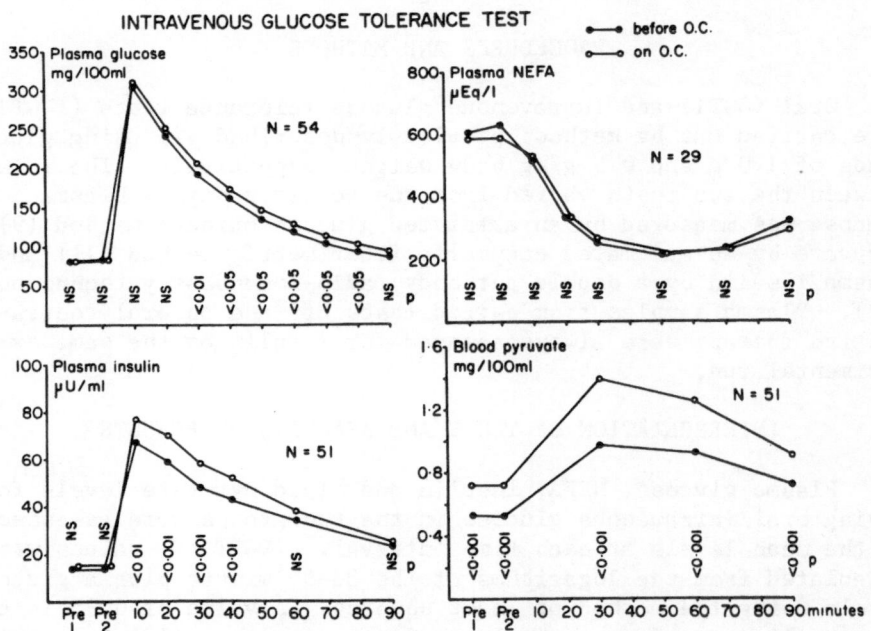

Fig. 2. IVGTT mean plasma glucose, NEFA, insulin and blood pyruvate levels in Group A before and during therapy.

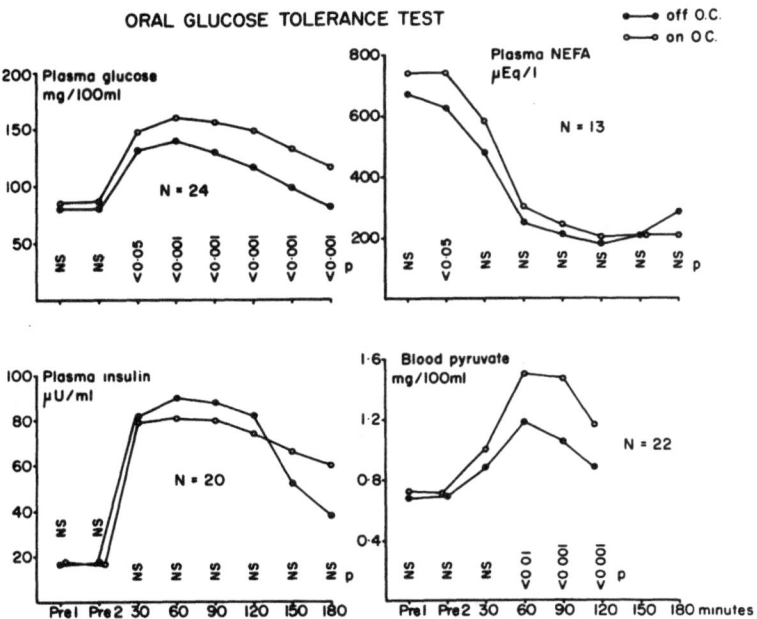

Fig. 3. OGTT mean plasma glucose, NEFA, insulin and blood pyruvate levels in Group B subjects during and after stopping therapy.

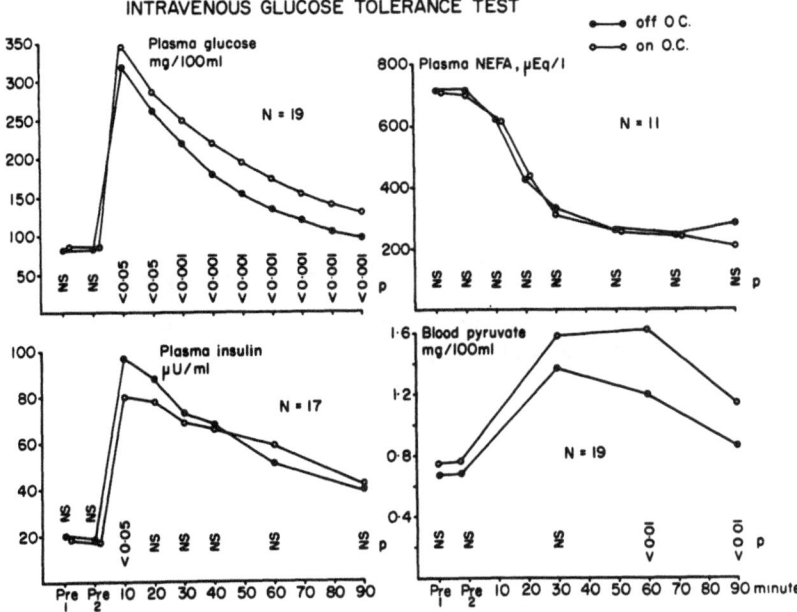

Fig. 4. IVGTT mean plasma glucose, NEFA, insulin and blood pyruvate levels in Group B subjects during and after stopping therapy.

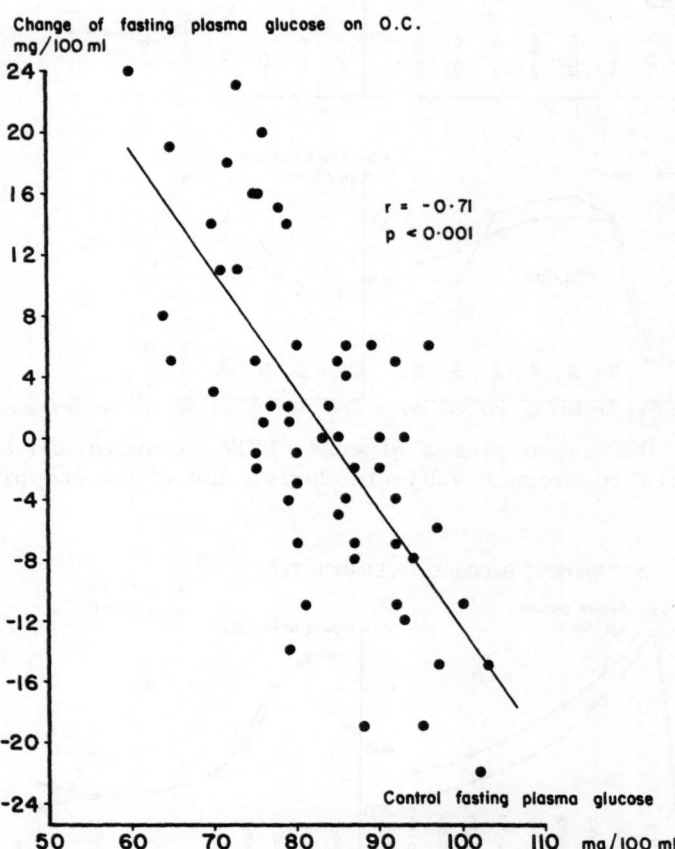

Fig. 5. Correlation between the control pre-therapy plasma glucose level and the change of plasma glucose level during therapy in Group A subjects.

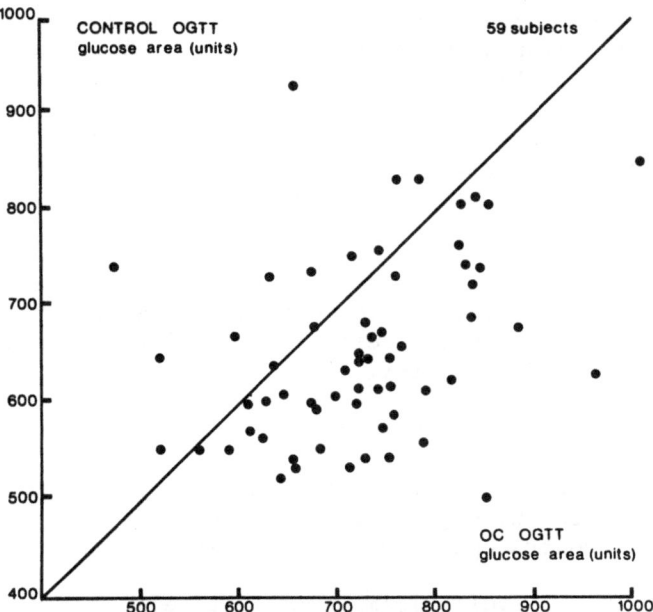

Fig. 6. Changes of OGTT total glucose area in Group A subjects
after starting therapy. A 45° line is shown.

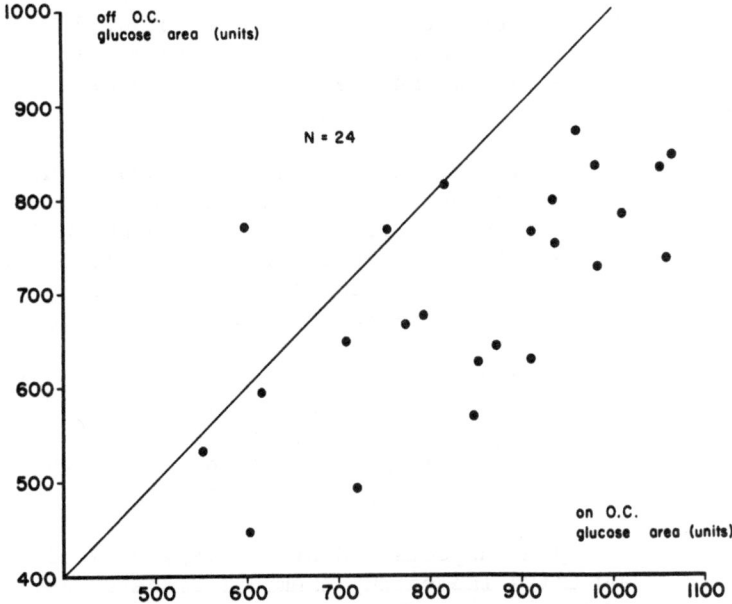

Fig. 7. Change of OGTT total glucose area in Group B subjects
after stopping therapy. A 45° line is shown.

the abscissa and the incremental area between the curve and a line
drawn horizontally through the fasting baseline. These areas were
calculated arithmetically in arbitrary units, assuming straight
lines between successive points. We have previously described the
use of the total area under the OGTT plasma glucose curve as a
graded criterion of oral glucose tolerance, and currently regard a
value of 800 units as the upper limit of normal in women of the age
group 20-40 years (2).

The significance of differences of means was assessed by the
paired 't' test, and the correlation between pairs of variables by
the product moment correlation coefficient. Calculations were performed by an Elliott 803 computer.

RESULTS

Mean plasma glucose, NEFA, insulin, and blood pyruvate levels
during oral and intravenous glucose tolerance tests in Groups A and
B on and off oral contraceptive therapy are shown in Figures 1-4.

OGTT and IVGTT Plasma Glucose Levels

The mean fasting plasma glucose level was not significantly
changed by oral contraceptive therapy in Groups A or B. A striking
negative correlation (r = -0.71, P<0.001) was found, however,
between the control fasting plasma glucose level and the change of
the fasting plasma glucose level during therapy in Group A subjects
(Fig. 5). A similar negative correlation (r = -0.56, P<0.01) was
found in Group B subjects between the fasting plasma glucose level
off therapy and change in fasting plasma glucose level when therapy
was discontinued.

In both groups, a significant impairment of oral glucose
tolerance was found during therapy. The changes of OGTT total
glucose area in each subject of Groups A and B are shown in Figures
6 and 7. Oral glucose tolerance was relatively impaired by oral
contraceptive therapy in 46 of 59 subjects (78%) in Group A and
improved after oral contraceptive therapy was discontinued in 22
of 24 subjects (92%) in group B. The mean OGTT glucose area during
therapy in 59 Group A subjects (724 ± 102 units*) was significantly
greater than their mean control value before therapy (657 ± 98,
P<0.001). The mean OGTT glucose area after stopping therapy in
24 Group B subjects (698 ± 116) was significantly less than the
mean value during therapy (846 ± 156, P<0.001).

Seven of 59 Group A subjects had pre-therapy OGTT glucose areas
of greater than 800 units indicating chemical diabetes mellitus.
In one of these subjects, the OGTT glucose area improved markedly

---

*mean ± SD

on treatment, and, in another, there was considerable deterioration. The remaining five cases were little affected (Fig.6). Nine of the remaining 52 Group A subjects (17%) developed evidence of chemical diabetes mellitus (OGTT) glucose area > 800 units) during therapy (Fig. 6).

Fifteen of 24 (63%) Group B subjects had OGTT glucose areas above 800 units when tested during therapy. All improved after therapy was discontinued, although only ten of the 15 achieved areas of less than 800 units (Fig. 7).

The mean IVGTT plasma glucose levels during oral contraceptive therapy were significantly greater than the respective control values during the greater part of the curve in both Groups A and B (Figs. 2 and 4). Abnormally low (<0.95) 'K' values were found in one of 54 Group A subjects before and in five subjects (9%) during therapy. Two of 19 (11%) Group B subjects had abnormal 'K' values during therapy and one of these remained abnormal after therapy was discontinued. The mean increase of 'K' value (0.57 ± 0.82, P<0.01) in Group B after stopping therapy was greater than the mean decrease of 'K' value found in Group A during therapy (0.06 ± 0.67, NS).

The IVGTT plasma glucose curves were also assessed in terms of the total area under the curve. The mean IVGTT glucose area during therapy in Group A (1521 ± 245 units) was significantly greater than the mean control value (1440 ± 254 units, P<0.03) and the mean value after stopping therapy in Group B (1587 ± 290) was significantly less than the mean vlue during therapy (1869 ± 209 units, P<0.001). The IVGTT glucose area increased in 34 of 54 (63%) Group A subjects during therapy and decreased in all 19 (100%) Group B subjects tested after therapy had been discontinued.

No significant correlation was found between the change of OGTT or IVGTT glucose tolerance area during therapy and age, degree of obesity, parity or duration of therapy in Group A subjects. Similar changes of glucose tolerance occurred in subjects receiving various oestrogen-progestagen combinations. The mean change of OGTT glucose area was similar in Group A subjects with (51 ± 110 units) and without (87 ± 126, NS) a family history of diabetes mellitus. A significant negative correlation was found between the change of OGTT glucose area during therapy and the control OGTT glucose area in Group A subjects (r = -0.54, P<0.001, Fig. 8). This correlation remained significant (r = -0.42, P<0.01) when four subjects with marked changes of OGTT glucose area of greater than 250 units were excluded from the series. A similar negative correlation was found between the change of IVGTT glucose area and control IVGTT glucose area in 54 Group A subjects (r = -0.53, P<0.001). In Group B subjects, a significant negative correlation

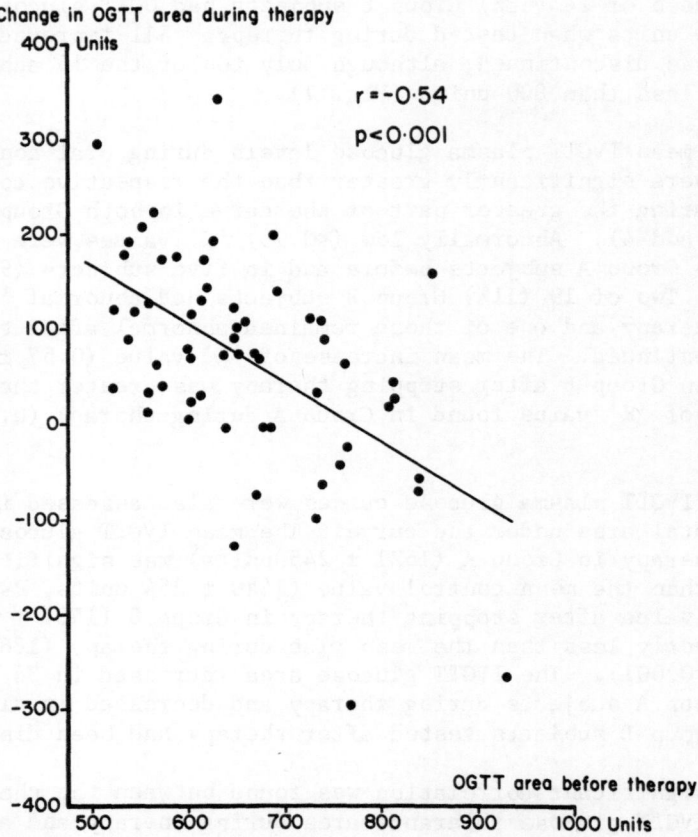

Fig. 8. Correlation between the control pre-therapy OGTT
total glucose area and the change of OGTT total glucose area during
therapy in Group A subjects.

was found between the IVGTT glucose area off therapy and the
decrease of IVGTT glucose area after therapy was stopped (r = -0.69,
P<0.001), but not between the OGTT glucose area off therapy and
the decrease of OGTT glucose area after therapy was stopped
(r = -0.12, NS).

OGTT and IVGTT Plasma NEFA Levels

Neither the mean fasting plasma NEFA level, nor the changes
following oral/intravenous glucose differed significantly in
Groups A and B during oral contraceptive therapy from the mean
respective control values (Figs. 1-4). No significant correlation
was found between the change of total area under the plasma NEFA
curve and the change of area under the plasma glucose curve in
oral or intravenous glucose tolerance tests in Group A and B subjects off and during oral contraceptive therapy.

OGTT and IVGTT Venous Blood Pyruvate Levels

The mean fasting venous blood pyruvate level was significantly
(P<0.001) elevated during oral contraceptive therapy in Group A
(Figs. 1 and 2). In Group B, however, the decrease after stopping
therapy was small and not significant. A significant negative
correlation (r = -0.35, P = 0.01) was found between the control
fasting blood pyruvate level and the increase of the fasting blood
pyruvate level during therapy. Mean OGTT and IVGTT pyruvate incremental areas were increased during therapy in both Groups A and
B (Table 3), although the changes were only significant for the
IVGTT in Group A and the OGTT in Group B.

It is of interest that certain subjects in Group B were found
to have abnormal venous blood pyruvate levels as long as six months
after oral contraceptive therapy had been discontinued.

Table 3

MEAN OGTT AND IVGTT PYRUVATE INCREMENTAL AREAS

IN GROUPS A AND B SUBJECTS

	mean OGTT pyruvate incremental area (units)	P	mean IVGTT pyruvate incremental area (units)	P
Group A before therapy	1.02 ± 0.52	NS	0.94 ± 0.46	<0.001
during therapy	1.26 ± 0.75		1.29 ± 0.54	
Group B during therapy	2.04 ± 0.93	<0.001	1.87 ± 1.11	NS
off therapy	1.16 ± 0.61		1.32 ± 0.60	

OGTT and IVGTT Plasma Insulin Levels

Mean fasting plasma insulin levels were not significantly different on and off contraceptive therapy in either Group A or Group B. During oral contraceptive therapy, however, mean plasma insulin levels after oral/intravenous glucose administration were significantly elevated above control levels in Group A but not in Group B (Figs. 1-4). The total area under the OGTT plasma insulin curve increased in 36 of 47 (77%) Group A subjects during therapy and decreased in ten of 20 (50%) Group B subjects after stopping therapy. The total area under the IVGTT plasma insulin curve increased in 33 of 51 (65%) Group A subjects and decreased in six of 17 (35%) Group B subjects after therapy was stopped.

Significant correlations were found in Group A subjects between the change in area under the plasma glucose curve and the change in area under the plasma insulin curve for both oral (r = 0.47, P<0.001) and intravenous (r = 0.64, P<0.001) glucose tolerance tests. These correlations were not significant in Group B subjects.

Body Weight

A small but significant increase in mean body weight (1.27 ± 3.15 kg, P<0.01) occurred in 67 Group A subjects during oral contraceptive therapy. The reduction of body weight in 24 Group B subjects after stopping oral contraceptive therapy (0.50 ± 3.15 kg), however, was not significant. Forty-seven of 67 (70%) Group A subjects gained weight during therapy and 11 of 24 (46%) Group B subjects lost weight after therapy was discontinued.

DISCUSSION

In a previous cross-sectional study of 105 women taking oral contraceptives and a control group of 78 women, we found impaired oral and intravenous glucose tolerance, elevated fasting plasma NEFA levels, and elevated venous blood pyruvate levels both before and after oral/intravenous glucose administration (2). The present study confirms the majority of these findings in longitudinal studies with the exception that mean plasma NEFA levels before and after glucose administration were not affected by oral contraceptive therapy. In addition, we have found mean plasma insulin levels to be elevated during oral contraceptive therapy after oral/intravenous glucose administration though the mean fasting plasma insulin level was unchanged. The majority of these metabolic changes were reversed after oral contraceptive therapy had been discontinued.

The mean fasting plasma glucose level did not change sig-

nificantly during oral contraceptive therapy confirming findings
of previous investigators (3,4,6,14,15). The total area under the
OGTT plasma/glucose curve, however, increased during therapy in
46 of 59 (78%) Group A subjects. Nine of 52 (17%) Group A subjects
developed chemical diabetes during therapy, an incidence similar
to that found in our previous study (2). With one notable exception (16), impairment of oral glucose tolerance during oral contraceptive administration has been found by other workers (1,15,17,18).
Plasma glucose levels were slightly but significantly elevated in
Group A subjects during therapy for the greater part of the IVGTT
plasma glucose curve. While no significant change of the mean
'K' value was found, five subjects (9%) developed abnormal values
(<0.95) during therapy. The total area under the IVGTT plasma
glucose curve was significantly increased during therapy and this
index increased in 34 of 54 (63%) Group A subjects.

The discrepancy between the analysis of results of 'K' values
and IVGTT glucose areas in Group A subjects before and during
therapy confirms a longstanding suspicion that the 'K' value is
not a satisfactory index of glucose tolerance. Its derivation
assumes glucose removal from the vascular compartment to be a first
order reaction and that the rate of entry of glucose into this
compartment is reduced to zero after intravenous glucose administration. Both of these assumptions are probably untrue (19,20).
Furthermore, it is clearly possible to have a whole range of dis-
similar IVGTT plasma glucose curves with identical 'K' values.
The use of the total area between the IVGTT plasma glucose curve
and the abscissa or the incremental area between the curve and a
line drawn horizontally through the fasting baseline is likely to
be a more sensitive index of changes of intravenous glucose
tolerance in longitudinal studies.

The results of previous longitudinal studies of the effects
of oral contraceptive therapy on intravenous glucose tolerance are
conflicting. Posner et al (3,4) found progressive impairment of
intravenous glucose tolerance in women receiving 'Enovid,' tested
two and four to six months after starting therapy. Spellacy et al,
using the same drug, noted relatively impaired intravenous glucose
tolerance during the first (5) and twelfth cycles (6) but not
during the sixth cycle of treatment (7). Starup et al (14), using
a combination of mestranol and megestrol acetate, found no impairment of intravenous glucose tolerance after treatment for one
year. These differences may result from differences of experimental
design.

No significant correlation was found between the changes of
oral or intravenous glucose tolerance area off and on therapy, and
the subjects' age, degree of obesity, parity or duration of therapy.
The present study, however, was unsuitable for analysis of the

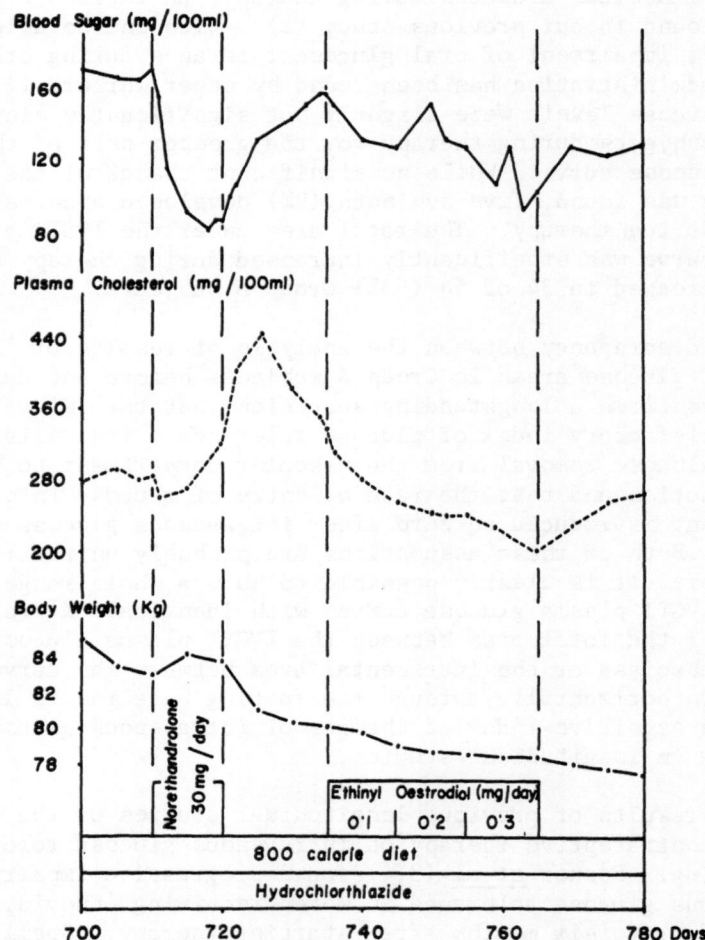

Fig. 9. Effect of ethinyl oestradiol on the fasting blood sugar level of a 49-year-old woman with maturity onset diabetes mellitus.

effects of duration of therapy, as this was similar in a large
proportion of the Group A subjects. No difference of the mean
changes of these indices of glucose tolerance was found in subjects
with and without a family history of diabetes, and similar changes
of glucose tolerance were observed in subjects receiving various
oestrogen-progestagen combinations. Of particular interest were
the findings of negative correlations between the change of total
area under the plasma glucose curve during therapy and control
oral glucose tolerance area (r = -0.54, P<0.001) and intravenous
glucose tolerance area (r = -0.53, P<0.001) in Group A subjects.
Javier et al (17) have previously noted that oral glucose tolerance
may be unchanged or even improved during oral contraceptive therapy
in subjects with mild chemical diabetes mellitus. These negative
correlations are largely due to a similar negative correlation
between the change of the fasting plasma glucose level during
therapy and the control fasting plasma glucose level (r = -0.71,
P<0.001). Analysis of fasting blood sugar data in 27 subjects
studied by Spellacy et al (21) before and during 'Enovid' therapy
showed a similar negative correlation (r = -0.46, P<0.05). We
have also observed a marked reduction of the fasting blood sugar
levels in two obese subjects during oestrogen therapy, one of which
is shown in Figure 9. A similar reduction of the fasting blood
sugar level has been observed in normal subjects during methandienone therapy (22), and again the magnitude of the change was
inversely related to the control fasting blood sugar level.
Whether these changes of fasting plasma glucose levels result from
altered rates of production and/or removal of glucose is not clear
and will not be further discussed at present.

There have been no detailed studies of the reversibility of
these changes of glucose tolerance after stopping oral contraceptive therapy. The improvement of oral and intravenous tolerance
in Group B subjects after therapy was discontinued is, therefore,
of interest. The total area under the oral glucose tolerance
curve decreased in 22 of 24 Group B subjects and the total area
under the intravenous glucose tolerance curve decreased in all
19 Group B subjects tested. While the magnitude of these changes
was greater than that found in Group A subjects tested before and
on therapy, the two groups are not comparable. In general, Group
B subjects were older, more obese, and more parous than Group A
subjects. Furthermore, they had received oral contraceptive
therapy for a longer period.

Neither the mean fasting plasma NEFA level nor the mean levels
following oral/intravenous glucose were affected by oral contraceptive therapy in the present series. While it has been suggested
that elevated plasma NEFA levels may contribute to the impaired
glucose tolerance of diabetes mellitus, thyrotoxicosis and acromegaly (23), the changes of glucose tolerance observed during oral

contraceptive therapy clearly cannot be accounted for by this
mechanism.

A striking finding was the elevation of venous blood pyruvate
levels during oral contraceptive therapy, both in the fasting state
and following oral/intravenous glucose administration. In certain
subjects, an abnormally great blood pyruvate increment above the
fasting level was noted following glucose. These results confirm
our previous observations (2). Occasional Group B subjects continued to have abnormally elevated venous blood pyruvate levels
during glucose tolerance tests for as long as six months after
stopping therapy, suggesting that certain of the metabolic changes
induced by oral contraceptives persist for at least this length of
time. Indirect studies of pyruvate metabolism using sodium L(+)
lactate infusions suggest that the increased fasting blood pyruvate
levels found in some subjects during oral contraceptive therapy are
likely to be due to an increased rate of formation rather than impaired degradation. This aspect is further discussed in a separate
communication (24).

Most (5,6,14,17), but not all (7,25), previous workers have
found the fasting plasma insulin level to be unchanged during oral
contraceptive therapy. Spellacy et al (5,6,7) observed plasma
insulin levels to be higher than pre-therapy levels during intravenous glucose tolerance tests, but Starup et al (14) found no
change. There have been few studies of plasma insulin levels
during oral glucose tolerance tests in subjects receiving oral
contraceptives. Javier et al (17) found higher plasma insulin
levels early in treatment but, with prolonged therapy, insulin
levels tended to be lower in some subjects as glucose tolerance
became further impaired. In the present study, no significant
change of mean fasting plasma insulin levels was found in Group A
or B subjects off and during oral contraceptive therapy. Plasma
insulin levels were significantly elevated above control values
during oral and intravenous glucose tolerance tests in Group A
Subjects during treatment. No significant change of mean plasma
insulin levels, however, occurred in Group B subjects after
stopping therapy in spite of improved oral and intravenous glucose
tolerance. These results are difficult to interpret but are compatible with increased peripheral resistance to the actions of
insulin in the Group A subjects. In Group B subjects who had
received oral contraceptive therapy for a longer period of time,
however, the similar mean insulin levels suggest impaired pancreatic
release of insulin.

The present findings and those of previous workers raise
several important questions. First, are the metabolic changes observed due to the oestrogen and/or progestagen? Second, are they
due to a direct effect of one or both of these steroids or secondary

to induced elevations of other circulating hormones such as cortisol, thyroxine or growth hormone? Third, will the changes become progressively greater when therapy is prolonged for many years? Fourth, do the metabolic changes regress permanently after therapy is discontinued? Fifth, are some subjects more liable to be affected than others?

Only some of these questions can be partly answered at the present time. There have been few studies of glucose tolerance in subjects treated with oestrogen or progestagen alone. Javier *et al* (17) found the one and two hour blood glucose levels to increase in nine of 12 subjects who had received mestranol for one month. While we have noted no significant change of OGTT or IVGTT plasma glucose levels in six women treated with mestranol for three months (unpublished observations), Pyörälä *et al* (26) found intravenous glucose tolerance to be significantly impaired after two weeks' treatment with ethinyl oestradiol. Oral glucose tolerance improved in ten of 18 women with endometrial carcinoma or hyperplasia following 17α-hydroxyprogesterone caproate administration (27).

Elevated circulating levels of plasma cortisol (28), thyroxine (29) and growth hormone (21) have been noted during oral contraceptive therapy and the possibility exists that one or more of these may be responsible for the observed metabolic changes. The elevated plasma levels of cortisol and thyroxine are due to increased levels of the respective binding proteins, and the free non-protein bound hormone concentrations are probably unchanged. Nevertheless, the possibility exists that the protein bound hormone, in general thought to be biologically inactive (30), may affect certain specific tissues such as the liver. We have been struck by the similarity of the abnormalities of plasma glucose and blood pyruvate levels during glucose tolerance tests in subjects receiving oral contraceptives to those found during glucocorticoid therapy. In a separate communication, we have discussed the similarity of these changes to those found during glucose tolerance tests performed in obese subjects, another situation in which the liver is probably exposed to excessive amounts of glucocorticoid.

Prolonged longitudinal studies will be necessary to determine whether the metabolic changes associated with oral contraceptive therapy become more marked with time. It should be noted, however, that Spellacy *et al* (31) carried out oral glucose tolerance tests in 31 subjects who had received combined oral contraceptives for more than eight years. Twelve subjects (39%) had borderline abnormal curves and a further 12 subjects (39%) had abnormal curves. While we have shown an early marked improvement of oral and intravenous glucose tolerance shortly after stopping oral contraceptive therapy, we do not know whether this improvement will continue or even be maintained. Indeed, in a small number of subjects retested at intervals following cessation of treatment, glucose tolerance has again become impaired after an early initial improvement.

The ability to predict which subjects will develop marked impairment of glucose tolerance during oral contraceptive therapy would be of great value. In the present study, however, no one patient characteristic was found to be useful in this respect.

The mechanism of the metabolic changes occurring during oral contraceptive therapy cannot even be postulated at the present time. Although many detailed in vitro studies of the effects of oestrogens and progesterone on the metabolism of the uterus have been described, there is a lack of data of the effects of these compounds on biochemical pathways in other tissues such as liver and muscle.

The most important question of all, namely whether the changes of glucose tolerance, increased plasma insulin levels, and increased fasting serum lipid and lipoprotein levels during oral contraceptive therapy will accelerate the rate of development of atherosclerosis, requires extremely careful consideration. The evidence will be difficult to obtain and the answer may only become apparent in 20-30 years' time.

SUMMARY

Longitudinal studies of plasma glucose, NEFA, insulin and blood pyruvate levels during oral and intravenous glucose tolerance tests are described in two groups of women treated with combined oral contraceptive preparations. Group A consisted of 67 subjects tested before and during therapy and Group B contained 24 subjects initially tested during therapy and again after this had been discontinued.

While the mean fasting plasma glucose level was unchanged during therapy, a significant correlation was observed in both groups between the fasting plasma glucose level off therapy and the change of the fasting plasma glucose level during therapy. Both oral and intravenous glucose tolerance became relatively impaired during therapy in 78% and 63% of Group A subjects respectively. In Group B, oral glucose tolerance improved in 92% and intravenous glucose tolerance improved in 100% of subjects after therapy was stopped.

Mean plasma NEFA levels, both before and after oral/intravenous glucose administration, were unchanged during therapy in both groups. During therapy the mean fasting blood pyruvate level was elevated in Group A subjects and mean blood pyruvate levels were also higher in both groups during oral and intravenous glucose tolerance tests.

The mean fasting plasma insulin level was unchanged during therapy in both groups. Significant elevation of plasma insulin levels during therapy, however, occurred in Group A subjects after oral and intravenous glucose administration. Mean plasma insulin levels during oral and intravenous glucose tolerance tests in Group B subjects, however, were not significantly different on and off therapy.

The mechanism and possible significance of these findings is discussed.

REFERENCES

1. Gershberg, H., Javier, Z. and Hulse, M.: Glucose tolerance in women receiving an ovulatory suppressant. Diabetes 13:378 (1964).

2. Wynn, V. and Doar, J.W.H.: Some effects of oral contraceptives on carbohydrate metabolism. Lancet i:715 (1966).

3. Posner, N.A., Silverstone, F.A., Pomerance, W. and Baumgold, D.: Oral contraceptives and intravenous glucose tolerance. I. Obst. and Gyn. 29:79 (1967).

4. Posner, N.A., Silverstone, F.A., Pomerance, W. and Singer, N.: Oral contraceptives and intravenous glucose tolerance. II. Obst. and Gyn. 29:87 (1967).

5. Spellacy, W.N. and Carlson, K.L.: Plasma insulin and blood glucose levels in patients taking oral contraceptives. Am. J. Obst. & Gynec. 95:474 (1966).

6. Spellacy, W.N., Carlson, K.L., Birk, S.A. and Schade, S.L.: Glucose and insulin alterations after one year of combination-type oral contraceptive treatment. Metabolism 17:496 (1968).

7. Spellacy, W.N., Carlson, K.L. and Birk, S.A.: Carbohydrate metabolic studies after six cycles of combined type oral contraceptive tablets. Diabetes 16:590 (1967).

8. Keen, H., Rose, G., Pyke, D.A. Boyne, D., Chlouverakis, C. and Mistry, S.: Blood sugar and arterial disease. Lancet ii:505 (1965).

9. Cramp, D.G.: New automated enzymatic method for measuring glucose by glucose oxidase. J. Clin. Path. 20:910 (1967).

10. Dole, V.P. and Meinertz, H.: Microdetermination of long-chaing fatty acids in plasma and tissues. J. Biol. Chem. 235: 2595 (1960).

11. Cramp, D.G.: Automated enzymatic fluorimetric method for the determination of pyruvic and lactic acids in blood. J. Clin. Path. 21:171 (1968).

12. Samols, E. and Bilkus, D.: A comparison of insulin immunoassays. Proc. Soc. Exp. Biol. Med. 115:79 (1964).

13. Lundback, K.: Intravenous glucose tolerance as a tool in definition and diagnosis of diabetes mellitus. Br. Med. J. 1:1507 (1962).

14. Starup, J., Date, J. and Deckert, T.: Serum insulin and intravenous glucose tolerance in oral contraception. Acta Endocr. 58:537 (1968).

15. Halling, G.R., Michals, E.L. and Paulsen, C.A.: Glucose intolerance during ethynodiol diacetate-mestranol therapy. Metabolism 16:465 (1967).

16. Danowski, T.S., Sabeh, G., Alley, R.A., Robbins, T.J., Tsai, C.T. and Sekaran, K.: Glucose tolerance prior to and during therapy with contraceptive steroids. Clin. Pharm. & Ther. 9:223 (1968).

17. Javier, Z., Gershberg, H. and Hulse, M.: Ovulatory suppressants, estrogens, and carbohydrate metabolism. Metabolism 17:443 (1968).

18. Peterson, W.F., Steel, M.W., Jr. and Coyne, R.V.: Analysis of the effect of ovulatory suppressants on glucose tolerance. Am. J. Obst. & Gynec. 95:484 (1966).

19. Park, C.R., Morgan, H.E., Henderson, M.J., Regan, D.M., Cadenas, E. and Post, R.L.: The regulation of glucose uptake in muscle as studied in the perfused rat heart. Recent Prog. Hormone Res. 17:493 (1961).

20. de Bodo, R.C., Steele, R., Altszuler, N., Dunn, A. and Bishop, J.S.: On the hormonal regulation of carbohydrate metabolism. Recent Prog. Hormone Res. 19:445 (1963).

21. Spellacy, W.N., Carlson, K.L. and Schade, S.L.: Human growth hormone levels in normal subjects receiving an oral contraceptive. J. Amer. Med. Ass. 202:451 (1967).

22. Landon, J., Wynn, V., Cooke, J.N.C. and Kennedy, A.: Effects of anabolic steroid, methandienone, on carbohydrate metabolism in man. Metabolism 11:501 (1962).

23. Randle, P.J.: Endocrine control of metabolism. Ann. Rev. Physiol. 25:291 (1963).

24. Doar, J.W.H., Wynn, V. and Cramp, D.G.: Studies of venous blood pyruvate and lactate levels during oral and intravenous glucose tolerance tests in women receiving oral contraceptives. This volume (1969).

25. Starup, J., Date, J., and Deckert, T.: Plasma insulin and intravenous glucose tolerance in oral contraception. Acta Endocr. (Kbh.) Suppl. 119:157 (1967).

26. Pyörälä, K., Pyörälä, T. and Lampinen, V.: Sequential oral contraceptive treatment and intravenous glucose tolerance. The Lancet ii:776 (1967).

27. Benjamin, F. and Casper, D.J.: Alterations in carbohydrate metabolism induced by progesterone in cases of endometrial carcinoma and hyperplasia. Am. J. Obst. & Gynec. 94:991 (1966).

28. Pulkkinen, M.O. and Pekkarinen, A.: The levels of 17-hydroxycorticosteroids in the plasma of users of oral contraceptives. Acta Endocr. (Kbh.) Suppl. 119:156 (1967).

29. Roman, W. and Bockner, V.: Paper at the 2nd Asia and Ociana Congress of Endocrinology, Sydney, 1963.

30. Matsui, N. and Plager, J.E.: In vitro physiological activity of protein-bound and unbound cortisol. Endocrinology 78:1159 (1966).

31. Spellacy, W.N., Buhi, W.C., Spellacy, C.E., Moses, L.C. and Goldzieher, J.W.: Carbohydrate studies in long-term users of oral contraceptives. Diabetes 17, Suppl. 1:344 (1968).

STUDIES OF VENOUS BLOOD PYRUVATE AND LACTATE LEVELS DURING
ORAL AND INTRAVENOUS GLUCOSE TOLERANCE TESTS IN WOMEN
RECEIVING ORAL CONTRACEPTIVES

J.W.H. Doar, V. Wynn and D.G. Cramp

Alexander Simpson Laboratory for Metabolic Research
St. Mary's Hospital Medical School, London

Pyruvate occupies a key position in intermediary metabolism being situated on both the glycolytic and gluconeogenetic
pathways. Unlike the majority of the phosphorylated intermedi-
airies, appreciable amounts of pyruvate diffuse across cell
membranes and it is assumed that blood pyruvate levels to some
extent reflect intracellular events.

We have previously found both the fasting blood pyruvate
level (throughout this paper blood pyruvate and lactate levels
refer to the concentrations in peripheral venous blood) and/or the
maximum blood pyruvate increment above the fasting level to be in-
increased in certain women receiving oral contraceptives (1). It
has yet to be determined whether these changes are due to a primary effect of the oestrogen and/or progestagen or are secondary
to elevations of other hormones such as plasma cortisol, thyroxine and growth hormone.

We have noted the resemblance of the changes in glucose tolerance and blood pyruvate levels during oral contraceptive therapy
to those found in subjects receiving glucocorticoid drugs (1). Recently, however, we have found a similar elevation of blood pyruvate levels both before and after oral/intravenous glucose administration in a group of obese women (2). It is not known whether
the increased blood pyruvate levels in these three conditions are
due to an increased rate of pyruvate production and/or impaired
pyruvate removal.

The present study attempts to answer some of these questions.

178

STUDY GROUPS AND METHODS

Oral and intravenous glucose tolerance tests were carried out by methods previously described (1) in 129 control women (control group) and 129 women receiving oral contraceptive therapy. Twenty-nine subjects in each group exceeded their ideal body weight (3) by more than 20% and were classified as obes´e. Details of both groups are shown in Table 1. Any subject with a diabetic parent, child, sibling, grandparent, uncle or aunt was considered to have a family history of diabetes. The interval between tests varied from one to seven days. All subjects consumed at least 200 g carbohydrate for three days before each test.

Table 1

COMPOSITION OF CONTROL AND TEST GROUPS

	Control group	Test group
Mean age (yrs) non-obese subjects	26 (100)	28(100)
obese subjects	26 (29)	29(29)
Mean weight of non-obese subjects	98	99
% 'ideal body weight of obese subjects	146	141
Positive family history of diabetes mellitus (%)	41	44
Mean duration of therapy in test group (months)		18.4 (range 2-156)

% of test group subjects receiving:

Ovulen	40
Anovlar/Gynovlar	18
'Step-Up'*	9
Lyndiol	8
Orthonovum	8
Norinyl	5
C-Quens	5
Conovid/Conovid	4
Volidan	3

Figures in parentheses refer to numbers of subjects.
*'Step-Up' (0.1 mg mestranol and 0.1 mg ethynodiol diacetate for 16 days, 0.1 mg mestranol and 0.5 mg ethynodiol diacetate for seven days).

The control group was largely derived from women taking part
in a longitudinal study of glucose tolerance. None were suffering
from any endocrine or metabolic condition (excepting the obesity
of the overweight group) known to affect glucose tolerance and no
subject of either group was taking any drug known to affect plasma
glucose of blood pyruvate levels (excepting oral contraceptives).
Venous plasma glucose levels were estimated by an automated glucose oxidase method (4) and venous blood pyruvate and lactate
levels by automated enzymatic fluorimetric techniques (5).

Sodium L (+) lactate (pH 5.1) infusions were carried out with
the subject fasting and at rest. An intravenous load of 35 mg/kg
body weight sodium L (+) lactate was followed by an intravenous
infusion of 2.5 mg/kg/min for forty minutes. Venous blood
samples were taken from a separate indwelling cannula for blood
lactate and pyruvate estimations before, during and for forty
minutes after the infusion.

ANALYSIS OF RESULTS

Oral glucose tolerance curves were assessed in terms of the
total area between the plasma glucose curve and the abscissa (1).
Intravenous glucose tolerance curves were evaluated by the 'K'
value, calculated from the expression $K = 69.3/T\frac{1}{2}$, where $T\frac{1}{2}$
represents the half life calculated from the logarithms of the 30-
60 minute plasma glucose levels by the method of least squares.
Blood pyruvate curves during oral and intravenous glucose tolerance tests were assessed in terms of the fasting level, the total
area between the curve and abscissa and the incremental area between the curve and a line drawn horizontally through the fasting
level. All areas were calculated assuming straight lines between
consecutive points. The significance of differences of means was
assessed by Student's 't' test, of ratios of variances by the "F"
test, and the correlation between variables by the product moment
correlation coefficient.

Results of intravenous sodium L(+) lactate infusions were
analysed in terms of a single compartment model (appendix) to
obtain the lactate rate removal constant (K_L), the endogenous
production rate of lactate (a_L) and the volume of distribution
(V_L). It was assumed that the distribution of infused lactate
was instantaneous and that the endogenous production rate of
lactate did not change during the test.

RESULTS

Mean blood pyruvate levels during oral and intravenous
glucose tolerance tests in non-obese and obese subjects of the
control and test groups are shown in Figures 1 and 2. The
mean blood pyruvate levels are higher in the non-obese and

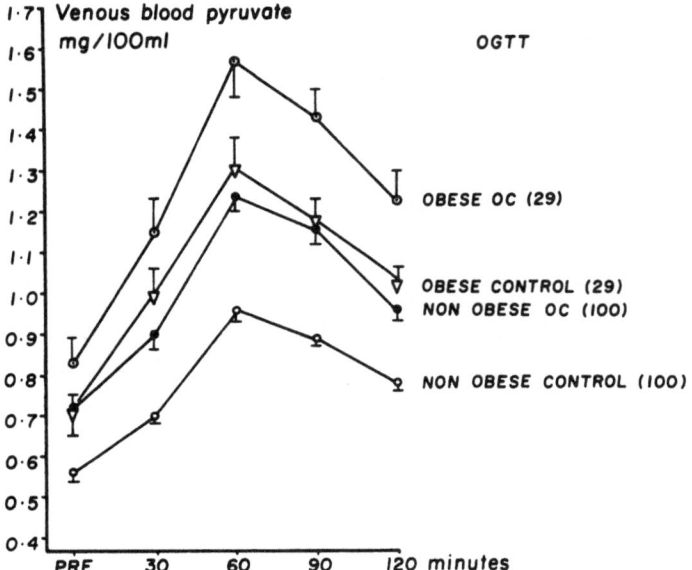

Fig. 1.   Mean OGTT venous blood pyruvate levels in control
and test group subjects.   In this and subsequent figures vertical
bars represent one standard error of the mean.

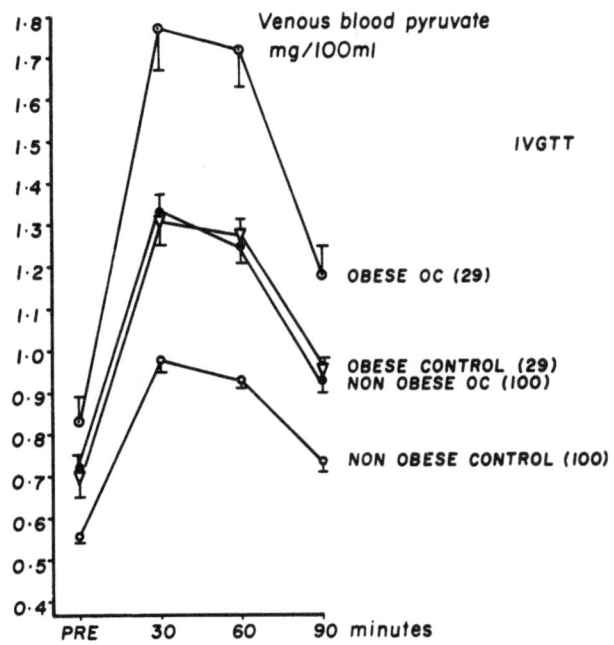

Fig. 2.   Mean IVGTT venous blood pyruvate levels in control
and test group subjects.

Table 2.

	NON-OBESE CONTROL GROUP	NON-OBESE TEST GROUP	OBESE CONTROL GROUP	OBESE TEST GROUP	WHOLE CONTROL GROUP	WHOLE CONTROL GROUP
NUMBER OF SUBJECTS	100	100	29	29	129	129
MEAN FASTING BLOOD PYRUVATE MG/100 ML.	0.56+0.15	0.72+0.28	0.71+0.31	0.83+0.32	0.60+0.21	0.74+0.29
t	5.06, P<0.001		1.45, NS		4.45, P<0.001	
F	3.30, P<0.01		1.03, NS		1.91, P<0.01	
MEAN OGTT PYRUVATE* INCREMENTAL AREA (UNITS)	96.2+56.8	127.4+79.7	139.6+78.9	197.5+86.7	106.0+64.7	143.2+86.2
t	3.19, P<0.001		2.67, P<0.01		3.92, P<0.001	
F	1.96, P<0.01		1.21, NS		1.77, P<0.01	
MEAN IVGTT PYRUVATE† INCREMENTAL AREA (UNITS)	89.3+43.8	122.5+64.1	120.2+64.4	191.2+99.6	96.2+50.6	137.9+78.6
t	4.28, P<0.001		3.22, P<0.01		5.07, P<0.001	
F	2.13, P<0.01		2.39, P<0.05		2.42, P<0.01	

*Oral glucose tolerance test
†Intravenous glucose tolerance test

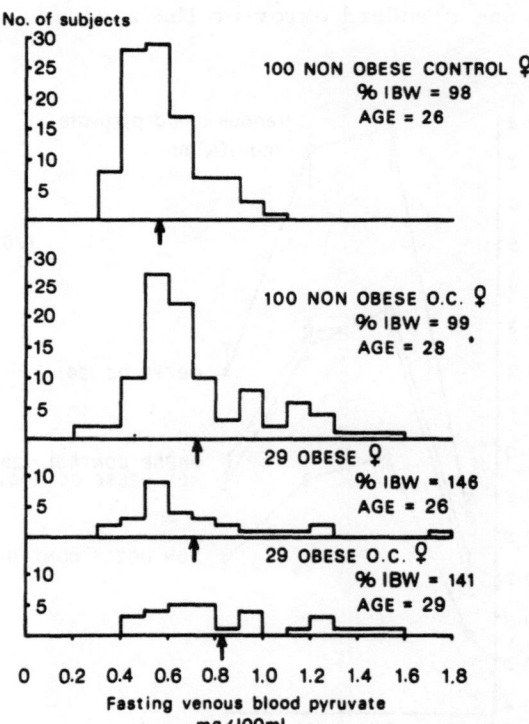

Fig. 3. Frequency distributions of fasting venous blood pyruvate levels in control and test group subjects.

obese test groups compared with the respective control groups. Of note is the close similarity between mean venous blood pyruvate levels in the non-obese test group and the obese control group.

Table 2 shows these results analysed in terms of the fasting blood pyruvate level, and oral and intravenous glucose pyruvate incremental areas. The mean levels and variances of these three indices are significantly greater in the test group as a whole.

Figure 3 shows the frequency distribution of fasting blood pyruvate levels in control and test groups. The increased variance of fasting blood pyruvate levels in the test group may have been due to two factors. First, endogenous variation of the test group may have resulted in elevation of the fasting blood pyruvate levels in some subjects but not in others. Endogenous variables considered were age, degree of obesity, family history of diabetes and glucose tolerance. The first two do not apply to the non-obese test group whose mean age and degree of obesity were very similar to those of the non-obese control group. No significant difference was found between the mean fasting blood pyruvate levels of subjects with and without a family history of diabetes in the control or test groups. There was no significant correlation between the fasting blood pyruvate levels and oral or intravenous glucose tolerance in the control or test groups. Second, exogenous variations of treatment in the test group may have resulted in a greater elevation of the fasting blood pyruvate level in some subjects than others. While no relation was found between the fasting blood pyruvate level and the nature of the oestrogen-progestagen combination, duration of therapy, or day of cycle in the test group (Fig. 4), the possibility cannot be excluded that the increased variance of fasting blood pyruvate levels in the non-obese test group was caused by a combination of two or more of these variables. It is of interest that the variance of the fasting blood pyruvate levels and OGTT and IVGTT pyruvate incremental areas in the non-obese test group did not differ significantly from those of the obese control group.

The correlation between fasting blood pyruvate levels in oral and intravenous glucose tolerance tests was similar for the control (r = 0.66, P<0.001) and test groups (r = 0.69, P<0.001). Figure 5 shows the correlation between OGTT and IVGTT pyruvate incremental areas in the test group (r = 0.48, P<0.001). A similar degree of correlation (r = 0.48, P<0.001) was found in the control group.

Venous blood lactate levels are also elevated in some women during oral contraceptive therapy. Figure 6 shows the mean ven-

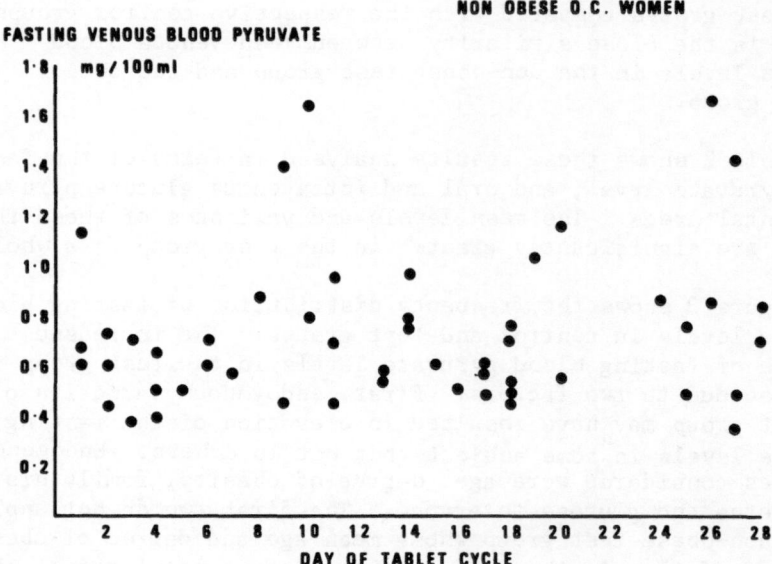

Fig. 4. Relation of fasting venous blood pyruvate levels to the day of tablet cycle in non-obese test group subjects.

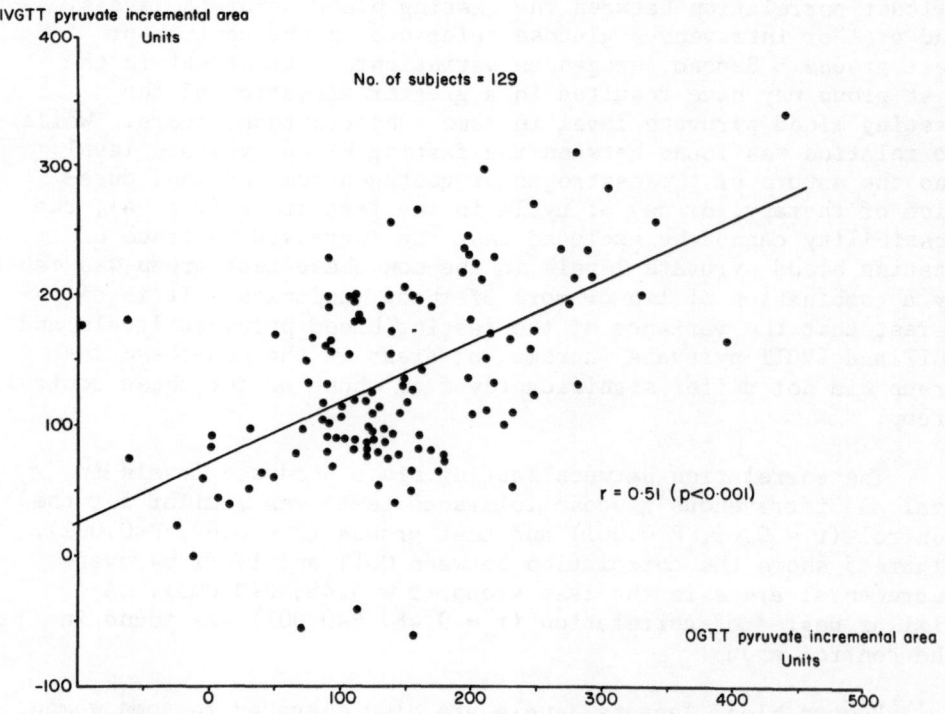

Fig. 5. Correlation between OGTT and IVGTT pyruvate incremental areas in 129 test group subjects.

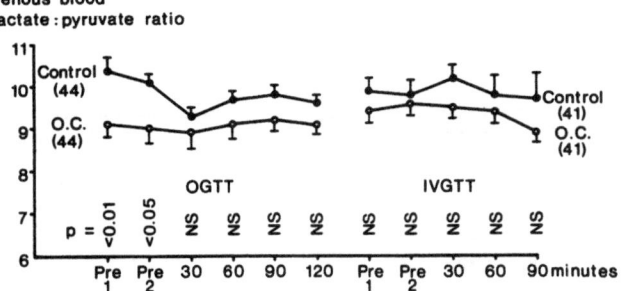

Fig. 6.   OGTT and IVGTT mean venous blood lactate/pyruvate ratios in control and test group subjects.

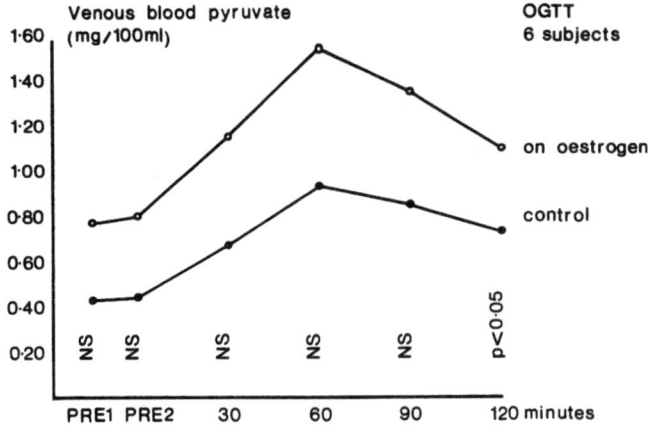

Fig. 7.   Mean OGTT venous blood pyruvate levels in six women before and during mestranol therapy.

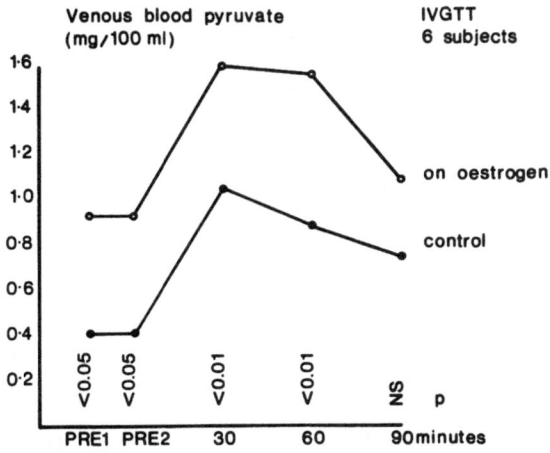

Fig. 8.   Mean IVGTT venous blood pyruvate levels in six women before and during mestranol therapy.

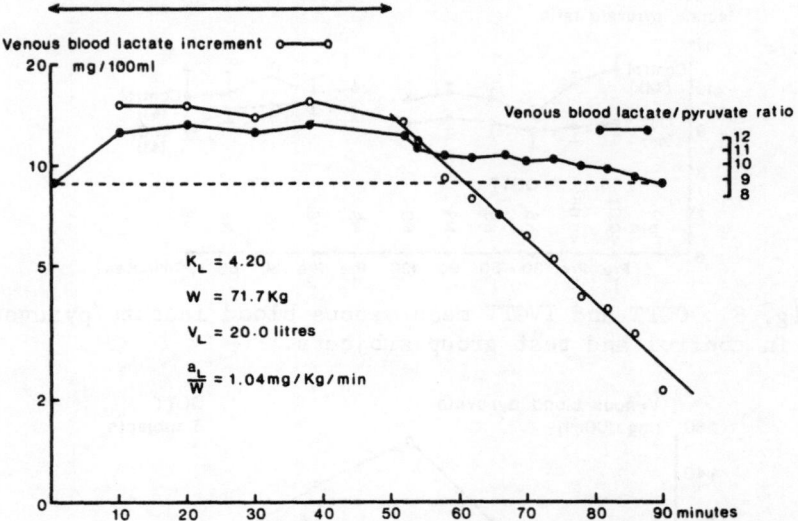

Fig. 9.   Results of a typical intravenous sodium L(+) lactate infusion.

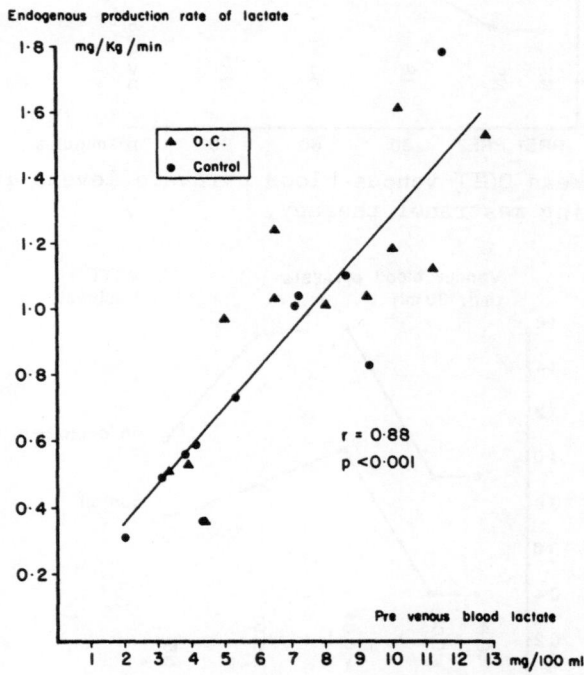

Fig. 10. Correlation between the fasting blood lactate level and endogenous production rate of lactate in control women and subjects receiving oral contraceptive therapy.

ous lactate/pyruvate ratio to be similar in a group of subjects
receiving oral contraceptives and a control group matched for
age, sex and degree of obesity.

It is not known whether the oestrogen and/or progestagen
result in elevation of blood pyruvate levels. A small longitudinal study of six women treated with mestranol for three months,
however, showed a similar elevation of venous blood pyruvate
levels.

Direct studies of L (+) lactate metabolism have been devised
to determine whether the elevated venous blood pyruvate and
lactate levels found in some subjects during oral contraceptive
therapy are due to an increased rate of formation of pyruvate and
lactate and/or an impairment od degradation of these metabolites.
The results of a typical sodium L (+) lactate infusion are shown
in Figure 9. Values for K_L, the rate constant of lactate removal,
V_L, the volume of lactate distribution and a_L/W, the endogenous
rate of production of lactate (mg/kg body weight/min.) were calculated from the results of sodium L (+) lactate infusions carried
out in 11 control women and 12 subjects receiving oral contraceptives.

The number of subjects studied is small and the results are
therefore only preliminary. While no significant correlation was
found between the fasting blood lactate e level and K_L, ($r = 0.28$,
NS), a significant correlation ($r = 0.88$, $P < 0.001$) was found
between the fasting blood lactate level and a_L/W the endogenous
rate of lactate production (Fig. 10). Urine losses of lactate during the infusion were small averaging less than 1% of the administered load.

DISCUSSION

The present study of venous blood pyruvate levels in 129
control female subjects (control group) and 129 women receiving
oral contraceptive therapy (test group) extends our previous observations (1). Twenty-nine subjects in each group were obese.

Mean venous blood pyruvate levels were significantly elevated
in both obese and non-obese subjects of the test group in the
fasting state and during oral and intravenous tolerance tests.

Certain similarities were noted between the obese subjects
of the control group and the non-obese subjects of the test
group. First, the mean blood pyruvate levels during oral and
intravenous glucose tolerance tests were virtually identical.
Second, the variance of the fasting blood pyruvate levels was
markedly increased in the non-obese subjects of the test group

compared with that of the control non-obese subjects. The
variance of the fasting blood pyruvate levels of the obese
control group was also significantly (P<0.01) greater than
that of the non-obese control group and did not differ significantly from that of the non-obese test group.

While the increased variance of fasting blood pyruvate
levels in the non-obese test group may have resulted from variations of treatment within this group, no relation between the
fasting blood pyruvate level and type of oestrogen-progestagen
combination, duration of therapy, or day of cycle was found.
It is, therefore, probable that this increased variance
results from a variable response of the fasting blood pyruvate
level of individual subjects to oral contraceptive therapy.
Age, family history of diabetes, and the plasma glucose responses to oral and intravenous glucose administration were
not found to be relevant in this respect. In a separate longitudinal study (6) of 51 women tested before and during oral
contraceptive therapy, however, we have found a significant
negative correlation between the control pre-therapy fasting
blood pyruvate level and the change of fasting blood pyruvate
level during therapy (r = 0.35, P =0.01). The explanation of
this finding in not clear.

The mean increase of blood pyruvate levels above the fasting
level, expressed as the area between the blood pyruvate curve
and the fasting baseline, was significantly greater in the test
group for both oral and intravenous glucose tolerance tests.
It is not known whether this represents an increased rate of
pyruvate formation from glucose or impaired pyruvate degradation
during oral contraceptive therapy. Of interest, however, was
the significant correlation between oral and intravenous
pyruvate incremental areas in both control and test group suggesting that the proportion of the glucose load converted to
pyruvate during oral and intravenous glucose tolerance tests
is similar in all subjects and that the rate of pyruvate degradation for a given subject is relatively constant over a short
period of time.

Similar elevations of blood pyruvate levels were found in a
longitudinal study of six women treated with oestrogen alone. It
is not known, however, whether progestagen therapy alone alters
blood pyruvate levels. Furthermore, it has not been determined
whether these changes result from a direct effect of the oestrogen
and/or progestagen or are secondary to increased levels of other
circulating hormones such as cortisol, growth hormone and thyroxine.

The fasting blood pyruvate level is neither increased in
thyrotoxicosis, (7) nor in control subjects after L-triiodothyronine

administration, (8). Similarly, we have found no elevation of blood pyruvate levels above control values during oral and intravenous glucose tolerance tests in acromegalic subjects (9),nor during intravenous glucose tolerance tests performed after administration of human growth hormone to control subjects (9). The elevated blood pyruvate levels during oral contraceptive therapy resemble those found during glucocorticoid therapy (10) and also those found in obesity (2). The elevation of plasma cortisol levels during oral contraceptive therapy (11) probably involves only the transcortin bound fraction which is thought to be biologically inactive (12). It is possible, however, that this fraction may have biological activity in certain tissues, such as the liver, and may be responsible for the changes of glucose tolerance and blood pyruvate levels found during oral contraceptive therapy. While plasma cortisol levels are normal in obesity, the cortisol production rate is often increased (13). The hepatic clearance of cortisol must therefore be increased and it is possible that this may be responsible for the impaired oral glucose tolerance and elevated blood pyruvate levels commonly found in this condition.

Initial attempts to study pyruvate metabolism by infusing sodium pyruvate solution met with difficulty. The sodium pyruvate solutions were unstable and certain subjects developed nausea and vomiting during the test. Aqueous sodium L (+) lactate solutions are stable and conversion of lactate to pyruvate is obligatory for lactate metabolism, infusion of sodium L (+) lactate solutions should provide information about pyruvate metabolism in vivo.

Preliminary results of whole body lactate metabolism in control women and subjects receiving oral contraceptives showed a significant correlation between the fasting blood lactate level and the calculated endogenous production rate of lactate (r = 0.88, P<0.001). A similar correlation using infusion of sodium C-14-lactate has been found in sheep (14). No significant correlation, however, was found between K_L, the rate removal constant for lactate, and the fasting blood lactate level. These findings suggest that the elevated fasting blood pyruvate and lactate levels found in some subjects receiving oral contraceptive therapy are due to increased rates of production rather than impaired removal of these metabolites.

Certain difficulties in interpretation of the results of sodium L(+) lactate infusions have arisen, including the choice of the model, lack of knowledge of rates of transfer of lactate and pyruvate across cell membranes and the effects of altered lactate/ pyruvate ratios on intracellular metabolic conversions.

Despite these problems we feel that the present results indicate that the elevated venous blood lactate and pyruvate levels found during oral and intravenous glucose tolerance tests in some subjects receiving oral contraceptive therapy are probably due to the oestrogen component of the drug and may result from increased amounts of glucose passing down the glycolytic pathway to pyruvate.

SUMMARY

We have previously observed elevation of the fasting venous blood pyruvate level and/or the maximum blood pyruvate increment above the fasting level following oral/intravenous glucose administration in certain women receiving oral contraceptives.

The present study extends these observations in 129 control women and 129 women receiving oral contraceptives. Twenty-nine subjects in each group were obese. Mean blood pyruvate levels in the control obese group were similar to those of the non-obese group receiving oral contraceptives. The variance of certain indices of the blood pyruvate curves was significantly increased in the group receiving oral contraceptives and possible explanations for this are discussed. Similar elevations of blood pyruvate levels occurred in women receiving oestrogen alone. It has yet to be determined, however, whether these changes result from a direct effect of oestrogen and/or progestagen or are secondary to increases of other circulating hormones such as cortisol, thyroxine or growth hormone.

The venous blood lactate/pyruvate ratio was found to be similar in oral contraceptive and control groups during oral and intravenous glucose tolerance tests. Preliminary studies of whole body lactate turnover rates suggest that the elevated blood pyruvate and lactate levels during oral contraceptive therapy may be due to increased rates of production rather than impaired degradation of pyruvate and lactate.

REFERENCES

1. Wynn, V., and Doar, J.W.H.: Some effects of oral contraceptives on carbohydrate metabolism. Lancet $\underline{ii}$:715 (1966).

2. Doar, J.W.H., Wynn, V., and Cramp, D.G.: Blood pyruvate and plasma glucose levels during oral and intravenous glucose tolerance tests in obese and non-obese women. Metabolism $\underline{17}$:690 (1968).

3. Documenta Geigy, 1956.

4. Cramp, D.G.: New automated method for measuring glucose by glucose oxidase. J. Clin. Path 20:910 (1967).

5. Cramp, D.G.: Automated enzymatic fluorimetric method for the determination of pyruvic and lactic acids in blood. J. Clin. Path. 21:171 (1968).

6. Wynn, V., and Doar, J.W.H.: Longitudinal studies of the effects of oral contraceptive therapy and plasma glucose, non-esterified fatty acid, insulin, and blood pyruvate levels during oral and intravenous glucose tolerance tests. This volume (1969).

7. Doar, J.W.H., Stamp, T.C.B., Wynn, V., and Audhya, T.K.: Effects of oral and intravenous glucose loading in thyrotoxicosis. Studies of plasma glucose, free fatty acid, plasma insulin and blood pyruvate levels. Submitted for publication.

8. Stamp, T.C.B., Doar, J.W.H., and Wynn, V.: Observations on some effects of L-triiodothyronine on carbohydrate and lipid metabolism in man. J. Clin. Path. (In press).

9. Doar, J.W.H., Maw, D.S.J., Simpson, R.D., Audhya, T.K., and Wynn, V.: The effects of growth hormone on plasma glucose, NEFA, insulin and blood pyruvate levels during intravenous glucose tolerance tests. (In press).

10. Hennes, A.R., Wajchenberg, B.L., Fajans, S.S., and Conn, J.W.: The effect of adrenal steroids on blood levels of pyruvic and alphaketoglutaric acids in normal subjects. Metabolism 6: 339 (1957).

11. Pulkkinen, M.O., and Pekkarinen, A.: The levels of 17-hydroxy-corticosteroids in the plasma of users of oral contraceptives. Acta endocr. (Kbh.) Suppl. 119:156 (1967).

12. Matsui, N., and Plager, J.W.: In vitro physiological activity of protein bound and unbound cortisol. Endocrinology 78:1159 (1966).

13. Schteingart, D.E., and Conn, J.W.: Characteristics of the increased adrenocortical function observed in many obese patients. Ann. N.Y. Acad. Sci. 131:388 (1965).

14. Annison, E.F., Lindsay, D.B., and White, R.R.: Metabolic interrelations of glucose and lactate in sheep. Biochem. J. 88: 243 (1963).

APPENDIX

a = endogenous production rate of lactate
b = rate of infusion of lactate
c_0 = blood lactate concentration prior to infusion
c_∞^0 = blood lactate concentration at new steady state level during lactate infusion
V = volume of distribution of lactate
K = rate constant of lactate removal from the compartment

Since the system is in a steady state both prior to and during the infusion:

$$a_L = K_L \cdot c_0 \cdot V_L \qquad\qquad (1)$$
$$b + a_L = K_L \cdot c_\infty \cdot V_L \qquad\qquad (2)$$

When the lactate infusion is stopped: $\quad dc = \dfrac{-(c \cdot K_L \cdot V_L - a_L) dt}{V_L}$

Integrating: $\quad \dfrac{1}{K_L V_L} \log_e (c \cdot K_L V_L - a_L) = \dfrac{-t}{V_L} + D \qquad\qquad (3)$

where D is an integration constant

From equations (1) and (3)

$$\frac{1}{K_L V_L} \log_e K_L V_L (c - c_0) = \frac{-t}{V_L} + D$$

if $t = 0$, $c = c_\infty$

$$\therefore \quad \frac{1}{K_L V_L} \log_e K_L V_L (c_\infty - c_0) = D$$

$$\therefore \quad \log_e \frac{(c - c_0)}{(c_\infty - c_0)} = -K_L \cdot t$$

$$\log_e (c - c_0) = -K_L \cdot t + \log_e (c_\infty - c_0) \qquad\qquad (4)$$

K_L can be obtained from a semilogarithmic plot of the blood lactate increment above the fasting baseline level against time.

From equations (1) and (2)

$$b = K_L \cdot V_L (c_\infty - c_0)$$

$$\therefore \quad V_L = \frac{b}{K_L (c_\infty - c_0)} \qquad\qquad (5)$$

and a_L may then be obtained from equation (1).

ACQUIRED SUBCLINICAL DIABETES MELLITUS IN WOMEN

RECEIVING ORAL CONTRACEPTIVE AGENTS

R. K. Kalkhoff, H. J. Kim and F. J. Stoddard

Department of Medicine, Department of Obstetrics and
Clinical Research Center, Marquette School of Medicine
and Milwaukee County General Hospital, Milwaukee,
Wisconsin

Although several conflicting observations have been reported
concerning the effects of oral contraceptive agents on standard
glucose tolerance tests, there is little doubt that the frequency
of abnormal steroid-provocative glucose tolerance tests (GTT) is
extraordinarily high among subjects on this regimen. diPaola and
co-workers (1) and Gershberg and associates (2) have observed
independently that the incidence of positive steroid tests in
women receiving agents containing mestranol ranges from 45 to 85
percent or 10 to 20-fold greater than a general population. These
findings imply that oral contraceptives induce an acquired form of
subclinical diabetes mellitus. Possible etiologies of this defect
and its reversibility after discontinuation of birth control medications are the subjects of this presentation.

METHODS AND RESULTS

Thirty women were studied initially (Table 1). Group 1 was
composed of ten subjects with negative family histories of diabetes
mellitus who were on no medications and who had normal standard and

This study was supported by United States Public Health Service Grant AM 10305 from the National Institute of Arthritis and
Metabolic Diseases and Grant 5 M01 FR-00058. Statistical analyses
were performed by Dr. Alfred Rimm, Department of Preventive Medicine. The technical assistance of Mrs. Linda Burns is gratefully
acknowledged.

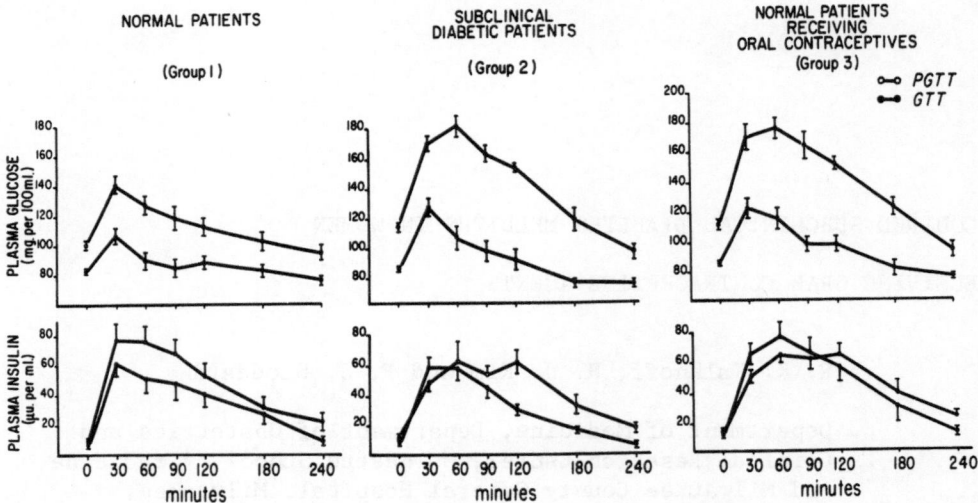

Fig. 1.   Plasma glucose and insulin responses during oral glucose (GTT) and prednisolone glucose (PGTT) tolerance tests in 10 control patients (Group 1), 10 subclinical diabetic patients (Group 2), and 10 normal women receiving oral contraceptive agents (Group 3).   Values are mean ± standard error of the mean.

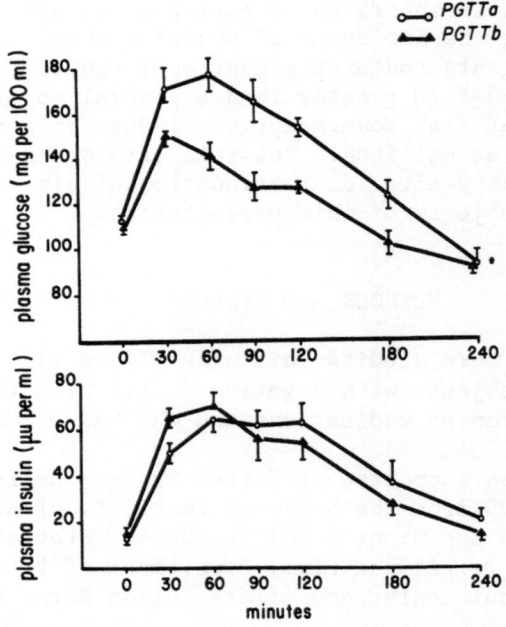

Fig. 2.   Plasma glucose and insulin responses during prednisolone glucose tolerance tests in Group 3 during administration of oral contraceptives (PGTTa) and 4-8 weeks after their withdrawal (PGTTb).   Values are mean ± standard error of the mean (S.E.M.).

steroid glucose tolerance tests. Group 2 was comprised of ten
women with known subclinical diabetes mellitus who had normal
oral glucose tolerance tests but diabetic responses to the steroid
glucose tolerance test. These patients were not taking any medications at the time of study. The ten women in Group 3 also had
negative family histories of diabetes mellitus and were similar to
Group 1 except they had been receiving an oral contraceptive for
an average period of nine months (range, 6 to 17 months) and had
abnormal steroid (prednisolone) glucose tolerance test while receiving this agent. The birth control pill contained 0.1 mg of
mestranol combined with 2 mg of norethindrone. All patients were
in good nutrition, of comparable age and within ten percent of
their ideal body weight.

Table 1

AGES AND WEIGHTS OF PATIENTS

Group	Age	Weight	I.B.W.	% from I.B.W.
1	23 ± 1	123 ± 5	120 ± 3	+ 3%
2	31 ± 2	141 ± 5	136 ± 4	+ 4%
3	29 ± 1	135 ± 8	129 ± 3	+ 5%

Group 1: Ten normal women on no medications.
Group 2: Ten subclinical diabetic women on no
            medications.
Group 3: Ten normal women receiving oral contra-
            ceptive agents.
I.B.W.: Ideal body weight.

Four hour 100 gram oral glucose tolerance tests were performed
after an overnight fast. Within two weeks the test was repeated
after the administration of prednisolone, 10 mg, 8½ and 2 hours
before the procedure which is equivalent to the dose and mode of
administration of cortisone acetate in the Fajans and Conn steroid
test (3). Their criteria for normal glucose curves were employed.
Plasma glucose was measured by an automated glucose oxidase
method (4) and plasma insulin by the immunoassay technique of
Morgan and Lazarow (5).

Effect of Oral Contraceptives on the Prednisolone Glucose Tolerance
Test

Figure 1 illustrates the plasma glucose and insulin responses

during standard and prednisolone glucose tolerance tests. Women
in each of the three groups had normal standard glucose tolerance
tests in association with brisk elevations of plasma insulin.
Following the administration of prednisolone, subjects in Groups
2 and 3 had diabetic plasma glucose responses while Group 1 retained normal carbohydrate tolerance. The glucose responses in
the control group during the prednisolone test, though normal,
were significantly higher than corresponding levels observed
during the control GTT (p value <0.05). These elevations were
associated with plasma insulin concentrations that were also significantly higher than control at 30, 60 and 90 minutes (p value
<0.05) and in phase with the elevated plasma glucose levels. The
abnormal prednisolone glucose tolerance test in Group 2, however,
was accompanied by an insulin response that was not significantly
above control hormonal levels until the second hour; and, in Group
3, essentially no differences existed between insulin levels before
and after steroid administration despite abnormal hyperglycemia
during the prednisolone test.

The data for the subclinical diabetic women in Group 2 confirm
a previously published report from our group (6) as well as from
Rull and co-workers (7) describing similar delayed insulin responses in subclinical diabetic subjects during prednisolone or
cortisone glucose tolerance tests.

Prednisolone Glucose Tolerance Test After Discontinuation of
Contraceptive Agents

To prove that the abnormal prednisolone GTT in women in Group
3 is an acquired abnormality that is related to the administration
of oral contraceptive agents, the birth control pills were discontinued and the prednisolone test was repeated between four and
eight weeks after withdrawal. Figure 2 reveals that in these patients, PGTT reverted to normal when the contraceptive agent was
withdrawn. Of major interest was the finding that the plasma insulin response was more briskly elevated and significantly higher
at 30 minutes (p value <0.05) after discontinuing birth-control
pills in association with the return of the glucose response to
normal.

In the present study, agents containing the estrogen, mestranol, enhance the diabetogenic effect of prednisolone in a fashion
that converts normal glucose and insulin curves to patterns resembling the subclinical diabetic individual. The combined mestra-
nol- prednisolone action is ostensibly the result of some form of
biological synergism. If this supposition is correct, then one
would predict that individuals not treated with oral contraceptive
agents may develop impaired carbohydrate tolerance with a defective
plasma insulin response if the dose of prednisolone is increased

during the 8½ hour period preceding glucose administration. This
hypothesis was subsequently tested.

Double Dose Prednisolone Glucose Tolerance Tests

    In this study seven normal untreated control subjects, Group
4, and five subclinical diabetic patients, Group 5, had three procedures performed: a standard glucose tolerance test, a prednisolone glucose tolerance test and a double dose prednisolone test.
Both Groups 4 and 5 were comparable in age and weight and all were
non-obese. Unlike the previous studies, these groups were comprised of males and females. Group 4 also had negative family
histories of diabetes mellitus (Table 2).

Table 2

AGES AND WEIGHTS OF PATIENTS

Group	Age	Weight	I.B.W.	% from I.B.W.
4	29 ± 3	153 ± 9	153 ± 6	0%
5	32 ± 3	146 ± 8	150 ± 11	- 1%

Group 4: Four male and three female normal patients.
Group 5: Three male and two female subclinical
          diabetic patients.
I.B.W.: Ideal body weight.

    Figure 3 depicts the plasma glucose and insulin levels during
each of the three tests in control Group 4. These subjects resembled normal patients studied previously (Group 1, Figure 1)
in that the single dose prednisolone test was associated with a
normal glucose curve, although significantly higher than the control response. Appropriate adaptation of the insulin response was
also evident since the fasting, 30, 60 and 90 minute levels were
higher than control (p value <0.05). However, when the double
dose test was performed one to two weeks later, a diabetic curve
was elicited. Although fasting insulin levels were elevated, the
30 and 60 minute values were not significantly different from standard GTT concentrations and the peak insulin response that was significantly higher than control was not observed until 90 minutes
(p value <0.05).

    Double dose prednisolone tests had even more striking effects
on the subclinical diabetic patients (Figure 4). As in Group 2
(Figure 1), the standard glucose tolerance test was normal in
association with a brisk release of plasma insulin, but the single

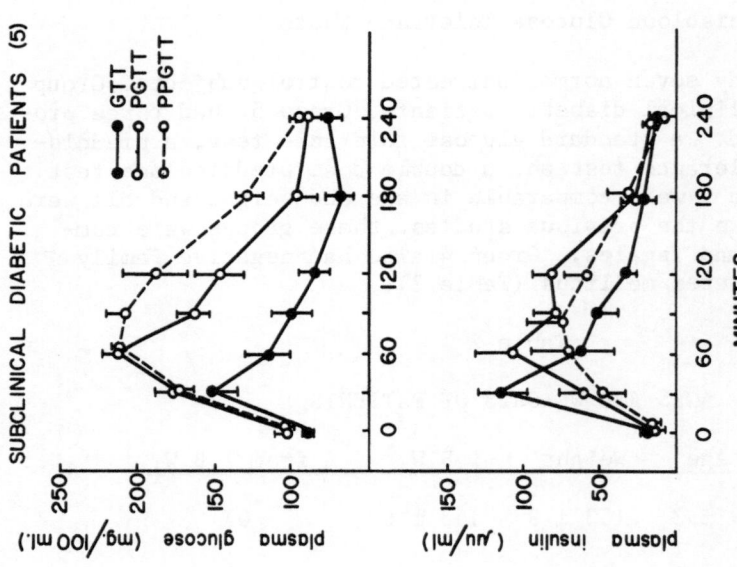

Fig. 4. Plasma glucose and insulin responses in five subclinical diabetic patients during oral glucose (GTT), prednisolone glucose (PGTT) and double dose prednisolone glucose (PPGTT) tolerance tests. Values are mean ± S.E.M.

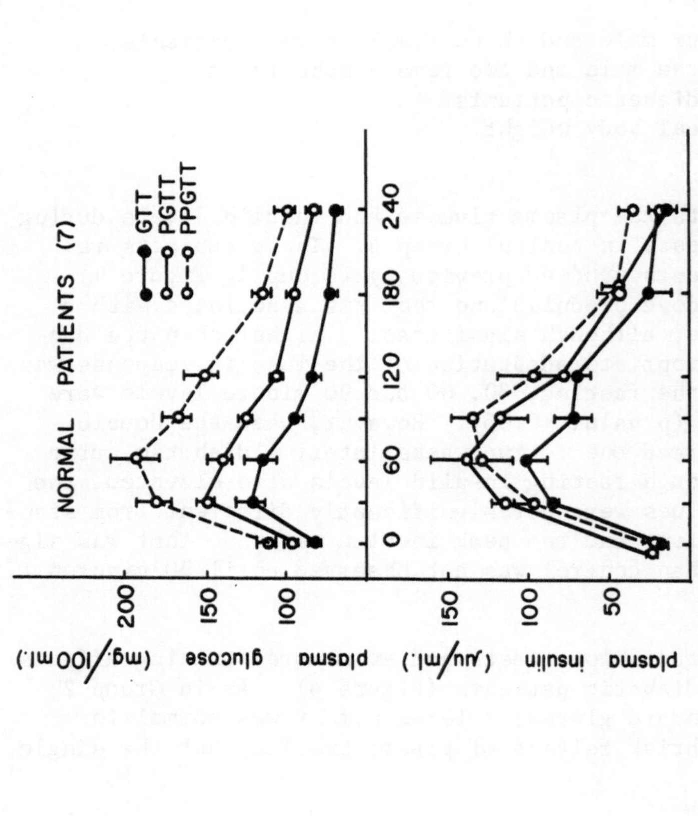

Fig. 3. Plasma glucose and insulin responses in seven normal patients (Group 4) during oral glucose (GTT), prednisolone glucose (PGTT) and double dose prednisolone glucose (PPGTT) tolerance tests. Values are mean ± S.E.M.

dose prednisolone test was abnormal and could be related to a delayed plasma insulin response. The double dose test resulted in a greater suppression of plasma insulin and carbohydrate tolerance was even more impaired.

Effects of Oral Contraceptive Agents on Tolbutamide Tolerance

Since there is little information concerning the effects of oral contraceptive agents on tolbutamide tolerance, the following additional study was performed on five women of normal body weight with negative family histories of diabetes mellitus. One gram of tolbutamide was administered in solution intravenously, and plasma samples were collected during a two hour period. Initial tests were done while these subjects were on an oral contraceptive regimen for an average period of eight months. Procedures were repeated six to eight weeks after discontinuation of the medication.

Figure 5 illustrates the percent fall of plasma glucose from fasting baseline levels together with plasma insulin responses. Tolbutamide tolerance during periods of birth control pill administration was normal since a nadir well below a 30 percent fall was achieved at 30 minutes. However, after withdrawal of these agents a small but significant improvement in the glucose lowering effect of tolbutamide was observed during the first half hour. Although the mean plasma insulin responses before and after discontinuation of contraceptives were not significantly different, four subjects had distinctly elevated hormonal levels while they were receiving these agents. Subsequent studies of larger groups of patients confirm this tendency in about 70% of the cases.

DISCUSSION

It is well known that gluco-corticoids promote hyperglycemia by augmenting hepatic glucose production (8) and impairing peripheral glucose utilization (9). Estrogens greatly potentiate this hormonal action. Ingle observed that certain doses of estrogen and cortisone, when administered separately to normal rats, had no effects on carbohydrate metabolism, but when given in combination, produced diabetes (10).

Similarly, Nelson and co-workers reported that subdiabetogenic doses of gluco-corticoids have minimal effects on control of human diabetic subjects but produce marked glycosuria when these individuals were treated concomitantly with estrogens (11). The greater incidence of impaired steroid glucose tolerance tests observed in pregnant women (12) and in individuals receiving agents containing

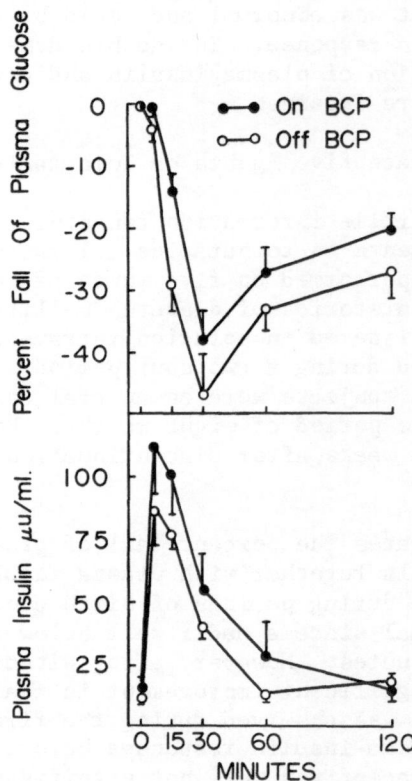

Fig. 5. Per cent fall of plasma glucose and plasma insulin response during intravenous tolbutamide tolerance tests in five normal women before and after withdrawal of birth control pills (BCP). Values are mean ± S.E.M.

synthetic estrogens (1,2) is consistent with these reports, but the nature of this diabetogenic synergism remains obscure.

Since estrogen treatment retards the plasma disappearance of administered cortisol in human subjects (13), it is possible that a greater plasma level of biologically active gluco-corticoid and, consequently, a more intense metabolic stress, may be achieved in mestranol-treated women as opposed to control subjects with similar doses of prednisolone. This effect alone could explain the greater frequency of impaired steroid tests in the former group.

There is also some evidence that estrogens enhance endogenous glucocorticoid activity. Plager and co-workers have reported elevated plasma free cortisol in subjects exposed to these hormones (14), and others have observed increased cortisol secretory rates under similar conditions of estrogen treatment (15). It should be pointed out, however, that reports from other laboratories have not confirmed these findings (12). Nevertheless, alterations of pyruvate metabolism (16), slight elevations of plasma glucose and insulin during standard glucose tolerance tests (17), as well as subtle changes in tolbutamide tolerance (Figure 5) among women receiving oral contraceptives may be consistent with an enhanced cortisol-like effect promoted by these agents. Such individuals would have a greater tendency to exhibit impaired steroid glucose tolerance tests following the additional diabetogenic stress imposed on them by oral prednisolone administration.

Mestranol also may alter the metabolic disposition of glucose in a manner that complements the contra-insulin effects of glucocorticoids. But until the action of synthetic estrogens on carbohydrate metabolism is defined more completely, particularly in liver and skeletal muscle, this also remains a speculation.

The data in the present report focus more attention on the possible effects mestranol-prednisolone interactions may have on pancreatic islet function. The impaired steroid glucose tolerance tests observed frequently in women treated with this estrogen can be related to a defective plasma insulin response similar to that observed in untreated subclinical diabetic patients (Figure 1). In overtly diabetic patients this hormonal defect also is observed during standard glucose tolerance tests according to previous reports of Yalow and Berson (18), Perley and Kipnis (19) and Seltzer and co-workers (20). In each instance the characteristic subnormal insulin increment observed during the initial 30 to 60 minutes of the procedure may explain the prompt establishment of abnormal hyperglycemia.

If mestranol induces abnormal steroid glucose tolerance solely by promoting higher plasma levels of gluco-corticoids after oral prednisolone administration, then the abnormality may be an artifact and more closely related to the impaired double dose prednisolone tests observed in control patients (Figure 3). However, it is equally possible that mestranol may create disturbances in pancreatic islet function that are unmasked by prednisolone stress. The latter supposition has some support from recent studies concerned with long term effects of contraceptive agents on carbohydrate tolerance. It was observed that as duration of treatment with combination type agents exceeded three or four years, the incidence of abnormal standard glucose tolerance tests steadily increased to 77 percent or more of this group (2,21). The impairment was associated with lowered plasma insulin responses. In this context, abnormal prednisolone tests elicited among women on relatively short term regimens may anticipate the future development of overt diabetes described by these investigators when administration is more prolonged. Further studies are warranted to test this possibility.

SUMMARY

An acquired form of subclinical diabetes mellitus is encountered frequently among women receiving mestranol-containing
oral contraceptive agents. The impaired prednisolone glucose
tolerance test observed in these instances is associated with a
defective plasma insulin response. The present study has established that 8½ hours of prednisolone administration has a basic
suppressive effect on the plasma insulin response to oral glucose.
Whether mestranol has a direct deleterious effect on pancreatic
islet secretion of insulin that is unmasked by prednisolone administration remains to be determined, but the condition appears
to be reversible in most cases when the contraceptive agent is
discontinued.

REFERENCES

1. diPaola, G., Puchulu, F., Robin, M., Nicholson, R., and
Marti, M.: Oral contraceptives and carbohydrate metabolism. Am.
J. Obst. and Gynec. 101:206 (1968).

2. Javier, Z., Gershberg, H., and Hulse, M.: Ovulatory suppressants, estrogens, and carbohydrate metabolism. Metabolism
17:443 (1968).

3. Fajans, S.S., and Conn, J.W.: The early recognition of
diabetes mellitus. Ann. N. Y. Acad. Sci. 82:208 (1959).

4. Hill, J.B., and Kessler, G.: An automated determination
of glucose utilizing a glucose oxidase-peroxide system. J. Lab.
Clin. Med. 57:970 (1961).

5. Morgan, C.R., and Lazarow, A.: Immunoassay of insulin:
two antibody system. Diabetes 12:115 (1963).

6. Kalkhoff, R.K., Richardson, B.L., and Stoddard, F.J.:
Defective plasma insulin response during prednisolone glucose
tolerance tests in subclinical diabetic mothers of heavy infants.
Diabetes 17:37 (1968).

7. Rull, J., Floyd, J.C., Jr., Fajans, S.S., and Conn, J.W.:
Insulin response to glucose in nondiabetic patients with negative
and positive cortisone glucose tolerance tests. Clin. Res.
13:419 (1965).

8. Welt, M.H., Stetten, D., Jr., Ingle, D.J., and Morley,
E.H.: Effects of cortisone on rates of glucose production and
oxidation in the rat. J. Biol. Chem. 197:57 (1952).

9. Riddick, F.A., Jr., Riesler, D.M., and Kipnis, D.M.: The
sugar transport system in striated muscle. Diabetes 11:171
(1962).

10. Ingle, D.J.: Effects of administering cortisone acetate and diethylstilbesterol to normal and force-fed rats. Am. J. Physiol. 172:115 (1953).

11. Nelson, D.H., Tanney, H., Mestman, G., Gieschan, V., and Wilson, L.P.: Potentiation of the biologic effect of administered cortisol by estrogen treatment. J. Clin. Endocr. 23:261 (1963).

12. Fajans, S.S., and Conn, J.W.: Comments on the cortisone-glucose tolerance test. Diabetes 10:63 (1961).

13. Peterson, R.E., Nokes, G., Chen, P.S., and Black, R.L.: Estrogens and adrenocortical function in man. J. Clin. Endocr. 20:495 (1960).

14. Plager, J.E., Schmidt, K.G., and Staubitz, W.J.: Increased unbound cortisol in plasma of estrogen-treated subjects. J. Clin. Invest. 43:1066 (1964).

15. Katz, F.H., and Kappas, A.: The effects of estradiol and estriol on plasma levels of cortisol and thyroid hormone-binding globulins and on aldosterone and cortisol secretion rates in man. J. Clin. Invest. 46:1768 (1967).

16. Wynn, V., and Doar, J.W.H.: Some effects of oral contraceptives on carbohydrate metabolism. Lancet ii:715 (1966).

17. Spellacy, W.N., and Carlson, K.L.: Plasma insulin and blood glucose levels in patients taking oral contraceptives. Am. J. Obst. and Gynec. 95:474 (1966).

18. Yalow, R.S., and Berson, S.A.: Plasma insulin concentrations in nondiabetic and early diabetic subjects. Diabetes 9:254 (1960).

19. Perley, M., and Kipnis, D.M.: Plasma insulin response to glucose and tolbutamide of normal weight and obese diabetic and nondiabetic subjects. Diabetes 15:867 (1966).

20. Seltzer, H.S., Allen, E.W., Herron, A.L., Jr., and Brennan, M.T.: Insulin secretion in response to a glycemic stimulus: relation of delayed initial release to carbohydrate intolerance in mild diabetes mellitus. J. Clin. Invest. 46:323 (1967).

21. Spellacy, W.N., Buhi, W.C., Spellacy, C.E., Moses, L.C., and Goldzieher, J.W.: Carbohydrate studies in long-term users of oral contraceptives. Diabetes 17: (supplement)344 (1968).

LIPID METABOLISM

ORAL CONTRACEPTIVES, LIPOPROTEINS,

AND LIPID TRANSPORT

Edwin L. Bierman

Department of Medicine, University of Washington
School of Medicine, Seattle, Washington

More than twenty-five years have elapsed since the obvious sex
difference in the prevalence of atherosclerosis before age 50 led
to the widely held view that gonadal hormones might affect plasma
lipids and hence influence the progression of atherosclerosis.
Further understanding awaited the development of methods of analysis
of the actual transport forms of lipid molecules in plasma, the
lipoproteins. A major insight into the problem was provided by
Russ, Eder and Barr (1) with the use of the precipitation method of
fractionation of lipoproteins into two major classes, "alpha" and
"beta" lipoproteins. By measurement of the cholesterol content of
these fractions they found that plasma from young women contained
more "alpha lipoprotein" and less "beta lipoprotein" than that from
men of comparable age. They also found that estrogen treatment of
males tended to eliminate this difference by decreasing the
"beta/alpha ratio".

Analysis of lipoproteins by ultracentrifugation (2,3) and by
electrophoresis (4) confirmed this difference in lipoprotein concentration between young men and women. Developments with these
techniques have led to our current understanding of the major lipoprotein transport forms in plasma (Fig. 1). There are three major
groups of lipoproteins which are important for this discussion and
they can be characterized both by flotation in the ultracentrifuge
and by migration on various electrophoretic media. The fraction
that contains most of the plasma cholesterol is the "beta" or low-
density lipoprotein fraction. Additional cholesterol and most of
the plasma phospholipid is carried in the alpha or high-density
lipoprotein fraction. The third important fraction is the triglyceride-rich, very low density ("pre-beta", or "alpha-2" migrating)
lipoprotein fraction, which has more recently come into prominence

Endogenous Plasma Lipids and Lipoproteins

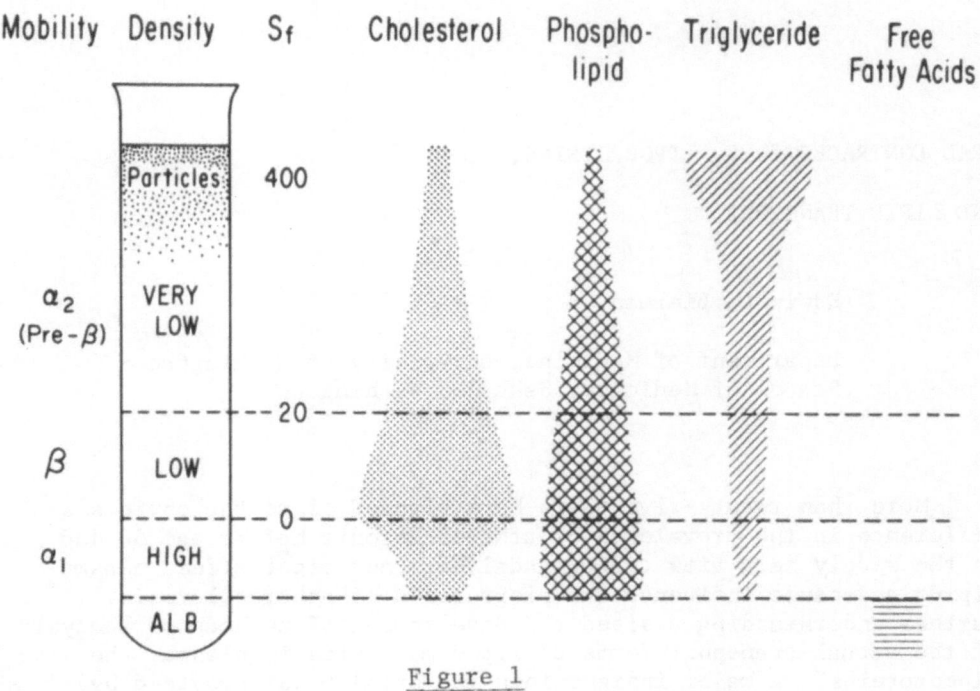

Figure 1

as a result of continuing examination of the effects of gonadal hormones and contraceptive steroids.

With any of these methods used to fractionate lipoproteins, it has become apparent that estrogen treatment, in a variety of subjects of either sex, affects the ratio of low density lipoproteins (LDL) to high density lipoproteins (HDL), both by decreasing LDL and increasing HDL (5,6). The effect of androgens is directly opposite; progestins have little or no effect on these lipoproteins (7). The estrogenic effect variably is reflected by a decrease in total plasma cholesterol concentration and, more consistently, by a decrease in the cholesterol:phospholipid ratio. As will be discussed further by Dr. Furman, the effect of estrogen appears to be both on the number of circulating lipoprotein aggregates and on the chemical composition of each lipoprotein class. These effects should be distinguished from each other. For example, estrogens might affect both the synthesis of alpha-lipoprotein protein, thereby increasing the number of lipoprotein particles, while at the same time reducing its cholesterol content by an effect on whole-body cholesterol metabolism.

I would like to examine in more detail the effect of gonadal
steroids on the transport of each of the major lipid classes;
cholesterol, phospholipid and triglyceride, and then try to summarize existing knowledge of the effects of oral contraceptives.
Undoubtedly the speakers today will elaborate on most of the salient
points and bring us up to date on current concepts.

Plasma cholesterol levels appear to be related to age, maleness, diet, and in epidemiological studies, to atherosclerosis.
In a typical United States white population there is a clear sex
difference before the age of 50 (Fig. 2) (8). On face value it
would appear that femaleness might cause the lower cholesterol
levels observed in young women. However, on closer examination,
the influence of this factor is relatively weak, since the sex
difference in cholesterol levels is not consistent in other populations and may be attenuated by a variety of environmental factors
(9). In contrast to the apparently minor influence of intrinsic
femaleness and physiological estrogen levels, pharmacological doses
of estrogen can reduce circulating cholesterol levels in both men
and women. How does estrogen lower plasma cholesterol levels, and
where does the cholesterol go? Does it leave the body, as evidenced

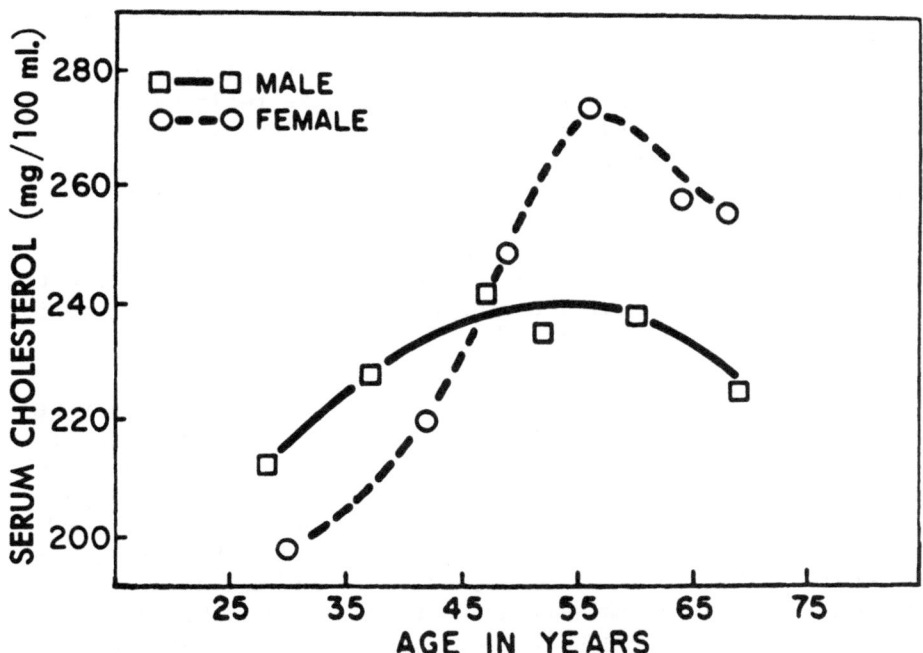

Figure 2. Change with age of serum cholesterol levels in
urban white adult males and females, from Schaefer (8).

by negative sterol balance? Or is cholesterol deposited in tissue
as a result of estrogen treatment (not necessarily a desirable
effect)? Does estrogen block the synthesis or alter the metabolism
of sterol in the liver and other tissues? These questions still
remain largely unanswered; however, some pertinent observations
have emerged. Nestel (10) has shown by isotopic methods that estrogen appears to increase the total turnover of cholesterol in man,
consistent with results of studies in rats showing that estrogens
increase cholesterol oxidation. However, alterations in synthesis
and accumulation of cholesterol in the liver also occur (11).
Little is known about the mechanism of action of gonadal steroids
on phospholipid metabolism. The major critical issue in regard to
estrogenic effect is whether the apparent decrease in circulating
cholesterol level and increase in circulating high density lipoproteins and phospholipids reflects a predominately deleterious or
beneficial effect on the whole organism.

     Plasma triglyceride levels also appear to be related to age,
maleness, atherosclerosis, and in addition, adiposity. This latter
effect may be responsible for the marked increase in average triglyceride levels of middle aged males seen in numerous population
studies (Fig. 3) (8,12,13). Thus a sex difference is also apparent
in triglyceride levels before the age of 50, perhaps partly due to
diet and other environmental factors as well as to intrinsic maleness. Furman and his associates (14) were among the first to call
attention to a major effect of estrogen on the triglyceride-rich
(very low density) lipoproteins. This effect is reflected by an increase both in triglyceride content of these lipoproteins and in
total circulating triglyceride levels. The cholesterol and phospholipid carried in this lipoprotein fraction appear to increase as
well. Again, the effect of androgens is opposite, and progestins
are relatively neutral. Prior to the impetus provided by the use
of contraceptive steroids, little investigative effort was directed
toward the mechanism by which estrogens altered plasma triglyceride
and very low density lipoproteins.

     Since metabolism of the different lipoprotein species may be
independently regulated, measurement of total plasma cholesterol,
triglyceride, and phospholipid concentrations may not necessarily
reflect specific estrogen-induced alterations made in each lipoprotein class. Changes in specific lipoproteins may relate more
closely to the development of atherosclerosis than do total plasma
lipid levels. Therefore, it is essential to examine hormonal
effects on lipoproteins as well as on total plasma lipid levels.
For example, as Dr. Furman will show, estrogen may lower cholesterol
concentration only in low density (beta) lipoproteins, while at the
same time increase cholesterol concentration in very low density
lipoproteins and produce only slight changes in high density (alpha)

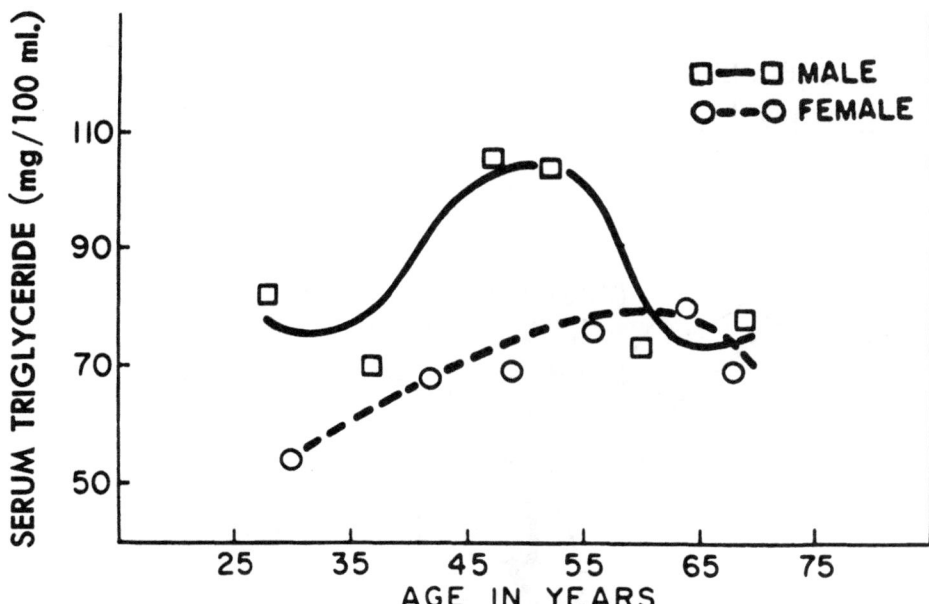

Figure 3.   Change with age of serum triglyceride levels, as in Figure 2.

lipoproteins. Thus, the effect of estrogen on the total plasma cholesterol concentration may be highly variable.

Few studies of the effect of contraceptive steroids per se on specific lipoproteins have been reported thus far, so only inferences can be made from knowledge of changes in total plasma lipids. When the use of contraceptive steroids was established, the first lipid measurement reported was plasma cholesterol. After Pincus (15) and others observed that the agents used had little or no effect on total circulating cholesterol levels, it was suspected that all the effects on lipid transport of pharmacological doses of estrogen might be neutralized by the progestational components. It soon became clear that this was not the case. Oral contraceptives were found to cause consistent increases in plasma triglyceride concentration, first observed by Aurell (16) and Wynn and Doar (17), and amply confirmed by ourselves and others. It also became clear that oral contraceptives elevated plasma phospholipid concentrations, particularly lecithin, as observed by Svanborg and associates (18). These observations were consistent with a major effect of contraceptive steroids on very low density and high density lipoproteins, and in accord with the historical evidence that relative hypertriglyceridemia is common in human and animal pregnancy (19,20). These effects of contraceptive agents all appear to result from their estrogenic component, since they can be reproduced in part by

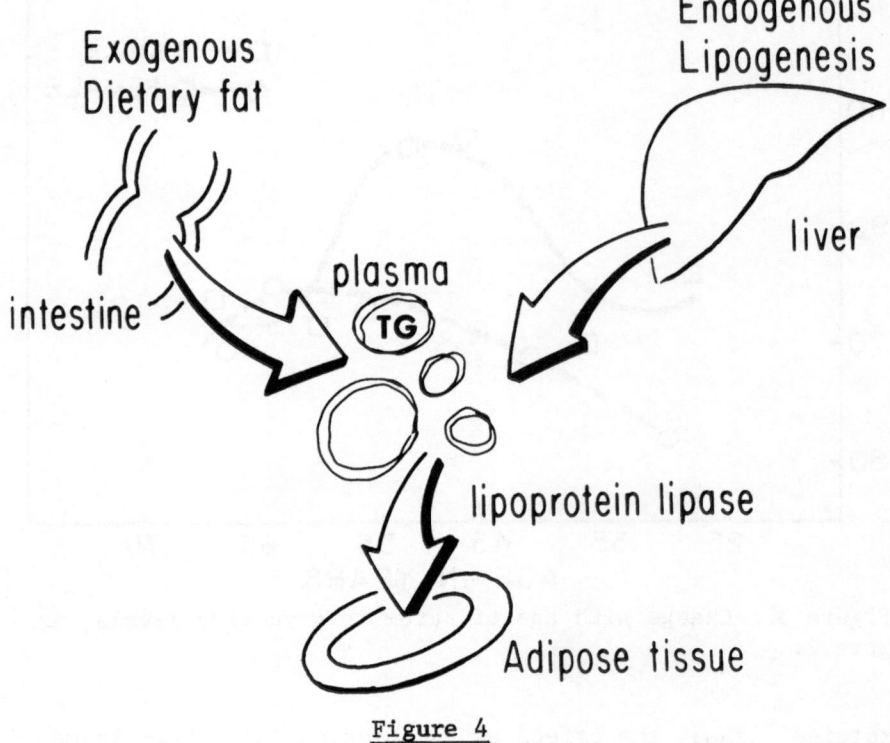

Figure 4

the administration of the estrogen alone, but not by the progestin alone.

The observation that contraceptive steroids consistently produce hypertriglyceridemia has focused attention in our laboratory on the mechanism of action of these agents on triglyceride transport. Briefly, there are only two tissues in the body, liver and intestine, that can synthesize and secrete triglyceride into the circulation and one major removal process, predominately localized in adipose tissue (Fig. 4). The contraceptive steroids could affect triglyceride transport by either accelerating triglyceride-rich lipoprotein production in the liver (by increased triglyceride synthesis or the production of additional carrier very low density lipoprotein), or impairing removal. It is unlikely that the input of fat from the diet, via intestinal synthesis and secretion of chylomicrons with subsequent transport from lymph into the circulation, is affected, since we have observed effects of contraceptives in subjects on fat-free diets (Fig. 5). In such a subject who was studied because of her hyperlipemia, estrogen administration in usual clinical dosage (0.625 mg Premarin/day) was associated with

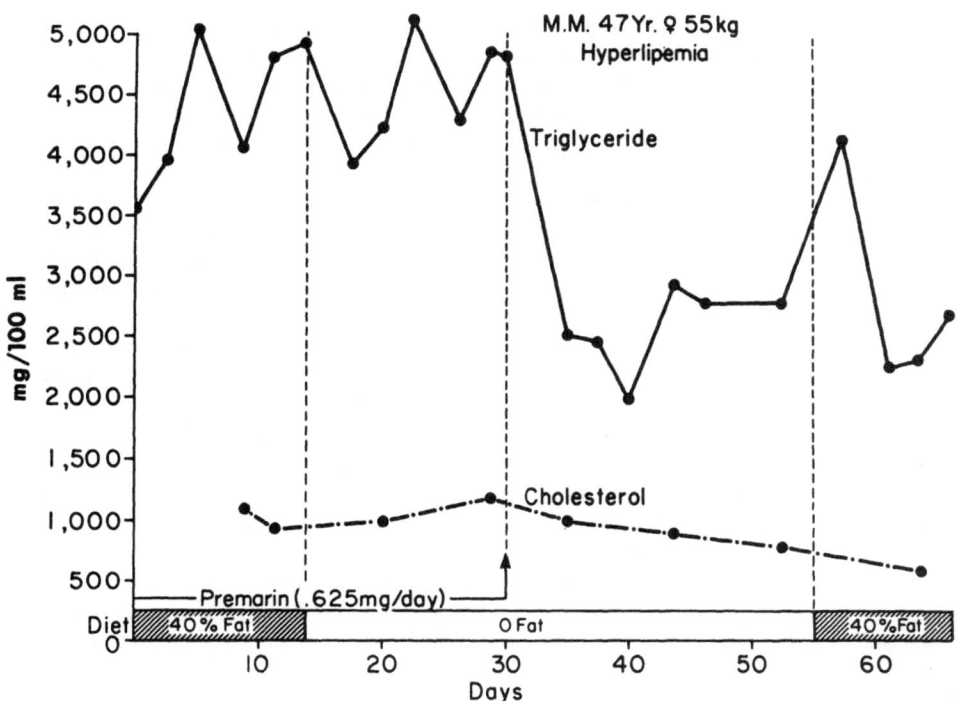

Figure 5. Plasma triglyceride and cholesterol levels in a 47-year old female with hyperlipemia maintained on normal fat and fat-free formula diets before and after withdrawal of oral Premarin therapy, .625 mg /day.

higher triglyceride levels despite a fat-free diet. This subject is one of several tested who demonstrate that estrogen or contraceptive steroids may aggravate pre-existing hyperlipemic states, perhaps by the same mechanism involved in the estrogen-induced elevation of triglyceride levels in all subjects.

If contraceptives affect either triglyceride or lipoprotein synthesis, the action is likely to be localized to the liver. Triglycerides are normally formed by simple esterification of both circulating fatty acids from adipose tissue stores and newly produced fatty acids derived from carbohydrate (lipogenesis). Lipogenesis requires insulin, and hence the degree of exposure of the liver to insulin presumably can influence the rate of triglyceride synthesis (21). Thus the known effects of contraceptives on insulin suggest a role in the alterations of triglyceride transport as well as in the observed alterations of carbohydrate tolerance.

Triglyceride removal appears to involve the action of an enzyme, lipoprotein lipase, located at or near adipose tissue capillaries. The activity of this enzyme appears to be critical for the assimilation of circulating lipoprotein triglycerides. Other hormones influence lipoprotein lipase activity. For example, insulin deficiency (22) and thyroid deficiency (23) impair the activity of this enzyme resulting in hypertriglyceridemia which can be reversed by appropriate hormonal replacement. Studies in animals have shown that this enzyme activity also decreases in late pregnancy, and this decrease has been associated in part with the hypertriglyceridemia of pregnancy in animals (20). These observations have led to a closer examination in our laboratory of this removal mechanism as influenced by contraceptive steroids, and results of these studies will be described by Dr. Hazzard. In general, the competence of this triglyceride removal mechanism can be assessed in several ways. For example, challenge with an oral fat load will accentuate any functional impairment in removal capacity and lead to an accumulation of circulating chylomicrons. Another method has been the measurement of activity of the enzyme directly, since it can be released into the circulation by the intravenous administration of charged molecules, such as heparin. An example of this assay in the normal state and in the presence of impaired enzyme activity is illustrated in Figure 6. Fabian and co-workers (24) have shown that post-heparin lipolytic activity was decreased after estrogen administration, consistent with the decrease observed by Sandhofer et al in late human pregnancy (25).

Published work to date on the effects of oral contraceptives on individual plasma lipid levels is summarized in Figure 7. Prior to the use of contraceptive steroid hormone combinations, it was apparent that estrogen alone in pharmacologic doses reduced total plasma cholesterol concentration and consistently elevated phospholipid and triglyceride concentrations. Progestational compounds alone uniformly have had little or no effect, variability perhaps due in part to differences in "estrogenicity" of various progestins (26). These agents may also differ in their interaction with estrogens. Thus, not all estrogen-progestin combinations are alike in their effect on plasma lipid levels. For example, in Anovlar, the progestational agent interacts, in a manner different from other compounds, with ethinyl estradiol to produce an alteration in the pattern of responses. In general, the progestin appears to neutralize the effect of estrogen on circulating cholesterol, resulting in essentially no change in cholesterol levels, whereas these compounds do not appear to affect the estrogen-induced increase in phospholipid and triglyceride levels. This suggests that contraceptive steroids do not have much effect on the cholesterol-rich, low density (beta) lipoproteins, while exerting profound effects on the triglyceride-rich, very low density lipoproteins and perhaps the high density lipoproteins as well. It is hoped that some light will soon be shed on the nature of changes in specific lipoprotein classes.

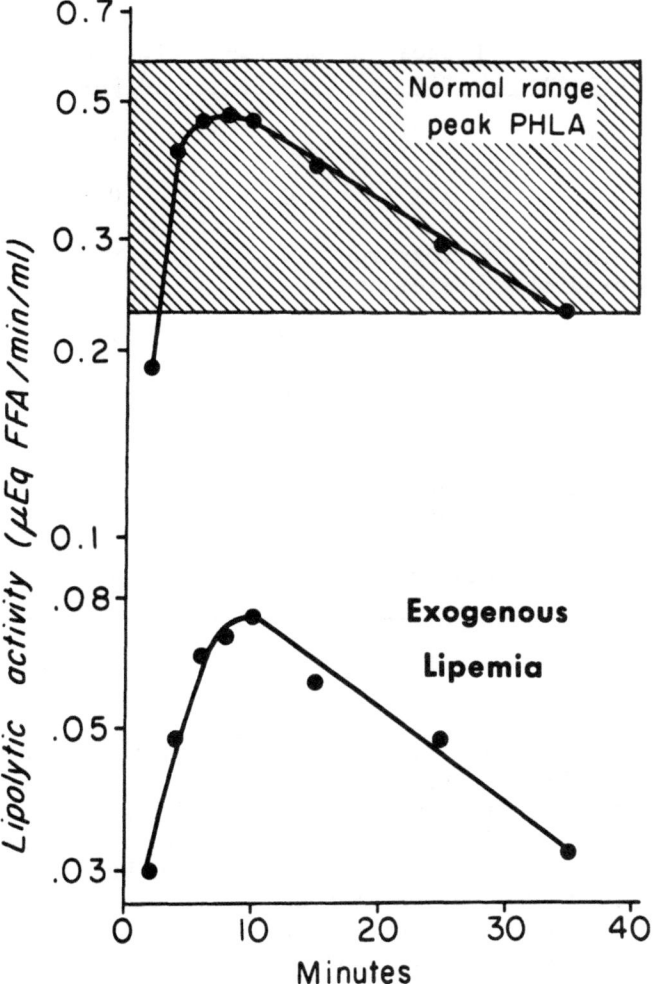

Figure 6. A semilogarithmic plot of the lipolytic activity in plasma after the rapid intravenous injection of heparin, approximately 0.1 mg/kg at 0 time. Subjects: Normal, above; hyperlipemic with impaired triglyceride removal, below. Normal range of peak post-heparin lipolytic activity is indicated in the shaded zone.

SUMMARY

ORAL CONTRACEPTIVES AND PLASMA LIPIDS   (Dec. 1968.)

	Estrogen	Progestin	Cholesterol	Phospholipid	Triglyceride
	All	--	↓	↑	↑
	--	All	0	0	0
(Provest)	Ethinyl Estradiol	Medroxyprogesterone	0	↑	↑
(Volidan)	"	Megestrol	0	↑	↑
(Anovlar)	"	Norethistrone	↓	sl↓	?↑
(Enovid)	Mestranol	Norethynodrel	0		↑
(Ovulen)	"	Ethynodiol	0	↑	↑

Figure 7

A major unanswered question that will remain with us for some
time is: what is the long-term result of these changes in lipid
transport induced by contraceptive steroid administration? Alterations such as these could conceivably be beneficial or detrimental
in isolated disorders of lipoprotein metabolism, but what of normal
young women? Can a combination of gonadal steroid hormones be developed that will remain effective as an oral contraceptive, but
not perturb lipoprotein homeostasis? I am sure the discussants
will direct some of their attention to these issues.

REFERENCES

1. Russ, E.M., Eder, H.A. and Barr, D.P.: Influence of
gonadal hormones on protein-lipid relationships in human plasma.
Amer. J. Med. 19:4-24 (1955).

2. Gofman, J.W., Jones, H.B., Lindgren, F.T., Lyon, T.P.,
Elliott, H.A. and Strisower, B.: Blood lipids and human
atherosclerosis. Circulation 2:161-178 (1950).

3. Havel, R.J., Eder, H.A. and Bragdon, J.H.: The distribution and chemical composition of ultracentrifugally separated lipoproteins in human serum. J. Clin Invest. 34:1345-1353 (1955).

4. Nikkila, E.: Studies on the lipid-protein relationships in normal and pathological sera and the effect of heparin on serum lipoproteins. Scand. J. Clin. & Lab. Invest. 5 (Suppl. 8) 1-101 (1953).

5. Furman, R.H., Howard, R.P., Norcia, L.N. and Keaty, E.C.: The influence of androgens, estrogens and related steroids on serum lipids and lipoproteins. Amer. J. Med. 26:80-97 (1958).

6. Marshall, N.B.: Gonadal hormones and lipid metabolism. In Lipid Pharmacology, ed. by R. Paoletti. (Chapter 8) Academic Press, New York, 1964.

7. Oliver, M.F. and Boyd, G.S.: Influence of the sex hormones on the circulating lipids and lipoproteins in coronary sclerosis. Circulation 13:82-91 (1956).

8. Schaefer, L.E.: Serum cholesterol-triglyceride distribution in a "normal" New York City population. Amer. J. Med. 36:262-268 (1964).

9. Walden, R.T., Schaefer, L.E., Lemon, F.L., Sunshine, A. and Wynder, E.L.: Effect of environment on the serum cholesterol-triglyceride distribution among Seventh Day Adventists. Amer. J. Med. 36:269-276 (1964).

10. Nestel, P.J., Hirsch, E.A. and Couzens, E.A.: Effect of chlorophenoxyisobutyric acid and ethinyl estradiol on cholesterol turnover. J. Clin. Invest. 44:891-896 (1965).

11. Aftergood, L., Alfin-Slater, R.B., and Hernandez, H.J.: Effect of large doses of the oral contraceptive Enovid on cholesterol metabolism in the rat. J. Lipid Res. 9:447-452 (1968).

12. Carlson, L.A.: Serum lipids in normal men. Acta Medica Scand. 167:Fasc. 5, 377-397 (1960).

13. New, M.I., Roberts, T.N., Bierman, E.L. and Reader, G.G.: The significance of blood lipid alterations in diabetes mellitus. Diabetes 12:208-212 (1963).

14. Furman, R.H., Alaupovic, P. and Howard, R.P.: Effects of androgens and estrogens on serum lipids and the composition and concentration of serum lipoproteins in normolipemic and hyperlipidemic states. Progr. Biochem. Pharmacol. 2:215-249 (1967).

15. Pincus, Gregory: The Control of Fertility. Academic Press, New York, 1965., pp. 276-277.

16. Aurell, M., Cramer, K. and Rybo, G.: Serum lipids and lipoproteins during long-term administration of an oral contraceptive. Lancet, 1:291-293 (1966).

17. Wynn, V. and Doar, J.W.H.: Some effects of oral contraceptives on serum-lipid and lipoprotein levels. Lancet 2:720-723 (1966).

18. Brody, S., Kerstell, J., Nilsson, L. and Svanborg, A.: The effects of some ovulation inhibitors on the different plasma lipid fractions. Acta Medica Scand. 183:1-7 (1968)

19. Peters, J.P., Heineman, M. and Man, E.B.: The lipids of serum in pregnancy. J. Clin. Invest. 30:388-394 (1951).

20. Otway, S. and Robinson, D.S.: Significance of changes in tissue clearing-factor lipase activity in relation to the lipaemia of pregnancy. Biochem. J. 106:677-682 (1968).

21. Reaven, G.M., Lerner, R.L., Stein, M.P. and Farquhar, J.W.: Role of insulin in endogenous hypertriglyceridemia. J. Clin. Invest. 46:1756-1767 (1967).

22. Bagdade, J.D., Porte, D., Jr. and Bierman, E.L.: Diabetic lipemia: a form of acquired fat-induced lipemia. New Eng. J. Med. 276:427-433 (1967).

23. Porte, D., Jr., O'Hara, D.D. and Williams, R.H.: The relation between post-heparin lipolytic activity and plasma triglyceride in myxedema. Metabolism 15:107-113 (1966).

24. Fabian, E., Stork, A., Kobilkova, J. and Sponarova, J.: The activity of the lipoprotein lipase and estrogens. Enzym. Biol. Clin. 8:451-455 (1967).

25. Sandhofer, von F., Sailer, S., Braunsteiner, H. and Braitenberg, H.: Post-heparin lipoproteinlipase und schwangerschaft. Untersuchunger uber die lipoproteinlipase II. 73:392-393 (1961).

26. Paulsen, C.A., Leach, R.B., Lanman, J., Goldston, N., Maddock, W.O. and Heller, C.G.: Inherent estrogenicity of norethidrone and norethynodrel: comparison with other synthetic progestins and progesterone. J. Clin. Endocrin. & Metab. 22:1033-1039 (1962).

FASTING SERUM TRIGLYCERIDE AND CHOLESTEROL

LEVELS DURING ORAL CONTRACEPTIVE THERAPY

V. Wynn and J. W. H. Doar

Alexander Simpson Laboratory for Metabolic Research
St. Mary's Hospital Medical School, London, W2

We have previously found elevated serum triglyceride, cholesterol, and low density and very low density lipoprotein levels in a cross-sectional study of 102 women receiving oral contraceptive therapy (1). While changes of serum triglyceride levels were marked, only slight elevations of serum cholesterol levels were observed.

It is known that serum lipid and lipoprotein levels differ in premenopausal women compared with men of the same age, but after the menopause tend to become similar (2). The incidence of clinical manifestations of atherosclerosis is less frequent in premenopausal women than in men, but after the menopause the incidence approximates in the two sexes (3). In view of the possible relevance of elevated serum lipid and lipoprotein levels to the development of clinical manifestations of atherosclerosis, the effects of oral contraceptive drugs on these indices are of importance.

Although elevation of serum lipid and lipoprotein levels during oral contraceptive therapy has now been found by many workers (1,4-7), several questions remain unanswered. Do all oestrogen-progestagen combinations cause elevation of serum lipid and lipoprotein levels? Is the oestrogen and/or progestagen responsible? Are the changes reversible? Are the changes pro-

This work has been supported by Contract No. PH-43-67-1344 of the United States National Institutes of Health.

We gratefully acknowledge the assistance of Miss G. Robertson and Miss T. Stokes in carrying out the analyses, and of Dr. R. Sharp, Mr. P. Samuel and Mr. G. Randall of Hatfield College of Technology for computing aid.

TABLE 1

DETAILS OF GROUP A AND B SUBJECTS

	Group A	Group B
No. of women	68	23
Mean age (yrs)	26(range 17-46)	32(range 23-49)
Mean body weight as % 'ideal body weight'	103(range 74-148)	120(range 87-196)
Obese women (%)	13	48
Mean parity	1.0(range 0-5)	2.2(range 0-7)
Positive family history of diabetes mellitus (%)	49	50
Mean time (months) on (group A) and off (group B) OC therapy	6.7(range 3-48)	5.7(range 2-19)
Mean duration of OC therapy in group B (months)		24.1(range 2-48)

TABLE 2

DRUG THERAPY OF GROUP A AND B SUBJECTS

	Group A	Group B
Ovulen	33	12
'Step-Up'*	11	0
Anovlar/Gynovlar	9	4
Norinyl	8	0
Lyndiol/Lyndiol 2.5	4	2
Volidan	1	3
Orthonovum	1	1
C-Quens	1	1

*'Step-Up' (0.1 mg mestranol and 0.1 mg ethynodiol diacetate for 16 days, 0.1 mg mestranol and 0.5 mg ethynodiol diacetate for seven days).

TABLE 3

FASTING SERUM LIPID LEVELS

Group A (68 subjects)

	Triglyceride (mg/100 ml)		Cholesterol (mg/100 ml)	
	before oc*	on oc	before oc	on oc
Mean	67.5±20.2	100.6±30.9	179.8±36.2	178.5±30.7
P	<0.001		NS	

Group B (23 subjects)

	Triglyceride (mg/100 ml)		Cholesterol (mg/100 ml)	
	on oc	off oc	on oc	off oc
Mean	135.2±44.4	85.2±29.0	210.1±40.1	188.0±37.6
P	<0.001		<0.01	

Mean fasting serum lipid levels ± SD in Group A and B subjects.
*Oral contraceptives

gressively greater with prolonged therapy? Do the changes occur
only in certain subjects? Are the changes due to increased rates
of lipoprotein entry into or decreased rates of lipoprotein
removal from the vascular compartment?

The present longitudinal study of serum triglyceride and
cholesterol levels off and during oral contraceptive therapy
attempts to answer some of these questions.

SUBJECTS

Two groups of women were studied. Sixty-eight women in group
A were tested before and again while receiving oral contraceptive
therapy. Twenty-three women in group B were initially tested
during therapy and again after this had been discontinued. No
subject was taking any drug known to affect lipid metabolism
(excepting oral contraceptives). Details of the two groups of
subjects are shown in Table 1. The nature of the oestrogen-
progestagen combinations used is shown in Table 2.

METHODS

Samples of venous blood were taken after an overnight fast
of at least 12 hours, care being taken to standardize the effects
of posture and hydrostatic pressure on serum lipid levels (8).
Thus, the subjects were in the horizontal position for at least
30 minutes before blood was taken and cuff pressure was avoided.
Serum cholesterol was estimated by the method of Zlatkis et al. (9)
as modified by Henly (10) and serum triglyceride by a semi-automated fluorimetric technique (11). The significance of differences of means was assessed by the paired 't' test and of the
correlation between two variables by the product moment correlation coefficient. Calculations were performed by an Elliott 803
computer. The ratio of variances was assessed by the 'F' test.
Oral glucose tolerance tests were also carried out in the majority
of these subjects.

RESULTS

Mean serum triglyceride and cholesterol levels off and on
oral contraceptive therapy for groups A and B are shown in
Table 3.

Serum Triglyceride Levels

The mean control fasting serum triglyceride level in Group A
subjects (67.5 ± 20.2 mg /100 ml) increased during therapy (100.6

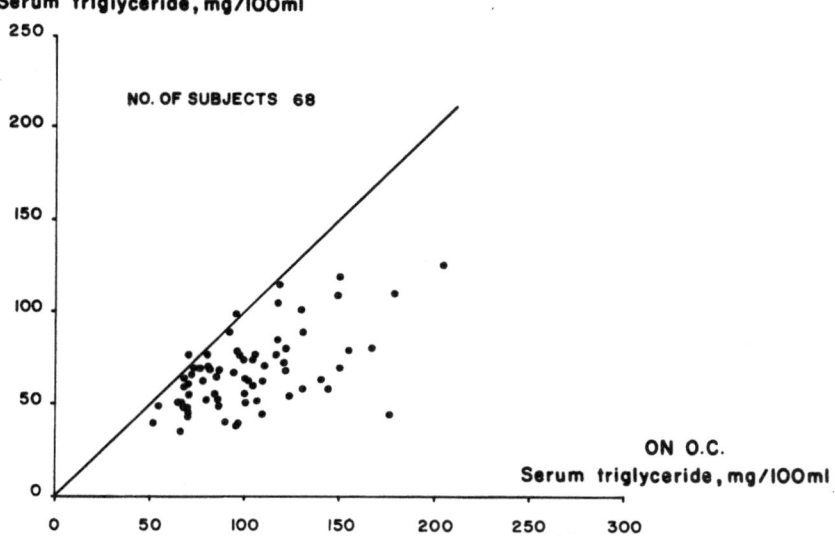

Fig. 1.   Changes of fasting serum triglyceride levels in
Group A subjects before and during therapy.

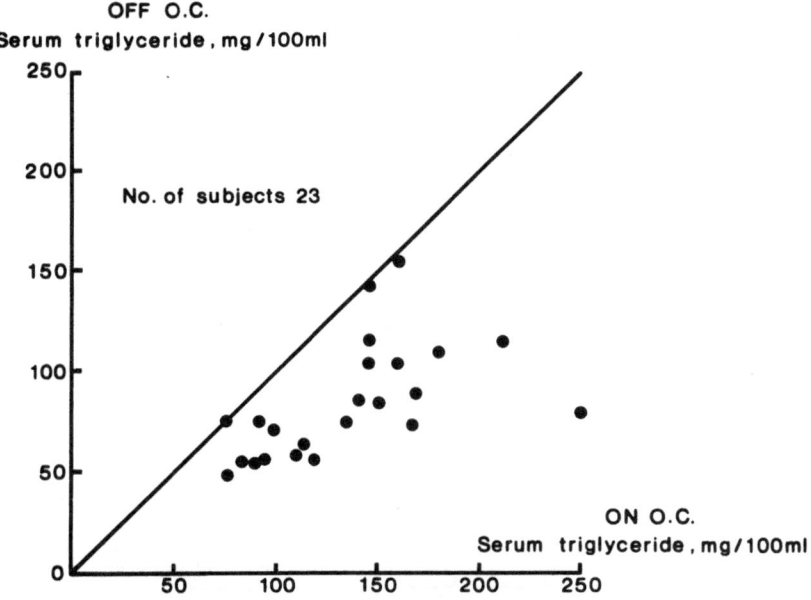

Fig. 2.   Changes of fasting serum triglyceride levels in
Group B subjects during and after stopping therapy.

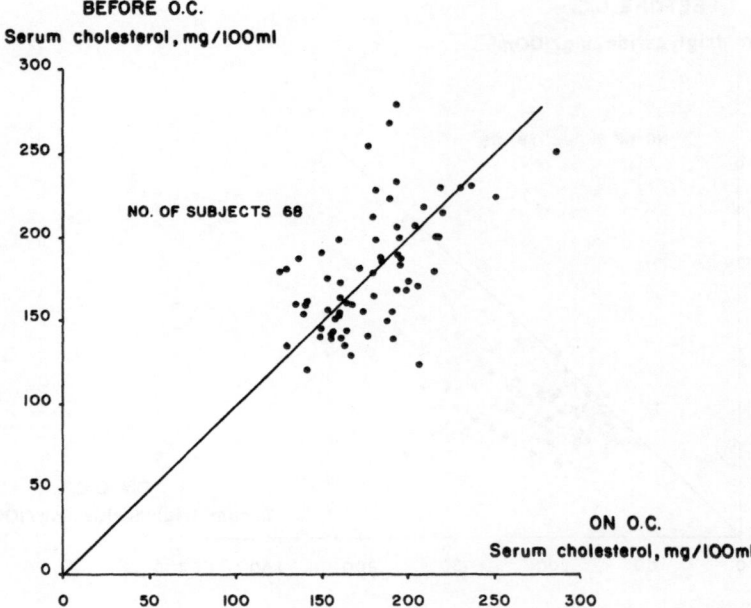

Fig. 3.   Changes of fasting serum cholesterol levels in
Group A subjects before and during therapy.

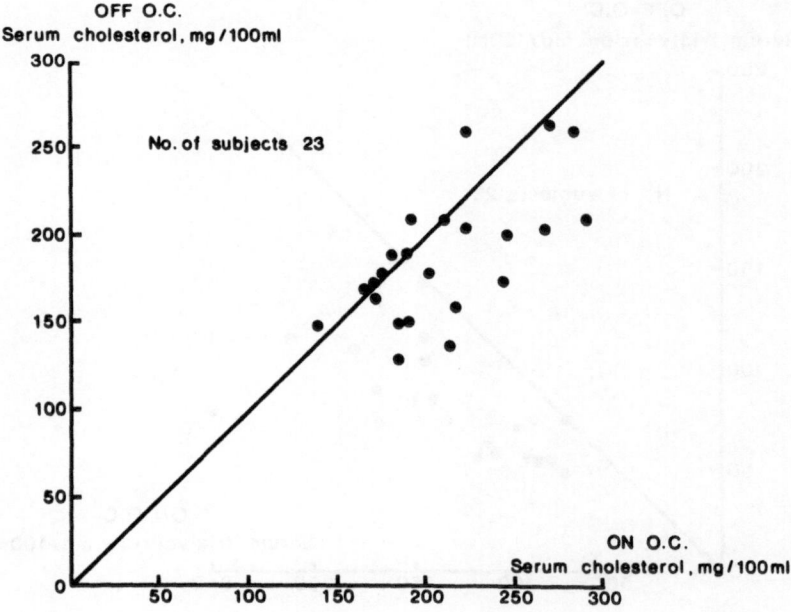

Fig. 4.   Changes of fasting serum cholesterol levels in
Group B subjects during and after stopping therapy.

± 30.9 mg /100 ml., P < 0.001). The mean fasting serum triglyceride level in Group B subjects during therapy (135 ± 44.4 mg /
100 ml) fell after therapy was discontinued (85.2 ± 29.0 mg /
100 ml , P < 0.001). The changes in individual subjects are shown
in Figures 1 and 2. Serum triglyceride levels rose in 66 of 68
(97%) Group A subjects during therapy and decreased in 22 of 23
(96%) Group B subjects after stopping therapy. We have previously defined our upper limit of normal serum triglyceride in
women of this age group as 131 mg./100 ml (1). Control values
for Group A subjects were all below this level but during oral
contraceptive therapy abnormally elevated levels occurred in
12 of 68 (18%) subjects. Thirteen of 23 (57%) Group B subjects
had abnormal serum triglyceride levels during therapy and of these
all but two returned to within the normal range after therapy was
discontinued. The variance of serum triglyceride levels was
significantly increased (P < 0.01) in both groups during therapy
indicating that some subjects were affected more than others.
No relation was found between the change of serum triglyceride
level and duration of therapy, nature of oestrogen-progestagen
combination or the day of treatment cycle. Similar mean changes
of fasting serum triglyceride levels during therapy were noted in
Group A subjects with (31.1 ± 29.4 mg /100 ml) and without (20.5
± 24.2 mg /100 ml) a family history of diabetes mellitus. A
similar finding was noted in Group B subjects. Weak negative
correlations existed in Group A subjects between the change of
fasting serum triglyceride level during therapy and the change in
fasting plasma glucose level (r = -0.31, P < 0.05) and the change
in total area under the oral glucose tolerance (OGTT) plasma glucose curve (r = -0.28, P < 0.05). No significant correlation in
Group A subjects was found between the change of serum triglyceride level during therapy and the control serum triglyceride
level, the control area under the oral glucose tolerance plasma
glucose curve, the change of fasting plasma insulin level or the
change of total area under the oral glucose tolerance test (OGTT)
plasma insulin curve during therapy. A significant correlation
(r = 0.31, P < 0.05) was found between the pre-therapy control
fasting plasma glucose level during therapy in Group A subjects.

Serum Cholesterol Levels

The mean control fasting serum cholesterol level in 68 Group
A subjects (179.8 ± 36.2 mg /100 ml.) did not change significantly
during oral contraceptive therapy (178.5 ± 30.7 mg /100 ml , NS).
The mean level in 23 Group B subjects (210.1 ± 40.1 mg /100 ml),
however, fell after therapy was discontinued (188.0 ± 37.6 mg /
100 ml , P < 0.01). The changes in individual subjects are shown
in Figures 3 and 4. The fasting serum cholesterol level increased
in 36 of 68 (53%) Group A subjects during therapy and decreased in
14 of 23 (61%) Group B subjects after therapy was discontinued.

Fasting Serum Lipid Levels During Mestranol Therapy

Fasting serum lipid levels in 6 subjects before and after
3 months treatment with mestranol 0.1 mg /day are shown in Table 4.
While a significant elevation of the fasting serum triglyceride
level was noted, the fasting serum cholesterol level was not
changed significantly.

DISCUSSION

We have found the fasting serum triglyceride level to be
increased during oral contraceptive therapy in 66 of 68 Group A
subjects. No significant change of the fasting serum cholesterol
level was found during therapy. These observations confirm the
findings of our previous cross-sectional study of 75 control women
and 102 women receiving oral contraceptives (1).

In addition, we have found significant decreases of both
fasting serum triglyceride and cholesterol levels in 23 women
(Group B) after oral contraceptive therapy was discontinued. The
two groups of women were not comparable in that Group B subjects
were on average older, more parous, more obese, and had received
oral contraceptive therapy for a longer period of time.

Until recently, there have been few studies of the effects of
gonadal steroids and their synthetic analogues on serum lipid and
lipoprotein levels in premenopausal women. Oestrogens, in general,
decrease serum low density lipoprotein (LDL) and serum total cholesterol and increase serum high density lipoprotein (HDL) levels
in postmenopausal women (12). Conjugated equine oestrogens were
found to increase serum triglyceride levels in postmenopausal women
(13) and Gershberg et al (6) found a similar effect with mestranol
therapy (7). In the present study, we observed the serum triglyceride level to rise in all six women treated with mestranol alone
for 3 months, though the serum cholesterol levels were not significantly changed.

Progesterone administration, either as the natural hormone or
as 17α-hydroxyprogesterone caproate, had no significant effect on
serum lipid levels in oophorectomized women (14). Brody et al (5)
found serum triglyceride levels in three oophorectomized women to be
unchanged during therapy with the synthetic progestagens, megestrol
acetate and norethisterone acetate, but serum cholesterol levels
fell during treatment with the latter.

The effects of androgens on serum lipid levels are of relevance
in view of the chemical similarity between certain synthetic progestagens and methyl testosterone. Androgens usually increase serum
LDL and decrease serum HDL levels while serum cholesterol levels

TABLE 4

MEAN FASTING SERUM LIPID LEVELS IN SIX WOMEN
BEFORE AND DURING MESTRANOL THERAPY

	Fasting serum tri-glyceride (mg/100 ml) mean ±SD	Fasting serum chol-esterol (mg/100 ml) mean ±SD
Before therapy	61.5±20.9	176.7±22.7
During therapy	107.8±26.4	185.2±29.5
P	0.02	NS

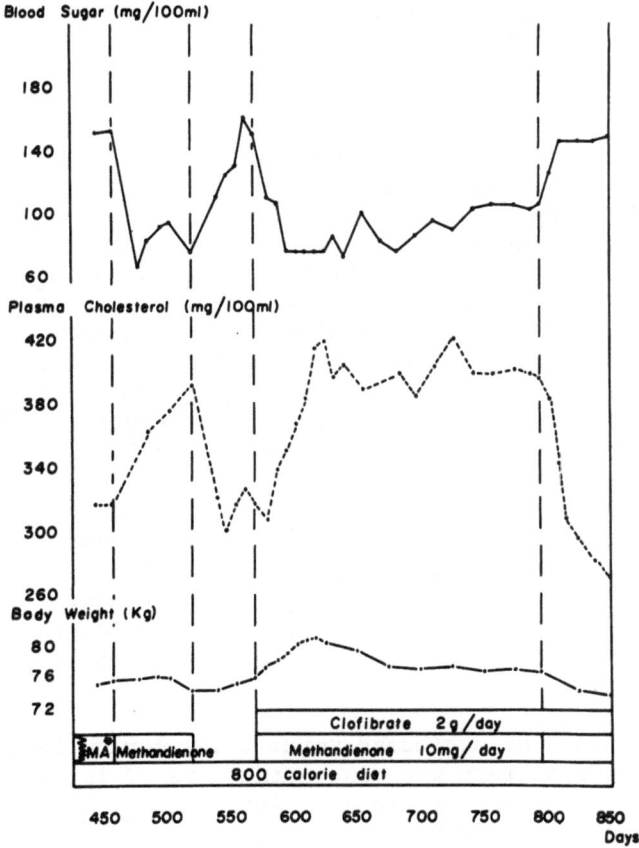

Fig. 5. Fasting blood sugar and plasma cholesterol levels
during methandienone therapy in a 50 year old woman with maturity
onset diabetes mellitus.

remain unchanged (12). In general, greater changes are found with
the synthetic orally active androgens. Of note is the observation
that administration of synthetic androgen during a period of
oestrogen therapy may not only reverse the effect of oestrogen on
serum lipid levels but may result in markedly elevated serum LDL
and cholesterol levels (15). It is therefore possible that administration of a combination of synthetic steroids may result in
effects on serum lipid levels which cannot be accounted for by the
effects of these steroids administered singly. Furthermore, the
response of serum lipid and lipoprotein levels to gonadal steroid
administration may differ in various subjects. Thus, we have
noted a striking increase of serum cholesterol levels during administration of methandienone to six subjects with maturity onset diabetes mellitus one of which is illustrated in Figure 5.

Longitudinal studies of the effects of combined oral contraceptives on serum lipid and lipoprotein levels have produced somewhat conflicting results. Pincus (16) found no change of serum
cholesterol or β-lipoprotein levels in 41 premenopausal women
treated with 'Enovid' for 1 year. Aurell et al (4) however, found
elevated serum triglyceride and cholesterol levels in eight subjects
during treatment with 'Anovlar' for 1 year, though Brody et al (5)
found no significant change of either plasma lipid level in nine
women treated with the same drug combination for a similar period.
The same group, however, noted a significant elevation of plasma
triglyceride levels during treatment with 'Ovulen', though the rise
of plasma cholesterol was not significant. Gershberg et al (6)
noted elevated (>110 mg /100 ml) plasma triglyceride levels in 23
of 38 (61%) women receiving 'Enovid' but plasma cholesterol levels
were normal. In a previous cross-sectional study, we found serum
triglyceride levels above the upper limit of normal (131 mg /100 ml)
in 32 of 102 (31%) women receiving oral contraceptives (1). Using
the same criterion, 18% of Group A subjects and 57% of Group B
subjects had abnormally elevated serum triglyceride levels during
therapy. The difference between the two groups may partly be related to the longer mean duration of therapy in Group B subjects,
since Gershberg (6) has noted a significant correlation between
the serum triglyceride level and duration of therapy. While this
correlation did not hold for Group A subjects in the present study,
the majority of subjects had received therapy for a similar period,
i.e., 3-6 months.

Our observation of decreased serum triglyceride levels after
oral contraceptive therapy was discontinued is of importance and
confirms the previous observations of Gershberg et al (6). It
will be important to determine whether this improvement is maintained after a longer period of time.

It is not known whether the effects of oral contraceptive

therapy on serum lipid and lipoprotein levels are due to a primary
effect of the oestrogen and/or progestagen or secondary to elevated
levels of circulating hormones such as thyroxine, cortisol and
growth hormone. It is clear, however, that similar changes of
serum lipid levels occur during treatment with oestrogen alone.
Nor is it known whether the elevated serum triglyceride levels are
due to an increased rate of production or impaired removal from the
circulation. In this respect, the finding (7) that plasma post-
heparin lipolytic activity is decreased during oral contraceptive
therapy is of interest, since lipoprotein lipase is thought to be
important in the removal of circulating triglyceride from the vascular compartment (17). Little is known of the relation of rates
of synthesis of lipoprotein apoproteins, the protein moieties of
lipoproteins, to rates of lipoprotein synthesis by the liver and
release into the circulation. Oestrogen therapy, however, is known
to be associated with increased serum levels of certain carrier
proteins including transcortin, thyroxine binding globulin and
caeruloplasmin (18). It has been stated that the α and β lipoproteins during oestrogen therapy contain a greater percentage of
protein than normal (19) and the possibility exists that increased
lipoprotein levels during oral contraceptive therapy may be secondary to increased rates of lipoprotein apoprotein synthesis by the
liver.

In view of the known association of elevated serum lipid and
lipoprotein levels with the development of clinical manifestations
of atherosclerosis (20), the changes of serum lipid and lipoprotein
levels in subjects treated with oral contraceptives cannot be viewed
with equanimity. While all subjects may not develop serum lipid
levels outside the normal range, it is possible that any elevation
of any serum lipoprotein level may increase the risk of development
of atherosclerosis. It will be many years before the answers to
these questions are resolved.

SUMMARY

The effects of oral contraceptive therapy on fasting serum
triglyceride and cholesterol levels have been assessed by longitudinal studies of two groups of women. Group A consisted of 68
subjects tested before and during therapy, while Group B consisted
of 23 women initially tested while receiving oral contraceptive
medication and again after this had been discontinued. In Group A,
the mean fasting serum triglyceride level was increased during oral
contraceptive therapy, but the mean fasting serum cholesterol level
was unchanged. In Group B, however, both the mean fasting serum
cholesterol and triglyceride levels fell significantly after oral
contraceptive therapy was discontinued.

The relationships of the changes of serum lipid levels to degree of obesity, family history of diabetes, glucose tolerance, nature of oestrogen-progestagen combination, duration of therapy and day of menstrual cycle are analyzed for both groups.

Results of serum lipid changes in a small longitudinal study of six women receiving oestrogen therapy alone are described.

Possible mechanisms for the changes of serum lipid levels during oral contraceptive therapy and their significance are discussed.

REFERENCES

1. Wynn, V., Doar, J.W.H. and Mills, G.L.: Some effects of oral contraceptives on serum-lipid and lipoprotein levels. The Lancet 1:720 (1966).

2. De Lalla, O.F., Gofman, J.W. in Methods of Biochemical Analysis (edited by D. Glick). Vol. 1, p. 459 (1954), New York.

3. Kannel, W.B., Kagan, A., Revotskie, N. and Stokes, J.: Factors of risk in the development of coronary heart disease. The Framingham study. Ann. Intern. Med. 55:33 (1961).

4. Aurell, M., Cramer, K. and Rybo, G.: Serum lipids and lipoproteins during long-term administration of an oral contraceptive. The Lancet 1:291 (1966).

5. Brody, S., Kerstell, J., Nilsson, L. and Svanborg, A.: The effects of some ovulation inhibitors on the different plasma lipid fractions. Acta Medica Scand. 183:1 (1968).

6. Gershberg, H., Hulse, M. and Javier, Z.: Hypertriglyceridemia during treatment with estrogen and oral contraceptives: an alteration in hepatic function? Obst. and Gyn. 31:186 (1968).

7. Hazzard, W.R., Spiger, M.J., Bagdade, J.D. and Bierman, E.L.: Mechanisms for hypertriglyceridemia induced by oral contraceptives. Excerpta Medica International Congress Series No. 157, 39 (1968).

8. Stoker, D.J., Wynn, V. and Robertson, G.: Effect of posture on plasma cholesterol level. Br. Med. J. 1:336 (1966).

9. Zlatkis, A., Zak, B. and Boyle, A.J.: New method for the determination of serum cholesterol. J. Lab. Clin. Med. 41:486 (1953).

10. Henly, A.A.: The determination of serum cholesterol. Analyst Lond. 82:286 (1957).

11. Cramp, D.G. and Robertson, G.: The fluorometric assay of triglyceride by a semi-automated method. Anal. Biochem. (In press).

12. Furman, R.H., Howard, R.P., Norcia, L.N. and Keaty, E.C.: The influence of androgens, estrogens and related steroids on serum lipids and lipoproteins. Am. J. Med. 24:80 (1958).

13. Robinson, R.W. and Lebeau, R.J.: Effect of conjugated equine estrogens on serum lipids and the clotting mechanism. J. Atheroscler. Res. 5:120 (1965).

14. Svanborg, A. and Vikrot, O.: The effect of estradiol and progesterone on plasma lipids in oophorectomized women. Acta Medica Scand. 179:615 (1966).

15. Hood, B. and Cramer, K.: Effects on serum lipoprotein cholesterol of estrogen in combination with Δ4 - androstenedione, testosterone and methyltestosterone. Acta Med. Scand. 165:459-466 (1959).

16. Pincus, G. in Control of Fertility, p. 277 (1965) New York.

17. Havel, R.J.: Metabolism of lipids in chylomicrons and very low density lipoproteins. In Handbook of Physiology, Section 5: Adipose tissue. Edited by A.E. Renold and G.F. Cahill, Jr. p. 499 (1965). Waverly Press Inc., Baltimore.

18. Doe, R.P., Mellinger, G.T., Swaim, W.R. and Seal, U.S.: Estrogen dosage effects on serum proteins: a longitudinal study. J. Clin. Endocr. 27:1081 (1967).

19. Furman, R.H., Alaupovic, P., Bradford, R.H. and Howard, R.P.: Gonadal hormones, blood lipids and ischemic heart disease. International Symposium on Recent Advances in Atherosclerosis, Athens (1966), p. 20.

20. Kannel, W.B., Dawber, T.R., Friedman, G.D., Glennon, W.E. and McNamara, P.M.: Risks in coronary heart disease. Ann. Intern. Med. 61:888 (1964).

STUDIES ON THE MECHANISM OF HYPERTRIGLYCERIDEMIA

INDUCED BY ORAL CONTRACEPTIVES

W.R. Hazzard, M.J. Spiger and E.L. Bierman

Department of Medicine, University of Washington School
of Medicine, Seattle, Washington

We have heard convincing evidence this morning of the
alterations in plasma lipids induced by a broad range of oral
contraceptive preparations. Because of the epidemiological association between atherosclerotic cardiovascular disease and hyperlipo-
proteinemia, hypertriglyceridemia as well as hypercholesterolemia
(1), and the possibility that progestational agents may therefore
limit the relative immunity from atherosclerosis enjoyed by premenopausal women, we have begun to explore the mechanism of the
hypertriglyceridemia of oral contraceptive therapy. These studies,
then, evaluate the altered balance between triglyceride (TG) input
and removal which result in a raised plasma TG concentration in
women given oral progestational agents.

We have studied 12 normal young women, aged 20-33 years,
before and after 14 days of treatment with ethinyl estradiol, 0.05
mg--medroxyprogesterone acetate, 10 mg (Provest). Both before and
during treatment, we measured three parameters which relate to
plasma triglyceride balance: 1) Basal plasma triglyceride after
an overnight fast; 2) Post-heparin lipolytic activity (PHLA), a
measure of heparin-releasable lipoprotein lipase activity, and
indirectly, of plasma triglyceride removal capacity; and 3) Basal
serum immunoreactive insulin (IRI), a possible index of endogenous
triglyceride synthesis and plasma input.

_____

This work was supported in part by NIH Grants T07-AM-01000,
and 5R01-AM-06670. Patient studies were performed in the Clinical
Research Center, University of Washington Hospital (NIH Grant FR-37).

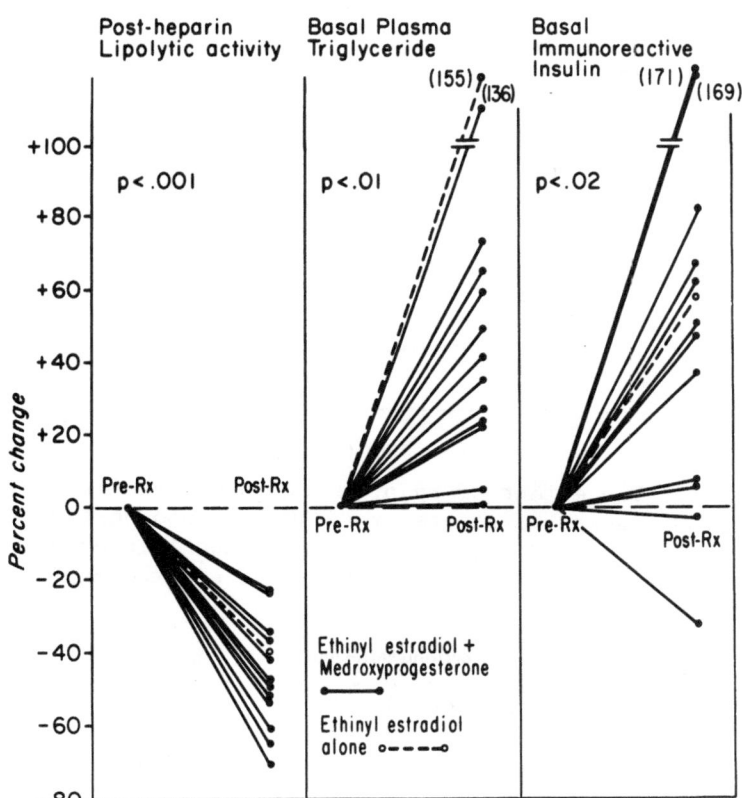

Fig. 1.   The effect of an oral contraceptive upon post-heparin lipolytic activity, basal plasma triglyceride, and basal serum immunoreactive insulin.

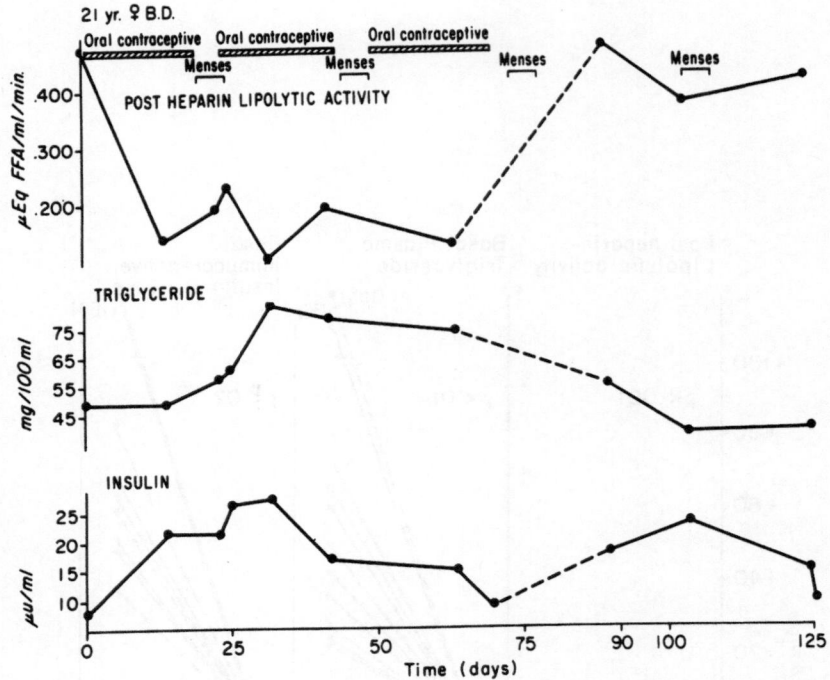

Fig. 2.   The effect of an oral contraceptive (ethinyl estradiol,.05 mg–medroxyprogesterone 10 mg) upon post–heparin lipolytic activity and basal triglyceride and immunoreactive insulin during three cycles of therapy and eight weeks after its discontinuation.

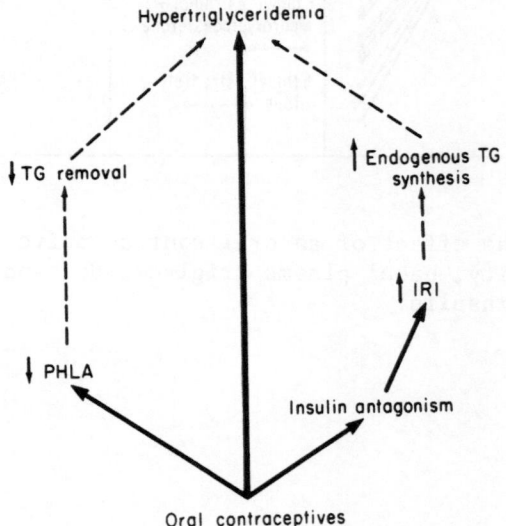

Fig. 3.   A possible scheme for the mechanism of the hypertriglyceridemia induced by oral contraceptives.

In Figure 1, we see the relative (percent) changes in the three parameters associated with two weeks of contraceptive therapy. Basal TG increased in 11 of 12 subjects by a mean for the entire group of 18.3 $\pm$ 3.8 mg% (S.E.M.), or 45% (p < .001). During the same treatment interval, basal IRI increased in 10 of 12 subjects by a group mean of 4.4 $\pm$ 1.7 µU/ml, or 56% (p < .02).

One subject, whose results are indicated by broken lines in Figure 1, was treated with ethinyl estradiol alone. She too showed an increase in basal TG, decline in PHLA, and increase in basal IRI. Her result would seem to indicate that the estrogen is by itself sufficient to cause the observed changes; however, our studies have not been designed to evaluate the relative contributions of estrogen vs. progestin, and I offer this single result only as an isolated observation.

In one subject, we followed these same three parameters at periodic intervals during 3 cycles of therapy and for six weeks following its discontinuation (Fig. 2). As can be seen in Figure 2, her basal TG increased to approximately twice pretreatment levels by the middle of the second cycle and remained at this plateau until after the drug was discontinued, when it returned to baseline levels once again. Post-heparin lipolytic activity declined promptly and remained depressed until therapy was terminated. Basal IRI was elevated but showed considerable fluctuation both during and after treatment, ultimately, however, returning to the pre-treatment value. Of particular significance in this study was the failure of the three parameters to return to pre-treatment levels between treatment cycles, no significant changes being evident 96 hours after the last dose.

Thus, our studies confirm in a prospective manner the relative hypertriglyceridemia of oral contraceptive therapy. Although the TG levels recorded lay well within the broad range of normal reported for large population groups (< 150 mg%), the trend was definite and, in the one subject followed longitudinally, persistent.

As in all forms of hypertriglyceridemia, the increase in TG levels may relate to increased plasma TG input from dietary or endogenous (hepatic) sources, impaired TG removal, mediated primarily by the heparin-releasable enzyme, lipoprotein lipase, or a combination of both. The exact mechanism of the TG increase of oral contraceptive therapy remains conjectural at this time, but the other two findings in these studies may be relevant. First, the decline in PHLA suggests an impairment in triglyceride removal (Fig. 3). A similar decline in PHLA has been reported by Fabian et al in post-menopausal women treated for 5 days with estradiol (2). A similar depression of PHLA has been reported in a physiological state of relative lipemia and hyperestrogenism, i.e., late

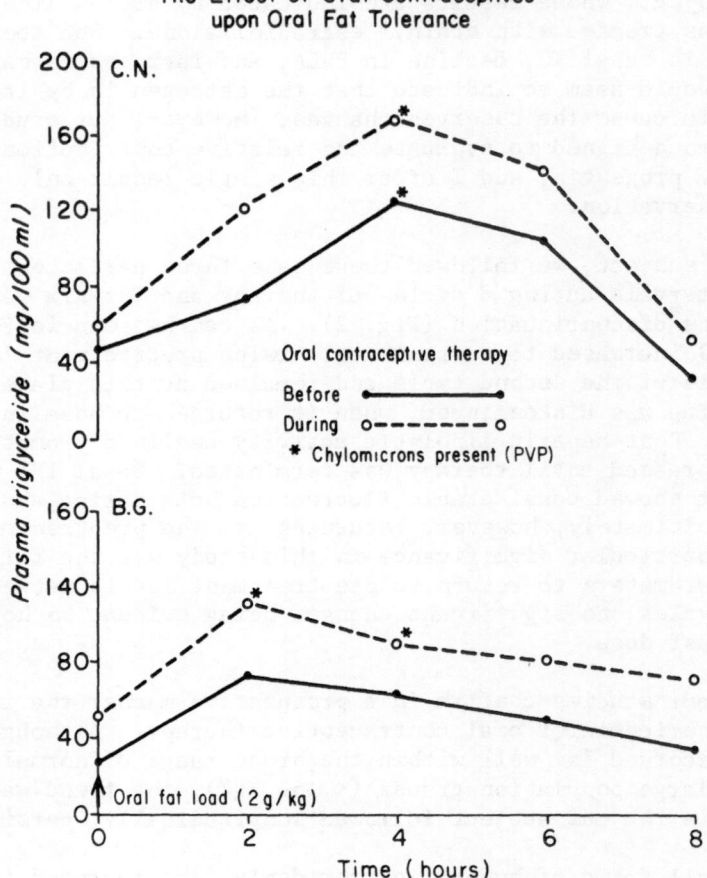

Fig. 4. The effect of ethinyl estradiol-medroxyprogesterone
upon oral fat tolerance (2 g/kg butterfat as whipping cream).

pregnancy (3). Animal studies have shown depressed tissue levels of lipoprotein lipase in late pregnancy as well (4).

However, before concluding that oral contraceptives produce a profound impairment in plasma TG removal capacity, we must note the discrepancy between the relative mildness of the TG elevation and the remarkably low absolute levels of PHLA recorded in our subjects. Several of the individuals developed PHLA values in the range of those reported in the gross exogenous lipemia of uncontrolled diabetes (5,6), myxedema (7) and familial, fat-induced lipemia (8).

Because of this discrepancy, we administered oral fat loads (2 g butter fat/kg) to six of the 12 subjects before and during therapy and followed TG and chylomicron levels for eight hours thereafter. For, although the oral fat tolerance test is an imperfect measure of TG clearing capacity (9), abnormalities in this test are evident not only in homozygous subjects with fat-induced lipemia but also in their heterozygous siblings whose basal TG levels are normal but whose tissue lipoprotein lipase activity is significantly depressed (10). The results of two of these fat tolerance tests are illustrated in Figure 4. As might be predicted, the peak TG levels recorded were higher during oral contraceptive therapy than before, but the increment above basal was not significantly increased, nor was the incremental area above basal for the entire curve appreciably altered. Thus, for the entire group of six subjects, there was no significant increase in either peak or area increment above basal. These results suggest that removal capacity for exogenous fat is not grossly impaired during oral contraceptive treatment and that the total increase in TG recorded after a fat load (basal plus increment above basal) is primarily dependent upon expansion of the basal plasma TG pool.

Thus, we are left with a depressed PHLA in the face of essentially normal removal capacity for exogenous fat. This decline in PHLA is not attributable to the presence of a circulating inhibitor of in vitro lipolysis: in three experiments no inhibition was introduced by the addition of plasma collected during oral contraceptive treatment to post-heparin plasma drawn prior to therapy.

Nor was insulin insufficiency the cause of the low PHLA, as has been shown to be responsible for the lipemia of uncontrolled diabetes (5,6). Not only were basal insulin levels increased but the administration of exogenous insulin to 3 subjects over a 24-hour period in doses sufficient to cause mild hypoglycemia failed to reverse the PHLA deficiency.

One other series of tests does provide a clue to the discrepancy between PHLA and oral fat tolerance, however. In one subject we performed heparin-PHLA dose-response tests before and

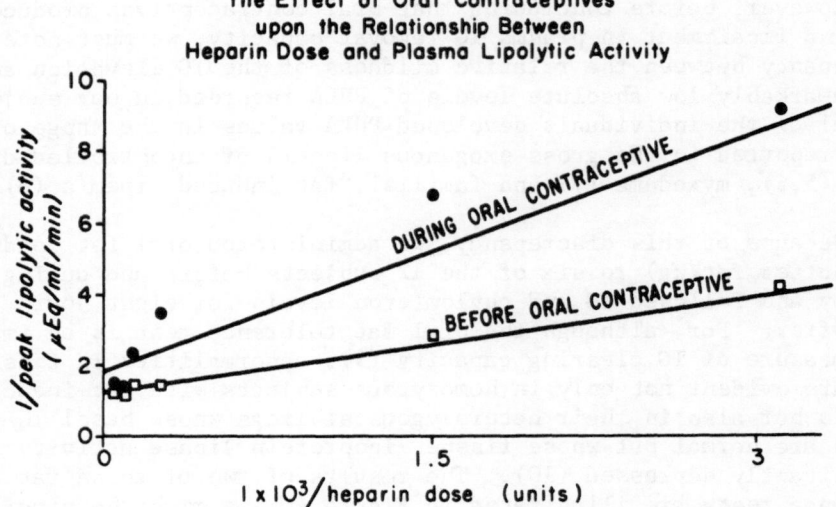

Fig. 5. Heparin-dose vs. post-heparin lipolytic activity
response before and during ethinyl estradiol-medroxyprogesterone
therapy. Before therapy, r = .970; during therapy, r = .993.

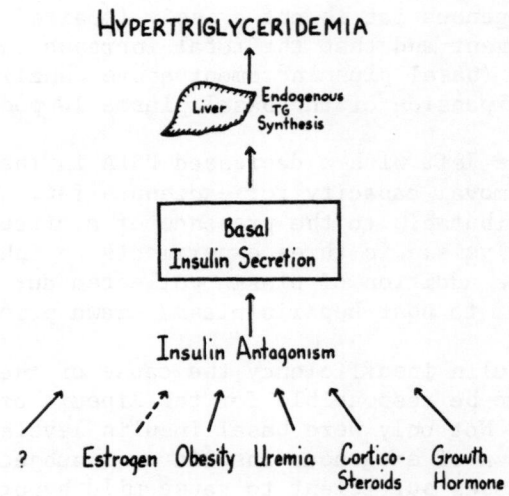

Fig. 6. Hypothesis for a mechanism of increased endogenous
triglyceride synthesis in states of peripheral insulin antagonism.

during ethinyl estradiol-medroxyprogesterone therapy. As can be seen in Figure 5, we evaluated the responses from the standpoint of the Lineweaver-Burk plot, usually applied to substrate-enzyme relations (11), but here applied to the dose-response relationship assuming an analogous interaction. We plotted the reciprocal of the velocity (of lipolysis) vs. the reciprocal of substrate concentration (in this case, heparin dose). An index of the validity of this approach is the statistical significance ($p < .001$) of the correlation coefficients in both the pre- ($r = .970$) and post-treatment ($r = .993$) states, and, more importantly, by the virtually identical lipolytic activities ("V_{max}") achieved with maximal doses of heparin in both conditions.

Thus, it is clear that with the administration of adequate doses of heparin, the apparent PHLA deficiency was overcome. Another way of expressing this conclusion is that oral contraceptive therapy seems to result in competitive inhibition of the release of lipoprotein lipase by heparin. These intriguing results suggest that a form of heparin insensitivity is induced by oral contraceptives, at least insofar as the ability to release clearing factor is concerned.

The role of endogenous heparin in plasma TG removal is uncertain but may possibly be physiologically important (12). Thus, despite the normal fat tolerance of women taking oral contraceptives and reversibility of their apparent PHLA deficiency with added heparin, a degree of limitation in TG removal capacity not detectable by the oral test may well be present. This limitation might be insignificant in the normal subject whose TG input does not saturate TG removal capacity and yet be critical in the individual with an already marginal removal ability. We are at present investigating this possibility in lipemic women whose hypertriglyceridemia has been aggravated by estrogen therapy.

The other finding which may relate to the mechanism of oral contraceptive-induced hypertriglyceridemia is the elevation in basal insulin noted after two weeks of Provest therapy. The elevated insulin levels may stimulate increased hepatic lipogenesis, an unproved but reasonable hypothesis (13,14) which receives support from the significant correlation between IRI and TG levels, both in the basal (15) and glucose-stimulated (16) states, as well as from the association reported by Farquhar et al (13) between the degree of hypertriglyceridemia induced by fat-free feedings in normal and hyperlipemic subjects and the insulin response to those feedings.

The elevated basal IRI levels induced by Provest confirm the hyperinsulinism of oral contraceptive therapy noted by Spellacy et al (17). The cause of the elevated IRI levels remains unclear, but by analogy with the hyperinsulinism of obesity (18) and other

states of insulin antagonism such as those in Figure 6, may relate
to peripheral insulin resistance conferred by the oral contraceptive and compensatory, increased insulin secretion in an attempt
to maintain euglycemia. This insulin resistance cannot be accounted
for by a change in weight per se, since weight gain was minimal in
our subjects (mean 0.9 kg), and the elevation in basal IRI exceeded
that which could be attributed to the change in weight. Of possible
relevance in accounting for insulin antagonism is the increase in
growth hormone levels reported in association with oral contraceptive therapy (19).

Thus, the relative hypertriglyceridemia of oral contraceptive
therapy may arise from impaired TG removal, as suggested by decreased PHLA, increased TG synthesis and plasma input, consistent
with the elevated basal IRI levels, or a combination of both. Our
studies at this point must be considered preliminary in that our
measurements represent indirect indices of TG input and removal.
We are currently investigating triglyceride balance by direct measurements of TG turnover in women receiving estrogens. We hope
through these studies to arrive at more definitive conclusions as
to which factor, increased input or impaired removal, is primarily
responsible for the hypertriglyceridemia of oral contraceptive
therapy.

REFERENCES

1. Albrink, M.J.: Triglycerides, lipoproteins, and coronary
artery disease. Arch. Int. Med. 109:345-359 (1962).

2. Fabian, E., Stork, A., Kobilkova, J., and Sponarova, J.:
The activity of the lipoprotein lipase and estrogens. Enzym.
Biol. Clin. 8:451-455 (1967).

3. Sandhofer, F., Sailer, S., Braunsteiner, H. and
Braitenberg, H.: Post-heparin lipoproteinlipase and schwangerschaft. Wien. Klin. Wschr. 73:392-393 (1961).

4. Otway, W., and Robinson, D.S.: The significance of
changes in tissue clearing-factor lipase activity in relation to
the lipemia of pregnancy. Biochem. J. 106:677-682 (1968).

5. Bagdade, J.D., Porte, D., Jr., and Bierman, E.L.: Diabetic
lipemia: a form of acquired fat-induced lipemia. New Eng. J. Med.
276:427-433 (1967).

6. Bagdade, J.D., Porte, D., Jr. and Bierman, E.L.: Acute
insulin withdrawal and the regulation of plasma triglyceride removal
in diabetic subjects. Diabetes 17:127-132 (1968).

7. Porte, D.,Jr., O'Hara, D.D. and Williams, R.H.: The relation between postheparin lipolytic activity and plasma triglyceride in myxedema. Metabolism 15:107-113 (1966).

8. Fredrickson, D.S., Ono, K., and Davis, L.L.: Lipolytic activity of post-heparin plasma in hypertriglyceridemia. J. Lipid Res. 4:24-33 (1963).

9. Fredrickson, D.S., Levy, R.I. and Lees, R.S.: Fat transport in lipoproteins--an integrated approach to mechanisms and disorders. Part III. New Eng. J. Med. 276:148-156 (1967).

10. Harlan, W.R., Winesett, P.S. and Wasserman, A.J.: Tissue lipoprotein lipase in normal individuals and individuals with exogenous hypertriglyceridemia and the relationship of this enzyme to assimilation of fat. J. Clin. Invest. 46:239-247 (1967).

11. Riggs, D.S.: The Mathematical Approach to Physiological Problems, Williams and Wilkins Co., Baltimore, 1963, Chapter 11, pp 272-298.

12. Robinson, D.S.: The clearing factor lipase and its action in the transport of fatty acids between the blood and the tissues. Adv. Lipid Res. 1:133-182 (1963).

13. Farquhar, J.W., Frank, A., Gross, R.C. and Reaven, G.M.: Glucose, insulin, and triglyceride responses to high and low carbohydrate diets in man. J. Clin. Invest. 45:1648-1656 (1966).

14. Bierman, E.L. and Porte, D., Jr.: Carbohydrate intolerance and lipemia. Ann. Int. Med. 68:926-933 (1968).

15. Bagdade, J.D., Porte, D., Jr. and Bierman, E.L.: Hypertriglyceridemia: a metabolic consequence of chronic renal failure. New Eng. J. Med. 279: 181-185 (1968).

16. Ford, S., Bozian, R.C. and Knowles, H.C.: Interactions of obesity, and glucose and insulin levels in hypertriglyceridemia. Amer. J. Clin Nutr. 21:904-910 (1968).

17. Spellacy, W.N., Carlson, K.L., Burk, S.A., and Schade, S.L.: Glucose and insulin alterations after one year of combination-type oral contraceptive treatment. Metabolism 17:496-501 (1968).

18. Bagdade, J.D.: Basal insulin and obesity. Lancet ii: 630-631 (1968).

19. Spellacy, W.N., Carlson, K.L. and Schade, S.L.: Human growth hormone levels in normal subjects receiving an oral contraceptive. J. Amer. Med. Assoc. 2:115-118 (1967).

POSSIBLE RELATIONSHIP BETWEEN PLASMA LIPIDS

AND HORMONAL STEROIDS

A. Svanborg

Department of Medicine, Vasa Hospital, University of
Göteberg, Gothenburg, Sweden

In order to investigate a possible influence of hormonal
steroids on plasma lipids, we have simultaneously analysed plasma
lipid concentration and the urinary excretion of 11-desoxy-17-
ketosteroids and estrogens in healthy individuals. In addition,
plasma neutral steroid sulphates were analyzed in patients with
essential hereditary hypercholesterolemia.

Table 1 shows the analyses performed. The individual phospholipids were determined by thin layer chromatography. All steroid
analyses except for the estrogen estimations were made using gas-
liquid chromatographic procedures tested as to their specificity by
combined gas-liquid chromatography-mass spectometry in the laboratories of Dr. H. Adlercreutz and of Dr. R. Vihko in Helsinki,
Finland.

The first studies were carried out on three normally menstruating women who were nulliparas. Blood specimens were drawn in the
morning every third to fourth day and 24-hour urine samples were
collected on the same days (1).

The second study was performed on another healthy woman from
the day of ovulation, during the whole pregnancy and the first
weeks after delivery. During the first 6 weeks blood and urinary
sampling was performed twice a week, later on generally every
second week (2).

The third study (3) is not yet completed and the observations
presented here are preliminary. Nine patients, four females and
five males, 39 to 64 years old, were studied once a week for three

242

Table 1

```
+---------------------------------------------------------------+
|                                                               |
|        POSSIBLE RELATIONSHIP BETWEEN PLASMA                   |
|                                                               |
|        LIPIDS AND HORMONAL STEROIDS                           |
|                                                               |
|                                                               |
|                   Analyses                                    |
|                                                               |
| Total and free cholesterol, triglycerides, free fatty acids, |
| total phospholipids, lecithin, lysolecithin, sphingomyelin and|
| cephalin.                                                     |
|                                                               |
| Plasma levels of the monosulfates of androsterone, dihydroepiandro-|
| sterone, epiandrosterone, androst-5-ene-3β, 17β-diol, pregnenolone,|
| pregn-5-ene-3β, 20α-diol, pregn-5-ene-3β, 17α, 20α-triol, the di-|
| sulphates of androst-5-ene-3β, 17α-diol, androst-5-ene-3β,    |
| 17β-diol and pregn-5-ene-3β, 20α-diol.                        |
|                                                               |
| Urinary excretion of androsterone, etiocholanolone, dehydroepi-|
| androsterone, pregnanediol, estrone, estradiol and estriol.   |
|                                                               |
+---------------------------------------------------------------+
```

to four weeks. Two of the women were still menstruating at 44 years of age. Two were postmenopausal, 54 and 60 years old. The males were 39 to 64 years old. All patients had been on a diet containing 25-35 percent caloric fat for six months to eight years. Four of these patients had subjective and objective symptoms of coronary insufficiency.

In the study of the hormonal variations during the menstrual cycle, the percentage of lecithin was correlated ($p < 0.01$) with the excretion of estrone, estradiol and total estrogens. The percentage of lysolecithin bore a slight inverse correlation ($p < 0.05$) to these hormones. Cyclic variations in the level of plasma free cholesterol was correlated ($p < 0.01$) to the temporal course on variations in pregnanediol. The plasma level of total phospholipids and total cholesterol showed a slight inverse correlation ($p < 0.05$) to the dehydroepiandrosterone excretion.

The analyses on the woman before, during and after pregnancy (Fig. 1) showed that at about the 11th week the relative and absolute level of lysolecithin started to decrease. At the same time, the excretion of estrogens had risen to above nonpregnancy levels. At about the 15th to 18th week, the increase in cholesterol, total phospholipid level and triglycerides started, corresponding in time with rapidly increasing placental activity as judged from urinary estriol determinations.

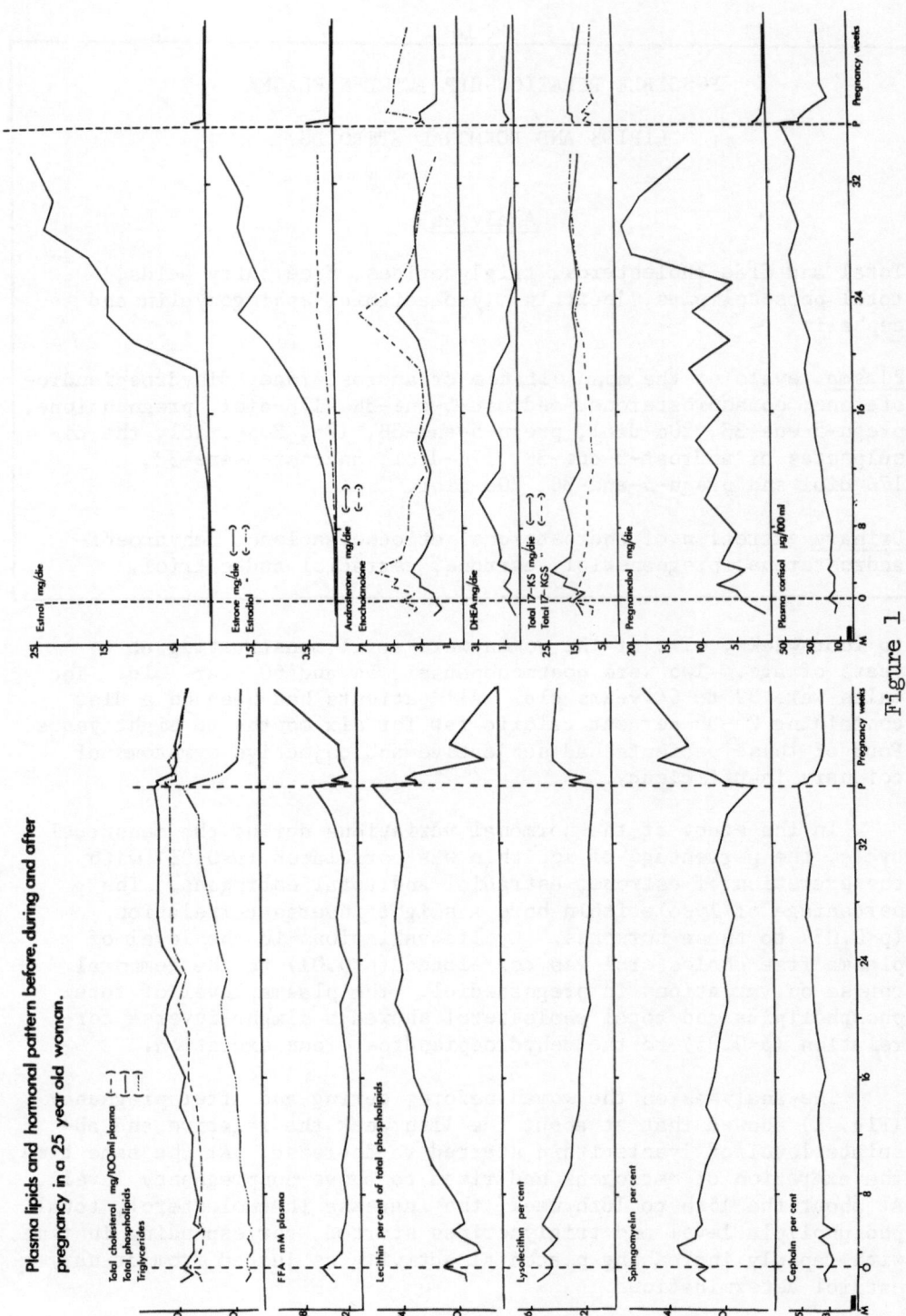

Plasma lipids and hormonal pattern before, during and after pregnancy in a 25 year old woman.

Figure 1

The patients with essential hypercholesterolemia showed that, although the homeostasis of cholesterol and phospholipids in plasma is abnormal, no gross abnormalities in the hormonal steroids have hitherto been observed. As in the healthy individuals studied, an inverse correlation seems to exist in these patients between the total phospholipid level in plasma and the dehydroepiandrosterone excretion as well as the dehydroepiandrosterone sulphate level in plasma.

These studies and other studies performed in our laboratories on pregnant women (8) on oophorectomized women treated with estradiol, progestational steroids (7), or androgenic steroids as well as studies on the influence of different anti-ovulatory drugs (4) have shown that the absolute and relative level of lysolecithin in plasma is a good indication of the balance between the estrogen activity and the androgen activity. Increased estrogen activity lowers the lysolecithin level. Norethisterone acetate and methylandrostenediol have the opposite effect. Progesterone derivatives do not seem to influence the composition of the plasma phospholipid fraction.

Various oral contraceptive preparations differ in respect to the effect on the plasma phospholipids. The combination of estradiol and a progestagen of the 17-α-hydroxy progesterone series produced marked changes similar to those seen during the last trimester of pregnancy. A combination of estradiol and a progestagen of the 19-nortestosterone series produced relatively small changes in the plasma lipids. The overall effects on the plasma lipids of combined oral contraceptives seem to reflect the competitional effects of the respective estrogenic and progestogenic components.

It seems reasonable to assume that it should be possible to make combined oral contraceptives with a wholly balanced hormonal effect on the plasma lipids. As evident from many of the reports during this conference and from our data, I think that we should stop talking about anti-ovulatory drugs as a unit but instead define the individuality of the components.

In oophorectomized women, with a lowered secretion of all ovarian steroid hormones, no significant change in the plasma phospholipid composition has been observed. The plasma lipids including the individual phospholipids were investigated in nine menopausal and ten menstruating 48-year old women selected at random in a population study (6). The percentage distribution of the phospholipids was the same in the two groups. In the clinical work we have found that the analyses of the plasma phospholipids can be used to indicate a desired good balance between administered estrogens and androgens at the treatment of oophorectomized women and postmenopausal women.

REFERENCES

1. Adlercreutz, H., Kerstell, J. and Svanborg, A.:
Simultaneous estimation of plasma cholesterol, total and individual
phospholipids, triglycerides, free fatty acids and cortisol, and
urinary estrogens, total 17-ketosteroids, individual 11-desoxy-17-
ketosteroids, total 17-ketogenic steroids and pregnanediol during
the menstrual cycle and in early pregnancy. Ann. Med. exp. Fenn.
45:285-292 (1967).

2. Adlercreutz, H., Kerstell, J. and Svanborg, A.: Plasma
lipids and hormonal steroids before, during and after pregnancy.
To be published.

3. Adlercreutz, H., Kerstell, J., Svanborg, A. and Vihko, R.:
Studies in plasma neutral steroid sulphates, urinary 11-desoxy-17
ketosteroids and estrogens, and plasma lipids in patients with
hypercholesterolemia. To be published.

4. Brody, S., Kerstell, J., Nilsson, L. and Svanborg, A.:
The effects of some ovulation inhibitors on the different plasma
lipid fractions. Acta Medica Scand. 183:1-7 (1968).

5. Felt, V. and Starka, L.: Metabolic effects of dehydroepiandrosterone and atromid in patients with hyperlipaemia.
Cor Vasa 8:40-48 (1966).

6. Hallberg, L., Högdahl, A-M., Svanborg, A. and Vikrot, O.:
Individual plasma phospholipids in women. A comparison of menstruating and menopausal 48 year old women. Acta Medica Scand.
181:143 (1967).

7. Svanborg, A. and Vikrot, O.: The effect of estradiol and
progesterone in plasma lipids in oophorectomized women. Acta
Medica Scand. 179:615-622 (1966).

8. Svanborg, A. and Vikrot, O.: Plasma lipid fractions,
including individual phospholipids at various stages of pregnancy.
Acta Medica Scand. 178:615 (1965).

GONADAL STEROID EFFECTS ON SERUM LIPIDS

R. H. Furman

Oklahoma Medical Research Foundation and the University
of Oklahoma Medical Center, Oklahoma City

The effects of gonadal hormones on serum lipids have been of
great interest to the physician because of the considerably greater
vulnerability of men to coronary heart disease in comparison with
women, whose lesser vulnerability to coronary artery disease has
been, until recently, popularly attributed to a presumed cholesterol-lowering effect of ovarian estrogen.

Attention has been focused on estrogens, especially so-called
"natural estrogens" in respect to their possible value in the
secondary prophylaxis of myocardial infarction and cerebral infarction ("stroke"). The use of estrogens in the prevention of recurrent myocardial infarction in men has yielded negative or, at
best, equivocal results. In survivors of stroke, estrogens have
been either of no prophylactic value or have tended to enhance the
likelihood of recurrent cerebral infarction. In the Veterans
Administration cooperative study of estrogen (diethylstilbestrol)
in the therapy of prostatic carcinoma, experience to date indicates
an increased incidence of thromboembolic events during estrogen
administration.

The belief is widespread that the decline in the ratio of male
to female deaths from coronary heart disease, beginning early in

Studies cited in this report as emanating from the author's
laboratory were supported in part by USPHS grants-in-aid HE-02528,
HTS-5403, HE-6915, HE-6221 and HE-07005. Support has also been
provided by the American Heart Association, the Oklahoma Heart
Association and Ayerst Laboratories, New York.

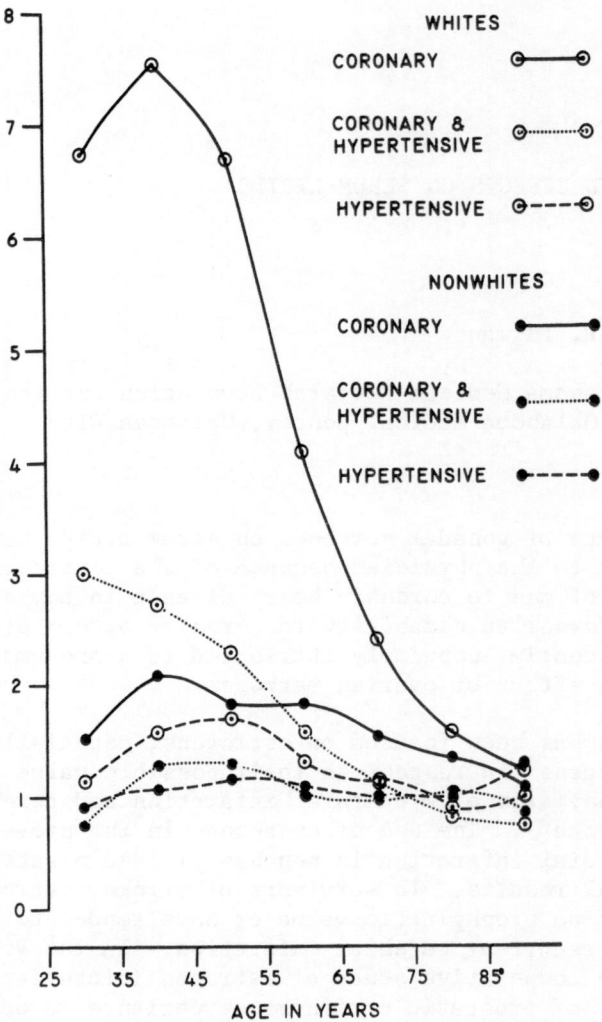

Fig. 1. Curves depicting values for the ratio of male:female
age-specific death rates for coronary heart disease and hypertension
in the United States for 1955. The male:female ratio reaches a peak
at about the 40th year, in advance of the time of the menopause, and
the high ratio is largely limited to the U.S. white population. (The
author is indebted to Dean E. Krueger of the Biometrics Research
Branch of the National Heart Institute, U.S.P.H.S., for these data
and the data depicted in Figure 2). (From Furman, R.H., et al:
Progress in Biochemical Pharmacology, Vol. 4, C.J. Miras, A.N.
Howard and R. Paoletti, editors. S. Karger, Basel/New York, 1968,
pp. 334-350.)

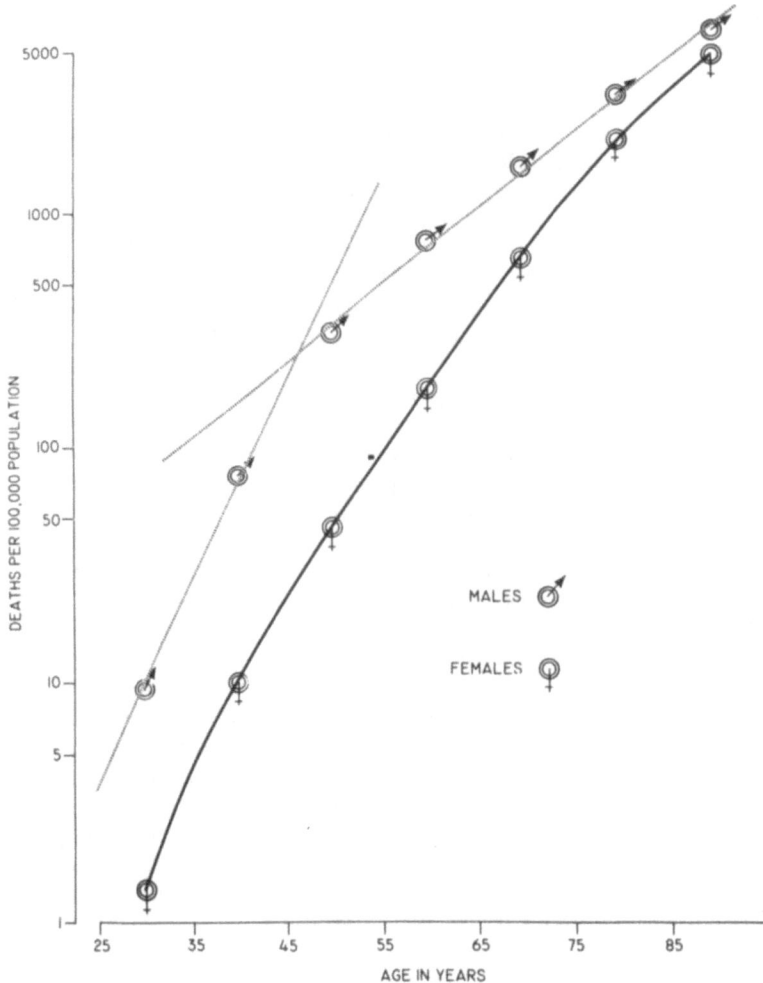

Fig. 2. Male and female mortality rates, coronary artery
disease, U.S. population for 1955. The curve for women shows no
change in slope in relation to the menopause. However, the rate of
acceleration of male mortality is sharply attenuated early in the
fifth decade, the time when the male:female ratio of deaths from
coronary artery disease begins to fall. (From Furman, R.H.: Ann.
N.Y. Acad. Sci. 149:822-933, 1968.)

the fifth decade, is due to an increased death rate from ischemic heart disease among women as a result of the menopause. Serum cholesterol levels increase with age in women, and both the increasing coronary heart disease mortality rates and the increasing serum cholesterol levels are popularly ascribed to postmenopausal decrease in ovarian estrogen production (Fig. 1).

The facts of the matter are, first, in the United States, the decline in the ratio of male to female death rates from coronary heart disease, first evident early in the fifth decade, is due to a relative flattening of the curve depicting coronary heart disease mortality rates in men as a function of age, rather than to any menopause-induced change in the coronary heart disease mortality curve for women (Fig. 2). Secondly, the effect of estrogen administration on serum cholesterol levels is too variable to support the presumption that increasing serum cholesterol levels with age in women beyond the menopause are due to estrogen deficiency. The subject has been reviewed recently by the author (1).

Serum cholesterol and phospholipid levels in women are reported to be similar to, or higher than, those of men (2-5) and to show different age-sex trends. In women, in contrast to men, average serum cholesterol concentrations increase steadily with age, without evidence of a menopause-related change. In men in the United States, mean serum cholesterol levels rise with age until about age 50. Thereafter, they plateau for a few years and then diminish with advancing age.

Serum lipid concentrations are reported to vary with the menstrual cycle. Oliver and Boyd (6) reported that serum cholesterol and phospholipid concentrations are lowest at about the time of ovulation, i.e., when estrogen production is maximal; however, Adlercreutz and Tallqvist (7), using a different technique for determining the time of ovulation, observed highest lipid values at the time of ovulation (10th to 14th day) with lowest values occurring over the succeeding four or five days.

Serum lipids increase during pregnancy (8) (although Masai women appear to be an exception in this respect (9)). During the 15th to 18th week of pregnancy serum cholesterol, phospholipid and triglyceride concentrations begin to increase, along with increased placental estrogen synthesis, as evidenced by urinary estriol excretion (10).

Estrogen administration has been reported to diminish the cholesterol: phospholipid ratio (11-23) by increasing serum phospholipid concentrations and/or lowering serum cholesterol concentrations, and to increase serum triglyceride concentrations (24).

Androgen administration lowers serum triglyceride and phospholipid concentrations, while the effect on serum cholesterol is variable (25). The triglyceride-lowering effect of androgens may be of value in the management of certain hyperlipemic states (24), as is noted below.

As various physical-chemical methods for lipoprotein analysis became available, sex-differences were demonstrated in the distribution of serum lipoproteins. Russ, Eder and Barr (15-18,26) observed that in plasma from young women there was relatively more cholesterol in Cohn fractions IV + V + VI (α-lipoproteins), and relatively less in fractions I + III (β-lipoproteins) in comparison with men. Lewis, Green and Page (27-29) noted higher concentrations of high density lipoproteins (HDL α-lipoproteins, d 1.063-1.21 g/ml) and lower concentrations of low density lipoproteins (LDL, β-lipoproteins d 1.006-1.063 g/ml, S_f 0-20) in women in comparison with men. Gofman, Jones, Lindgren, Lyon, Elliott and Strisower (30) noted lower concentrations of S_f 10-20 lipoproteins in serum from young women than in serum from men of comparable age. Havel, Eder, and Bragdon (31) similarly noted that a greater proportion of the plasma lipids were transported as HDL in women. Using paper electrophoretic techniques, Nikkila (32) and Antonini, Piva, Salvini and Sordi (33) observed that relatively more serum lipid was present as α-lipoprotein in young women than in young men. Furman, Howard and Imagawa (34), in a study of male castrates, observed that serum HDL concentrations were greater in eunuchs than in noncastrated control subjects.

Barclay and associates (35) observed that the concentration of HDL in the sera of 10 of 11 premenopausal women increased at or near the 14th day of the menstrual cycle.

An increase in the cholesterol content of HDL and a decrease in LDL cholesterol, during estrogen administration, were first observed by Barr, Russ and Eder (15-18). The effect of androgens was reported to be opposite to that of estrogens (16,18,36). No change in serum lipids or LDL was observed by Engelberg, Glass, and Marcus (37,38), during the administration of estradiol for periods as long as four months, although a slight increase in S_f 12-100 lipoproteins was observed during testosterone administration. Robinson and associates (23), utilizing paper electrophoresis, noted a diminished beta/alpha lipoprotein ratio in subjects treated with estrogens. Oliver and Boyd (39), also utilizing paper electrophoresis, noted that estrogen administration diminished the beta/alpha lipoprotein ratio, β cholesterol, serum cholesterol and C/P ratios in men with coronary artery disease whose serum cholesterol levels were greater than 260 mg %. Methyltestosterone administration was stated to have an opposite effect.

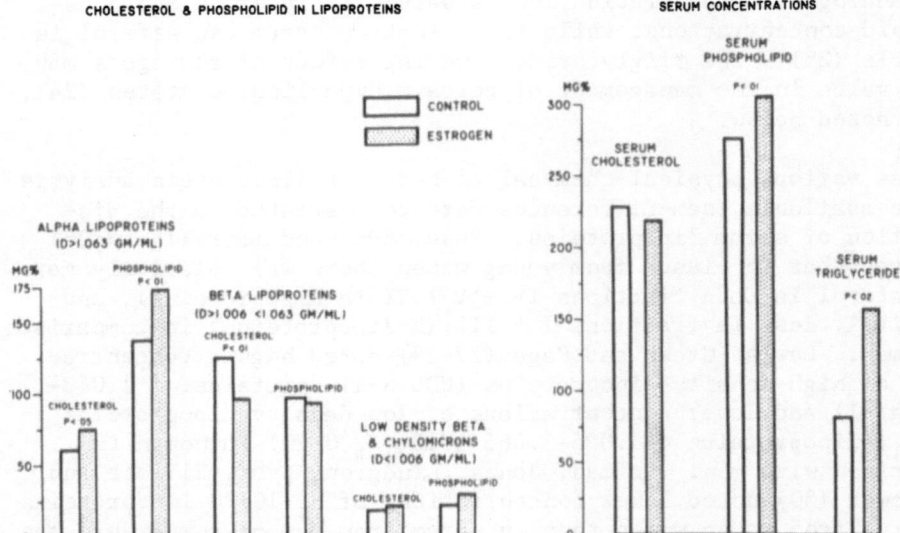

Fig. 3. Effects of estrogen administration in seven normolipemic, hypoestrogenic women. Significant increases in serum and
α lipoprotein phospholipid and serum triglyceride are noted, while
β lipoprotein cholesterol diminished. (From Furman, R.H., et al:
Progress in Biochemical Pharmacology, Vol. 2, D. Kritchevsky, R.
Paoletti and D. Steinberg, editors. S. Karger, Basel/New York, 1962,
pp. 215-249.)

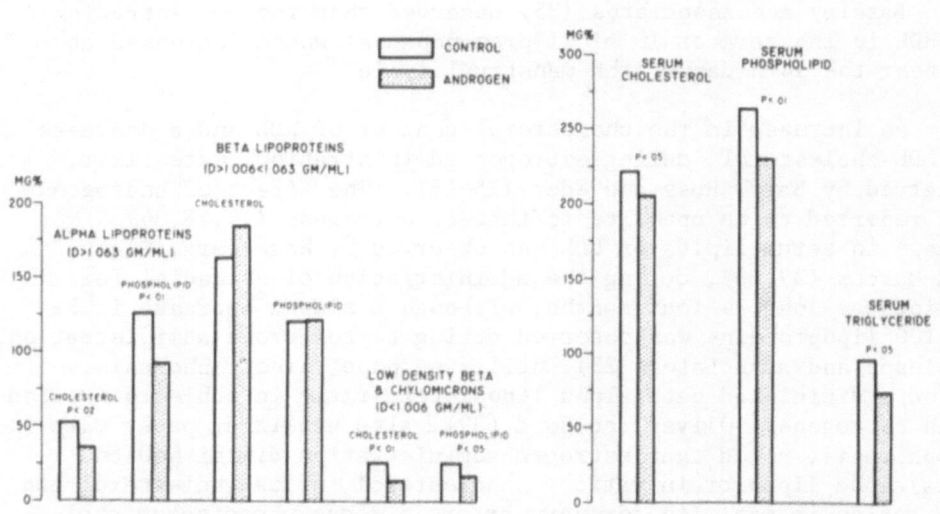

Fig. 4. Effects of androgen administration in five normolipemic men. Significant decreases of α lipoprotein lipids, VLDL
lipids and serum lipids are noted. (From Furman, R.H., et al:
Progress in Biochemical Pharmacology, Vol. 2, D. Kritchevsky, R.
Paoletti and D. Steinberg, editors. S. Karger, Basel/New York, 1962,
pp. 215-249.)

Utilizing analytical ultracentrifugation at solvent density
1.210 g/ml, Furman, Howard, Norcia and Keaty (25) observed that
estrogens promptly and consistently increased HDL concentrations
while androgens lowered them. The LDL concentrations either did
not change, or changed in a direction opposite to that of HDL,
when gonadal steroids were administered. When the concentrations
of HDL and LDL varied inversely, serum cholesterol concentrations
showed little or no change. When LDL concentrations failed to
change during gonadal steroid administration, serum total cholesterol and phospholipid levels varied with HDL concentrations.
Serum phospholipid concentrations vary with HDL concentrations because of the relatively high phospholipid content of HDL. The
high solvent density (1.210 g/ml) employed in these studies (25)
made it virtually impossible to detect changes in the triglyceride-
rich VLDL fraction (very low density lipoproteins, d<1.006 g/ml),
since the high triglyceride content VLDL imparts a density so low
that most of these particles had undergone flotation during acceleration of the rotor.

Subsequently, utilizing preparative ultracentrifugation, the
administration of androgenic anabolic steroids was noted to lower
triglyceride-rich VLDL as well as HDL (40), and estrogenic steroids
to increase them (24) (Figs. 3,4).

In normolipemic subjects, estrogen administration increases
HDL and VLDL lipids (24). Since HDL is rich in phospholipid (C/P
ratio approximately 0.4 (41)) and VLDL is rich in triglyceride,
the net effect of estrogen administration on serum lipid concentrations is an increased concentration of serum phospholipid and
triglyceride and a diminished C/P ratio.

While the effect of estrogen administration on the serum
total cholesterol concentration is relatively slight in normolipemic women, due to the tendency for changes of HDL and LDL
concentrations to be reciprocal, it is noteworthy that serum triglyceride concentrations (VLDL) increase, although rarely to
grossly abnormal levels (24).

The tendency for LDL concentrations to diminish during estrogen administration is best observed in women with familial hypercholesterolemia (hyperbetalipoproteinemia, "type II hyper-
lipidemia"). In such subjects significant lowering of serum
cholesterol concentrations may be noted, although serum triglyceride and HDL concentrations increase (24).

Progestational steroids (progesterone in oil intramuscularly
or sublingual progesterone, and allopregnanolone orally) had
little or no effect on serum lipids and lipoproteins in six subjects, although oral progesterone produced significant reduction
of HDL in one (25), i.e., had an "androgenic" effect.

The decreases in HDL and VLD1 concentrations characteristic
of androgen administration impart to this gonadal steroid serum
lipid lowering properties, one of which may prove useful in the
management of certain hyperlipidemic conditions in man. In respect
to the latter, the administration of methyltestosterone or methyl-
androstanopyrazole (Winstrol) has proved effective in achieving
prolonged lowering of serum lipid concentrations in subjects with
carbohydrate-accentuated or "mixed" hyperlipemia (24). One possibly disadvantageous side effect of androgen administration is a
slight to moderate increase in hematocrit values resulting from
androgen stimulation of hematopoiesis. Occasionally, the administration of C-17 alkylated androgenic-anabolic steroids may result
in markedly increased serum lipid levels, due to increased LDL and
VLDL lipid. These lipid changes may herald occult or manifest
intrahepatic cholestasis (e.g., "methyltestosterone jaundice")
which they accompany.

The lowering of serum HDL concentrations characteristic of
androgen administration accounts for the remarkable cholesterol-
lowering effect of testosterone derivatives in such species as the
dog (42) in which approximately 70% of the serum cholesterol and
80% of the serum phospholipid can be accounted for as HDL (43).
Similar lipid-lowering effects have been observed in the rat
(44,45) and in chickens (46). Dogs on a diet high in fat may
develop increased serum lipid levels when given methyltestosterone
(47) in spite of lowered HDL concentrations, due to an increased
lipid content of LDL under these conditions.

It might be anticipated that estrogen would increase serum
lipid concentrations in the dog because of the characteristic
HDL-elevating and triglyceride-elevating effect of estrogen. We
have observed increased serum cholesterol and phospholipid concentrations, but no changes in the serum triglyceride levels, in
dogs given estrogen (Premarin) for periods of ten weeks.

In adult healthy subjects, differences related to age and sex
are evident in respect to the serum cholesterol, phospholipid and
triglyceride concentrations, and in respect to the relative amounts
of the serum lipids present in the major lipoprotein fractions.
Postmenopausal women and adult men differ from premenopausal women
in that the latter have a smaller proportion of serum lipid present
in the form of VLDL. Since VLDL are rich in triglyceride, men and
postmenopausal women have higher average serum triglyceride concentrations. Additionally, postmenopausal women have more lipid
present in the HDL and VDL fractions than do either men or premenopausal women (Fig. 5).

It is thus evident that, in women, the lipid content of all
lipoprotein fractions increases with age with the result that the

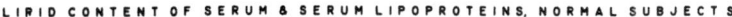

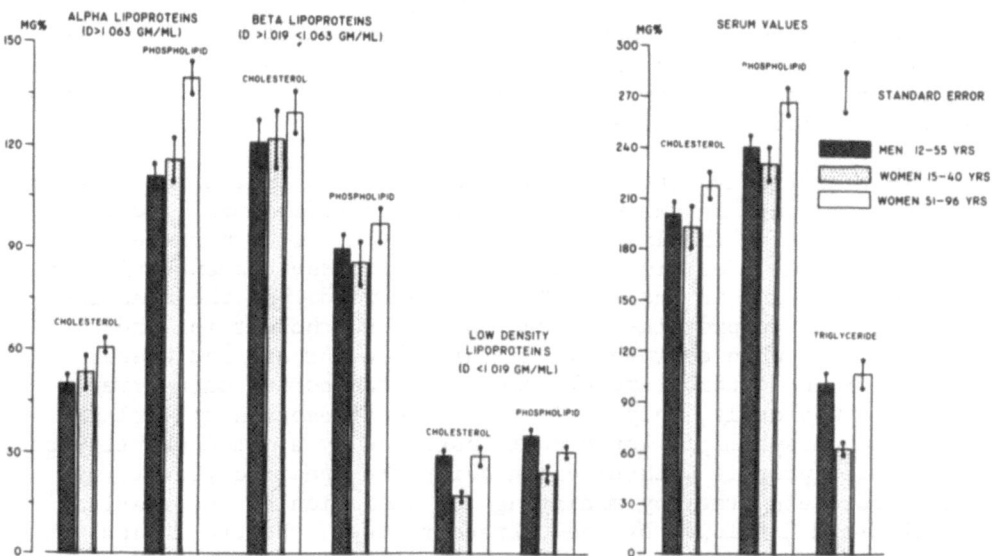

Fig. 5.   Cholesterol and phospholipid content of serum and
α, β and VLD (d < 1.019 g/ml) lipoproteins observed in 18 men, 11
premenopausal women and seven postmenopausal women. Postmenopausal
women have significantly more cholesterol in α lipoprotein (HDL)
than men and more phospholipid in α lipoprotein and in serum than
either men or premenopausal women. Premenopausal women have significantly less VLD (d < 1.019 g/ml) lipoprotein cholesterol and
phospholipid, and. significantly lower serum triglyceride concentrations, than men or postmenopausal women. (From Furman, R.H.,
et al: Progress in Biochemical Pharmacology, Vol. 2, D. Kritchevsky,
R. Paoletti and D. Steinberg, editors. S. Karger, Basel/New York,
1962, pp. 215-249.)

average serum concentrations of cholesterol, phospholipid and triglyceride are highest, in the older age group, in postmenopausal
women. The differences between the serum lipid concentrations and
the serum lipoprotein patterns of premenopausal and postmenopausal
women are often ascribed to differences in ovarian estrogen production. However, the administration of estrogenic hormones to estro-
gen-deficient women does not produce changes in the serum lipid and
lipoprotein pattern such that the pattern comes to resemble that of
the younger premenopausal women. Thus, it seems unlikely that the
effects of gonadal hormones on serum lipids can be offered by way
of explanation of the increased susceptibility of men to coronary
heart disease.

The effects of gonadal steroid administration on serum lipoprotein concentrations have been determined, classically, by

measurement of the lipid content of various lipoprotein fractions isolated by ultracentrifugal, electrophoretic, macromolecular or other physical-chemical techniques, before and after the administration of hormone. Comparison of the serum cholesterol, phospholipid or total lipid content with the sum of these lipids in the serum lipoprotein fractions indicates good "recovery" of serum lipoprotein lipid, i.e., 90% or better.

No quantitative studies have been reported indicating whether or not any change in the protein content of individual lipoproteins accompanies the lipid changes observed during hormone administration, i.e., is there any change in the concentration of "carrier protein" in the serum? In other words, is there an increase in HDL apoprotein-A as well as in HDL cholesterol and phospholipid, when estrogen is administered, or are increased amounts of cholesterol and phospholipid transported on carrier protein? Obviously, only limited additional amounts of cholesterol and phospholipid could be transported by a fixed quantity of HDL carrier protein without diminishing the specific gravity of the lipoprotein, thereby modifying its flotation in the gravitational field developed by the ultracentrifuge. However, since the density range of HDL extends from approximately 1.25 to 1.063 g/ml, and it consists of 49% protein, changes of some magnitude in the cholesterol and phospholipid content of HDL could occur without altering HDL density to the degree whereby the lipoprotein would no longer possess an ultracentrifugal flotation rate within the range characteristic of HDL.

A preliminary study of this problem has been made in this laboratory (24,48). Estrogen administration was observed to diminish the content of cholesterol relative to the content of protein in both HDL (α) and LDL (β) (Fig. 6). The change was more marked in HDL. The phospholipid content changed relatively little, as a result, while the cholesterol/protein ratio was diminished, the phospholipid/protein ratio was diminished to a much lesser degree. In these studies, the subjects received equilin sulfate, 10 mg per day or conjugated equine estrogens (Premarin) 15 mg per day. In two subjects who were given smaller doses of estrogen, a diminished content of protein and an increased content of cholesterol and phospholipid were observed in the VLDL fraction. However, the smaller estrogen dose employed in this study had no effect on the composition of HDL or LDL in one subject, although it diminished HDL cholesterol relative to protein in the other. It is of interest that, in the subject in whom VLDL phospholipid increased significantly during the administration of small doses of estrogen, there was, however, no increase in serum triglyceride concentration or VLDL triglyceride content (24).

The effects of methyltestosterone administration on HDL and

EFFECTS OF ESTROGEN ON THE CHOLESTEROL/PROTEIN RATIOS OF SERUM LIPOPROTEINS

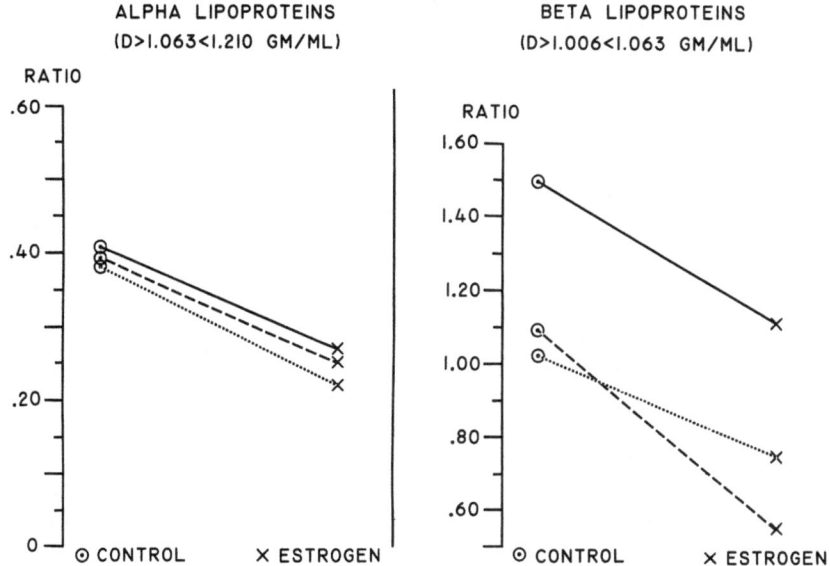

Fig. 6.   Cholesterol:protein ratios in purified HDL (alpha
lipoprotein) and LDL (beta lipoprotein) during estrogen administration.   The cholesterol:protein ratios fell in both lipoprotein
fractions during estrogen administration.   (From Furman, R.H.,
et al: Progress in Biochemical Pharmacology, Vol. 2, D. Kritchevsky,
R. Paoletti, and D. Steinberg, editors.   S. Karger, Basel/New York,
1962.)

LDL have been studied in three men. The effect on HDL composition
was observed to be opposite that noted during estrogen administration in other subjects. The effect on LDL content was not uniform
and the variability of the response and the preliminary nature of
these studies do not permit conclusions in respect to androgen
effects on lipoprotein composition at this time. No analysis of
VLDL composition has been made in respect to the effects of androgen administration.

     These studies suggest that estrogen administration diminishes
the cholesterol content of the HDL particle relative to the phospholipid and protein content, and increases the concentration of
HDL particles in the serum. The latter conclusion is based on the
fact that during estrogen administration relatively and absolutely
more of the serum cholesterol can be accounted for in the HDL
fraction. The relative constancy of the ratio of phospholipid to
protein in HDL during estrogen administration is consistent with
the suggestion that the HDL carrier protein is a phospholipoprotein
(24). Estrogen thus may be regarded as a cholesterol-lowering

hormone in respect to the cholesterol content of the HDL particle
(and to a lesser extent of the LDL particle), while it increases
the concentration of HDL particles in the blood.

Conversely, these studies suggest that the effect of androgen
administration is to diminish the concentration of HDL particles
in the blood, each particle containing more cholesterol relative
to HDL protein than it did prior to androgen administration.

The parallelism in the changes of HDL and VLDL (triglyceride)
concentrations when either estrogen or androgen is administered is
worthy of note.

Thus, when estrogens are administered, triglyceride-rich
VLDL and phospholipid and protein-rich HDL increase. Conversely,
androgen administration diminishes HDL and VLDL. The role of HDL
in the transport of triglyceride (as VLDL), while as yet largely
unknown, may prove to be an extremely important one. The high
phospholipid and protein content of HDL might stabilize the VLDL
particle, act as a cofactor for triglyceride lipolysis, possibly
by providing some conformational requirement, or facilitate lipoprotein transport across membranes. That HDL plays an essential
role in the transport of VLDL in the serum of healthy subjects is
suggested by the observation that in hyperglyceridemic (hyperlipemic) syndromes HDL deficiency, both absolute and relative, is
invariably present. Furthermore, there is evidence that HDL particles are contained in the VLDL fraction (41,49,50).

The mechanism whereby gonadal hormones bring about such
extraordinary changes in the content and composition of serum
lipids and lipoproteins is largely unknown. It is of interest to
note that estrogens appear to be without effect on the serum lipid
and lipoprotein pattern in individuals whose diets lack protein
(51,52). On the other hand, testosterone administration during
dietary protein deprivation not only abolishes the protein anabolic
effect of testosterone but, additionally, causes marked decreases
in the concentrations of LDL and HDL with the result that the
serum lipid level falls to extraordinarily low values (e.g., cholesterol concentrations below 30 mg %). Testosterone diminishes
the incorporation of C^{14} acetate into serum cholesterol (mainly
free cholesterol) in dogs (43), diminishes the concentration of
HDL particles in the serum and reduces the incorporation of C^{14}-
lysine into HDL protein (53).

Postheparin lipoprotein lipase activity is diminished in
women during estrogen administration. It seems unlikely that this
is the principal mechanism whereby estrogens elevate serum triglyceride concentrations, since we have observed subnormal levels
of postheparin lipoprotein lipase activity in women on estrogen

therapy in whom increased concentrations of serum triglycerides
did not occur.

The administration of clofibrate (ethyl ester of chlorophen-
oxy-isobutyric acid) will lower serum triglyceride levels in
subjects with estrogen-induced increases in serum triglyceride
concentrations.

The increased serum triglyceride levels accompanying estrogen
administration may result from an increased hepatic synthesis of
endogenous triglyceride (fatty acids), released to the blood
stream in the form of triglyceride-rich VLDL. Estrogen-stimulated
release of growth hormone impairs the insulin response to a
glucose load and the resulting high insulin levels and elevated
blood glucose concentrations would increase hepatic fatty acid
synthesis. This situation would appear similar to the increased
hepatic synthesis of VLDL observed in certain moderately obese,
hyperlipemic subjects with impaired carbohydrate tolerance and
exaggerated insulin responses to glucose loads.

It seems probable that the increased concentrations of serum
triglycerides, cholesterol and phospholipids, along with impaired
carbohydrate tolerance and increased levels of insulin and growth
hormone, observed during the administration of oral contraceptives,
are due to the estrogen component of the contraceptive pill.

Noteworthy in this respect is the observation of Aurell,
Cramer and Rybo (54) that five of eight women on an oral contraceptive (containing 50 micrograms of 17-ethynyl-estradiol and 4
milligrams of 17 α-ethynyl-19-nortestosterone acetate) who were
followed with repeated serum lipid determinations over a period of
one year developed increased serum triglyceride concentrations.
Although knowledge of the effects of progestational agents on serum
lipids and lipoproteins, and on glucose tolerance and levels of
human growth hormone and insulin is limited, it would appear unlikely that the progestational agent in the oral contraceptive
mixture plays a significant role in the genesis of the changes,
unless that agent is itself an androgenic-anabolic steroid, or
metabolized to a derivative with a testosterone-like action. In
our experience, the combined administration of androgen and estrogen in "physiologically equivalent" amounts results in an effect
on serum lipoproteins which is characteristic of androgen (25).

Acknowledgments: The author wishes to point out that the studies
reported herein as originating in this laboratory represent the
efforts of several collaborators including P. Alaupovic, R. H.
Bradford, J. Drake, R. P. Howard and M. McDearmon. The manuscript
was prepared by Mrs. L. Stansberry.

REFERENCES

1. Furman, R.H.: Are gonadal hormones (estrogens and androgens) of significance in the development of ischemic heart disease?
Ann. New York Acad. Sci. 149:822-833 (1968).

2. Kornerup, V.: Concentrations of cholesterol, total fat
and phospholipid in serum of normal men. Arch. Int. Med. Exp.
85:398-415 (1950).

3. Peters, J.P. and Van Slyke, D.D.: Quantitative Clinical
Chemistry. Interpretations, Vol. 1 (Williams and Wilkins Co.,
Baltimore, 1946).

4. Block, W.J., Barker, N.W. and Mann, F.D.: Effect of
small doses of heparin in increasing the transluscence of plasma
during alimentary lipemia. Studies in normal persons and patients
having atherosclerosis. Circulation 4:674-678 (1951).

5. Moore, F.E. and Gordon, T.: Serum cholesterol levels of
adults. United States 1960-1962, U.S. Department of Health,
Education and Welfare, National Center for Health Statistics,
Series 11, Number 22, United States Government Printing Office,
Washington, D.C. (1967).

6. Oliver, M.F. and Boyd, G.S.: Changes in the plasma
lipids during the menstrual cycle. Clin. Sci. 12:217-222 (1953).

7. Adlercreutz, H. and Tallqvist, G.: Variations in the
serum total cholesterol and hematocrit values in normal women
during the menstrual cycle. Scand. J. Clin. Lab. Invest. 11:1-9
(1959).

8. Peters, J.P., Heineman, M. and Man, E.B.: The lipids of
serum in pregnancy. J. Clin. Invest 30:388-394 (1951).

9. Mann, G.V. and Shaffer, R.D.: Cholesteremia in pregnant
Masai women. J. Am. Med. Assoc. 197:1071-1073 (1966).

10. Adlercreutz, H., Kerstell, J. and Svanborg, A.:
Simultaneous estimation of plasma cholesterol, total and individual phospholipids, triglycerides, free fatty acids and cortisol,
and urinary estrogens, total 17-ketosteroids, individual 11-deoxy-
17-ketosteroids and pregnanediol during the menstrual cycle and in
early pregnancy. Ann. Med. Exp. Fenn. 45:285-292 (1967).

11. Eilert, M.L.: The effects of estrogens upon the partition of the serum lipids in female patients. Amer. Heart J.
38:472 (1949).

12. Eilert, M.L.: The effect of estrogens upon the partition of the serum lipids in female patients. Metabolism 2:137-145 (1953).

13. Oliver, M.F. and Boyd, G.S.: The effect of estrogens on the plasma lipids in coronary artery disease. Amer. Heart J. 47:348-359 (1954).

14. Oliver, M.F. and Boyd, G.S.: The influence of the sex hormones on the circulatory lipids and lipoproteins in coronary sclerosis. Circulation 13:82-91 (1956).

15. Barr, D.P., Russ, E.M. and Eder, H.A.: Influence of estrogens on lipoproteins in atherosclerosis. Trans. Assoc. Amer. Physicians 65:102-113 (1952).

16. Barr, D.P.: Some chemical factors in the pathogenesis atherosclerosis. Circulation 8:641-654 (1953).

17. Barr, D.P., Russ, E.M. and Eder, H.A.: Section VII of Blood cells and plasma proteins; in Tullis' Protein-lipid relationships in plasma, Ch. 4 (Academic Press, New York 1953).

18. Russ, E.M., Eder, H.A. and Barr, D.P.: Influence of gonadal hormones on protein-lipid relationships in human plasma. Amer. J. Med. 19:4-24 (1955).

19. Steiner, A., Payson, H. and Kendall, F.E.: Effect of estrogenic hormone on serum lipids in patients with coronary atherosclerosis. Circulation 11:784-788 (1955).

20. Marett, W.C. and Vivas, J.R.: The effect of oral estrogens on serum cholesterol and total lipids. U.S. Armed Forces Med. J. 4:1439-1448 (1953).

21. Gitman, L. and Greenblatt, I.J.: Effect of intravenously administered estrogen in cardiovascular disease. Angiology 4:502-509 (1953).

22. Gertler, M.M., Hudson, P.B. and Jost, H.: Effects of castration and diethylstilbestrol on the serum lipid pattern in man. Geriatrics 8:500-503 (1953).

23. Robinson, R.W., Higano, N., Cohen, W.D., Sniffen, R.C. and Sherer, J.W., Jr.: Effects of estrogen therapy on hormonal functions and serum lipids in men with coronary atherosclerosis. Circulation 14:365-372 (1956).

24. Furman, R.H., Alaupovic, P. and Howard, R.P.: Effects of androgens and estrogens on serum lipids and the composition and concentration of serum lipoproteins in normolipemic and hyperlipidemic states. Prog. Biochem. Pharmacol. 2:215-249 (Basel/New York 1967).

25. Furman, R.H., Howard, R.P., Norcia, L.N. and Keaty, E.C.: The influence of androgens, estrogens and related steroids on serum lipids and lipoproteins. Observations in hypogonadal and normal human subjects. Amer. J. Med. 24:80-97 (1958).

26. Russ, E.M., Eder, H.A. and Barr, D.P.: Protein-lipid relationships in humn plasma. I. In normal individuals. Amer. J. Med. 11:468-479 (1951).

27. Lewis, L.A., Green, A.A. and Page, I.H.: Ultracentrifuge lipoprotein patterns of serum of normal, hypertensive and hypothyroid animals. Amer. J. Physiol. 171:391-400 (1952).

28. Lewis, L.A., Green, A.A. and Page, I.H.: The alpha and beta lipoprotein pattern of normal and pathological human sera. Fed. Proc. 10:84 (1951).

29. Lewis, L.A. and Page, I.H.: Electrophoretic and ultracentrifugal analysis of serum lipoproteins of normal, nephrotic and hypertensive persons. Circulation 7:707-717 (1953).

30. Gofman, J.W., Jones, H.B., Lindgren, F.T., Lyon, T.P., Elliott, H.A. and Strisower, B.: Blood lipids and human atherosclerosis. Circulation 2:161-178 (1950).

31. Havel, R.J., Eder, H.A. and Bragdon, J.H.: The distribution and chemical composition of ultracentrifugally separated lipoproteins in human serum. J. Clin. Invest. 34:1345-1353 (1955).

32. Nikkila, E.: Studies on the lipid-protein relationships in normal and pathological sera and the effect of heparin on serum lipoproteins. Scand. J. Clin. Lab. Invest. (Suppl. 8) 5:1-101 (1953).

33. Antonini, F.M., Piva, G., Salvini, L. and Sordi, A.: Lipoproteine ed eparina nel guardo umorale della chemiopatogenesi dell'arterosclerosi. Gior. Gerontol. (Suppl. 1), 1-96 (1953).

34. Furman, R.H., Howard, R.P. and Imagawa, R.: Serum lipid and lipoprotein concentrations in castrate and noncastrate institutionalized male subjects. Circulation 14:490-491 (1956).

35. Barclay, M., Barclay, R.K., Skipski, V.P., Terebus-Kekish, O., Mueller, E.S. and Elkins, W.L.: Fluctuations in human serum lipoproteins during the normal menstrual cycle. Biochem. J. 96:205-209 (1965).

36. Barr, D.P.: Influence of sex and sex hormones upon the development of atherosclerosis and upon the lipoproteins of plasma. J. Chron. Dis. 1:63-85 (1955).

37. Glass, S.J., Engelberg, H., Marcus, R., Jones, H.B. and Gofman, J.: Lack of effect of administered estrogens in the serum lipids and lipoproteins of male and female patients. Metabolism 2:133-136 (1953).

38. Engelberg, H. and Glass, S.J.: Influence of physiologic doses of sex steroid hormones on serum lipids and lipoproteins in humans. Metabolism 4:298-301 (1955).

39. Oliver, M.F. and Boyd, G.S.: Endocrine aspects of coronary sclerosis. Lancet 2:1273 (1956).

40. Howard, R.P. and Furman, R.H.: Metabolic and serum lipid effects of methylandrostane and methylandrostene pyrazoles. J. Clin. Endo. and Metab. 22:43-51 (1962).

41. Furman, R.H., Howard, R.P., Lakshmi, K. and Norcia, L.N.: The serum lipids and lipoproteins in normal and hyperlipidemic subjects as determined by preparative ultracentrifugation. Effects of dietary and therapeutic measures. Changes induced by in vitro exposure of serum to sonic forces. Amer. J. Clin. Nutr. 9:73-102 (1961).

42. Furman, R.H., Norcia, L.N., Robinson, C.W., Jr. and Gonzalez, I.E.: Influence of testosterone, methyltestosterone and dl-ethionine on canine liver lipids, serum lipids and lipoproteins. Amer. J. Physiology 191:561-572 (1957).

43. Furman, R.H., Robinson, C.W., Jr., Bradford, R.H., Alaupovic, P. and Norcia, L.N.: Methyltestosterone effect on serum cholesterol radioactivity in dogs given C^{14}-acetate. Proc. Soc. Exper. Biol. and Med. 113:789-794 (1963).

44. Mosbach, E.H., Abell, L.L. and Kendall, F.E.: In Drugs Affecting Lipid Metabolism. Elsevier Publishing Company, The Netherlands. pp. 119-131 (1961).

45. Abell, L.L. and Mosbach, E.H.: Hypocholesterolemic effect of methyltestosterone in rats. J. Lipid Res. 3:88-91 (1962).

46. Raiford, R.L. and Wong, H.Y.C.: In vivo incorporation
of acetate-1-C^{14} into cholesterol and fatty acids following
testosterone propionate administration. Circulation Res. 11:752-
757 (1962).

47. Abell, L.L., Mosbach, E.H. and Kendall, F.E.: Influence
of diet on the hypocholesterolemic action of methyltestosterone
in dogs. J. Nutrition 87:285-292 (1965).

48. Alaupovic, P., Howard, R.P. and Furman, R.H.: Effect of
estrogens and androgens on the alpha and beta lipoprotein composition in human subjects. Circulation 28:647 (1963).

49. Furman, R.H., Sanbar, S.S., Alaupovic, P., Bradford, R.H
and Howard, R.P.: Studies of the metabolism of radioiodinated
human serum alpha lipoprotein in normal and hyperlipidemic subjects. J. Lab. Clin. Med. 63:193-204 (1964).

50. Levy, R.I., Lees, R.S. and Fredrickson, D.S.: A
functional role for plasma alpha$_1$ lipoproteins. J. Clin. Invest.
44:1068 (1965).

51. Furman, R.H., Howard, R.P. and Norcia, L.N.: In
Hormones and Atherosclerosis, G. Pincus, Editor, Academic Press,
New York, Ch. 25, pp. 349-370 (1958).

52. Furman, R.H., Howard, R.P. and Norcia, L.N.: Modification of the responses of serum lipids, lipoproteins, and urinary
creatine excretion to androgen and estrogen administration
following isocaloric substitution of carbohydrate for dietary
protein. J. Lab. Clin. Med. 52:813-814 (1958).

53. Crider, Q.E., Bradford, R.H. and Furman, R.H.: Effect of
methyltestosterone on the protein moiety of canine serum alpha-
lipoproteins. Circulation 32 (II):8 (1965).

54. Aurell, M., Cramer, K. and Rybo, G.: Serum lipids and
lipoproteins during long term administration of an oral contraceptive. Lancet 1:291-293 (1966).

EFFECT OF AN ORAL CONTRACEPTIVE STEROID MIXTURE ON SOME ASPECTS OF LIPID METABOLISM IN THE RAT

Lilla Aftergood and Roslyn B. Alfin-Slater

School of Public Health, University of California,
Los Angeles

Despite the widespread use of oral contraceptives only some of the metabolic effects of these drugs have been thoroughly investigated. Their role in lipid metabolism remains relatively obscure.

For many years, we have been concerned with the relationship between sex hormones and various aspects of lipid metabolism in the rat. Some of the effects appear to be quite significant. The majority of investigations support the results obtained with human subjects where decreased plasma cholesterol levels follow estrogen administration (1). Not only does the concentration of cholesterol esters decrease but also fatty acids combined with the cholesterol are affected by administration of sex hormones. For instance, Oliver and Boyd (2) observes in humans that the ratio of linoleate:oleate:palmitate in the cholesterol ester fraction was markedly influenced by estrogen administration changing from a ratio of 46:25:15 to 30:20:22. Fewster et al (3) also reported that the percentage of cholesterol oleate increased in the plasma cholesterol ester fraction of estrogen-treated rats.

A recent publication from our laboratory (4) reports the results of the administration of unphysiological doses of the oral contraceptive Enovid-E to the mature female rat. The recommended human daily dose of this drug is 2.6 mg which consists of a progestogen-estrogen mixture of 2.5 mg. of norethynodrel and 0.1 mg of mestranol. The rats were given orally one mg of this mixture in 0.5 ml. sesame oil daily, corresponding to approximately 1/2 of the human dose, 40 times greater than the minimal estrogenizing dose in rats and approximately three times the minimal

progestational dose based on a comparison of the weight of the
rat with a woman weighing 125 lbs. These high levels of hormones
were used to emphasize and hasten the appearance of any effects
which might result from the use of smaller doses over a longer
period of time. The control group received sesame oil only.
Rats were treated for a period of seven days; in later studies
comparable results were obtained after four days of hormone administration.

Table 1 presents total cholesterol content of plasma, liver,
adrenals, and ovaries of control and Enovid-treated rats. In
this experiment, we had 8-10 rats per group. Enovid administration

Table 1

CHOLESTEROL CONTENT OF PLASMA, LIVER, ADRENALS,
AND OVARIES IN CONTROL AND ENOVID-TREATED FEMALE RATS

	Control (8)	Enovid Treated (10)	Change %
Plasma, mg chol /100 ml	$49.9 \pm 9.3^{1/}$	10.5 ± 3.7	-79
% free	38.8	42.9	
Liver, mg chol/g	2.24 ± 0.22	3.02 ± 0.33	+35
mg chol/rat	16.8	35.5	+111
% free	89.0	75.5	
Adrenals, mg chol/g	33.0 ± 7.2	7.0 ± 3.3	-79
mg chol/rat	2.19	0.42	-81
% free	9.1	29.7	
Ovaries, mg chol/g	6.5 ± 0.2	5.0 ± 1.2	-23
mg chol/rat	0.38	0.17	-56
% free	27.0	31.0	

Numbers in parentheses represent the number of animals and the
number of analyses. 1/ Standard Deviation

results in a marked decrease in the level of total cholesterol in
plasma and adrenals. The decrease in adrenals is expressed primarily in the esterified cholesterol fraction. Part of the
decrease in ovarian cholesterol reflects the fact that there is
a decrease in ovarian size and weight as a result of hormone
treatment. Cholesterol in the liver of Enovid-treated rats is
significantly elevated when calculated either per gram of liver
or per total liver.

Major fatty acids of plasma adrenal and ovarian sterol esters

of control and Enovid-treated rats are shown in Tables 2 and 3.
In the plasma, the most striking change is a decrease in arachidonate (20:4) content. The amount of linoleate present is also

Table 2

MAJOR FATTY ACIDS OF PLASMA STEROL ESTERS
IN CONTROL AND ENOVID-TREATED FEMALE RATS

	16:0 %	16:1 %	18:0 %	18:1 %	18:2 %	20:4 %
C(7)	11.3+2.3[1/]	6.6+1.9	4.4+1.3	9.7+2.3	16.6+1.9	41.4+6.1
E(9)	18.0+4.6	12.4+2.0	8.8+1.5	21.8+1.5	10.8+1.3	8.9+2.2

Table 3

MAJOR FATTY ACIDS OF ADRENAL AND OVARIAN STEROL
ESTERS IN CONTROL AND ENOVID-TREATED FEMALE RATS

Adrenals

	16:0 %	16:1 %	18:0 %	18:1 %	18:2 %	20:4 %	22:4 %
C(6)	11.1+1.0[1/]	4.8+1.4	4.2+0.9	16.7+3.0	6.6+1.0	15.9+1.9	25.4+3.3
E(7)	14.4+1.9	10.7+1	8.2+1.9	22.2+2.7	7.2+0.9	8.2+1.3	11.0+4.5

Ovaries

	16:0 %	16:1 %	18:0 %	18:1 %	18:2 %	20:4 %	22:4 %
C(6)	17.8+5.7	10.7+1.6	9.3+1.8	18.1+2.0	4.0+1.9	4.3+0.6	11.0+1.1
E(7)	18.0+3.8	11.4+2.2	10.5+0.7	20.2+2.8	4.3+1.5	4.3+0.8	7.0+1.3

Numbers in parentheses represent number of animals and the number
of analyses. 1/ Standard Deviation

lowered. These changes are compensated by significant increases
in palmitoleate, oleate, and stearate content. In adrenals and
ovaries, the decrease in cholesterol content is reflected by the
decreased content of 20:4 and 22:4 (docosatetraenoic acid) in the
adrenals and the 22:4 acid in the ovaries.

Following these experiments, we undertook a series of studies
on cholesterol biosynthesis in liver, adrenals, and ovaries in control and Enovid-treated female rats for four days with either
sesame oil alone or with 1.04 mg of Enovid-E in sesame oil.

Table 4

STUDY ON CHOLESTEROL BIOSYNTHESIS FROM ACETATE-1-^{14}C

Organ	Wt. (g)		Total Cholesterol mg/g tissue		Cpm/g Tissue [1]		Cpm/mg Cholesterol [1]		% Incorporation	
	C	E	C	E	C	E	C	E	C	E
Liver	7.22	7.76	2.30	3.74	9,480(7) [2] ±3,700	3,490(9) [2] ±1,100	4,180 ±2,070	970 ±400	5.20	1.96
Ovaries (pr)	0.0450	0.0375	9.92	5.72	22,980 ±16,200	82,160 ±27,250	2,570 ±2,000	17,300 ±5,000	0.52	3.00
Adrenals (pr)	0.0427	0.0514	42.5	9.53	1,210 ±577	3,080 ±940	31 ±14	322 ±215	0.07	0.32

[1] = Mean ± Standard Deviation.
[2] = Number of organs incubated separately in duplicate analyses.

Table 4 presents the results of this study.

In all three tissues, significant differences were obtained in the weight of the tissues, the cholesterol content of the tissues and the amount of cholesterol biosynthesized. As previously observed, total cholesterol per g of tissue increased in liver, and markedly decreased in both ovaries and adrenals. Cholesterol biosynthesis was depressed in liver but significantly enhanced in ovaries and adrenals. Since there is a simultaneous increase in hepatic cholesterol concentration and it is known that hepatic cholesterol biosynthesis is depressed under these conditions, the hormone effect of biosynthesis may be a secondary effect. However, the stimulation of biosynthesis in adrenals and ovaries, organs from which cholesterol appears to be removed very rapidly, probably through a transformation into other steroids (steroid hormones), indicates an increased requirement for cholesterol by these organs. It has been suggested (5) that sterol esters rather than free sterol are the starting material for steroid biosynthesis.

Our investigations on the effect of anovulatory drugs on cholesterol metabolism have been extended by studying cholesterol excretion. As previously, four doses of 1.04 mg of Enovid-E were employed. Feces were collected three days prior to treatment, during treatment, and for three days following the treatment. Total cholesterol was determined on extracts of dried feces. Table 5 presents the results obtained in this study. Although the cholesterol content per g feces did not change during the experimental period and there was no difference between the control and experi-

Table 5

STUDY OF CHOLESTEROL EXCRETION

| | | | | Days | | | | |
Group	1-3	4	5	6	7	8	9	10
				Cholesterol, mg/g feces				
Control	3.43	3.31	3.49	3.57	3.31	3.36	3.30	3.27
Enovid	3.28	3.35	3.63	3.20	3.33	4.01	3.78	3.29
				Cholesterol, total excreted, mg/day				
Control	10.68	7.06	8.18	10.16	10.36	10.49	8.29	7.00
Enovid	8.87	7.78	4.29	3.71	4.02	6.36	6.71	7.10

mental group, the amount and therefore the weight of feces excreted was much less in the hormone treated group. When the results
were expressed as total mg. of cholesterol excreted per day it
became obvious that less cholesterol was excreted during the
Enovid treatment. This occurred as early as one day after the
administration of the first dose and returned to normal two days
after cessation of treatment. It should be pointed out that the
treated rats also ate less food and lost weight. Pincus (6)
has suggested that an inhibition of growth promoting stimulation
(perhaps by pituitary somatotropin) takes place when rats are
given large doses of Enovid. In this experiment, the average
change in weight during the four days of treatment was +5 g for
the control animals and -22 g for the Enovid-treated rats. At
the same time the food consumption averaged 16 g/day/rat and
8 g/day/rat respectively.

Finally we have set up an experiment in which we have tested
the recovery of the female rat following the cessation of Enovid
treatment and the effect of a repeated treatment. The plan of
this experiment is shown in Table 6.

Table 6

PLAN OF EXPERIMENT

Group I   - 1 dose/day for 4 days - Enovid E (1.0 mg norethynodrel
            and 0.04 mg mestranol) (E4).

Group II - As I but killed 3 days after the last dose (E4 + 3).

GroupIII - As I but killed 30 days after the last dose (E4 + 30).

Group IV - As I, kept 30 days without dosing, then 1 dose/day for
            4 days (E4 +30 + E4).

Table 7 presents changes in body weight and plasma cholesterol levels resulting from hormone administration and withdrawal. Enovid-treated rats lost weight as a result of drug
administration, did not recover in three days, but did recover
completely after 30 days. The second Enovid treatment again
resulted in a substantial weight loss. Plasma cholesterol levels
are well on the way to recovery three days following cessation of
treatment and again are affected similarly by repeated treatment. Table 8 presents changes in liver cholesterol levels. The
four day treatment results in an increase of hepatic cholesterol level; recovery takes place within three days and is
maintained over the 30 day period. The second treatment with
Enovid gives results similar to those observed after the first
series of hormone administration. Changes in adrenals resulting

Table 7

CHANGES IN BODY WEIGHT, AND PLASMA CHOLESTEROL
RESULTING FROM HORMONE ADMINISTRATION AND WITHDRAWAL

Group #	Change in Body Weight g	Plasma Cholesterol mg/100 ml	% F
Control	+16	55.5	32.2
I (E4)	-11	12.1	41.3
II (E4 + 3)	-10	35.9	34.1
III (E4 + 30)	+17	60.6	32.1
IV (E4 + 30 + E4)	-25	13.3	37.2

(6 rats per group)

Table 8

CHANGES IN LIVER RESULTING FROM HORMONE
ADMINISTRATION AND WITHDRAWAL

Group #	Weight g	Cholesterol mg/g	mg/liver
Control	7.57	1.94	14.7
I (E4)	7.37	3.03	22.4
II (E4 + 3)	6.97	1.84	12.8
III (E4 + 30)	8.06	1.71	13.8
IV (E4 + 30 + E4)	7.24	2.73	19.8

from hormone administration and withdrawal are presented in Table 9. Again, some recovery from the effects of drug administration is achieved after three days and complete return to control values is apparent after 30 days. A second administration of hormone yields results similar to those observed after the first series.

Table 10 shows some of the major fatty acids of plasma cholesteryl esters. As expected, the most striking change resulting from Enovid administration is the decrease in arachidonic acid.

Table 9

CHANGES IN ADRENALS RESULTING FROM HORMONE ADMINISTRATION AND WITHDRAWAL

Group #	Wt. mg	mg/g	Cholesterol mg/total organs	%F
Control	50.3	32.9	1.64	12.5
I (E4)	48.0	10.0	0.48	20.5
II (E4 + 3)	58.2	18.5	0.84	14.4
III (E4 + 30)	44.3	34.7	1.54	14.5
IV (E4 + 30 + E4)	50.7	15.4	0.78	18.5

Table 10

SOME OF THE MAJOR FATTY ACIDS OF PLASMA CHOLESTERYL ESTERS OF CONTROL AND ENOVID-TREATED RATS

	18:1 %	18:2 %	20:4 %
Control	13.3	17.4	32.2
I (E4)	20.7	13.5	12.3
II (E4 + 3)	15.0	16.2	27.5
III (E 4 + 30)	12.5	17.8	34.9
IV (E4 + 30 + E4)	26.5	8.5	7.5

Apparently cholesteryl arachidonate is being selectively removed and further metabolized. After cessation of treatment, the fatty acids approach control values after three days and reach control level after 30 days. A second hormone treatment results in a response similar to the first series.

In the case of adrenal cholesteryl esters (Table 11) arachidonic and docosatetraenoic (adrenergic) acids are most affected by the treatment. The response of these acids to the experimental procedure is analogous to other previously mentioned indices. In other words, a partial recovery is evident three

Table 11

SOME OF THE MAJOR FATTY ACIDS OF ADRENAL CHOLESTERYL ESTERS

	16:1 %	18:1 %	20:4 %	22:4 %
Control	4.8	12.9	14.1	25.0
I (E4)	11.5	17.4	5.3	14.3
II (E4 + 3)	6.4	17.4	12.9	17.2
III (E4 + 30)	5.8	12.2	14.6	29.7
IV (E4 + 30 + E4)	9.1	21.5	8.7	14.0

days after the cessation of treatment, complete recovery after
30 days, and repeated treatment yields reoccurrence of the
initial response. We must emphasize, however, that these were
short term experiments. We do not know how long it would take
for the animals to recover following long term treatment.

In summary, the administration to rats of the anovulatory
drug, Enovid-E, in doses containing 1.0 mg of norethynodrel
and 0.04 mg of mestranol results in decreases in plasma and
adrenal cholesterol levels, increases in liver cholesterol
content and decreases in the polyunsaturated fatty acids of
cholesteryl ester fraction in plasma and adrenals. A return to
control values is achieved rapidly after cessation of hormone
administration. Further hormone treatment yields effects
qualitatively and quantitatively similar to the initial results.
In addition, we have observed that while less cholesterol is
excreted, a marked stimulation of adrenal and ovarian cholesterol
biosynthesis and a depression of hepatic cholesterol biosynthesis
takes place. These findings indicate that several aspects of
cholesterol metabolism are affected. There may be a hormone
induced redistribution as well as anabolic and catabolic changes.
Cholesterol accumulation in liver could be caused by liver damage
resulting from toxic effects of the hormones or impaired transport due to an inhibition of phospholipid and lipoprotein synthesis resulting from the relative unavailability of polyunsaturated fatty acids.

REFERENCES

1. Boyd, G.S.: Effect of linoleate and estrogen on cholesterol metabolism. Federation Proc. 21:86-92 (1962).

2. Oliver, M.F., and Boyd, G.S.: Influence of reduction of serum lipids on prognosis of coronary heart disease. Lancet ii:499-505 (1961).

3. Fewster, M.F., Pirrie, R.E., and Turner, D.: Effect of estradiol benzoate on lipid metabolism in the rat. Endocrinology 80:263-271 (1967).

4. Aftergood, L., and Alfin-Slater, R.B.: Effect of large doses of the oral contraceptive Enovid on cholesterol metabolism in the rat. J. Lipid Res. 9:447-452 (1968).

5. Riley, G.: Lipids of human adrenals. Biochem. J. 87:500-507 (1963).

6. Pincus, G.: Experimental studies of fertility control by hormonal steroids in mammals. Proceedings IInd Intern. Congress on Hormonal Steroids, Excerpta Med. Found., Intern. Congress Series, p. 100-110 (1967).

PROTEIN AND AMINO ACID METABOLISM

EFFECTS OF GONADAL AND CONTRACEPTIVE HORMONES ON PROTEIN AND AMINO ACID METABOLISM

U. S. Seal and R. P. Doe

Metabolic Research Laboratory, Veterans Administration
Hospital and Departments of Biochemistry and Medicine,
University of Minnesota, Minneapolis, Minnesota.

The literature on androgens and anabolic steroids has been reviewed extensively (5, 49, 57, 101, 112, 128, 214). The actions of estrogens and progestins on nonsexual organs have also been reviewed with general emphasis on their catabolic effects (7, 70, 107, 112, 128) except in the veterinary literature where attention has focused on growth-promoting or weight-gaining and meat "finishing" effects (10, 51, 52, 72, 140, 150, 153, 206). Most of the recent laboratory investigation has been devoted to sites and mechanisms of action particularly in target tissues with mechanisms being sought within the framework of the Jacob-Monod hypothesis at the level of transcription (57, 100, 183, 214).

This review is primarily directed at bringing together recent literature on non-target tissue effects of gonadal hormones on protein and amino acid metabolism with especial emphasis on blood. Much of this is a recording of in vivo occurring alterations in distribution and concentration of constituents since only a small fraction of studies report data using isotopically-labeled materials, or are directed at mechanisms in supposedly "non-target" tissues. The effect of estrogen treatment and pregnancy on serum nonprotein-bound cortisol is documented in detail in view of the potential metabolic significance of an increase in the available active fraction of serum cortisol.

These studies were supported in part by PHS Research Grant AM-11376-07 from the National Institute of Arthritis and Metabolic Diseases and the V.A. Cooperative Urological Research Project.

TABLE 1. Total plasma amino acids in young and
old adults and with testosterone

Group	Men (N)	Women (N)
Young	2261 ± 175 (16)	2279 ± 124 (17)
Old		
Before	2035 ± 101 (17)	2040 ± 122 (17)
After*	2140 ± 92 (17)	2148 ± 94 (17)

* Testosterone propionate in oil 35 mg, twice
weekly, intramuscular for 3 months. Data are
from Ackermann and Kheim (1964) and are given
as micromoles per liter ± standard deviation.

Plasma and Urinary Amino Acids

Quantitative comparisons of plasma amino acids in young and
elderly adult males and females have been reported by Ackermann
and Kheim and they have also recorded the effects of testosterone
propionate treatment in elderly adult males and females (2). They
found significantly lower total amino acids in the older groups of
both sexes (Table 1). The concentrations of serine, alanine,
valine, isoleucine, phenylalanine and lysine were lower in both
older groups. Tyrosine was lower in the older male group and glycine, methionine, and arginine were lower in the older female group.
Testosterone treatment of the older groups resulted in a significant
increase in total amino acids. Serine was increased in both groups
and isoleucine and lysine were significantly increased in the male
group.

Comparison of prepubertal with pubertal and young adult males
(219) yielded inconclusive results on plasma amino acids except
when the data were analyzed in terms of testosterone excretion.
Then higher plasma levels of methionine, isoleucine, phenylalanine
and leucine were found in the high testosterone group. There were
no significant differences in muscle amino acids between the
groups; however, the data were scanty.

We have measured by ion-exchange chromatography the plasma amino
acids and urinary amino acid excretion in a group of young adult,
healthy males before and after 14 days of testosterone treatment
(100 mg testosterone cyclopentylpropionate i.m. on day 0 and day 7)
and found no statistically significant changes either in the total
amino acid excretion or in the excretion of any single amino acid.
Analysis by the method of paired variates indicated a significant

increase in the plasma levels of proline and glutamic acid and a significant decrease in tyrosine.

Testosterone in high doses (50-200 mg/day x 4) significantly reduced the urinary excretion of hydroxyproline according to Katz and Kappas (91, 92, 93). Estradiol (5-20 mg/day) and estriol (8-40 mg/day) also reduced the urinary hydroxyproline output, usually after a delay of 3-10 days, in 11 of 13 subjects and 9 of 14 subjects, respectively.

The effects of androgens on protein synthesis and amino acid incorporation by nonsexual tissues include observations on muscle (26, 40, 54, 218), liver (29, 103, 119), brain (184, 209), and other tissues (3, 43, 44, 78, 79, 86, 87, 96, 97, 99, 127, 157). The work on kidney includes several species (3, 32, 95, 96) but has centered on certain mouse strains since these are very responsive or dependent (56, 85, 94, 98, 147).

Landau and Lugibihl reported that administration of progesterone (50 mg/day) to men resulted in an immediate 2-5 gm increase in urinary nitrogen in the form of urea per day (105, 106, 107). There was also a decrease in the plasma concentrations of ten amino acids (threonine, proline, glycine, alanine, lysine, arginine, ornithine, citrulline, cystine and serine) in 4 subjects studied 4 days (105). We found statistically significant decreases in plasma levels of threonine, alanine, valine, ornithine and arginine and an increase in phenylalanine in 5 male subjects treated with 100 mg progesterone i.m. per day for 7 days (224). Decreases bordering on significance were observed for serine, glutamine, glycine and histidine. Thus, the reported changes in plasma amino acids are in substantial agreement. We also found a significant increase in the urinary excretion of taurine, cystine, phenylalanine and perhaps tyrosine (224). Human studies suggest that the catabolic effect of progesterone occurs by enhancement of liver utilization of amino acids from exogenous protein and endogenous amino acids. Animal studies suggest this may be by way of stimulation of gluconeogenesis (202, 203). Progesterone has also been said to increase the turnover of muscle proteins in rats (202), a result which should be confirmed by other techniques.

Estrogen (diethylstilbestrol 5 mg/day x 7) administration to normal males resulted in a significant decrease in plasma glutamic acid, tyrosine, and ornithine and an increase in threonine. The urinary excretion of tyrosine and histidine were decreased and 1-methyl histidine was increased (225). The results of these studies and the effects of an estrogen-progesterone combination are summarized in Tables 2 and 3. Recently Katz and Kappas (91, 92) have documented a reduction in urinary excretion of hydroxyproline in females during treatment with estradiol or estriol.

TABLE 2. Hormonal effects on the urinary excretion of free amino acids

Amino acid	Progesterone	Progesterone +estrogen	Estrogen	Cortisol	Pregnancy
Taurine	+	+	NS	NS	NS
Threonine	NS	NS	NS	+	+
Serine	NS	NS	NS	+	+
Asparagine/Glutamine	NS	NS	NS	+	+
Glutamic acid	NS	NS	NS	NS	NS
Glycine	NS	NS	NS	+	+
Alanine	NS	NS	NS	+	+
α-NH$_3$-n-butyric acid	NS	NS	NS	+	+
Valine	NS	+	NS	+	+
Cystine/2	+	NS	NS	+	+
Cystathionine	NS	+	NS	+	+
Methionine	NS	NS	NS	NS	NS
Isoleucine	NS	NS	NS	NS	NS
Leucine	NS	NS	NS	+	NS
Tyrosine	NS	NS	−	NS	+
Phenylalanine	+	NS	NS	+	NS
β-NH$_3$-isobutyric acid	NS	NS	NS	NS	NS
Ornithine	NS	−	NS	+	+
Ethanolamine	NS	NS	NS	+	+
Lysine	NS	NS	NS	+	NS
1-Methyl histidine	NS	NS	+	NS	NS
Histidine	NS	NS	−	+	+
3-Methyl histidine	NS	+	NS	NS	NS

(+) or (−) signifies statistically significant increase or decrease.
NS signifies no significant change.

The effect was significant, transitory and frequently delayed in appearance. The disappearance rate of injected ^{14}C-proline was increased (93) while that of ^{3}H-hydroxyproline was not affected. These results are consistent with the reported estrogen-stimulated changes in connective tissue metabolism (104, 123, 155, 192) including the increase in collagen synthesis (88, 185, 189), and collagen turnover by way of a proline-rich precursor (75) in aorta, skin and bone. They also are probably relevant to the dietary protein-dependent (187) production of aortic ruptures in turkeys by estrogens (14, 186).

Estrogen (DES) treatment of livestock being fed finishing diets before slaughter is very widespread in the U.S.A. Beef cattle receive implants of 16-24 mg yielding a release of about 1 mg per 100 kilo per week (140). This equals about 0.1 mg per day for man, which is a threshold dose for estrogen effects on serum proteins in man (47, 129). In beef cattle this treatment caused a reduction in the concentrations of threonine, valine, isoleucine, phenylalanine, lysine, tryptophane, arginine, glycine, proline, serine, and urea. Methionine, histidine and especially hydroxyproline were increased in concentration. These effects were in part diet-dependent, differing when corn was replaced by wheat, suggesting a possible interaction with rumen micro-organisms (140). The effects of this estrogen treatment in livestock include weight gain (mostly water), alteration of the connective tissue, and supposedly increased feed efficiency (10, 51, 52, 72, 112, 123, 150, 153, 206).

TABLE 3. Hormonal effects on the plasma concentration of free amino acids

Amino acid	Progesterone	Progesterone +estrogen	Estrogen	Cortisol	Pregnancy
Citrulline	NS	−	NS	NS	−
Taurine	NS	NS	NS	NS	NS
Threonine	−	−	+	NS	NS
Serine	NS	NS	NS	NS	NS
Asparagine/Glutamine	NS	NS	NS	NS	NS
Glutamic acid	NS	NS	−	NS	NS
Glycine	NS	−	NS	NS	−
Alanine	−	−	NS	NS	NS
Valine	−	−	NS	NS	NS
α-NH$_3$-n-butyric acid	NS	−	NS	NS	NS
Cystine/2	NS	NS	NS	NS	NS
Cystathionine	NS	NS	NS	NS	NS
Methionine	NS	NS	NS	NS	NS
Isoleucine	NS	NS	NS	NS	NS
Leucine	NS	NS	NS	NS	NS
Tyrosine	NS	NS	−	NS	−
Phenylalanine	+	NS	NS	NS	−
β-NH$_3$-isobutyric acid	NS	NS	NS	NS	NS
Ornithine	−	−	−	NS	−
Ethanolamine	NS	NS	NS	NS	NS
Lysine	NS	−	NS	NS	−
1-Methyl histidine	NS	NS	NS	NS	NS
Histidine	NS	NS	NS	NS	NS
3-Methyl histidine	NS	NS	NS	NS	NS
Arginine	−	−	NS	NS	−

(+) or (−) signifies statistically significant increase or decrease.
NS signifies no significant change.

The urinary aminoaciduria following estrogen treatment of women differs from that described for men (Table 4). The excretion of histidine and threonine was increased, suggesting the possibility of biologically significant increased nonprotein-bound cortisol (NPC) with estrogen treatment in women. This was borne out by measurements of NPC as shown in Tables 5 and 6. The statistical analysis of Table 6 indicates significantly elevated NPC at 9 AM in estrogen-treated women and in pregnant women at 9 AM and 9 PM. The pregnant women have significantly higher values than the estrogen-treated women at 9 PM. These data lend additional substance to the interpretation offered by Munro that some estrogen effects on protein metabolism are the consequence of increased adrenocortical activity (128, p. 453). This relationship between NPC and aminoaciduria is further illustrated in Fig. 1 where the relationship between the evening NPC and threonine and histidine excretion is shown for normal, estrogen-treated and pregnant women. A similar relationship is shown in Fig. 2 for normal, estrogen, and estrogen-cortisol treated women. The additional cortisol further increases the aminoaciduria.

Estrogen therapy with either ethinyl estradiol (65) or estradiol (90) does not increase cortisol secretion rate nor is the urinary excretion of free cortisol increased. The evidence for increased nonprotein-bound cortisol (66, 148, 182) in estrogen-treated and pregnant subjects is being extended in several laboratories with substantial agreement as to the phenomenon.

TABLE 4. Steroid Aminoaciduria in Females

Amino Acid	Pre	Estrogen[1]	Estrogen and Cortisol[2]
	μM/kg/24 hrs		
Group 1			
Histidine	12.9	+	+
Threonine	4.3	+	+
Alanine	5.8	NS	+
Asparagine/glutamine	9.5	NS	+
Serine	7.8	NS	+
Group 2			
Cystine/2	1.9	NS	NS
Lysine	2.9	NS	NS
Glycine	45.8	NS	NS
Phenylalanine	1.3	NS	NS
Cystathionine	0.7	NS	NS
Group 3			
Valine	1.5	NS	+
Ethanolamine	4.9	NS	NS
α-amino-n-butyric acid	0.2	NS	NS
Leucine	1.4	NS	NS
Ornithine	0.3	NS	NS
Group 4			
Taurine	5.8	NS	+
Glutamic acid	1.4	NS	NS
Isoleucine	0.7	NS	NS
Tyrosine	1.6	NS	+
β-aminobutyrate	1.7	NS	NS
1-methyl histidine	13.5	NS	NS
3-methyl histidine	4.1	NS	NS
Tryptophane	1.4	NS	NS
Arginine	0.4	NS	NS
Methionine	1.3	NS	NS

[1] Urine collected after 14 days on 200 μg/day of ethinyl estradiol

[2] Urine collected after 5-7 days on 200 μg/day of ethinyl estradiol and 100 mg of hydrocortisone every a.m.

TABLE 5. Cortisol-Binding Protein Relationships (Mean ± SD)

	9 AM				9 PM	
	17-OHCS µg%	NPC µg%	CBG mg/l	Alb gm%	17-OHCS µg%	NPC µg%
Normal ♂	16.5 ± 4.6	1.27 ± .51	38.4 ± 4.2	4.5 ± .4	6.3 ± 3.4	.36 ± .20
Normal ♀	19 ± 6	1.40 ± .40	38.7 ± 3.7	5 ± .4	7.4 ± 2.5	.43 ± .22
♀-Estrogen	51 ± 10	2.31 ± .72	99 ± 12.6	4.5 ± .5	19 ± 6.8	.56 ± .18
Pregnancy	42.7 ± 9.2	2.62 ± .34	80 ± 18	3.6 ± .4	24 ± 5	1.02 ± .23
Ca Prostate-Untreated	21.6 ± 4	2.21 ± .79	41.7 ± 5.5	4.2 ± .4	10.3 ± 1.3	.84 ± .24
Ca Prostate-Estrogen	53 ± 9	2.60 ± .70	119 ± 21	3.9 ± .5	33 ± 6.4	1.21 ± .40

Values obtained (mean ± S.D.) for the various interacting cortisol-binding components of serum.

TABLE 6. Nonprotein-Bound 17-OHCS -- Statistical Analysis

		t	p
Normal Female (Pre vs. Post Estrogen)	9AM	5.26	< 0.001
	9PM	1.84	< 0.1
Normal Female vs. Pregnancy	9AM	3.75	< 0.01
	9PM	5.85	< 0.001
Estrogen-Treated Female vs. Pregnancy	9AM	1.27	< 0.3
	9PM	4.94	< 0.01
Normal Male vs. Untreated Ca Prostate	9AM	3.30	< 0.01
	9PM	3.99	< 0.01
Normal Male vs. Estrogen-Treated Ca Prostate	9AM	5.06	< 0.001
	9PM	5.91	< 0.001
Ca Prostate (Pre vs. Post Estrogen)	9AM	1.09	< 0.3
	9PM	2.17	< 0.05

Statistical analysis (Student t test) of the values obtained between the various treatment groups in Table 5.

These relationships were further explored in terms of a dose-response relationship for the acute aminoaciduria response to an oral dose of corticoid. The steroid was given at 9 AM and the urine collected for 12 hours under a standard water intake regimen. Each person served as his own control. The curves are presented as linear plots of the increase in excretion of the particular amino acid, Figs. 3 and 4. An increase was observed at the lowest dose for threonine, serine, and asparagine. The responses were linear over the dosage range studied but were suggestive of different slopes to the response curve. It would appear that the threshold of response may be low since 35 to 60% of the response occurred at the lowest dosage of 30 mg. The sensitive response of plasma amino acid levels and urinary excretion to control mechanisms is further suggested by recent reports of circadian variations in plasma levels and urinary excretion (216).

Recent studies on steroid maintenance of pregnancy in protein-deficient rats have demonstrated that estrone and progesterone treatment (73) permits successful completion of pregnancy. The results indicated that maternal skeletal muscle furnished the protein for placental and fetal growth. More recently (19) prednisolone or ACTH treatment was found to be equally successful in maintaining pregnancy. The amino acid mobilizing effects of this

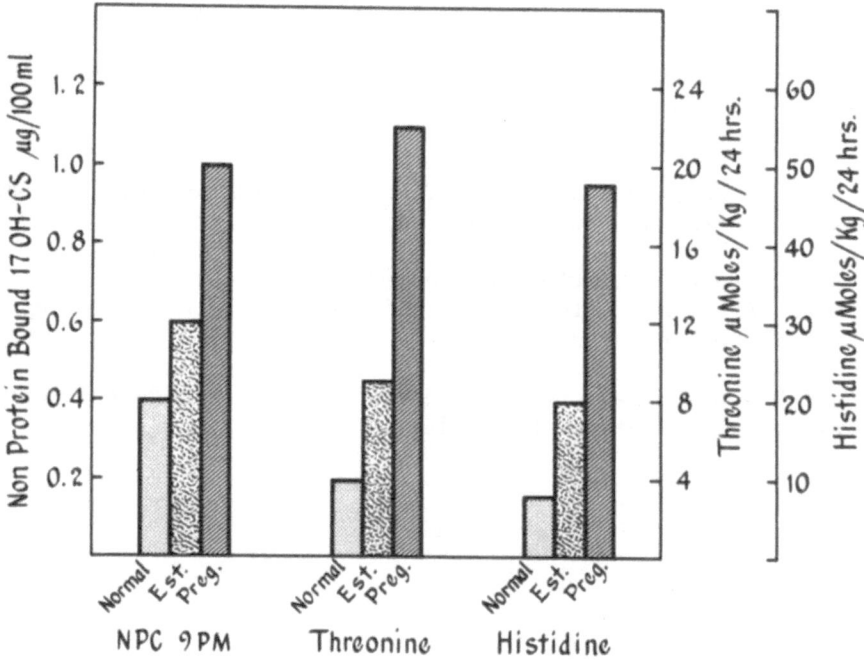

Fig. 1: Urinary amino acids and 9 PM NPC.

treatment were acknowledged. Hypoproteinemia in humans results in elevated NPC levels and a wasting syndrome similar to Cushing's disease (114). Mechanisms for these effects of estrogens (59), corticoids, and pregnancy (22, 141, 169, 170, 226) on amino acid and protein metabolism are being explored in terms of effects on the metabolism of specific amino acids (30, 67, 126, 154, 171, 221, 222), the effects of one altered amino acid on the entire pattern (80), amino acid transport (165, 183), effects on pyridine nucleotides (45, 46, 166) and in terms of effects on specific tissues (41, 62, 76, 102, 115, 117, 118, 120, 128, 132, 134, 151, 191, 209) or on specific proteins (34, 48, 63, 77, 136).

Blood Proteins

The effects of estrogens and more recently androgens on blood proteins in man and other mammals has occupied our attention for several years. The effects of anabolic and androgenic steroids on serum proteins have been well reviewed through 1962 by Krüskemper (101). He summarizes the protein metabolic effects of androgens or anabolic agents as follows:

"1.   Androgens and anabolic steroids effect an increased formation of tissue protein, both genitally and extragenitally.
This can be recognized by a lower excretion of nitrogen, phosphorus, potassium, calcium, and water in the urine; the balances of these substances become positive.

2.   The basal nitrogen content of the serum and the nitrogen
excretion in the feces remain unchanged.

3.   Nitrogen retention is lowered after a certain period of
time. After cessation of steroid treatment, the nitrogen
balance becomes negative.

4.   One essential condition for the anabolic effect is optimal protein intake with the diet."

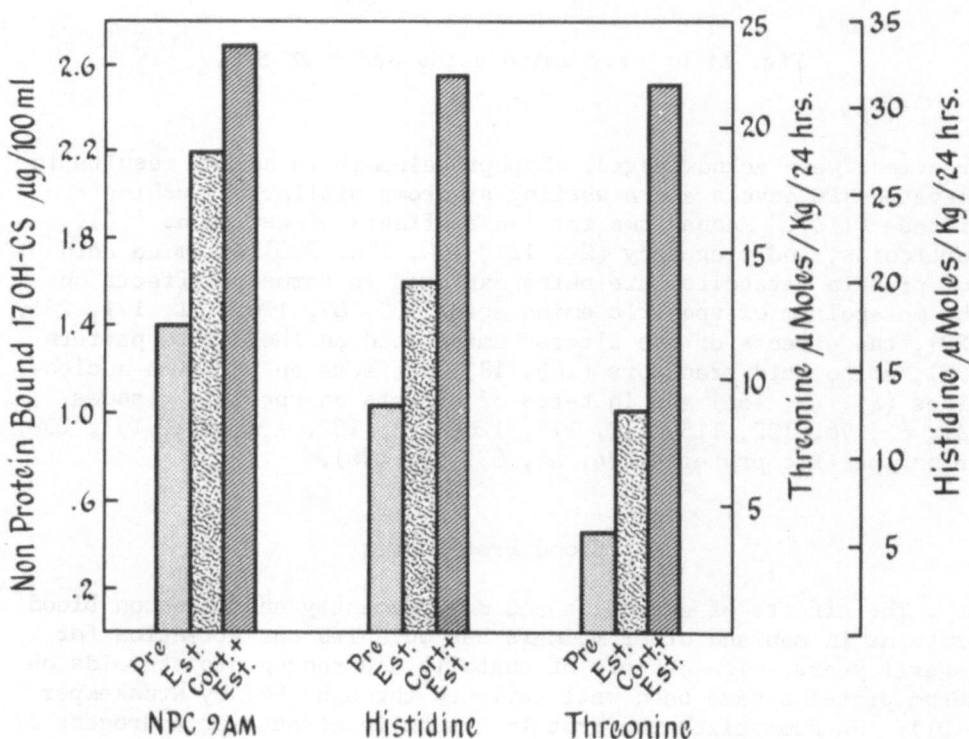

Fig. 2:   9 AM amino acid uria and NPC.

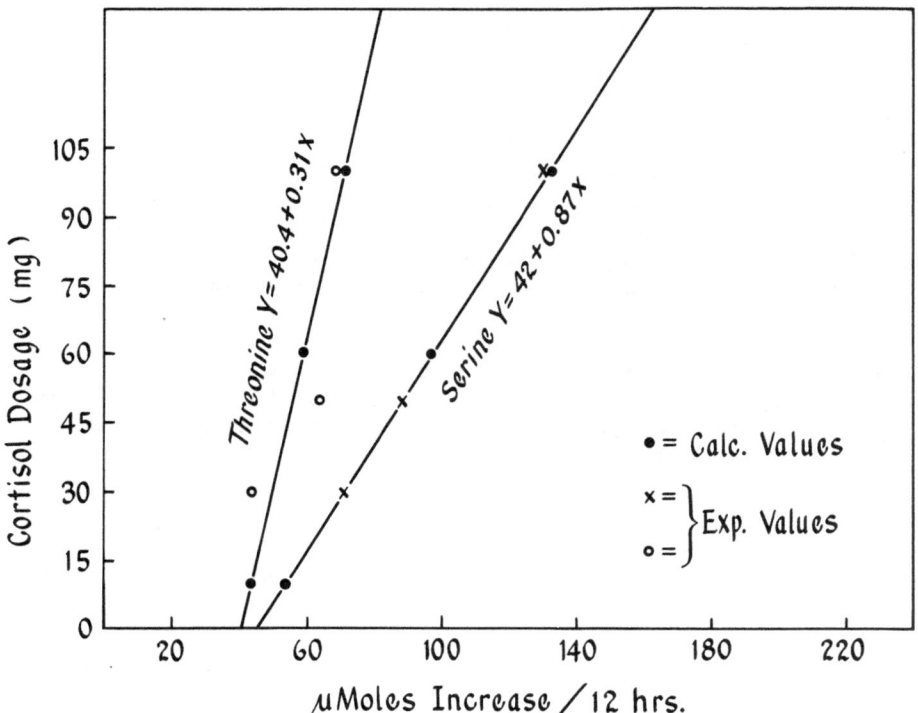

Fig. 3: Dose response (least squares).

The protein content of serum has not been useful for study of anabolic agents since it has been shown not to be altered in eunuchs or by replacement therapy. Also, the results in disease have been quite variable, both with respect to total protein and individual fractions determined by paper electrophoresis (1, 101, 138). As Krüskemper documented (101), the effects of androgens and anabolic agents on total serum proteins and albumin have been examined primarily in diverse disease states and the results have ranged from a decrease to an increase in values. Krüskemper studied a series of 20 healthy males (25-40 yrs) using an oral dose of 20 mg/day for 21 days of 1-methyl-17β-hydroxy-5a-androst-len-3-one. The total protein and electrophoretic patterns were normal. We also have made these measurements using testosterone cyclopentylpropionate, 100 mg IM twice at seven-day intervals. The only significant difference was a modest increase in alpha-one globulins, Table 7. This fraction primarily contains orosomucoid (acid alpha-one-glycoprotein) and the alpha-one trypsin inhibitor. Quantitation of the trypsin inhibitor indicated no significant change in this protein. The concentration of fibrinogen was also decreased by testosterone treatment, Fig. 5, whereas plasminogen was unaffected. Nonprotein-

bound cortisol was likewise unaltered. Measurements of specific
alpha globulins have suggested stimulation of haptoglobin formation
(173, 201), a finding which we could not duplicate in normal males
as shown in Table 8. We found instead a decrease in TBG (23, 24,
25, 81, 143), CBG (42) and in transferrin. The findings with CBG
and TBG confirm other reports but the transferrin decrease has not
been described. Ceruloplasmin and haptoglobin were unchanged. The
report describing an increase in haptoglobin was on 10 women with
unspecified diseases being treated with methylandrostenediol or
methyltestosterone, of whom 6 already had elevated haptoglobin
levels.

Studies of testosterone effects on blood proteins in other
species have yielded similar results. Three weeks' administration
of 10 mg/day of 17α-ethyl-19-nortestosterone to guinea pigs had
little effect on total serum proteins, albumin, or total globulins.
No difference in turnover of ^{131}I-labeled serum proteins was observed (162). A significant fall in β globulins (transferrin) was
found. Testosterone administration (5 mg on alternate days for
5 injections) to the tortoise (Testudo elegans) produced no effects

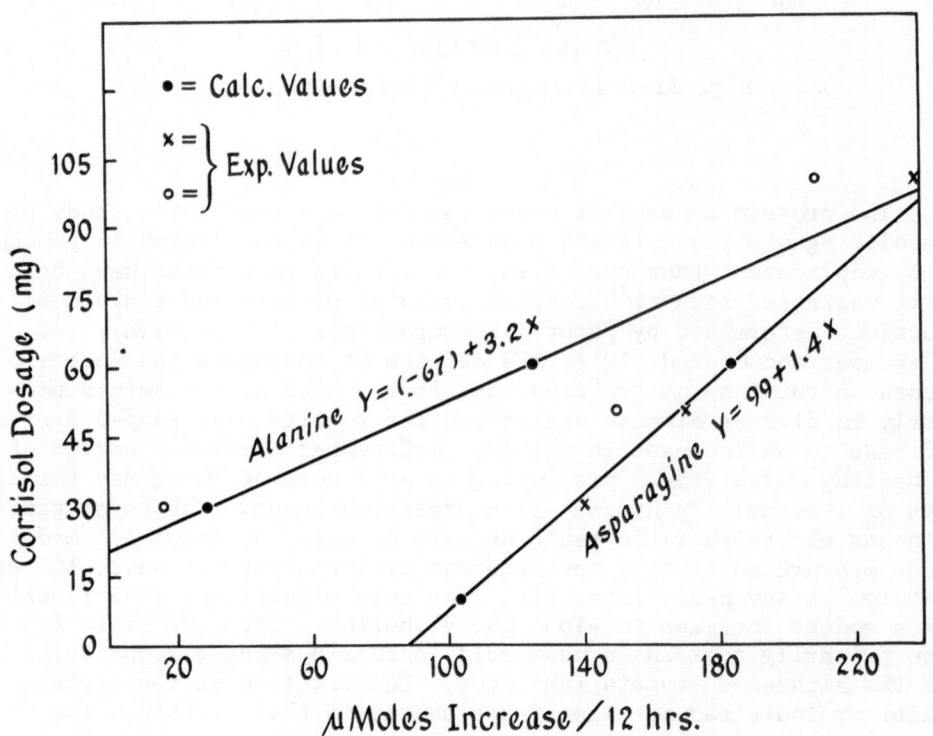

Fig. 4: Dose response (least squares).

TABLE 7. Effect of Testosterone on Paper Electrophoretic serum protein fractions.

| Protein* | Time of Sample | | | p value | |
	Day 0	Day 7	Day 14	0-7 days	0-14 days
Albumin	5.4 ± 0.7	5.1 ± 0.3	5.1 ± 0.5	0.3	0.2
α_1 globulins	0.23 ± 0.03	0.27 ± 0.05	0.26 ± 0.03	< .02	< .05
α_2 globulins	0.50 ± 0.10	0.49 ± 0.10	0.50 ± 0.08	0.9	1.0
β globulins	0.64 ± 0.10	0.60 ± 0.09	0.56 ± 0.32	0.2	0.1
γ globulins	1.02 ± 0.30	0.99 ± 0.22	0.93 ± 0.15	0.5	0.2
Total protein	7.8 ± 1.0	7.4 ± 0.5	7.3 ± 0.6	0.4	0.4

* All values are given as mean ± one standard deviation in gm/100 ml of serum.
  There were 10 subjects.

TABLE 8. Effect of Testosterone on Six Serum Proteins

Protein	Time of Sample			p Value	
	Day 0	Day 7	Day 14	0-7 days	0-14 days
TBG (μg/100 ml T$_4$ bound)	21 ± 2.8	17 ± 2.1	17 ± 1.6	< 0.01	0.001
TBPA (μg/100 ml T$_4$ bound)	133 ± 8.2	137 ± 6.5	138 ± 5.7	0.2	0.1
CBG (mg/1)	38 ± 5	36 ± 5	34 ± 5	0.2	< 0.05
Transferrin (μg Fe/100 ml bound)	399 ± 33	350 ± 28	346 ± 20	< .001	< 0.001
Ceruloplasmin (mg/100 ml)	27 ± 7	26 ± 4	25 ± 4	0.6	0.8
Haptoglobin (mg/100 ml)	68 ± 29	78 ± 22	68 ± 30	0.3	0.9

All values are given as means ± one standard deviation.

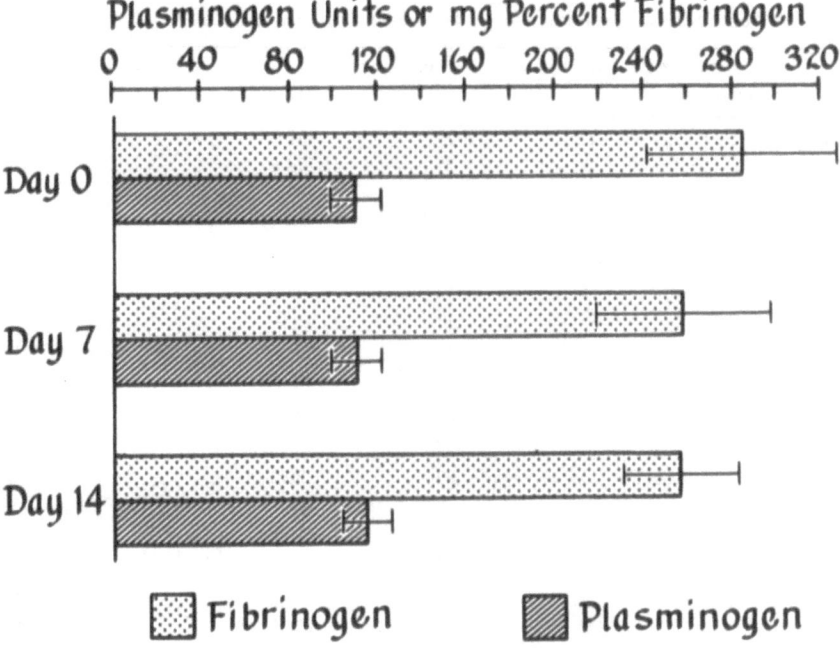

Fig. 5: Effect of 100 mg. i.m. of testosterone propionate at zero and seven days on the levels of fibrinogen and plasminogen.

on the total serum proteins or the electrophoretic pattern (158). This is in contrast to the effects of estrogen treatment which produced increases in total protein and a shift in the relative content of the fractions.

Studies of antibody formation (137) and reticuloendothelial system activity (131, 213) indicate that testosterone treatment has little if any effect except perhaps on interferon production (223), again in contrast to the results obtained with estrogens and corticosteroids. An increase in plasma arylesterase activity after castration in dogs with suppression by testosterone treatment (8) has been observed. In addition, a trace starch-gel fraction of normal dog plasma increased in concentration after castration and was suppressed with testosterone. These changes parallel the observations of Lederer (113) on serum iron in the castrated rabbit and its reduction with testosterone treatment. However, Planas (149) found no significant changes in iron-binding capacity following castration in several domestic livestock species. A prealbumin, PA, of BALB/C$^{\pm}$ mice disappears after castration and

Table 9. *Serum proteins before (0) and 6 months after use of megestrol-mestranol (S)*

Serum proteins		No. of Cases	Mean	P	Standard deviation
Prealbumin	O	29	171.0	> .05	30.7
(TBPA)	S	29	174.6		30.4
μg/100 ml					
Albumin	O	30	4.32	< .001	0.178
g/100 ml	S	30	3.79		0.202
Orosomucoid	O	30	83.6	< .001	20.6
% of normal mean	S	30	53.2		12.4
α_1-antitrypsin	O	30	106.3	< .001	15.1
% of normal mean	S	30	160.6		23.4
Ceruloplasmin	O	30	107.2	< .001	19.5
% of normal mean	S	30	308.4		45.7
Thyroxine-binding globulin	O	29	20.0	< .001	2.77
μg/100 ml	S	29	32.9		5.43
Haptoglobin	O	30	104.5	< .001	37.9
HbBC mg/100 ml	S	30	78.5		25.5
α_2-macroglobulin	O	30	115.6	< .01	26.2
% of normal mean	S	30	124.1		31.9
Plasminogen	O	30	101.6	< .001	11.5
% of normal mean	S	30	149.2		21.5
Transferrin	O	30	328.3	< .001	65.9
TIBC μg/100 ml	S	30	412.4		77.0
Immunoglobulins					
γA	O	29	88.0	< .001	41.3
	S	29	78.1		33.7
γM	O	27	93.1	> .05	31.4
	S	27	92.1		32.5
γG	O	29	102.1	< .05	23.0
% of normal mean	S	29	98.3		19.1
Total serum lipids	O	30	689.3	< .001	108.4
mg/100 ml	S	30	791.4		114.1
Serum cortisol	O	29	14.6	< .001	5.1
μg/100 ml	S	29	23.9		8.8
Glutamyltranspeptidase	O	30	31.4	> .05	10.3
units	S	30	27.5		12.4

Table modified from Laurell, C. B., S. Kullander, and J. Thorell. Scand.J.Clin.Lab.Invest., 21:337-343, 1968.

Pa_2 and PA decreases in concentration. Testosterone propionate injection re-established the normal male pattern (164). These effects differ from the reported 75% increase of thyroxine-binding prealbumin in human serum following norethandrolone (24, 25).

TABLE 10. Paper Electrophoresis of Serum Proteins.

	Total Protein*	Albumin	α_1-Globulin	α_2-Globulin	β-Globulin	γ-Globulin
Before Estrogen	7.33 ± .063	3.87 ± .13	.46 ± .042	.75 ± .060	.91 ± .075	1.35 ± .072
After Estrogen	6.75 ± .163	3.38 ± .12	.44 ± .033	.75 ± .081	.94 ± .069	1.24 ± .095
p**	< .01	< .01	.61	1.0	.65	.21

* All figures are grams/100 ml serum ± standard error of mean (N = 11).

**p is probability that difference between means before and after estrogen is due to chance (Student's t test of paired variables).

TABLE 11. Effect of estrogen on four specific plasma proteins.

	Ceruloplasmin (mg/100 ml)	Corticosteroid-Binding Globulin (mg/100 ml)	Thyroxine-Binding Globulin (μg Thyroxine bound/100 ml)	Haptoglobin (mg Hemoglobin bound/100 ml)
Before Estrogen	39.8 ± 4.7	4.3 ± .49	26.3 ± 2.2	88.2 ± 7.4
After Estrogen	73.5 ± 2.8	11.5 ± .34	35.0 ± 1.6	54.0 ± 3.2
% Change	+84.6	+166.3	+33.1	-38.3
p	< .01	< .01	< .01	< .01

TABLE 12. Effect of estrogen on four proteins as measured
on polyacrylamide electrophoresis.

	% Change (±S.E.M.)	p
G-c component	+94.8 ± 9.2	< 0.01
Ceruloplasmin	+84.1 ± 8.6	< 0.01
Transferrin	+ 8.5 ± 5.5	> 0.1
S-α_2-Globulin	+ 1.7 ± 4.3	> 0.2

Estrogen effects on human proteins have been studied in detail
by many investigators partly in an effort to rationalize the
changes occurring in pregnancy, partly to gain insight into sex
differences in heart disease, and partly because of the wide therapeutic use of estrogens in prostatic cancer and in women for contraception.

Some of the changes occurring in human blood proteins following estrogen treatment are tabulated in Table 9 taken from Laurell
et al (110) and in Tables 10, 11 and 12 taken from Musa et al (124).
These two studies using different methodologies are in good agreement where they overlap. Decreases in orosomucoid (108, 109),
haptoglobin, albumin (82, 193), and total serum proteins were
observed. Immunoglobulins were either unaffected or slightly
reduced in concentration in contrast to the results reported for
several rodent species (89, 131, 137), which include induction of
the wasting syndrome in fetal mice (163). Thyroxine-binding prealbumin was unaffected in one study (110) but has been shown to be
decreased by other methods which have demonstrated a reciprocal
relationship with TBG (25, 174). The estrogen-induced increases
in TBG and PBI (20, 43) have also been shown to be dose-dependent
(47), as shown in Fig. 6. TBG is also increased in pregnancy and
with estrogen treatment in monkeys of the genus Macacca (50, 199).
Proteins recently shown to be increased by estrogen treatment include plasminogen (18, 47, 110), the group specific components
(130), testosterone-and estrogen-binding proteins (145, 172), the
C-reactive protein (179), renin (37), factor VII (18), factor IX
(38), fibrinogen (4, 18, 195), naphthylamidase isozymes (6), and
arylesterase in dogs (8). Proteins decreased by estrogen include
lipoprotein lipase (53), cholinesterase (167), some components of
mouse prealbumins (164, 196), some components of mouse complement
(33, 212), and the sex-associated protein of rat liver (31).
Effects on clotting (133, 160, 178) and fibrinolysis (17) are

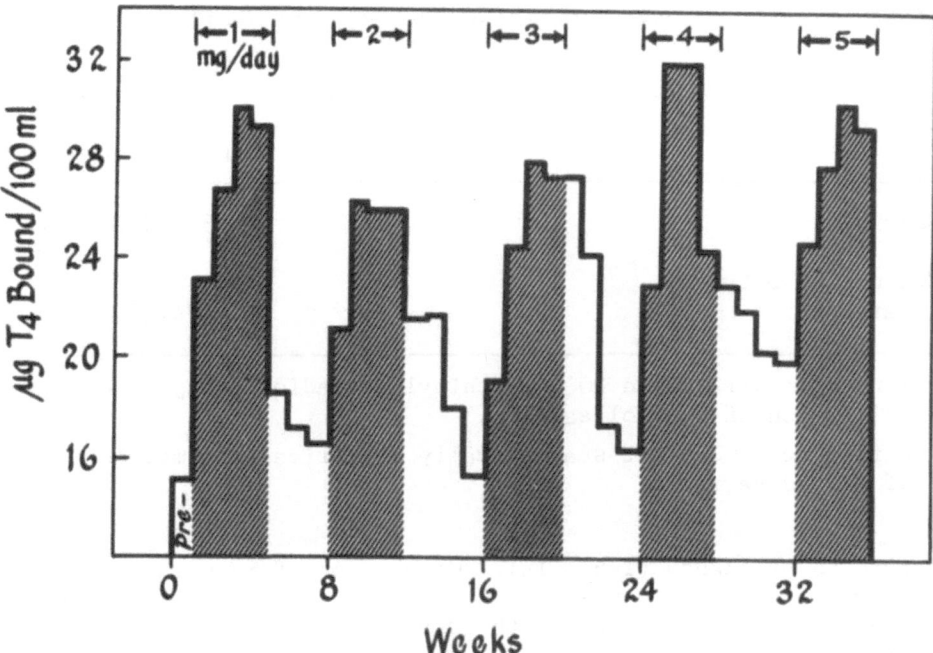

Fig. 6: Effect of alternating four week periods of varying dosage estrogen treatment and rest on plasma thyroxine-binding globulin.

discussed separately in this volume. Increased serum lipids in man and alterations in their distribution among the serum globulins have been repeatedly demonstrated in pregnancy and with estrogen treatment (9, 11, 14, 21, 110, 135, 205, 217, 220) with especial emphasis on the variability of the low-density lipoproteins. Effects on mammalian liver lipids (121) have also been documented. Changes apparently specific for pregnancy include an increase in alkaline phosphatase (16, 168) and several cystine amino peptidases (15, 168). These enzymes appear to be produced by the placenta as electrophoretically-recognizable isoenzymes. In contrast, leucine aminopeptidase can be induced by estrogen treatment (15, 168) as can the pregnancy-associated α_2-globulin (122, 168) and thus can no longer be considered pregnancy-specific.

The results reported on transferrin, the iron-binding protein, appear to conflict since Laurell et al (Table 9) describe a significant increase, whereas we found a small insignificant increase (Table 13), and certainly nothing comparable to the changes

TABLE 13. Lack of effect of estrogen treatment on transferrin concentration.

Treatment	N	Mean μg/100 ml	Range μg/100 ml
Control	10	402	312-504
Two weeks' estrogen treatment*	10	410**	294-477

* Ten women were given 200 μg ethinyl estradiol daily after collection of control samples.

**Differences were not statistically significant by method of paired variates.

observed in pregnancy (Table 14). Comparison of results shows lower control values in the Laurell study with increases to levels comparable to those we found with estrogen treatment. The treatment levels, even with a long-term study, do not approach those of pregnancy so we feel that further work on the induction of transferrin in pregnancy is needed.

Studies of blood proteins in other mammals have yielded widely diverging results when compared to the human picture (12, 13, 83). For example, ceruloplasmin increases about two-fold with estrogen and in pregnancy in man (28, 55, 142, 181) but is not changed in sheep (27), horse (200), swine (despite an increase in copper) (36, 181), black bear (Table 15) and other species (181). It is of interest that many other blood proteins which increased during human pregnancy are unaltered in other species such as the rat (207), sheep (190) and the bear and white-tailed deer shown in Tables 15 and 16. These non-domestic species clearly demonstrate that many alterations commonly associated with pregnancy are not a necessary accompaniment (182).

A comparison of the changes with testosterone or estrogen treatment and pregnancy (Table 17) shows that most of the changes in pregnancy can be mimicked by estrogen treatment with the exception of haptoglobin and transferrin. Other parallel changes reported by Laurell et al (110) include a 30-35% decrease in orosomucoid, a 50% (estrogen) and 100% (pregnancy) increase in α-1-antitrypsin, a 15% and 40% increase in lipoproteins, and a 7% and 40% increase in α-2-macroglobulin, respectively. Testosterone treatment decreases TBG, CBG, transferrin and fibrinogen, thus only partly producing changes opposite to those of the estrogens. Certainly the anabolic effects of androgens are not reflected by increases in the plasma proteins.

TABLE 14. Transferrin levels during pregnancy and with long-term estrogen treatment.

Group	Number	Mean*	Range	S.D.	p
Controls	10	371	286-446	48	> 0.1
Estrogen**	10	403	342-460	38	
Pregnancy***	9	587	495-720	78	< 0.001

* All values are as μg of iron bound per 100 ml serum.
** These women had been taking estrogen preparations for periods ranging from one month to five years with an average time of 1.8 years.
***Third trimester of pregnancy.

TABLE 15. Effects of pregnancy on blood proteins of the bear, deer and man.

	Hgb	Alb	Ceruloplasmin	Transferrin
Deer	NC	NC	NC	NC
Man	-	-	+	+
Bear	-	NC	NC	NC

TABLE 16. Effects of pregnancy on blood proteins of the bear, deer and man.

	PBI	CBG	β-glucuronidase	Fibrinogen
Deer	NC	NC	NC	+ ?
Man	+	+	+	+
Bear	NC	NC	NC	NC

TABLE 17. Contrasting effects of testosterone, ethinyl estradiol and pregnancy on plasma proteins.

Measurement	TREATMENT*		
	Testosterone	Estrogen	Pregnancy
Serum Proteins	0	-	-
TBPA	+	-	-
Albumin	0	-	-
Orosomucoid		-	-
TBG	-	+	+
Trypsin Inhibitor	0	+	+
CBG	-	+	+
Transferrin	-	0	+
Ceruloplasmin	0	+	+
Haptoglobin	0	-	0
Immunoglobulins	0	0	0
Plasminogen	0	+	+
Fibrinogen	-	+	+

* + = significant increase; 0 = no change; and - = significant decrease in concentration.

The increase in CBG and plasma 17-OHCS in pregnancy (Fig. 7) has served as a model for the study of estrogen action on a serum protein as well as offering a tantalizing problem concerning its significance (39, 58, 116, 175, 176, 180, 198). The elevation of CBG concentration can be induced by estrogen treatment (39, 129, 130, 176) and the response is dose-dependent (Fig. 8) for ethinyl estradiol, diethylstilbestrol and Premarin (129). The detectable threshold for the response to diethylstilbestrol is about 0.1 mg (Figs. 9 and 10). This dose-dependent response to estrogen treatment (47, 130) also occurs with ceruloplasmin, β-glucuronidase, TBG, plasminogen, and in part fibrinogen, as shown in Figs. 11 and 12. The dose-dependence was demonstrated in single individuals receiving the various DES dosages for 4-week periods alternating with 4-week periods of no treatment. However, CBG responds virtually only to estrogen treatment or pregnancy, whereas each of the other proteins is affected by other conditions.

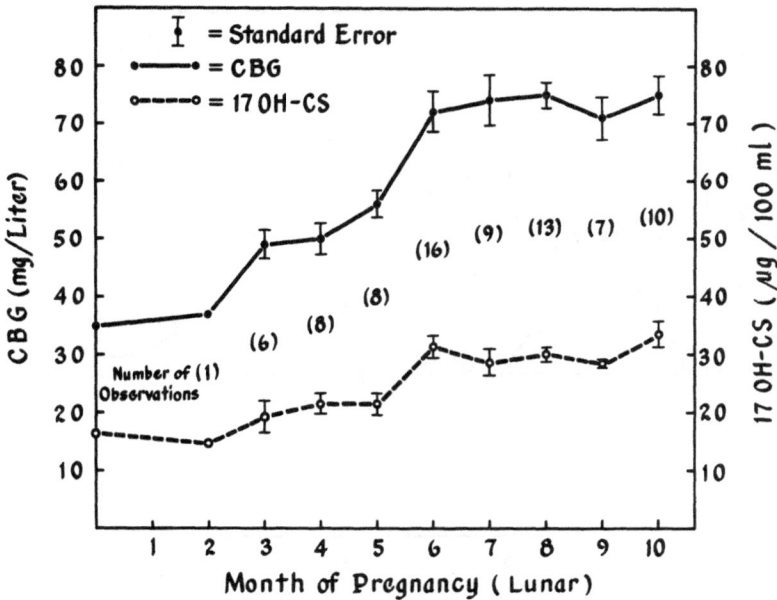

Fig. 7: Changes in CBG and plasma 17-OHCS in human pregnancy.

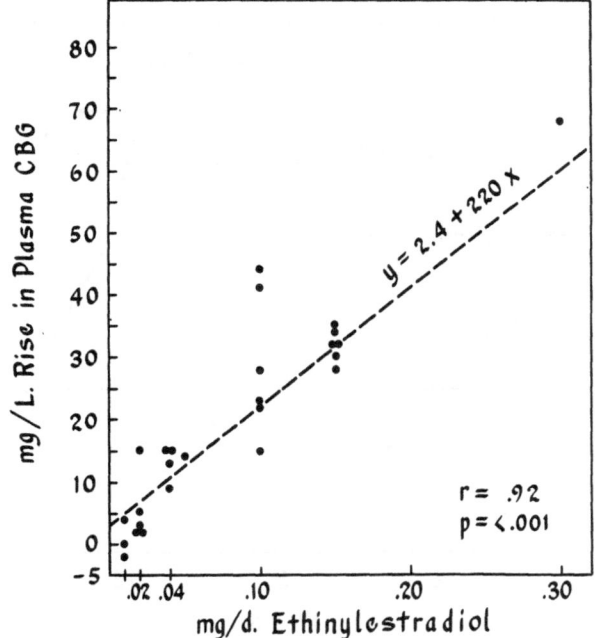

Fig. 8: Dose-response relationship of CBG increase following
six days' administration of graded doses of ethinylestradiol.

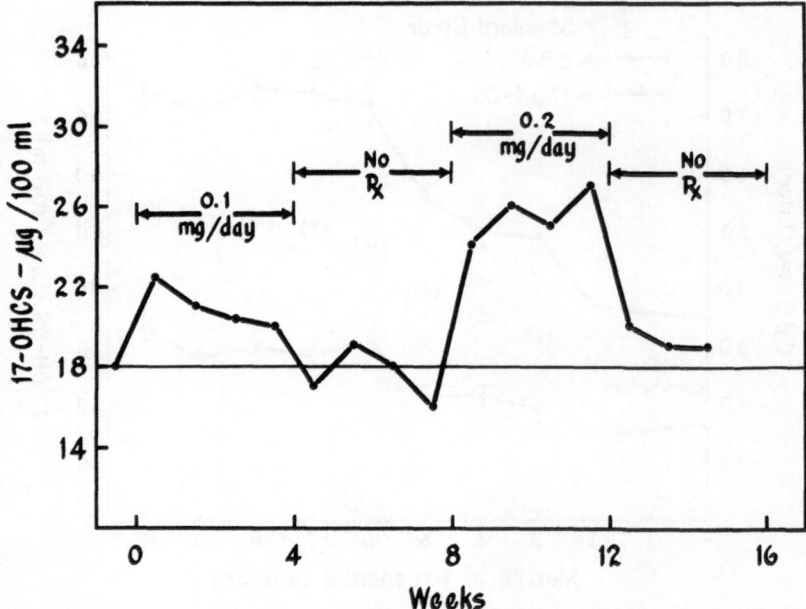

Fig. 9: Mean response in five individuals of plasma 17-OHCS to 0.1 and 0.2 mg./day doses of diethylstilbestrol over four-week periods separated by four weeks off medication.

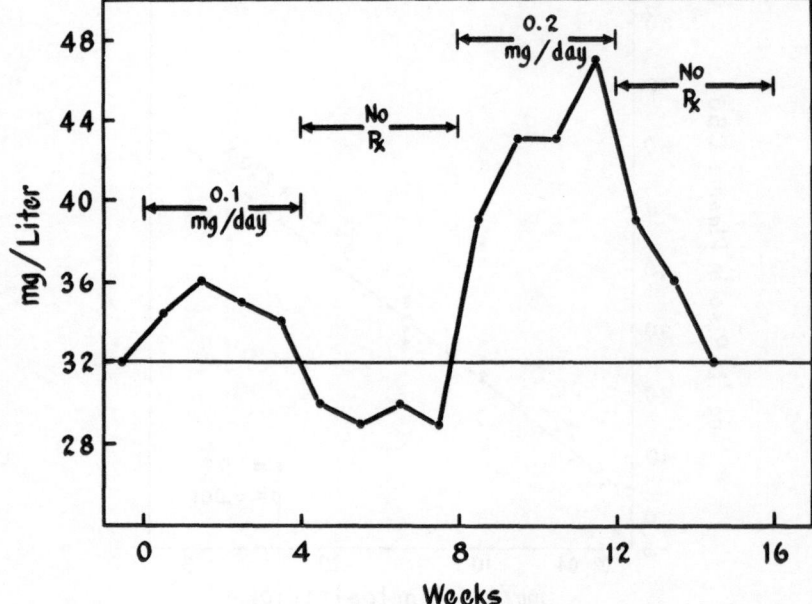

Fig. 10: Mean response in five individuals of CBG to 0.1 and 0.2 mg./day doses of diethylstilbestrol over four-week periods separated by four weeks off medication.

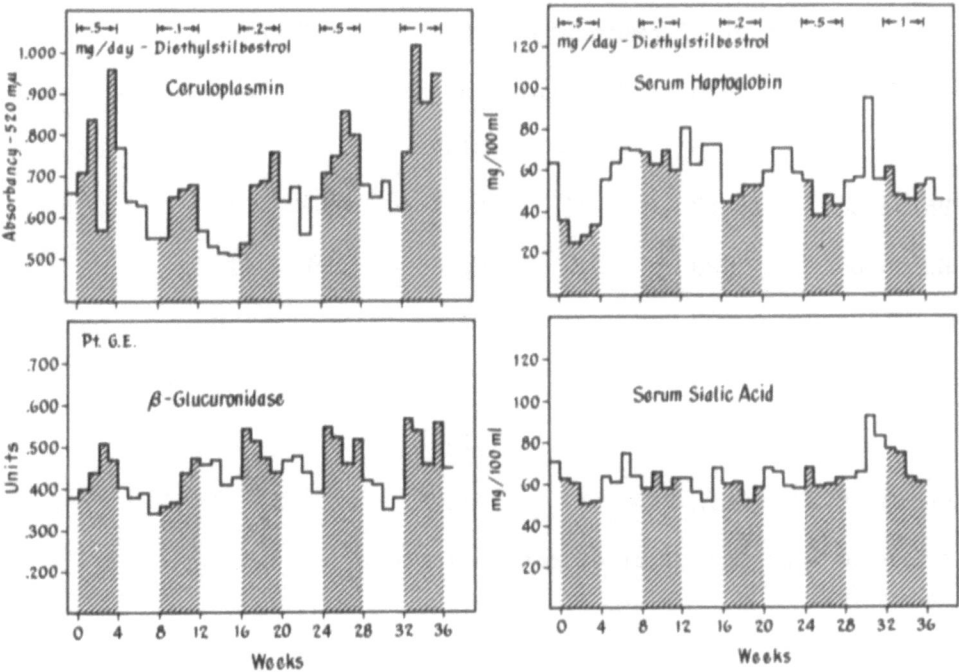

Fig. 11: Effect alternating four week periods of varying DES dosage treatment and rest on serum levels ceruloplasmin, haptoglobin, β-glucuronidase, and sialic acid.

The variable response of CBG to pregnancy (Table 18), or estrogen treatment in other mammals (Table 19) again illustrates the fact that the changes occurring in human pregnancy do not represent all placental mammals. We have not found such changes in samples from species representing the Carnivora, Pinnipedia, Proboscidea, Perissodactyla and Artiodactyla. Similar changes have been found in some species of Insectivora, Primates, Rodentia and Lagomorpha. Thus the direct measurement of nonprotein-bound cortisol and the assessment of effects attributable to increased corticosteroid activity will be essential for determining if the effects of pregnancy or estrogen treatment ascribed to increased corticoids apply to these species. Further, it will be interesting to explore what other estrogen-mediated changes of human pregnancy are present in these groups of mammalian species failing to show changes in transcortin (182).

The changes induced by estrogen treatment in nonmammalian vertebrates including birds (61, 68, 69, 74, 84, 111, 125, 144, 177, 181, 188, 194, 197), reptiles (35, 71, 156, 158, 159, 181, 204), amphibians (161, 181, 210, 211) and fish (64, 181, 208)

Table 18. Effect of pregnancy on CBG in the Carnivora.

Species	Normal	Pregnant	Species	Normal	Pregnant
Dog	6	6	Mink	12	12
Polar Bear	18	15	Striped Skunk	12	10
Brown Bear	20	17	Hognose Skunk	18	18
Asiatic Bear	20	21	Cat	5	4
Raccoon	100	120	Lion	6	6
Coatimundi	22	14	Tiger	40	40
Cacomistle	12	3	Hyena	18	?

All values as µg/100 ml of cortisol bound.

Table 19. Estrogen and pregnancy effects on CBG.

Species	Control (µg%)	Post Estrogen (µg%)	Pregnancy (µg%)
Man	22	70	55
Rhesus Monkey	20	16	14
Green monkey	28	90	72
Squirrel monkey	5	80	80
Slow Loris	24	16	15
Guinea Pig	15	200*	600
Dog	6	6	6
Raccoon	85	80	90
Cat	5	5	5

* Variable.

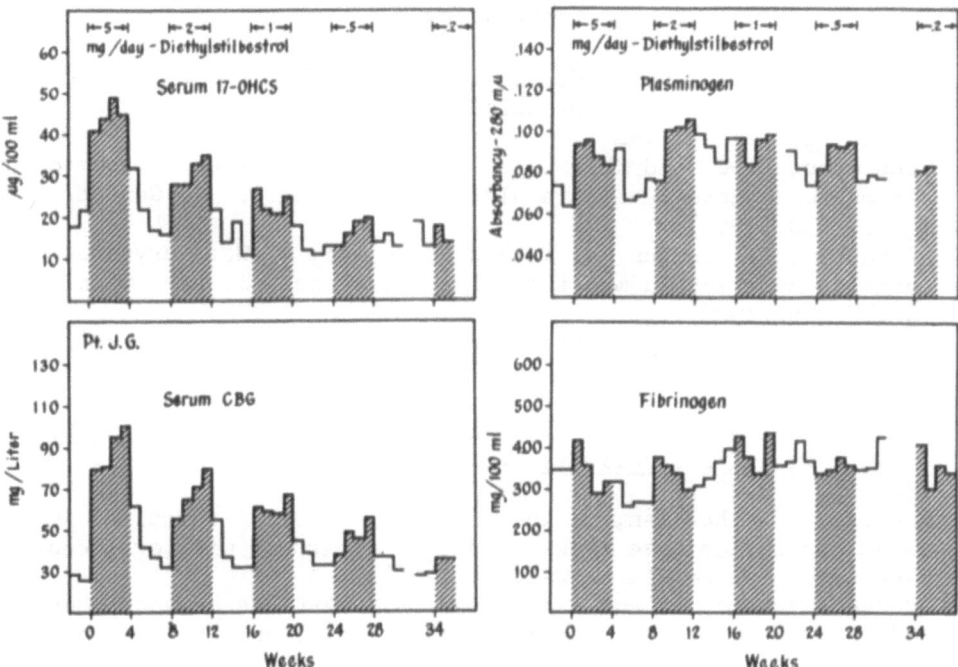

Fig. 12:   Effect of alternating four week periods of varying estrogen dosage and rest on fibrinogen, plasminogen, 17-OHCS and CBG.

focus attention on the liver as a target tissue for estrogen action (70). In general, the liver of these vertebrates synthesizes lipophosphoproteins which are then transported in the blood to the ovary for deposition in the yolk. The quantity depends upon the volume of yolk and is massive in groups such as the birds. Associated with these protein changes are increases in plasma calcium, iron and other components. The proteins have been demonstrated to be synthesized in the liver by egg-producing females (69, 70) and they can be induced by administered estrogen in both females and males (69, 74). The eutherian or placental mammals do not show these dramatic effects but some of the changes seen in human pregnancy including the alterations in serum lipids and lipoproteins, and other liver synthesized proteins (139) may represent a residual of our phylogenetic heritage. In contrast, it has been difficult to demonstrate in the nonmammalian species many of the specific blood changes found in humans (180, 181).

REFERENCES

1. Abels, J. C., Young, N. F. and Taylor, H. C.: Effects of testosterone propionate on protein formation in man. J. Clin. Endocr. 4:198-201 (1944).

2. Ackermann, P. G. and Kheim, T.: The effect of testosterone on plasma amino acid levels in elderly individuals. J. Geront. 19:207-210 (1964).

3. Alexanian, R., Vaughn, W. K. and Ruchelman, M. W.: Erythropoietin excretion in man following androgens. J. Lab. Clin. Med. 70:777-785 (1967).

4. Amundson, B. A. and Pilgeram, L. O.: Observations on a relationship between steroid metabolism and the concentration of plasma fibrinogen.

5. Arnold, A. and Potts, G. O.: Anabolic steroids, in New Methods of Nutritional Biochemistry, Vol. 2, Academic Press, New York, 1965, p. 403-431.

6. Arturson, G., Beckman, L. and Persson, B. H.: Alterations in serum naphthylamidase isozymes during treatment with oral contraceptives. Nature 214:1252-1253 (1967).

7. Aschkenasy-Lelu, P. and Aschkenasy, A.: Effects of androgens and oestrogens on the metabolism of proteins and the growth of tissues. World Rev. Nutr. Dietet. 1:29-60 (1959).

8. Augustinsson, K. B. and Henricson, B.: Effect of castration and of testosterone on arylesterase activity and protein content of blood plasma in male dogs. Acta Endocr. 50:145-154 (1965).

9. Aurell, M., Cramer, K. and Rybo, G.: Serum lipids and lipoproteins during long-term administration of an oral contraceptive (Anovlar). Lancet 1:291-293 (1966).

10. Baker, D. H., Jordan, C. E., Waitt, W. P. and Gouwens, D. W.: Effect of a combination of diethylstilbestrol and methyltestosterone, sex and dietary protein level of performance and carcass characteristics of finishing swine. J. Animal Sci. 26:1059- (1967a).

11. Barclay, M., Barclay, R. K., Skipski, V. P., Kerkish, O. T., Mueller, C. A., Shah, E. and Elkins, W. L.: Fluctuations in human serum lipoproteins during the normal menstrual cycle. Biochem. J. 96:205-209 (1965).

12. Baskakova, V. P.: Effect of courses of folliculin administration on the blood serum proteins of normal and castrated rabbits. Probl. Endokr. Gormonoter. 11:85-88 (1965).

13. Baskakova, V. P.: Conditioned reflex changes occurring in the blood serum proteins under the effect of folliculin, hexestrol, progestin and testosterone propionate. Farmakol. i. Tiksikol. 28:566-567 (1965).

14. Beall, C. W., Simpson, C. F., Pritchard, W. R. and Harms, R. H.: Aortic rupture in turkeys induced by diethylstilbestrol. Proc. Soc. Exp. Biol. Med. 113:442-443 (1963).

15. Beckman, L., Bjorling, G. and Christodoulou, C.: Pregnancy enzymes and placental polymorphism. II. Leucine aminopeptidase. Acta Genet., Basel 16:122-131 (1966).

16. Beckman, L., Bjorling, G. and Christodoulou, C.: Pregnancy enzymes and placental polymorphism. I. Alkaline phosphatase. Acta Genet., Basel 16:59-73 (1966).

17. Beller, F.K., Douglas, G. W., Morris, R. H. and Johnson, A. J.: The fibrinolytic enzyme system in pregnancy. Amer. J. Obstet. Gynec. 101:587-592 (1968).

18. Beller, F.K. and Porges, R. F.: Blood coagulation and fibrinolytic enzyme studies during cyclic and continuous application of progestational agents. Amer. J. Obstet. Gynec. 97: 448-459 (1967).

19. Berg, B. N., Sigg, E. B. and Greengard, P.: Maintenance of pregnancy in protein-deficient rats by adrenocortical steroid or ACTH administration. Endocrinology 80:829-834 (1967).

20. Bockner, V. and Roman, W.: Influence of oral contraceptives on the binding capacity of serum proteins. Med. J. Aust. 2: 1187-1194 (1967).

21. Borden, T. A., Wissler, R. W. and Hughes, R. H.: Physicochemical study of the lipoprotein system of the normal and estrogen-treated male rat in relation to atherosclerosis. J. Atheroscler. Res. 4:477-496 (1964).

22. Bourdel, M. G.: Attempts to reproduce the protein anabolism of pregnancy in castrated female rats by injection of progesterone. Proc. Fifth Int. Congr. Anim. Reprod. and A. I. (Trento, Italy 9/6-13/64), 3:298-303.

23. Braverman, L. E., Foster, A. E. and Ingbar, S. H.: Sex-related differences in the binding in serum of thyroid hormones. J. Clin. Endocr. 27:227-232 (1967).

24. Braverman, L. E. and Ingbar, S. H.: Effects of norethandrolone on the transport in serum and peripheral turnover of thyroxine. J. Clin. Endocr. Metab. 27:389-396 (1967).

25. Braverman, L. E., Socolow, E. L., Woeber, K.A. and Ingbar, S.H.: Effect of norethandrolone on the metabolism of ^{125}I-labeled thyroxine-binding prealbumin. J. Clin. Endocr. Metab. 28:831-835 (1968).

26. Breuer, C. B. and Florini, J. R.: Amino acid incorporation into protein by cell-free systems from rat skeletal muscle. 4. Effects of animal age, androgens and anabolic agents on activity of muscle ribosomes. Biochemistry 4:1544-1550 (1965).

27. Butler, E. J.: The influence of pregnancy on the blood, plasma and caeruloplasmin copper levels of sheep. Comp. Biochem. Physiol. 9:1-12 (1963).

28. Carruthers, M. E., Hobbs, C. B. and Warren, R. L.: Raised serum copper and caeruloplasmin levels in subjects taking oral contraceptives. J. Clin. Path. 19:498-500 (1966).

29. Cascone, O., Marletta, F. and Amaro, A.: Behavior of blood and liver proteins after administration of 4-chlorotestosterone. Boll. Soc. Ital. Biol. Sper. 40:1040-1042 (1964).

30. Chanarin, I., Rothman, D., Ardeman, S. and McLean, A.: Studies in histidine and urocanate metabolism in pregnancy. Clin. Sci. 28:377-384 (1965).

31. Chandra, P., Orii, H. and Wacker, A.: Studies on the regulation of a sex-associated protein in rat liver. Hoppe-Seyler Z. Physiol. Chem. 349:784-788 (1968).

32. Chesanow, R. L., Salvi, M. L. and Angeletti, P. U.: Androgen influence on protein and enzyme pattern of rat kidney. Experientia 20:212-214 (1964).

33. Churchill, W. H., Jr., Weintraub, R. M., Borsos, T. and Rapp, H. J.: Mouse complement: The effect of sex hormones and castration on two of the late-acting components. J. Exp. Med. 125:657-672 (1967).

34. Clausen, J. and Gerhardt, W.: Sequential inhibition of lactic dehydrogenase isozymes of human brain by Honvan (stilboestrol diphosphate). Acta Neurol. Scand. 39:305-322 (1963).

35. Clark, N. B.: Influence of estrogens upon serum calcium, phosphate and protein concentrations of fresh-water turtles. Comp. Biochem. Physiol. 20:823-834 (1967).

36. Cox, D. H. and Hale, O. M.: Dietary hormones and fat and serum cholesterol, transaminases and copper in swine. J. Nutr. 72:77-80 (1960).

37. Crane, M. G., Heitsch, J., Harris, J. J. and Johns, V. J., Jr.: Effect of ethinyl estradiol (Estinyl) on plasma renin activity. J. Clin. Endocr. Metab. 26:1403-1406 (1966).

38. Daniel, D. G., Bloom, A. L., Giddings, J. C., Campbell, H. and Turnbull, A.C.: Increased factor IX levels in puerperium during administration of diethylstilboestrol. Brit. Med. J. 1:801-803 (1968).

39. Daughaday, W. and Mariz, I. K.: Corticosteroid-binding globulin: Its properties and quantitation. Metabolism 10:936-950 (1961).

40. DeLoecker, W.: Effects of testosterone on the incorporation of glycine-U-C^{14} into the proteins and nucleic acids of skeletal muscle (rat). Arch. Int. Pharmacodyn. 153:69-78 (1965).

41. DeLoecker, W., Brooks, S. C. and DeWever, F.: Stimulation in vitro of protein synthesis in muscle microsomal supernatant by estradiol-3, 17β-disulfate (rats). Biochim. Biophys. Acta 119:655-657 (1966).

42. DeMoor, P., Steeno, O., Brosens, I. and Hendrikx: Data on transcortin activity in human plasma as studied by gel filtration. J. Clin. Endocr. 26:71-78 (1966).

43. Devalle, J. J., Curbelo, H. M., Houssay, A. B., Tocci, A. A. and Gamper, C. H.: Effect of testosterone propionate upon sialic content of salivary glands in mice. Acta Physiol. Lat. Amer. 18:42-46 (1968).

44. Diamond, L. K., Jacobson, W. and Sidman, R.: Increased thymidine incorporation in children's bone marrow under the influence of testosterone. J. Physiol. 185:40-1P (1966).

45. Dietrich, L. S. and Yero, I. L.: Endocrine involvement in the suppression of NAD synthesis produced by hyperphysiological levels of steroid hormones. Biochim. Biophys. Acta 97:385-388 (1965).

46. Dietrich, L. S.: Effect of hyperphysiological levels of steroid hormones on nicotinamide deamidase and NAD synthesis in mouse liver tissue. Biochem. Pharmacol. 14:467-472 (1965).

47. Doe, R. P., Mellinger, G. T., Swaim, W. R. and Seal, U. S.: Estrogen dosage effects on serum proteins: A longitudinal study. J. Clin. Endocr. Metab. 27:1081-1086 (1967).

48. Dohrmann, R. E. and Giffels, G.: Behavior of glutamic pyruvic transaminase, aldolase, β-glucuronidase and of the protein spectrum in the serum during action of an ovulation inhibitor. Med. Klin. 60:1844-1847 (1965).

49. Dorfman, R. I. and Shipley, R. A.: Androgens: Biochemistry, Physiology and Clinical Significance. John Wiley and Sons, Inc., New York (1956).

50. Dowling, J. T., Hutchinson, D. L., Hindle, W. R. and Kleeman, C. R.: Effects of pregnancy on iodine metabolism in the primate. J. Clin. Endocr. 21:779-791 (1961).

51. Ellington, E. F., Fox, C. W., Kennick, W. H. and Sather, L. A.: Feedlot performance and carcass characteristics of lambs receiving cortisone and diethylstilbestrol. J. Anim. Sci. 26:462-465 (1967).

52. Ellison, T. and Scott, G. C.: The effects of a plant steroid on body weight and feed efficiency of broilers. Poult. Sci. 42:530-531 (1963).

53. Fabian, E., Stork, A., Koblilkova, J. and Sponarova, J.: Activity of the lipoprotein lipase and estrogens. Enzymol. Biol. Clin. 8(6):451-455 (1967).

54. Fazzini, G. and Fonnesu-Severi, C.: In vitro incorporation of leucine-1-C14 into heart proteins of intact and castrated rats treated with testosterone and 4-chlorotestosterone. Sperimentale 115(2):104-112 (1965).

55. Feher, L., Sipos, J. and Hevizy, H. E.: Correlation of ceruloplasmin and the neuro-endocrine system. 2. The effect of estrogens on the ceruloplasmin and CU content of the blood serum. Relationship between the estrogen effect and thyroid effect. Magy. Balorv. Arch. 15:214-216 (1962).

56. Frieden, E. H. and Harper, A. A.: Some characteristics of the steroid-sensitive amino acid incorporating system of mouse kidney (testosterone). Endocrinology 72:465-469 (1963).

57. Frieden, E. H.: Sex hormones and the metabolism of amino acids and proteins, in Actions of Hormones on Molecular Processes, John Wiley and Sons, Inc., New York, 1964, p. 509-559.

58. Gala, R. R. and Westphal, U.: Corticosteroid-binding activity in serum of mouse, rabbit, and guinea pig during pregnancy and lactation: Possible involvement in the initiation of lactation. Acta Endocr. 55:47-61 (1967).

59. Galand, P., Rodesch, F., Leroy, F. and Chretien, J.: Altered duration of DNA synthesis and cell cycle in non-target tissues of mice treated with oestrogen. Nature 216:1211-1212 (1967).

60. Gawienowski, A. M., Knoche, H. W. and Moser, H. C.: The metabolism of ^{14}C- and ^{3}H-labeled diethylstilbestrol in the rat. Biochim. Biophys. Acta 65:150-152 (1962).

61. Gilbert, A. B.: The effect of oestrogen and thyroxine on the blood volume of the domestic cock. J. Endocr. 26:41-47 (1963).

62. Gligore, V., Gozariu, L., Gherman, G., Lucaciu, O., Holan, T., Szantay, I. and Farcasan, M.: Changes in the function of hepatocellular uptake of S-35 labeled methionine in patients with hyperfolliculinism. Stud. Cercet. Endocr. 14:261-266 (1963).

63. Glucksohn-Waelsch, S., Greengard, P., Quinn, G. P. and Teicher, L. S.: Genetic variations of an oxidase in mammals. J. Biol. Chem. 242:1271-1273 (1967).

64. Gottfried, H.: The occurrence and biological significance of steroids in lower vertebrates, a review. Steroids 3:219-242 (1964).

65. Grant, S. D., Pavlatos, F. Ch. and Forsham, P. H.: Effects of estrogen therapy on cortisol metabolism. J. Clin. Endocr. 25:1057-1066 (1965).

66. Greaves, M. S. and West, H. F.: Cortisol and cortisone in saliva of pregnancy. J. Endocr. 26:189-195 (1963).

67. Green, J. P., Fram, D. H. and Kase, N.: Methylhistamine and histamine in the urine of women during the elaboration of estrogen. Nature 204:1165-1168 (1964).

68. Greengard, O., Mendelsohn, N. and Gordon, M.: Iron accumulation in cockerel plasma after estrogen: Relation to induced phosphoprotein synthesis. Science 147:1571-1572 (1965).

69. Greengard, O., Sentenac, A. and Acs, G.: Induced formation of phosphoprotein in tissues of cockerels in vivo and in vitro. J. Biol. Chem. 240:1687-1691 (1965).

70. Gruber, M.: Regulation of protein synthesis in chicken liver: The action of estradiol, in Regulation of Nucleic Acid and Protein Biosynthesis, Elsevier Publishing Co., Koningsberger and Bosch (eds.), 1967.

71. Hahn, W. E.: Estradiol-induced vitellinogenesis and concomitant fat mobilization in the lizard, Uta stansburiana. Comp. Biochem. Physiol. 23:83-93 (1967).

72. Harter, G. D. and Vetter, R. L.: Feeder lamb response to cortisone acetate and diethylstilbestrol. J. Anim. Sci. 26:1397-1403 (1967).

73. Hazelwood, R. L. and Nelson, M. M.: Steroid maintenance of pregnancy in rats in the absence of dietary protein. Endocrinology 77:999-1013 (1965).

74. Heald, P. J. and McLachlan, P. M.: Isolation of phosvitin from the plasma of the oestrogen-treated immature pullet. Biochem. J. 92:51-55 (1964).

75. Henneman, D. H.: Effect of estrogen on in vivo and in vitro collagen biosynthesis and maturation in old and young female guinea pigs. Endocrinology 83:678-690 (1968).

76. Hershberger, L. G., Thompson, C. R. and Clegg, M. T.: Myotrophic effects of estrogen in mice and lack of effect in rats. Proc. Soc. Exp. Biol. Med. 121:785-788 (1966).

77. Herzfeld, A. and Knox, W. E.: The properties, developmental formation, and estrogen induction of ornithine aminotransferase in rat tissues. J. Biol. Chem. 243:3327-3332 (1968).

78. Heuson, J. C. and Legros, N.: In vitro effect of testosterone and 17β-estradiol on protein metabolism of human breast cancer. Cancer Chemother. Rep. 16:277-278 (1962).

79. Heuson, J. C. and Legros, N.: In vitro effect of testosterone and 17β-estradiol on L-leucine-C^{14} incorporation into human breast cancer tissue. Cancer 16:404-407 (1963).

80. Holton, J. B.: The effect of a histidine load on plasma levels and renal clearances of other amino acids. Clin. Chim. Acta 21:241-245 (1968).

81. Holvey, D. N., Cutler, R. E. and Dowling, J. T.: Thyroxine-binding by the thyroxine-binding globulin as a measure of the anabolic activity of congeners of testosterone. Metabolism 14:891-898 (1965).

82. Honger, P. E.: Albumin metabolism in normal pregnancy. Scand. J. Clin. Invest. 21:3-9 (1968).

83. Houssay, A. B. and Blumenkrantz, N.: Changes in glycoproteins in serum, urine and aqueous humor after gonadectomy or sex hormone injections in rats. Endocrinology 74:825-832 (1964).

84. Hunsaker, W. G.: Blood volume of geese treated with androgen and estrogen. Poult. Sci. 47:371-376 (1968).

85. Ide, H. and Fishman, W. H.: De Novo synthesis of endoplasmic reticulum glycoprotein; androgen-stimulated mouse renal β-glucuronidase. J. Cell. Biol. 35(2,ii):60A (1967).

86. Jacobson, W., Sidman, R. L. and Diamond, L. K.: Effect of testosterone on the uptake of tritiated thymidine by the bone marrow of children. Ann. N. Y. Acad. Sci. 149:389-405 (1968).

87. Jepson, J. H. and Lowenstein, L.: The effect of testosterone, adrenal steroids and prolactin on erythropoiesis. Acta Haemat. 38:292-299 (1967).

88. Kao, K. Y. T., Hitt, W. E. and McGavack, T. H.: Connective tissue. 13. Effect of estradiol nenzoate upon collagen synthesis by sponge biopsy connective tissue (rats). Proc. Soc. Exp. Biol. Med. 119:364-367 (1965).

89. Kappas, A., Jones, H. E. H. and Roitt, I. M.: Effects of steroid sex hormones on immunological phenomena. Nature 198:902 (1963).

90. Katz, F. H. and Kappas, A.: The effects of estradiol and estriol on plasma levels of cortisol and thyroid hormone-binding globulins and aldosterone and cortisol secretion rates in man. J. Clin. Invest. 46:1768-1777 (1967).

91. Katz, F. H. and Kappas, A.: Influence of estradiol and estriol on urinary excretion of hydroxyproline in man. J. Lab. Clin. Med. 71:65-74 (1968).

92. Katz, F. H. and Kappas, A.: Effect of natural estrogens on hydroxyproline excretion in man. J. Clin. Invest. 44:1063 (1965).

93. Katz, F. H.: Effects of oestradiol and oestriol on the disposition of injected radio-active proline, hydroxyproline and tyrosine in man. Acta Endocr. 58:664-672 (1968).

94. Kochakian, C. D., Hill, J. and Anouma, S.: Regulation of protein biosynthesis in mouse kidney by androgens. Excerpta Medica Fdn., Int. Congr. Series No. 51 (1962).

95. Kochakian, C. D.: Androgen regulation of rate of incorporation of leucine-$1C^{14}$ in tissues of guinea pig. Fed. Proc. 22:408 (1963).

96. Kochakian, C. D., Hill, J. and Costa, G.: Amino acid composition of the proteins of the muscles and organs of the normal, castrated and testosterone-treated guinea pig. Acta Endocr. 45:613-622 (1964).

97. Kochakian, C. D.: Effect of castration and testosterone on protein biosynthesis in guinea pig tissue preparations. Acta Endocr. 46:Suppl. 92 (1964).

98. Kochakian, C. D. and Hama, T.: Regulation of ribonucleic acid and protein biosynthesis in the mouse kidney by androgens. Excerpta Medica Fdn., Int. Congr. Series No. 111:76 (1966).

99. Kochakian, C. D., Tanaka, R., Hill, J. and Harrison, D. C.: Regulation of amino acid activating enzymes and nucleic acids of guinea pig tissues by androgens. Proc. Fifth Int. Congr. Biochem. 29:315 (1963).

100. Korner, A.: RNA and hormonal (including LH, androgens, estrogens) control of protein synthesis, in Progress in Biophysics and Molecular Biology, Vol. 7, Pergamon Press, 1967, p. 63-98.

101. Kruskemper, H. L.: Anabolic Steroids, Academic Press, New York, 1963.

102. Kuchler, R. J., Arnold, N. J. and Grauer, R. C.: Estradiol-cellular interaction in tissue culture. Proc. Soc. Exp. Biol. Med. 8:798-804 (1962).

103. Kulpmann, W. R. and Mosebach, K.-O.: Influence of testosterone on the incorporation of L-histidine-^{14}C into the proteins of some sexual and other organs of starving immature rats. Acta Endocr., Suppl. 100:128 (1965).

104. Kvarstein, B., Nordbo, H. and Schultz-Haudt, S. D.: Effect of estrogen on chondroitin sulphate of rat skin connective tissue. Acta Endocr. 44:209-215 (1963).

105. Landau, R. L. and Lugibihl, K.: The effect of progesterone on the concentration of plasma amino acids in man. Metabolism 16:1114-1122 (1967).

106. Landau, R. L. and Lugibihl, K.: The effect of progesterone on amino acid metabolism. J. Clin. Endocr. Metab. 21:1355-1363 (1961).

107. Landau, R. L. and Lugibihl, K.: The catabolic and natriuretic
     effects of progesterone in man. Recent Progr. Hormone Res.
     17:249-292 (1961).
108. Laurell, C. B.: Orosomucoid and α_1-antitrypsin in maternal
     and fetal sera at parturition. Scand. J. Clin. Lab. Invest.
     21:136-138 (1968).
109. Laurell, C. B. and Skanse, B.: Estrogens and plasma oroso-
     mucoid. J. Clin. Endocr. 23:214-215 (1963).
110. Laurell, C. B., Kullander, S. and Thorell, J.: Effect of
     administration of a combined estrogen-progestin contraceptive
     on the level of individual plasma proteins. Scand. J. Clin.
     Lab. Invest. 21(4):337-343 (1968).
111. Leach, R. M., Jr., Norris, L. C. and Scott, M. L.: The effect
     of diethylstilbestrol on choline deficiency in the chick.
     Poult. Sci. 41:1828-1832 (1962).
112. Leathem, J. H.: Some aspects of hormone and protein metabolic
     interrelationships, in Mammalian Protein Metabolism, Vol. 1,
     Academic Press, New York, 1964, p. 343-381 and 364-366.
113. Lederer, J.: Controle endocrinien du metabolisme du fer.
     Annales d'Endocrinologie 23:563-568 (1962).
114. Leonard, P. J. and D'Arbela, P. G.: The plasma concentrations
     of free and protein-bound cortisol in hypoproteinaemia.
     J. Endocr. 34:265-270 (1966).
115. Lewis, U. J., Cheever, E. V. and Vanderlaan, W. P.: Alter-
     ation of the proteins of the pituitary gland of the rat by
     estradiol and cortisol. Endocrinology 76:362-368 (1965).
116. Lindner, H. R.: Comparative aspects of cortisol transport:
     Lack of firm binding to plasma proteins in domestic ruminants.
     J. Endocr. 28:301-320 (1964).
117. Litteria, M. and Timiras, P. S.: Effects of estradiol on
     1-^{14}C-lysine uptake and incorporation into brain protein (rat).
     Fed. Proc. 26:365 (1967).
118. Litteria, M.: Effects of estradiol on uptake, incorporation
     and localization of 1-^{14}C-lysine in brain protein (rat).
     Diss. Abstr. 28:4629B (1968).
119. Little, B. and Lincoln, E.: Effect of estrogen, progesterone
     and testosterone on the incorporation of 1-valine-1-C^{14} into
     protein of the rat liver and uterus. Endocrinology 74:1-8
     (1964).
120. Lorincz, A. B. and Kuttner, R. E.: Comparative studies on
     free amino acids in female reproductive tissues. Amer. J.
     Obstet. Gynecol. 101:462-472 (1968).
121. Lyman, R. L., Hopkins, S. M., Sheehan, G. and Tinoco, J.:
     Effects of estradiol and testosterone on the incorporation and
     distribution of Me-^{14}C methionine in rat liver lecithins.
     Biochim. Biophys. Acta 152:197-207 (1968).
122. MacLaren, J. A., Reid, D. E., Konugres, A. A. and Allen, F. H.:
     Pa 1, a new inherited alpha-2-globulin of human serum. Vox
     Sang. 11:553-560 (1966).

123. McIntosh, E. N., Acker, D. C. and Kline, E. A.: Influence of orally administered stilbestrol on connective tissue of skeletal muscle of lambs fed varying levels of protein. Agricult. Food Chem. 9:418-421 (1961).

124. Mirand, E. A. and Gordon, A. S.: Mechanism of estrogen action in erythropoiesis. Endocrinology 78:325-332 (1966).

125. Moore, J. D. and Breitenbach, R. P.: The effects of estradiol-17β and/or progesterone on nitrogen balance values in studies on the castrated rooster. Gen. Comp. Endocr. 7:430-444 (1966).

126. Moriyama, I.: Influences of progesterone, estrogen and glucocorticoid on protein and amino acid metabolism. Folia. Endocr. Jap. 41:610-622 (1965).

127. Mosebach, K.-O. and Engels, T.: Einfluss von testosteron auf den DNA-stoffwechsel in vesikulardrusen unreifer ratten. Hoppe-Seyler Z. Physiol. Chem. 345:111-121 (1966).

128. Munro, H. N.: General aspects of the regulations of protein metabolism by diet and hormones, in Mammalian Protein Metabolism, Academic Press, New York, Vol. 1, 1964, p. 382-482.

129. Musa, B. U., Seal, U. S. and Doe, R. P.: Elevation of certain plasma proteins in man following estrogen administration: A dose-response relationship. J. Clin. Endocr. Metab. 25:1163-1166 (1965).

130. Musa, B. U., Doe, R. P. and Seal, U. S.: Serum protein alterations produced in women by synthetic estrogens. J. Clin. Endocr. Metab. 27:1463-1469 (1967).

131. Nicol, T., Bilbey, D. L. J., Charles, L. M., Cordingley, J. L. and Vernon-Roberts, B.: Oestrogen: The natural stimulant of body defence. J. Endocr. 30:277-291 (1964).

132. Notides, A. C.: Estrogen-induced synthesis of a specific uterine protein (rat). Diss. Abstr. 27:4103B (1967).

133. Nour-Eldin, F. and Lewis, F. J. W.: Hypo-or hypercoagulability of blood with high levels of clotting factors? Nature, 212: 417 (1966).

134. Novikova, M. A. and Chestukhin, A. V.: Control of protein synthesis in various tissues by steroid hormones. Excerpta Medica Fdn., Int. Congr. Series No. 111:321 (1966).

135. Novotny, A., Dvorak, V. and Opplt, J.: Dyslipoproteinaemia after surgical castration of women. Rev. Czech. Med. 13:151-159 (1967).

136. Oelkers, W. and Nolten, W.: Inhibition of tryptophane oxygenase activity with oestrone, sulphate and nonesterified oestrogen (rats). Hoppe-Seyler Z. Physiol. Chem. 338:(3-6) 105-112 (1964).

137. Oettgen, H. F., Binaghi, R. A. and Benacerraf, B.: The effect of various hormones on the serum level of anaphylactic antibody in the rat. Int.Arch. Allergy 29:131-139 (1966).

138. Oikonomides, M.: Observations on the behavior of serum protein fractions and amino acids under the influence of the deprivation and administration of androgenic hormones of the testis. Acta Microbiol. Hellen. 9:20-33 (1964).

139. Olson, J. P., Miller, L. L. and Troup, S. B.: Synthesis of clotting factors by the isolated perfused rat liver. J. Clin. Invest. 45:690-701 (1966).

140. Oltjen, R. R. and Lehmann, R. P.: Effect of diethylstilbestrol on the blood plasma amino acid patterns of beef steers fed finishing diets. J. Nutr. 95:399-405 (1968).

141. O'Malley, B. W.: In vitro hormonal induction of a specific protein (avidin) in chick oviduct. Biochemistry 6:2546-2551 (1967).

142. O'Reilly, S. and Loncin, M.: Ceruloplasmin and 5-hydroxyindole metabolism in pregnancy. Amer. J. Obstet. Gynecol. 97:8-12 (1967).

143. Oppenheimer, J. H.: Role of plasma proteins in the binding, distribution and metabolism of the thyroid hormones. New Eng. J. Med. 278:1153-1161 (1968).

144. Pavel, J. and Svozil, B.: The distribution of lactic dehydrogenase isoenzymes in the blood serum of surgically and hormonally castrated cockerels. Poult. Sci. 47:91-94 (1968).

145. Pearlman, W. H., Crepy, O. and Murphy, M.: Testosterone-binding levels in the serum of women during the normal menstrual cycle, pregnancy, and the post-partum period. J. Clin. Endocr. 27:1012-1018 (1967).

146. Perklev, T., Gassner, F. X., Martin, R. P., Huseby, R. A. and Shimoda, W.: Excretion of radioactivity by human subjects after ingestion of liver from cattle treated with labeled polydiethylstilbestrol phosphate. Proc. Soc. Exp. Biol. Med. 119:996-998 (1965).

147. Pettengill, O. S. and Fishman, W. H.: Influence of testosterone on glycine incorporation into mouse kidney β-glucuronidase. Exp. Cell. Res. 28:248-253 (1962).

148. Plager, J. E., Schmidt, K. G. and Staubitz, W. J.: Increased unbound cortisol in the plasma of estrogen-treated subjects. J. Clin. Invest. 43:1066-1072 (1964).

149. Planas, J.: Serum iron in normal and castrated mammals. Nature 197:186-187 (1963).

150. Plimpton, R. F., Jr., Cahill, V. R., Teague, H. S., Grifo, A. P., Jr. and Kunkle, L. E.: Periodic measurement of growth and carcass development following diethylstilbestrol implantation of boars. J. Anim. Sci. 26:1319-1324 (1967).

151. Pora, E., Gozariul, Toma, V. and Bedivan, M.: Experimental investigations of the influence of estrogens on hepatic metabolism of S-35 labeled methionine. Stud. Cercet. Endocr. 14:237-241 (1963).

152. Prellwitz, W. and Bassler, K. H.: Verandrungen an Proteinen der Leber und des Blutes bei experimenteller Lebercirrhose und nach Behandlung mit Decortin und einen anabolen steroid. Klin. Wschr. 41:1125 (1963).

153. Preston, R. L., Martin, J. E., Blakely, J. E. and Pfander, W. H.: Structural requirements for the growth response of

of certain estrogens in ruminants. J. Anim. Sci. 24:338-340 (1965).

154. Price, J. M., Thornton, J. J. and Mueller, L. M.: Tryptophan metabolism in women using steroid hormones for ovulation control. J. Clin. Nutr. 20:452-456 (1967).

155. Priest, R. E. and Koplitz, R. M.: Inhibition of synthesis of sulfated mucopolysaccharides by estradiol. J. Exp. Med. 116: 565-574 (1962).

156. Prosser, R. L., III. and Suzuki, H. K.: The effects of estradiol valerate on the serum and bone of hatchling and juvenile caiman crocodiles, Caiman sclerops. Comp. Biochem. Physiol. 25:529-534 (1968).

157. Quintarelli, G. and Dellovo, M. C.: Activation of glycoprotein biosynthesis by testosterone propionate on mouse exorbital glands. J. Histochem. Cytochem. 13:361-364 (1965).

158. Rao, C. A. P.: Effect of steroids on the serum protein fractions of the tortoise, Testudo elegans. Comp. Biochem. Physiol. 26:1119-1122 (1968).

159. Rao, C. A. P. and David, G. F. X.: Effect of certain steroids (including androgens, pregnenolone) on the serum protein concentrations of the female lizard, Uromastix hardwickii. Gen. Comp. Endocr. 9(2):227-233 (1967).

160. Rao, P. B. R., Paolucci, A. M. and Johnson, B. C.: Relationship of estrogen and vitamin K. Proc. Soc. Exp. Biol. Med. 112:393-396 (1963).

161. Redshaw, M. R. and Follett, B. K.: Effects of estrogens on protein and fat metabolism in Xenopus laevis. Gen. Comp. Endocr. 9(3):485 (1967).

162. Reed, M.: The effect of norethandrolone (Nilevar) on serum proteins in the female guinea pig. J. Endocr. 37:253-260 (1967).

163. Reilly, R. W., Thompson, J. S., Bielski, R. K. and Severson, C. D.: Estradiol-induced wasting syndrome in neonatal mice. J. Immunol. 98:321-330 (1967).

164. Reuter, A. M. and Kennes, F.: Influence of castration and of testosterone on prealbumin in mouse serum. Experientia 22: 840-841 (1966).

165. Riggs, T. R. and Walker, L. M.: Action of estrogen sulfates on accumulation of amino acids by Ehrlich (mouse) ascites tumor cells in vitro. Endocrinology 74:483-488 (1964).

166. Ritter, C.: NAD biosynthesis as an early part of androgen action. Molec. Pharmacol. 2:125-133 (1966).

167. Robertson, G. S.: Serum protein and cholinesterase changes in association with contraceptive pills. Lancet 1:232-235 (2/4/67).

168. Robinson, J. C., London, W. T. and Pierce, J. E.: Observations on the origin of pregnancy associated proteins. Amer. J. Obstet. Gynec. 96:226-230 (1966).

169. Rombauts, P. and DuMesnil DuBuisson, F.: Protein anabolism in

hysterectomized sow and role of progesterone in protein metabolism. Proc. Fifth Int. Congr. Anim. Reprod. & A. I., Vol. 2: 410-413 (1964).

170. Rombauts, P., Fevre, J. and DuMesnil DuBuisson, F.: Influence of exogenous progesterone on the protein metabolism of ovariectomized sows during estrous cycle or gestation. C. R. Acad. Sci. 258:5531-5533 (1964).

171. Rose, D. P.: The influence of oestrogens on tryptophane metabolism in man. Clin. Sci. 31:265-272 (1966).

172. Rosner, W., Kelly, W. G., Deakins, S. M. and Christy, N. P.: The binding of estrogens and testosterone in human plasma, p. 325-338, in Radioisotopes in Medicine: In Vitro Studies (Hayes, R. L., Goswitz, F. A. and Murphy, B. E. P., eds.) U. S. Atomic Energy Commission (Conf.-671111) Oak Ridge, Tenn. June 1968.

173. Sachs, B. A. and Wolfman, L.: Effect of anabolic steroids on plasma glycoproteins. Nature 216:297-298 (1967).

174. Sakurada, T., Saito, S., Inagaki, K., Tayama, S. and Torikai, T.: Polyacrylamide gel electrophoretic study on the effect of estrogen on human thyroxine-binding prealbumin. Tohoku J. Exp. Med. 93:339-362 (1967).

175. Sandberg, A. A., Woodruff, M., Rosenthal, H., Nienhouse and Slaunwhite, W. R.: Transcortin: A corticosteroid-binding protein of plasma. VII. Half life in normal and estrogen-treated subjects. J. Clin. Invest. 43:461-466 (1964).

176. Sandberg, A. A. and Slaunwhite, W. R.: Transcortin: A corticosteroid-binding protein of plasma. II. Levels in various conditions and the effects of estrogens. J. Clin. Invest. 38:1290-1297 (1959).

177. Schjeide, O. A. and Wilkens, M.: Parameters of oestrogen-stimulated protein synthesis (chick embryos). Nature 201:42-44 (1964).

178. Schrogie, J. J. and Solomon, H. M.: Estrogenic hormones and blood coagulation. J. Chron. Dis. 20:675-678 (1967).

179. Schumacher, G. F. B.: Acute phase protein in serum of women using hormonal contraceptives. Science 153:901-902 (1966).

180. Seal, U. S. and Doe, R. P.: Vertebrate distribution of corticosteroid-binding globulin and some endocrine effects on concentration. Steroids 5:827-841 (1965).

181. Seal, U. S.: Vertebrate distribution of serum ceruloplasmin and sialic acid and the effects of pregnancy. Comp. Biochem. Physiol. 13:143-159 (1964).

182. Seal, U. S. and Doe, R. P.: The role of corticosteroid-binding globulin in mammalian pregnancy. Excerpta Medica Int. Congr. Series No. 132, p. 697-706 (1966).

183. Segal, S.: Hormones (including oestradiol), amino acid transport and protein synthesis. Nature 203:17-19 (1964).

184. Sehe, C. T. and Clayton, R. B.: Control of utilization of H^3-uridine in the brain and other tissues by sex hormones

(including testosterone, oestradiol; rat). Gen. Comp. Endocr. 9(3):492 (1967).

185. Simmons, D. J.: Collagen formation and endochondral ossification in estrogen-treated mice. Proc. Soc. Exp. Biol. Med. 121: 1165-1168 (1966).

186. Simpson, C. F. and Harms, R. H.: Aortic ruptures in turkeys induced by diethylstilbestrol and dienestrol diacetate. Proc. Soc. Exp. Biol. Med. 123:604-606 (1966).

187. Simpson, C. F. and Harms, R. H.: Reduction of incidence of diethylstilbestrol induced aortic ruptures in turkeys by iodinated casein. Proc. Soc. Exp. Biol. Med. 128:863-867 (1968).

188. Simpson, C. F., Harms, R. H. and Kling, J. M.: The nature of inclusions in erythrocytes of turkeys treated with diethylstilbestrol. Exp. Molec. Pathol. 5:125-133 (1966).

189. Skosey, J. L. and Kappas, A.: Effect of estradiol on skin collagen turnover rate (rats). Fed. Proc. 26:426 (1967).

190. Slebodzinski, A. and Wojcik, K.: Protein level and trend of changes in serum protein fractions in sheep receiving estrone injections. Acta Physiol. Pol. 13:430-438 (1962).

191. Snell, R. S.: Effect of alpha M.S.H. and estrogen on melanin pigmentation in the albino. J. Invest. Dermatol. 44:17-21 (1965).

192. Sobel, H., Lee, K. D. and Hewlett, M. J.: Effect of estrogen on acid glycosaminoglycans in skin of mice. Biochim. Biophys. Acta 101:225-229 (1965).

193. Sobel, H., Kovacevic, A. M. and Ramelli, G.: Effect of estradiol on albumin-I^{131} in the skin of mice following intravenous injection. Proc. Soc. Exp. Biol. Med. 119:358-360 (1965).

194. Somes, R. G., Jr. and Smyth, J. R., Jr.: Effects of estrogen on feather phaeomelanin intensity in the fowl. Poult. Sci. 46:26-32 (1967).

195. Spellacy, W. N., Birk, S. A., Noer, K. A. and Schade, S. L.: Sedimentation rate in the normal menstrual cycle or with oral contraceptives. Minn. Med. 5/67:645-647.

196. Stabilini, R., Vergani, C., Agostoni, A. and Agostoni, R.P.V.: Influence of age and sex on prealbumin levels. Clin. Chim. Acta 20:358-359 (1968).

197. Starcher, B. and Hill, C. H.: Hormonal induction of ceruloplasmin in chicken serum. Comp. Biochem. Physiol. 15:429-434 (1965).

198. Steinetz, B. G., Beach, V. L., DiPasquale, G. and Battista, J. V.: Effects of different gestogenic steroid types on plasma-free corticosteroid levels in ACTA-treated rats. Steroids 5:93-108 (1965).

199. Stolte, L., Kock, H., van Kessel, H. and Kock, L.: Thyroxine utilization in non-pregnant, steroid-induced pseudopregnant, and pregnant monkeys. Acta Endocr. 52:383-390 (1966).

200. Stowe, H. D.: Effects of age and impending parturition upon serum copper of thoroughbred mares. J. Nutr. 95:179-183 (1968).

201. Studnitz, W. V. and Nyman, M.: Effects of androgens on α_2-globulins in women. J. Clin. Endocr. 17:910-912 (1957).

202. Sugawa, T. and Moriyama, I.: Observations on amino acid and protein metabolism with reference to the hormonal control in pregnancy. 1. Effect of progesterone and estrogen on the turnover of tissue protein. J. Jap. Obstet. Gynec. Soc. 13: 116-122 (1966).

203. Sugawa, T., Moriyama, I., Hirooka, C., et al: Observations on amino acid and protein metabolism with reference to their hormonal control in pregnancy. 2. Effect of steroid hormone on glucogenesis of amino acid. J. Jap. Obstet. Gynec. Soc. 14:59-66 (1967).

204. Suzuki, H. K. and Prosser, R. L., III: The effects of estradiol valerate upon the serum and bone of the lizard, Sceloporus cyanogenys. Proc. Soc. Exp. Biol. Med. 127:4-7 (1968).

205. Svanborg, A. and Vikrot, O.: Plasma lipid fractions, including individual phospholipids, at various stages of pregnancy. Acta Med. Scand. 178:615-630 (1965).

206. Teague, H. S., Plimpton, R. F., Jr. and Cahill, V. R.: Influence of diethylstilbestrol implantation on growth and carcass characteristics of boars. J. Anim. Sci. 23:332-338 (1964).

207. Varga, L., Tiboldi, T., Varga, G. and Hegedus, Z.: Effect of six months oestrogen and progesterone treatment on the serum proteins and protein-bound carbohydrate components in rats. Med. Pharmacol. Exp. 17(4):339-345 (1967).

208. Wainwright, S. D., Bright-Asare, P. and Campbell, J. C.: Exploratory studies of the liver glutamic dehydrogenase of the hagfish myxine glutinosa. Lack of regulation of activity by ADP and diethylstilbestrol in a physiological saline. Canad. J. Biochem. 45:614-618 (1967).

209. Wakabayashi, K., Ogiso, T. and Tamaoki, B.-I.: Acute effects of androgen and estrogen on the promotion of amino acid incorporation into LH and protein in the anterior pituitary glands of male rats. Endocrinology 82:721-730 (1968).

210. Wallace, R. A. and Jared, D. W.: Studies on amphibian yolk. 7. Serum phosphoprotein synthesis by vitellogenic females and estrogen-treated males of Xenopus laevis. Canad. J. Biochem. 46:953-959 (1968).

211. Wallace, R. A. and Jared, D. W.: Estrogen induced lipophosphoprotein in serum of male Xenopus laevis. Science 160:91-92 (1968).

212. Weintraub, R. M., Churchill, W. H., Jr., Crisler, C., Rapp, H. J. and Borsos, T.: Mouse complement: Influence of sex hormones on its activity. Science 152:783-785 (1966).

213. Wexler, W. M. and Kantor, F. S.: Reticuloendothelial function in pregnancy. Yale J. Biol. Med. 38:315-322 (1966).

214. Williams-Ashman, H. G., Liao, S., Hancock, R. L., Jurkowitz, L. and Silverman, D. A.: Testicular hormones and the synthesis of ribonucleic acids and proteins in the prostate gland.

Recent Prog. Horm. Res. 20:247-302 (1964).

215. Wodzicka-Tomaszewska, M.: Bioassay of oestrogen and recurring oestrus in ovariectomized ewes. Nature 198:299-301 (1963).

216. Wurtman, R. J., Rose, C. M., Chou, C. and Larin, F. F.: Daily rhythms in the concentrations of various amino acids in human plasma. New Engl. J. Med. 279:171-175 (1968).

217. Wynn, V., Doar, J. W. H. and Mills, G. L.: Effects of oral contraceptives on serum lipid and lipoprotein levels. Lancet 2:720-725 (1966).

218. Yuriev, V. A., Zhakhova, Z. N. and Lopatina, N. I.: Change of the protein composition of the skeletal, cardiac and smooth muscles after castration. Byull. Eksp. Biol. Med. 55:54-56 (1963).

219. Zachmann, M., Cleveland, W. W., Sandberg, D. H. and Nyhan, W. L.: Concentrations of amino acids in plasma and muscle. Amer. J. Dis. Child. 112:283-289 (1966).

220. Zappi, E. J., Perez, M. H., Colongo, F., Moreno, R. F. and de la Balze, F. A.: Modifications of lipids and serum lipoproteins by the action of androgens and estrogens in subjects of advanced ages. Medicina 22(1):9-14 (1962).

221. Zarkower, A.: Histamine in the cow: Pre-and postpartum histamine concentration in plasma, milk and tissue. Amer. J. Vet. Res. 28:1751-1755 (1967).

222. Zarkower, A.: Histamine in the cow: Effect of histamine and estradiol administration on protein concentrations in milk. Amer. J. Vet. Res. 28:1757-1762 (1967).

223. Zeitlenok, N. A., Roihel, V. M. and Gorbachkova, E. A.: Effects of testosterone analogues on interferon formation, induction of antiviral protein and synthesis of cell protein in tissue culture. Nature 219:978-979 (1968).

224. Zinneman, H. H., Seal, U. S. and Doe, R. P.: Urinary amino acids in pregnancy, following progesterone, and estrogen-progesterone. J. Clin. Endocr. 27:397-405 (1967).

225. Zinneman, H. H., Musa, B. U. and Doe, R. P.: Changes in plasma and urinary amino acids following estrogen administration to males. Metabolism 14:1214-1219 (1965).

226. Zuspan, F. P. and Goodrich, S.: Metabolic studies in normal pregnancy. 1. Nitrogen metabolism. Amer. J. Obstet. Gynec. 100:7-14 (1968).

METABOLIC INHIBITORS AND THE ANABOLIC ACTIONS OF TESTOSTERONE PROPIONATE

E.H. Frieden

Department of Chemistry, Kent State University, Kent, Ohio

The utility of the mouse kidney as a physiological tool for the study of the anabolic action of androgenic steroids is a reflection of the multiplicity of the metabolic responses of this organ to testosterone, its esters, and other androgens. These responses include increases in kidney weight, in nucleic acid content, and in the concentrations of a number of enzymes (1,2). In addition, acute effects of androgens upon the rates of incorporation of precursors into RNA and protein can be demonstrated.

In an attempt to study the detailed mechanism of these responses, a study was initiated of the effects of some metabolic inhibitors upon various responses of the mouse kidney to testosterone propionate (T.P). The first relevant observation was that although actinomycin D, an inhibitor of DNA - directed RNA synthesis, effectively inhibited androgen-induced increase in kidney β-glucuronidase activity, it failed to diminish the concomitant increase in rates of incorporation of several amino acids _in vitro_ (3). These studies have now been extended to include experiments with other inhibitors (DL-ethionine, cycloheximide, and puromycin) as well as other parameters of androgen action (increase in kidney arginase, incorporation _in vivo_ of labeled leucine and labeled orotic acid into kidney protein and kidney RNA, respectively).

The valuable assistance of Sandra S. Fishel and Chia-Chuan Ku is gratefully acknowledged. This work was supported by a research grant from the National Science Foundation (GB-5848).

METHODS

Cloudman female mice were obtained fron Jackson Laboratory, Bar Harbor, Maine. Most of the data reported here were obtained using animals which were six to ten weeks old at the beginning of the experiment, although in a few instances older (up to six months) animals were employed. Testosterone propionate, (T.P.), cyclohex-imide (CHX), DL-ethionine, and puromycin dihydrochloride were pur-chased from Nutritional Biochemicals; Actinomycin D was the generous gift of Merck, Sharpe, and Dohm. T.P. (one milligram in 0.1 ml. sesame oil) was injected once daily intramuscularly; the inhibitors were administered twice daily intraperitoneally. Methods for the determination of arginase and β-glucuronidase have been described previously (4).

The effects of DL-ethionine (50 mg /kg /day), actinomycin D (0.2 mg./kg./day), cycloheximide (30 mg /kg /day), and puromycin dihydrochloride (150 mg./kg./day) upon the responses of kidney arginase and β-glucuronidase to the administration of T.P. for five days are summarized in Figures 1-4.

In untreated animals, kidney arginase usually ranges between 11-14 units per gram, while kidney β-glucuronidase averages about 1100 units per gram*. After five daily injections of T.P., kidney arginase increases 2-4 fold, depending somewhat upon the age of the animal, while kidney β-glucuronidase increases 16-20 fold. DL-ethionine will inhibit the β-glucuronidase response by 85-90%, and completely abolishes the arginase response (Fig. 1). Both actino-mycin D (Fig. 2) and puromycin (Fig. 3) reduce the elevation of β-glucuronidase which occurs following T.P. administration; at least in the amounts used actinomycin D is the more effective in-hibitor. Neither actinomycin D nor puromycin diminishes the arginase response; puromycin, in fact, significantly potentiates the T.P. effect (150% vs. 80%).

In sharp contrast to the effects of actinomycin and puromycin, cycloheximide failed to diminish the β-glucuronidase response to T.P., even if treatment with cycloheximide was begun before the first T.P. injection. Indeed, the data suggest a slight potentia-tion of the response (1650% vs. 1320%). On the other hand, the increase in arginase concentration was reduced by 80% when cyclo-heximide was given during the last three days of a 5-day T.P. regi-men, and was diminished even more when treatment with the inhibitor was begun earlier.

---

*In one group of animals (Fig. 3) arginase concentrations in untreated animals were considerably lower than usual. The effect of T.P. was undiminished, however.

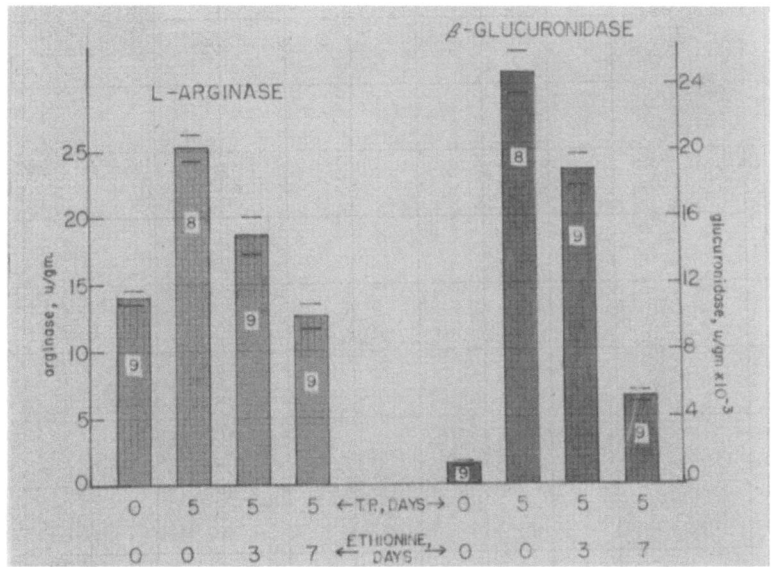

Fig. 1. Effect of **DL-ethionine** (50 mg/kg/day) upon mouse kidney arginase and β-glucuronidase. The number of animals in each group, and the standard errors (short horizontal lines) are indicated for each set of data. Ethionine injections were begun either two days before or two days after the first T.P. injection.

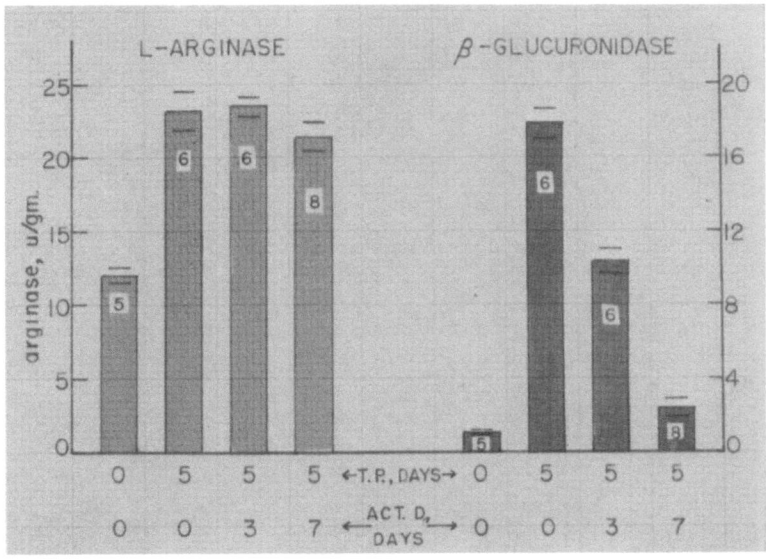

Fig. 2. Effect of actinomycin D (0.2 mg/kg/day) upon mouse kidney arginase and β-glucuronidase. Other details as in Fig. 1.

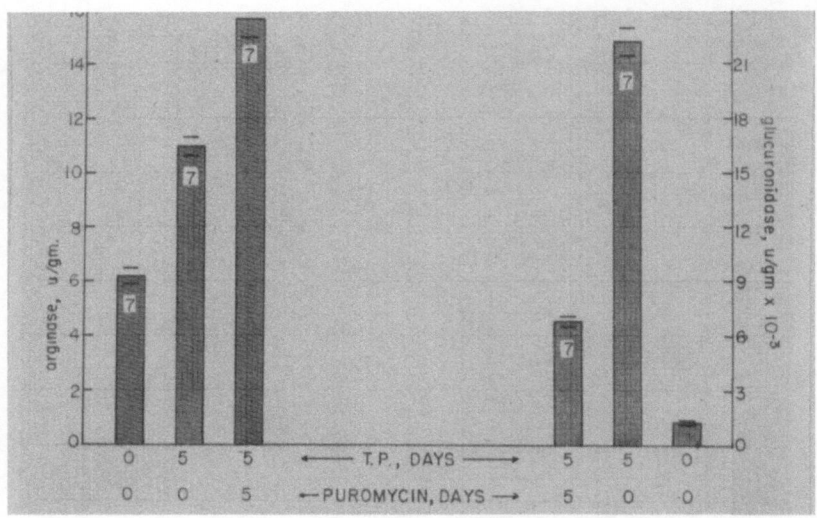

Fig. 3.   Effect of puromycin dihydrochloride upon mouse
kidney arginase and β-glucuronidase. T.P. and puromycin
(150 mg/kg/day) were both given for 5 days. Other details as
in Fig. 1.

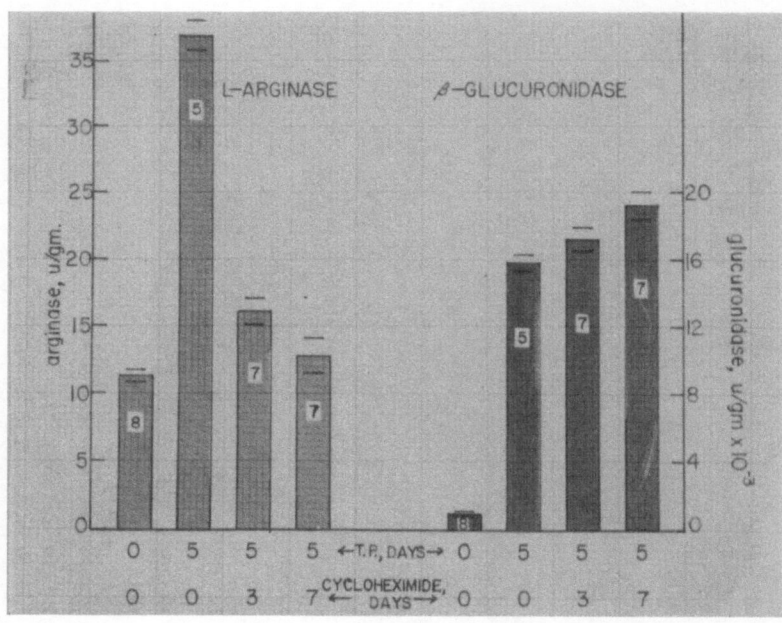

Fig. 4.   Effect of cycloheximide (30 mg/kg/day) upon mouse
kidney arginase and β-glucuronidase. Other details as in Fig. 1.

The enzymatic parameters of androgen action described above represent relatively slow responses to T.P. stimulation, since in order to demonstrate significant increased in enzyme concentration, treatment with the hormone for a minimum of three to five days is necessary. In addition to these responses to chronic androgen stimulation, it is also possible to show the existence of an acute and transitory phase of androgen action on the mouse kidney. For example, within 18-24 hours of a single injection of T.P., increases in the incorporation in vivo of labeled leucine into mixed kidney protein and of labeled orotic acid into kidney RNA can be demonstrated, as compared to untreated animals. It seemed of interest to explore the effects of the same group of inhibitors upon these metabolic parameters as well.

Each experimental group consisted of six animals; comparisons were made between treated and untreated animals of the same age and weight distribution. Food was removed 6 hours before termination of the experiment. Each animal received 2.5 μC of DL-leucine-1-^{14}C or 0.50 μC orotic acid-6-^{14}C, injected intraperitoneally in 0.20 ml. saline. In experiments with orotic acid, the animals were killed two hours later and the specific activities of kidney RNA determined after conversion to ribonucleotides using the procedure of Fleck and Munro (5). Animals which received DL-leucine were killed three hours after injection of the label, and the specific activities of kidney protein determined after precipitation with trichloroacetic acid. All data were corrected to a uniform body weight of 20 gm. Ethionine- and cycloheximide-treated animals received these substances for a total of five days preceding the injection of the labeled compounds, while actinomycin D was given for four days; the dose schedules were the same as those described above. Androgen-treated animals received a single injection of 1 mg. T.P. 20-22 hours before the label.

As shown in Figure 5, the specific activity of mouse kidney protein, isolated three hours after the injection of labeled leucine into T.P.-treated animals, increased 52% as compared to untreated controls. Cycloheximide and ethionine both effectively eliminated this difference. It seems clear, however, that the two inhibitors operate by different mechanisms, since ethionine reduces the effect in T.P.-treated animals essentially to the control level, whereas cycloheximide increases the latter to values characteristic of treated animals.

Figure 6 summarizes the data concerning effects on RNA synthesis. In otherwise untreated animals, T.P. increases the rate of RNA synthesis by approximately 80%. As expected, this difference is abolished quite completely in actinomycin-treated animals. Ethionine also eliminates most of the T.P. effect; in cycloheximide-treated animals, however, a substantial effect of T.P. on RNA turnover is retained.

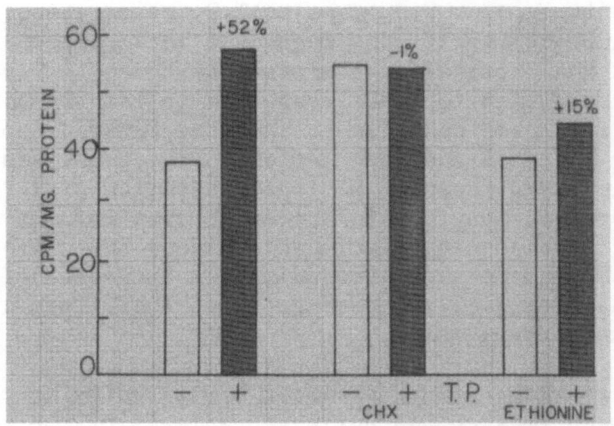

Fig. 5. Effects of cycloheximide (30 mg/kg/day) and
DL-ethionine (50 mg/kg/day) upon incorporation of labeled leucine
into mouse kidney protein in vivo. The shaded bars represent data
obtained for animals receiving 1 mg T.P. 20-22 hours before the
label. Unshaded bars represent control animals. For other
details, see text.

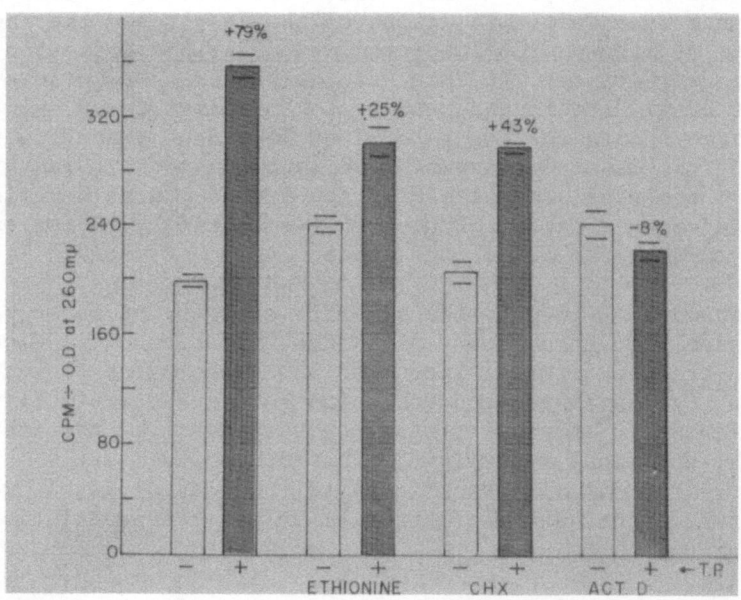

Fig. 6. Effects of DL-ethionine (50 mg/kg/day), cycloheximide (30 mg/kg/day) and actinomycin D (0.2 mg/kg/day) upon
incorporation of labeled orotic acid into mouse kidney RNA.
Shaded bars represent T.P.-treated animals. Ordinate: specific
activity (counts per minute/optical density at 260 mµ) of ribonucleotides. For other details, see text.

DISCUSSION

There is ample evidence (6) that the marked elevation in β-glucuronidase activity which occurs in the kidneys of mice receiving androgen is due to increased synthesis of enzyme protein. The fact that the stimulation of both enzymes by T.P. is abolished or reduced by ethionine, an agent which inhibits protein synthesis in mice as well as in other animals (7), suggests that a common mechanism is involved; the obvious corollary is that T.P. increases the rate of synthesis of arginase protein as well as glucuronidase protein.

Several authors have suggested that inhibition of protein synthesis by ethionine is due to its function as an ATP trap, as a consequence of the irreversible formation of S-ethionyl adenosine. Some such mechanism could readily account for the effects of ethionine upon T.P.-stimulated RNA synthesis reported here, since increased RNA synthesis might be limited by the available ATP supply.

Our data appear to offer general support to the hypothesis (2) that at least one of the mechanisms involved in the anabolic action of the androgens entails stimulation of DNA-directed RNA synthesis. Thus, the acute effects of T.P. upon orotic acid incorporation into RNA, as well as the sensitivity of the latter to actinomycin D are both consistent with this hypothesis. The failure of actinomycin D to affect the synthesis of arginase, in contrast to its ready inhibition of β-glucuronidase, might be explained by a difference in sensitivity of the two DNA primers to this agent (reflecting, perhaps, a difference in number or accessibility of guanosine residues).

It is clear from the data of Figure 5 that although the amounts of cycloheximide used in these experiments were quite high, significant inhibition of protein synthesis must have been confined to a relatively brief period immediately following injection of the drug. Jondorf (8) has reported that although the immediate (1-2 hours) consequence of CHX administration to rats is inhibition of the incorporation of leucine into liver microsomal protein, a modest increase can be demonstrated after 24 hours. In our experiments, the last injection of cycloheximide occurred some 15-16 hours before giving the label. It is quite possible, therefore, that an inhibitory phase of limited duration escaped observation. If it did occur, the inhibitory phase was apparently followed by a "rebound" phase similar to that observed by Jondorf (8).

The hypotheses that CHX inhibits protein synthesis for only a brief period may possibly explain the different effects of this agent upon T.P. induction of β-glucuronidase and arginase. Synthesis of new arginase protein in response to T.P. occurs at a much slower rate than does the synthesis of new β-glucuronidase protein. The slower process might be significantly more sensitive to periodic inhibition followed by stimulation, than the faster.

The failure of puromycin to inhibit the arginase response to T.P. was unexpected. In the absence of specific information concerning its effects upon protein metabolism in the mouse kidney, speculation as to the significance of this phenomenon seems unwarranted.

One rather curious feature of all the inhibitor-enzyme experiments is the failure of any of the inhibitors used (puromycin was not tested) to reduce the concentration of either enzyme to values lower than that of treated controls. Thus, while actinomycin D strongly suppresses the increase in β-glucuronidase characteristic of T.P.-treated animals, it does not diminish the concentration of this enzyme in otherwise untreated animals. This observation suggested the possibility that the enzyme synthesized in response to androgen represents, in fact, an isozyme of the protein normally present--a different protein with similar enzymatic properties. Some attempts have been made to gain support for this hypothesis by demonstrating a difference between 'endogenous' and stimulated β-glucuronidase. Several criteria were applied: the comparative susceptibility of different substrates, comparison of Michaelis constants, and the comparative rates of inactivation of the two forms at elevated temperatures. To date, however, all such efforts have been fruitless.

REFERENCES

1. Frieden, E.H. in: _Actions of Hormones on Molecular Processes_. G. Litwak and D. Krichevsky, Eds. John Wiley and Sons, New York (1964).

2. Kochakian, C.D., in: _Mechanisms of Hormone Action_, P. Karlson, Ed. Academic Press, New York (1965).

3. Frieden, E.H., Harper, A.A., Chin, F., and Fishman, W.H.: Steroids 4:777 (1964).

4. Frieden, E.H., and Fishel, S.S.: Biochem. Biophys. Res. Communica 31:515 (1968).

5. Fleck, A., and Munro, H.N.: Biochem. Biophys. Acta 55:571 (1962).

6. Pettengill, O.S., and Fishman, W.H.: Exper. Cell. Res. 28:248 (1962).

7.   Simpson, M.V., Farber, E., and Tarver, H.:   J. Biol. Chem. 182:81 (1950).

8.   Jondorf, W.R.:   Biochem. Pharmacol. 17:839 (1968).

ANDROGEN REGULATION OF MOUSE KIDNEY RNA

C. D. Kochakian

Laboratory of Experimental Endocrinology, University of Alabama, Birmingham

The anabolic effect of the androgens is observed in many tissues other than the secondary sex organs. The responsiveness of the extra sexual tissues varies widely with species of animals and the steroid hormone (1,2). The induction of growth by the steroids, however, utilizes the recognized protein biosynthetic systems. The amino acid incorporating activity of cell free preparations of these is decreased by castration and enhanced by androgen administration (2). These changes in rate of protein biosynthesis are accompanied by changes in the RNAs of the tissue (2). Since various forms of RNAs are essential for the protein biosynthetic system, this report will describe some of the recent information concerning the regulation of RNA in an androgen sensitive organ, the mouse kidney.

INTRACELLULAR SITES

Effect of Castration

The total and microsomal RNA was decreased at a greater rate than the weight of the kidney after castration (Table 1). The nuclear and soluble RNAs were decreased in proportion with the change in kidney weight and the mitochondrial RNA at a slightly lower rate. The decrease in DNA, as expected (3), was much less than the percentage decrease in weight. It should be noted that only a small amount of DNA was detected in the mitochondrial fraction and questionable amounts in the microsomal and soluble fraction.

Effect of Testosterone Propionate

The androgen produced the expected increase in kidney weight and the concomitant increase in RNA (2,3). The increase in the

Table 1

COMPARISON OF THE RNA CONCENTRATION IN THE VARIOUS

INTRACELLULAR FRACTIONS OF THE KIDNEYS OF NORMAL,

CASTRATED AND TESTOSTERONE PROPIONATE TREATED MICE*

	Ribonucleic Acid, mg/g		
	Normal	Castrate	TP-2 Days
Homogenate	4.19 ± 0.32	3.48 ± 0.35	4.08 ± 0.23
Nuclear	0.70 ± 0.12	0.63 ± 0.15	0.78 ± 0.18
Mitochondrial	0.48 ± 0.02	0.46 ± 0.06	0.48 ± 0.08
Microsomal	2.53 ± 0.08	1.91 ± 0.12	2.33 ± 0.09
Soluble	0.56 ± 0.10	0.52 ± 0.04	0.60 ± 0.06
Sum	4.28	3.51	4.18
Kidney	652 ± 91	426 ± 52	462 ± 45
DNA (mg/g)	3.29 ± 0.12	2.88 ± 0.17	3.77 ± 0.04

*The values and standard deviations are for four groups of
five mice each. Castration was performed at 31 days of age. The
testosterone propionate (TP) was implanted subcutaneously as a
15 ± mg pellet two days before autopsy. The amount absorbed was
0.5 ± 0.24 mg. The ages of the mice were 246 to 296 days. (From
Kochakian, C.D., unpublished).

total and intracellular RNA was evident within two days (Table 1).
The total RNA was increased to the normal level within two weeks
(Fig. 1). The microsomal (ms) RNA increased at a more rapid rate.
The normal level was attained between two (Table 1) and seven days
(Fig. 1). The mt-RNA increased in direct proportion with the increase in kidney weight. The increase in n-RNA was delayed but
attained the normal level. The s-RNA increased at a slightly
greater rate than the weight of the kidney. The increase, however,
was small and of questionable significance. In numerous other experiments the rate of increase of s-RNA was small in proportion to
the kidney weight.

A second implantation of testosterone propionate thirteen'
days before autopsy at the 44-day period did not significantly
modify the results. Maximal stimulation was being provided by the
original androgen pellet.

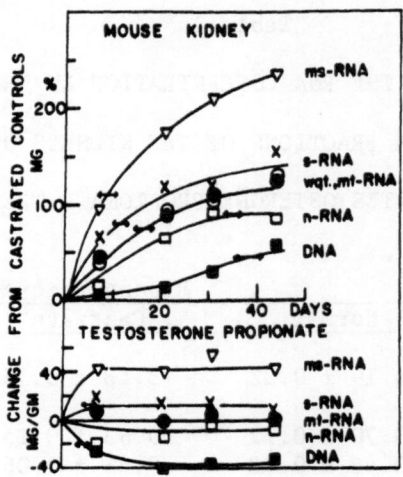

Fig. 1.   Effect of testosterone propionate on the nucleic acids in the various parts of the kidney cell.   The mice were castrated 26 to 28 days of age and 21 days later a pellet (approximately 15 mg.) of testosterone propionate was implanted subcutaneously.   The amount of androgen absorbed from the pellets was 1.1, 3.4, 5.1, and 5.5 mg. per respective period.   The mice were killed in groups of 5 at the indicated intervals.   The pooled kidneys of ten castrated control animals were analyzed simultaneously at each period.   The values of the forty castrated control mice were: kidney weight 358(320-420) mg., DNA 1.35(1.28-1.41) mg., n-DNA 1.18(1.07-1.36) mg., RNA 1.60 (1.49-1.71) mg., n-RNA 0.36(0.31-0.40) mg., mt-RNA 0.23(0.20-0.25) mg., ms-RNA 0.74(0.70-0.80) mg., s-RNA 0.21(0.19-0.21) mg.

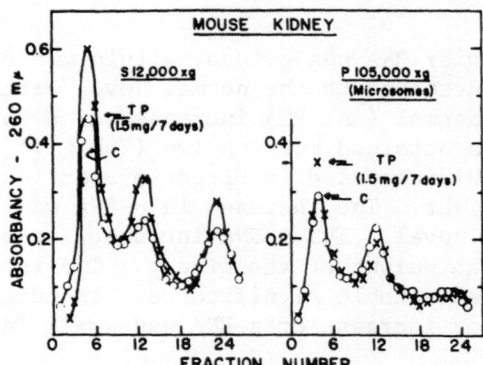

Fig. 2.   Sucrose gradient profile of RNA from mouse kidney. The mice were castrated at one month of age and a pellet of testosterone propionate was implanted three months later.   The sucrose gradient profile (4) was prepared in a Spinco SW39L rotor.   The RNA for the $S_{12,000}$xg fractions was: C = 150μg, TP = 167μg and microsomes 80μg for C and TP.   (From Kochakian, C.D. and Nishida, M., unpublished).

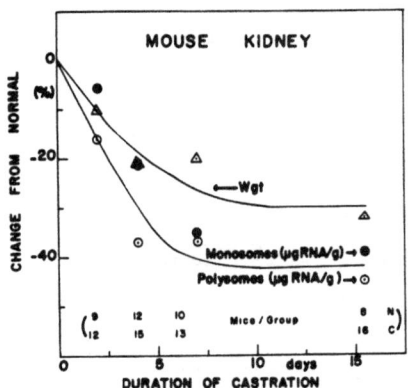

Fig. 3. Effect of castration on the concentration of mono- and
polysomes in the postmitochondrial fraction ($S_{12,000}$xg) of mouse
kidney. A group of three month old male mice were divided into sub-
groups as indicated. The average values for the four groups of
normal mice were polysomes 530 (486-581)μg RNA/g kidney with an
E260/280 = 1.74. (From Kochakian, C.D. and Nishida, M. unpublished.)

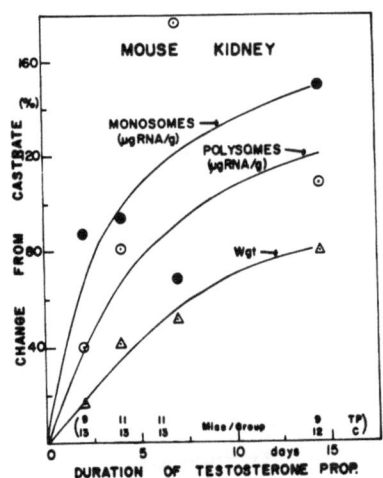

Fig. 4. Effect of testosterone propionate treatment on the
concentration of mono- and polysomes in the postmitochondrial
fraction of the kidneys of castrated mice. A group of mice were
divided into sub-groups as designated in the graph. Castration was
performed at 2.5 months of age; two weeks later a pellet of testosterone propionate was implanted subcutaneously. The average values
for the four groups of castrated control mice were: polysomes 342
(289-346)μg RNA/g kidney and E260/280 = 1.78; monosomes 64(47-91)μg
RNA/g kidney and E260/280 = 1.74. (From Kochakian, C.D. and
Nishida, M. unpublished.)

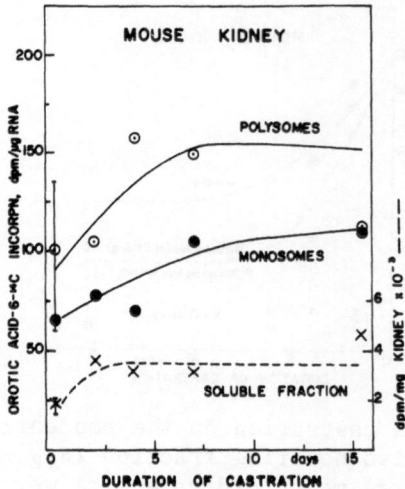

Fig. 5. Effect of castration on the incorporation of radioactivity of orotic acid-6-^{14}C in various ribosomal fractions. The
fractions were those of Figure 3. The mice were injected intraperitoneally with 3µc of orotic acid (34µc/µ mole) 20µc/ml two hours
before autopsy. (From Kochakian, C.D. and Nishida, M. unpublished.)

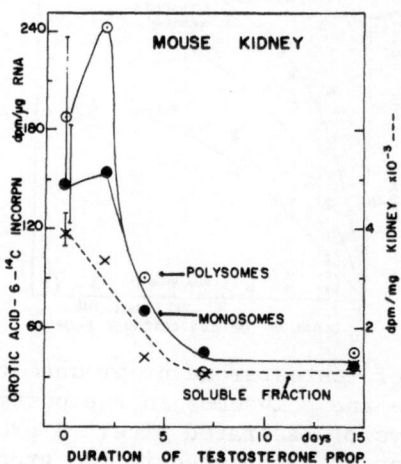

Fig. 6. Effect of testosterone propionate on the incorporation
of radioactivity of orotic acid-6-^{14}C in various ribosomal fractions.
The fractions were from those of Figure 4. The orotic acid was injected as in Figure 5. (From Kochakian, C.D. and Nishida, M.,
unpublished.)

RNA SPECIES

Phenol extraction and gradient centrifugation (4) of the RNA
in the postmitochondrial and microsomal fraction showed no differences in the RNA species from the kidneys of castrated and testosterone propionate treated mice (Fig. 2).

RIBOSOMES

Amount

Castration produced a decrease in the concentration of both
the monosomes and polysomes (5) in parallel with the decrease in
kidney weight but at a greater rate (Fig. 3). The administration
of testosterone propionate stimulated a rapid (within two days)
and progressive increase in both the mono- and polysomes (Fig. 4).

Electron Micrographs

The polysomes from the castrated mice appeared more linear
while those from the testosterone propionate treated mice were more
helical in structure.

Orotic Acid Incorporation

The incorporation of radioactivity from orotic acid-6-^{14}C injected intraperitoneally two hours before autopsy was progressively
increased after castration in the mono- and polysomes and also the
soluble fractions (Fig. 5). The increases were evident within two
days. The administration of testosterone propionate had no significant effect after two days but after four days produced a significant decrease in the incorporation of radioactivity in the
ribosomes and soluble fraction (Fig. 6). A maximal decrease was
attained after seven days of androgen treatment.

Sucrose Gradient Profiles

Castration did not change the gradient profile of the
polysomes. The incorporation of radioactivity, however, began to
increase in each of the peaks within two days after castration to
maximum levels within four days (Fig. 7).

The implantation of a pellet of testosterone propionate
produced a slight shift of the gradient profile from the monosomes
and light polysomes to the heavy polysomes (Fig. 8). The incorporation of radioactivity was not affected after two days, was
somewhat decreased after four days and restored to normal by seven
days (Fig. 7).

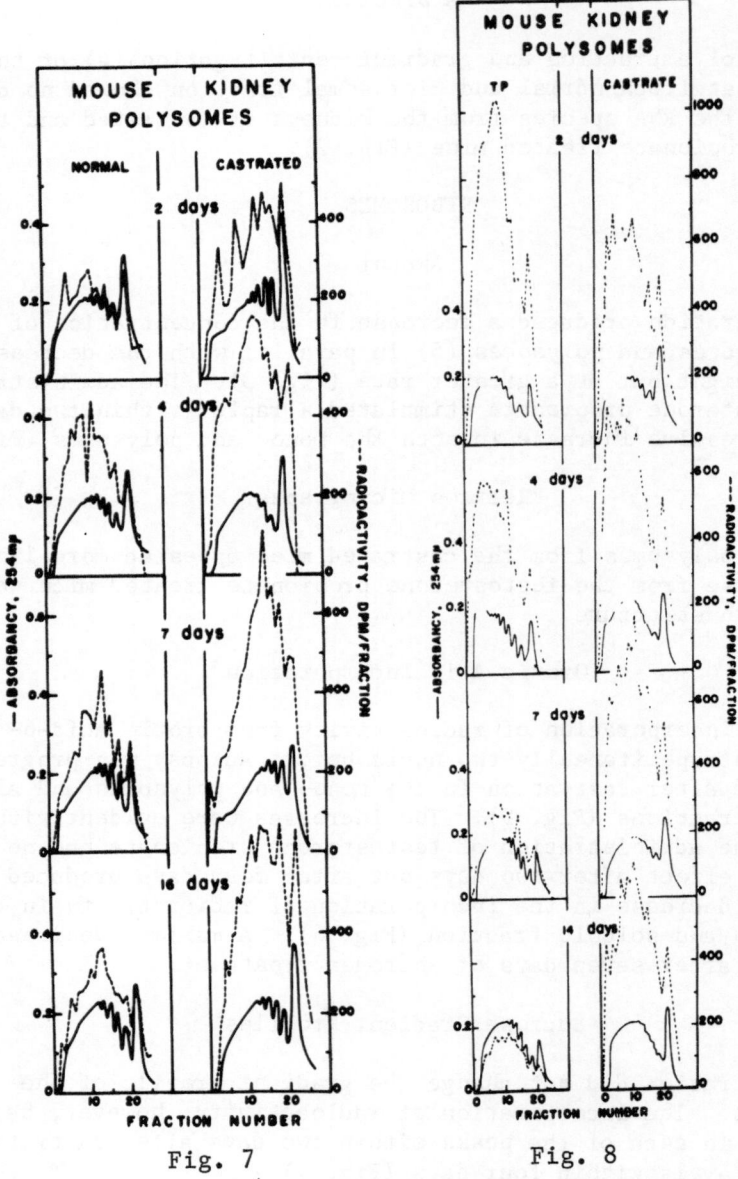

Fig. 7   Fig. 8

Figs. 7&8. Effects of castration and testosterone propionate on the sucrose gradient profile of the polysomes from mouse kidneys. The polysomes were prepared (5) from the castrated and testosterone-treated mice of Figures 5 and 6 respectively. An amount containing 200 μg RNA was centrifuged in a Spinco SW39L rotor for 45 minutes at 37,000 RPM. (From Kochakian, C.D. and Nishida, M., unpublished.)

The monosome profiles showed trace amounts of the lighter polysomes and incorporation of radioactivity similar to that shown by the polysomes after castration and testosterone propionate treatment.

Ribosomal RNA

The RNA was removed from the polysomes by phenol extraction and the sucrose gradient profiles determined (4). Two peaks of RNA characteristic of microsomal RNA were observed. The relative proportion of these RNAs was not changed by castration or testosterone propionate. The incorporation of radioactivity was greater in the slower moving species of RNA but both were proportionately increased after castration and decreased after androgen treatment.

RIBONUCLEASES

The total alkaline ribonuclease activity was not changed by castration. Thus, the concentration increased with the decrease in kidney weight. The "acid" ribonuclease activity, on the other hand, changed in proportion to the change in weight of the kidney after castration and testosterone propionate (7).

RNA POLYMERASES

The RNA polymerase activity was measured in the kidney nuclei by a procedure essentially the same as that of Weiss (8) and also by the addition of 0.5M $(NH_4)_2SO_4$ and Mn^{2+} (9) to the incubation mixture.

Effects of Castration

Castration produced an immediate and sharp decrease in the RNA polymerase activity of the nuclei which reached a minimum level within one week (Fig. 9). The addition of $(NH_4)_2SO_4-Mn^{2+}$ to the incubation system enhanced the RNA polymerase activity but nearly completely removed the effect of castration.

Effect of Testosterone Propionate

The subcutaneous implantation of a pellet of testosterone propionate produced an abrupt rise, after two days, in the RNA polymerase activity followed by a small but gradual further increase (Fig. 10). The increase was less pronounced after addition of $(NH_4)_2SO_4$ and Mn^{2+} were added to the system.

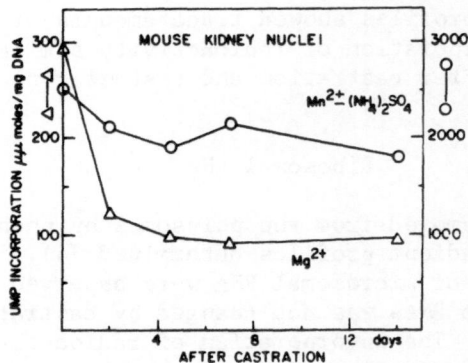

Fig. 9. Effect of castration on the RNA polymerase activity of mouse kidney nuclei. The mice were castrated at approximately two months of age and autopsied at the same time. The purified nuclei were incubated at 37° for 15 minutes in the following medium: 50 μmoles Tris-HCl (pH 8.1), 2.5 μmoles magnesium acetate, 37.5 μmoles KCl, 3.5 μmoles mercaptoethanol, 0.5 μmole each of ATP, CTP, GTP and UTP, 5 μCUTP-^{3}H (2.24c/μmole) and nuclei containing 100-200 μg DNA. In addition, determinations were made after the addition of 1 μmole $MnCl_2$ and 250 μmoles of ammonium sulfate (pH 8.1). The final volume was 0.5 ml. (From Avdalovic, N. and Kochakian, C.D., unpublished.)

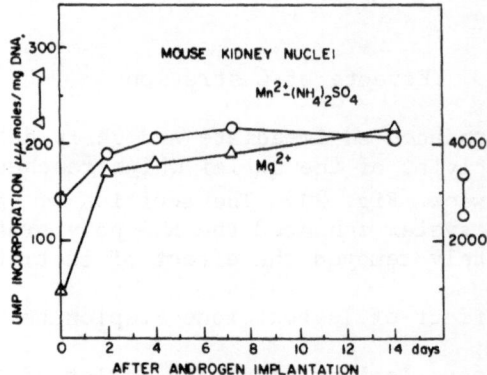

Fig. 10. The effect of testosterone propionate on the RNA polymerase activity of mouse kidney nuclei. The mice were castrated at approximately one month of age; thirty days later they were divided into groups by body weight and a testosterone propionate pellet was implanted so that the duration of treatment for all of the groups terminated at the same time. The determination of RNA polymerase activity was as in Figure 9. (From Avdalovic, N. and Kochakian, C.D., unpublished.)

DISCUSSION

The decrease after castration and the increase after androgen in the RNA of the different intracellular sites of the kidney is consistent with the changes in protein biosynthesis (2). Apparently all of the RNAs essential for protein biosynthesis are involved in the regulatory effect of the androgen. It is especially significant that not only the amount but also the concentration of the final assembly unit of the amino acids, the polysomes, are decreased after castration and increased after androgen administration.

The failure to detect any differences in the species of RNA or polysomes suggests that there is a uniform overall change in the elements concerned with protein biosynthesis. It is known, however, that certain enzymes (10) are greatly affected and in different degrees e.g., arginase is increased while alkaline phosphatase is decreased. Thus, more sophisticated methods may provide recognizable qualitative differences in the kidney RNA's and polysomes of normal, castrated and androgen-treated mice.

The course of incorporation of radioactivity from injected orotic acid-6-^{14}C into the RNA of the polysomes is in keeping with the previous studies (6). Furthermore, these experiments indicate that the incorporation is in the final functional unit. It is still not clear why there is such a long delay in the appearance of the effect of the androgen on the incorporation of radioactivity from the orotic acid into the RNAs. The androgen was ineffective after two days even though changes in the various RNAs had already been induced. Other precursors of RNA are being studied to obtain further insight into the regulation of the biosynthesis of the RNAs by androgens.

The amount of the RNAs is dependent on catabolic as well as anabolic processes. It is now apparent that there are a large number of nucleases in tissues. It was of interest that two categories of these enzymes responded differently to the absence and presence of the androgen. The exact significance of the role of these enzymes, however, is not apparent at this time. The changes in the activity of the RNA polymerase of the nuclei provide an explanation of the anabolic regulation of RNA biosynthesis by the androgen and is consistent with the changes in RNA. The very rapid (less than two hours) induction of an increase in the activity of this enzyme suggests that this is one of the early effects of the androgen. The induction of an increase in protein biosynthesis is not detected until 24 hours after androgen administration.

REFERENCES

1. Kochakian, C.D.: Protein anabolic property of androgens. Alabama J. Med. Sci. 1:24-37 (1964).

2. Kochakian, C.D.: Mechanism of anabolic action of androgens, Karlson, P. (ed.), Mechanisms of Hormone Action. Academic Press, New York, London, p. 192-213 (1965).

3. Kochakian, C.D. and Harrison, D.G.: Regulation of nucleic acid synthesis by androgens. Endocrinology 70:99-108 (1962).

4. Munro, A.J. and Korner, A.: Messenger ribonucleic acid of rat liver cytoplasm. Nature 201:1194-1197 (1964).

5. Wettstein, F.O., Staehlin, T. and Noll, H.: The ribosomal aggregate engaged in protein synthesis: characterization of the ergosome. Nature 197:430-435 (1963).

6. Kochakian, C.D. and Hill, J.: Effect of androgen on the incorporation of orotic acid-6-^{14}C into ribonucleic acids and free nucleotides of mouse kidney. Biochemistry 5:1696-1701 (1966).

7. Kochakian, C.D., Elsas, F., and Harrison, D.G.: Androgen regulation of mouse kidney ribonucleases. Acta Endocrinologica 46:179-184 (1964).

8. Weiss, S.B.: Enzymatic incorporation of ribonucleoside triphosphates into the interpolynucleotide linkages of ribonucleic acid. Proc. Natl. Acad. Sci. 46:1020-1030 (1960).

9. Widnell, C.C. and Tata, J.R.: Evidence for two DNA-dependent RNA polymerase activities in isolated rat liver nuclei. Biochem. Biophys. Acta 87:531-533 (1964).

10. Kochakian, C.D.: Mechanisms of androgen actions. Lab. Invest. 8:538-556 (1959).

PROGESTERONE: MECHANISM OF ACTION

B. W. O'Malley

Endocrinology Branch, National Cancer Institute,
National Institutes of Health, Bethesda, Maryland 20014

In 1672, Regner de Graaf first published a description of the corpus luteum and recognized that the presence of a corpus luteum is associated with a fetus in utero. The definitive experiments of Corner (1), Allen and Reynolds (2) showed that pregnancy in rabbits is controlled by a product of the corpus luteum -- the ovarian steroid progesterone. Nevertheless, at present there is no unifying concept which would define the major role of progesterone in animal tissues. Furthermore, the biochemical actions of this steroid at the molecular level of cell metabolism have been so elusive that it is difficult even to construct a good hypothetical mechanism of action. The biologic effects of progesterone may be grouped as follows: (1) uterine endometrial cells are transformed in such a way that they may receive the early embryo and facilitate its implantation; (2) myometric activity is suppressed, aiding in retention of the embryo during implantation and growth prior to normal parturition; (3) numerous and varied metabolic parameters may be altered which may have no direct impact on maintenance and termination of pregnancy.

The effects of progesterone on the myometrial cell have been studied and reviewed by Csapo (3). Uterine muscle functions normally only if its spindle-shaped cells possess, as a result of estrogen stimulation, sufficient concentrations of contractile proteins for adequate working capacity. The excitable membrane of the uterine muscle cell must also be capable of undergoing periodic changes between rest and activity. The spontaneous rhythmic activity of the individual cell membrane must be transmitted to the contractile system of the myoplasm through an effective excitation. Progesterone exerts a "blocking effect" so that an excitation wave

cannot spread from one region to another. This steroid has been
reported to increase the membrane potential to an extent where
spontaneous activity is suppressed (4) and a gradual reduction in
spike discharge occurs (5). The molecular mechanism for the inhibitory effect of progesterone on uterine muscle is not clear. Progesterone has been reported to inhibit incorporation of radiolabeled
glycine into protein in both control and estrogen treated uteri(6),
potassium ion influx and efflux through myometrial cell membranes
(7), and mitochondrial respiration (8). The relationship of these
inhibiting events to the progesterone "quieting" effect on uterine
myometrium can be only speculative.

Although progesterone is needed for alveolar development in
breast tissue of some species, the major new capacity which develops in animals in response to progesterone is the ability of the
uterine endometrial cells to accept and support the blastocyst.
Under the influence of estrogen the endometrium proliferates and
becomes dense. Progesterone inhibits further endometrial proliferation and the epithelium becomes secretory. The outline of the
endometrial glands becomes irregular and the nuclei become basally
prominent. The glycogen content of the epithelium increases, the
stroma becomes edematous, and an increase in perivascular alkaline
phosphatase occurs. The endometrium is now able to accept, hold,
and nourish the fertilized ovum. These cytobiological changes
probably reflect earlier intracellular biochemical events.

This cellular "transformation" may require gene activation
and transcription of chromosomal information, but few model systems
have been available to investigate specific progesterone mediated
changes in nucleic acid and protein metabolism. Over the past
three years, this laboratory has reported a series of studies on
the mechanism of action of progesterone in the chick oviduct, a
unique model system for investigation of progesterone regulation
of protein synthesis. Estrogenic substances are known to stimulate
oviduct growth in newborn and older chicks (9) and we have found
that estrogen markedly stimulates synthesis of oviduct DNA and RNA
and numerous tissue specific proteins, similar to other model
systems presently available (10). However, the administration of
a single dose of progesterone to estrogen-stimulated chicks results
in the induction of synthesis of a specific oviduct protein,
avidin (11,12). Unless otherwise indicated, avidin was determined
in all subsequent studies by the method of Korenman and O'Malley
(13), an assay utilizing the unique biological affinity of avidin
for biotin labeled with ^{14}C. In addition to the biological
assay, the experimental product has been rigorously identified as
avidin by two additional criteria. Rabbit antiserum to avidin was
utilized to precipitate an avidin-C^{14}-biotin complex and to demonstrate an increased rate of incorporation of labeled amino acids
into avidin during the incubation (14). The newly synthesized

avidin is also identical to authentic avidin standard run alone or
as an avidin-biotin complex on disc-gel electrophoresis.

The results of in vivo and in vitro induction of avidin synthesis by progesterone in the estrogen-stimulated chick oviduct are
seen in Table 1. After a single 5 mg dose of progesterone given
in vivo at zero time, the chicks are sacrificed at the indicated
times and avidin is measured in the oviducts. Synthesis is first
apparent at 10 hours and begins to plateau at 24 hours. No avidin
appears in the oviduct either before or after estrogen treatment
unless progesterone is administered.

TABLE 1

PROGESTERONE INDUCTION OF AVIDIN SYNTHESIS

(Total Avidin Produced)

Time (Hrs.) After Progesterone	In Vivo (µg/g. oviduct)	In Vitro-Mince (µg/g. oviduct)	In Vitro-Culture (µg/culture)
0	0	0	0
6	0	0.42	0
10	0.18	0.9	–
12	0.5	1.0	.05
24	6.0	4.0	0.5
48	7.2	5.5	0.63
72	–	6.0	0.69

A typical induction curve for avidin synthesis in vitro is
also shown in Table 1. Oviduct tissue was minced and incubated
under sterile conditions with 5 µg of progesterone in tissue culture medium. Avidin synthesis was first noted at six hours and
reached a maximum between 48 and 72 hours (15). The versatility of
this model system is even further demonstrated by results of tissue
culture experiments. Cell cultures have less intercellular orien-
tation and are composed of a more homogeneous cell population.
Table 1 shows the effect of steroid hormones on induction of specific proteins in monolayer cell cultures of chick oviduct tissue.
No measurable synthesis of avidin occurred in control cultures or
cultures treated with estrogen or glucocorticoids. However, avidin
induction began after introduction of progesterone into the culture
medium. The maximum stimulation occurred during the first 48 hours
and approached a plateau after the sixth day.

TABLE 2

LEVELS OF AVIDIN, OVALBUMIN, LYSOZYME AND GENERAL PROTEIN

SYNTHESIS DURING IN VITRO INCUBATION

Incubation Time (hours)	Avidin (µg/g. oviduct)	Ovalbumin (mg/g. oviduct)	Lysozyme (mg/g. oviduct)	Total Protein (cpm/100 mg. oviduct)
0	0	22	1.7	7,100
6	0.18	9	1.3	4,600
12	0.6	14	1.1	2,600
24	5.6	11	1.1	900
48	7.5	14	1.0	690

Methods have been described previously (B.W. O'Malley and W.L McGuire, J. Clin. Invest. 47:654, 1968).

The specificity of response of this cell culture induction
system is shown in Table 2 . During a 48 hour incubation with progesterone, no significant increases in ovalbumin or lysozyme were
noted. Table 2 shows that the specificity of this induction system
was also maintained in oviduct minces incubated with progesterone
in vitro. No increase in other major proteins such as ovalbumins
or lysozyme occurred during the incubation. We cannot absolutely
rule out induction of some unknown oviduct protein; however, general protein synthesis measured by successive pulses of ^{3}H-amino
acids into TCA precipitable protein showed a progressive fall over
the course of the incubation. These events are in contrast to the
increased rate of avidin synthesis occurring concomitantly.

TABLE 3

EFFECT OF VARIOUS STEROIDS ON INDUCTION OF AVIDIN

SYNTHESIS IN THE ESTROGEN-STIMULATED CHICK OVIDUCT

Compound*	Avidin (μg/g. oviduct)
No hormone	0.0
Progesterone	1.6
d-Aldosterone	0.0
Pregnenolone	0.0
Cortisol	0.0
Dehydroepiandrosterone	0.0
Androsterone	0.0
Estriol	0.0
Estradiol	0.0
17-Hydroxyprogesterone	0.1
Testosterone	0.3
20α-hydroxy-4-pregnen-3-one	0.7
19-Norprogesterone	0.9
17-Ethynyl-19-nortestosterone	2.0
Allopregnane-21-ol-3,20-dione	0.7

*Each steroid was administered as a single 5 mg. dose and oviducts
were removed and analyzed for avidin content 20 hours later.

The capacities of the various steroids to induce avidin synthesis are shown in Table 3.   Avidin was not detectable in control
glands from animals injected with propylene glycol:ethanol alone.

All but one of the steroids that stimulated avidin synthesis had a Δ^4-3-keto configuration in the A ring. The Δ^4-3-keto function was not an absolute requirement, as induction occurred with allo-pregnane-21-ol-3,20 dione. The presence of the Δ^4-3-keto group alone was not sufficient to induce synthesis, since cortisol and aldosterone were inactive. Significant activity was maintained after hydroxylation of progesterone at the 20α position, but hydroxylation at the 17 position caused loss of almost all activity. The 19-carbon is not required in the induction process, as shown by the significant activity of 19-norprogesterone. These data do not permit formulation of absolute structural requirements for avidin induction. Nevertheless, the correlation of ability to induce avidin synthesis and the biologic progestational activity of the various compounds is striking. All progestational steroids tested stimulated avidin synthesis and the more potent progestins such as progesterone, 17-ethynyl-19-nortestosterone, 19-norprogesterone, and 20α-hydroxy-4-pregnene-3-one were also the more potent inducers of avidin formation. Progestational activity, as defined by endo-metrial proliferation, cannot easily be separated from anti-uterotrophic or anti-estrogenic activity. At this time, we cannot categorically assume that intracellular alteration (e.g., hydroxy-lation) of the progesterone molecule does not occur before in-duction of avidin synthesis.

We attempted next to define the molecular mechanism of proges-terone induction of avidin synthesis. The presence of hydroxyurea, a known specific inhibitor of DNA synthesis, did not significantly affect progesterone induction of avidin synthesis during a 48 hour incubation of cultured oviduct (Table 4).

TABLE 4

EFFECT OF INHIBITORS ON AVIDIN SYNTHESIS

	Avidin (µg/g. oviduct)*
Progesterone alone	4.2
Progesterone + Hydroxyurea (.001 M)	4.0
Progesterone + Cycloheximide (0.5 µg/ml)	0.15
Progesterone + Actinomycin D (1.0 µg/ml)	0.9

*Minced oviduct was incubated for 48 hours in tissue culture media with progesterone and the above antibiotics added at zero time.

Hydroxyurea (.001 M) decreased ^{3}H-thymidine incorporation into
DNA 65% over controls at this concentration but did not affect RNA
or general protein synthesis. Addition of colchicine (25 mμg/ml)
to the incubation medium also had no effect on the induction
process. Addition of actinomycin D caused an 80% inhibition of
avidin synthesis without inhibiting general protein synthesis as
measured by incorporation of labeled amino acids into TCA precipitable material. The induction process was dependent on new
protein synthesis since addition of cycloheximide at any time
during the incubation prevented further synthesis of avidin.

TABLE 5

CHANGES IN OVIDUCT RAPIDLY-LABELED NUCLEAR RNA SYNTHESIS

AND RNA POLYMERASE ACTIVITY FOLLOWING PROGESTERONE

Hours After Progesterone	Nuclear RNA Synthesis ^{3}H-Uridine (cpm/mg RNA)	RNA Polymerase Action ^{3}H-UMP (cpm/mg DNA)	
		Estrogen-pretreated	Unstimulated
0	40,000 ± 3,000	72,000 ± 2,000	410 ± 80
2	27,000 ± 8,000	61,000 ± 5,000	----
6	24,000 ± 6,000	74,000 ± 2,000	440 ± 70
12	41,000 ± 4,000	83,000 ± 2,000	1250 ± 100
24	59,000 ± 3,000	90,000 ± 4,000	2400 ± 140
48	50,000 ± 3,000	70,000 ± 3,000	1350 ± 110
72	8,000 ± 8,000	----	----

Progesterone was administered at zero time and oviducts were homogenized and analyzed for ^{3}H-uridine incorporation into RNA and RNA
polymerase activity as previously described (16).

The rate of synthesis of rapidly labeled oviduct nuclear RNA
was studied at various times during in vitro avidin induction
utilizing 20 minute pulses of tritiated or ^{14}C-uridine. Extraction
and sucrose density purification of intact nuclei were carried out
and nuclear RNA specific activity was determined. A decrease (50%)
at two to six hours followed by a rise in nuclear RNA specific activity was consistently observed prior to avidin induction (Table 5).
The rise reached a maximum between 24 and 48 hours and generally
did not exceed the levels observed at zero time. Controls showed
neither the fall nor rise in nuclear RNA seen in the minces incubated with progesterone. A fall in the specific activity of
rapidly labeled nuclear RNA was noted after 48 hours which coin-
cided temporally with cessation of avidin synthesis. No change in

total oviduct RNA by either mass or precursor incorporation methods was noted. Analysis of RNA polymerase activity of isolated nuclei was noted which was quite similar to that seen with rapidly labeled nuclear RNA (Table 5). A fall from zero time levels occurred two hours after progesterone administration followed by a rise prior to induction of avidin synthesis (16). Stimulation of RNA polymerase activity also increased but from a low baseline when progesterone was administered to immature chicks (16).

The studies to this point indicated a primary nuclear action for progesterone. The mechanisms involved in this early decrease and then rise in nuclear RNA synthesis and RNA polymerase are not yet elucidated. Estrogen withdrawal cannot explain the initial drop in activity as controls are unchanged and estrogen stimulation of RNA polymerase lasts at least 48 hours after a single injection. This initial drop in nuclear RNA labeling and polymerase activity could represent a sudden change in precursor pool size but we must account for the fact that: (1) the results are identical using either labeled uracil, UTP or CTP; (2) similar curves can be obtained in vitro or in vivo; (3) early changes in RNA production have also been obtained using purified chromatin isolated at various times following progesterone administration and incubated in vitro with E. coli RNA polymerase and known amounts of precursor nucleotides. We must also consider that two populations of oviduct cells exist, one of which responds to progesterone and one of which is unresponsive or inhibited. Progesterone inhibition of cytoplasmic synthesis of all oviduct proteins except avidin could account for the initial fall in rapidly labeled nuclear RNA but would be unlikely. The progesterone-mediated changes in RNA metabolism are small but this would be expected if only one or a few new proteins were produced. We have subsequently discovered a qualitative change in the pattern of nuclear rapidly-labeled RNA using acrylamide-agarose electrophoresis, (Dingman, Aronow, Peacock and O'Malley, unpublished observations).

Since avidin was the only known new protein synthesized in response to progesterone, the changes in nuclear RNA synthesis and RNA polymerase activity would suggest a mechanism of action for this steroid at the transcription level of protein synthesis. However, if an interaction between steroid and the genome actually takes place, we might expect to see an early alteration in DNA-chromatin template directed RNA synthesis. In addition, the appearance of a new species of hybridizable RNA in the cell nucleus following progesterone but at no time prior to administration of the steroid would be a final evidence for a direct effect of progesterone on transcription.

A template assay was performed (17) on chick oviduct chromatin-DNA isolated at varying time periods following progesterone administration to estrogen pretreated chicks. An early

decrease, followed by a rise in template activity was present two
to four hours after in vivo progesterone (unpublished data, W.L.
McGuire and B.W. O'Malley). It should be emphasized that these
time points precede detectable avidin synthesis. We next attempted
to delineate a qualitative change in the RNA synthesized from
isolated chromatin after progesterone. The RNA's synthesized in
vitro from oviduct chromatin prepared from diethylstilbestrol
stimulated chicks before and four hours after progesterone administration were subjected to nearest neighbor frequency analysis.
A limited number of the dinucleotide pairs were different after
progesterone, e.g., CpA, ApG, UpG, UpU (W.L. McGuire and B.W.
O'Malley, unpublished data). We therefore conclude that progesterone, upon entering the cell, either directly or indirectly
interacts with the DNA chromatin complex. It then may alter the
level of pre-existing RNA, but perhaps more importantly it allows
new regions of the DNA to be transcribed which contain information
necessary for the synthesis of avidin.

The possibility existed then that the changes in nuclear RNA
metabolism described above were responsible for the production of
new species of mRNA. We chose to utilize the techniques of DNA-RNA
hybridization to detect new gene transcriptions. The experimental
results suggested that progesterone initiates the production of
new species of nuclear rapidly-labeled DNA-like RNA in the chick
oviduct.

The hybridization techniques were similar to those described
earlier (18). Competition experiments were performed by using
unlabeled oviduct nuclear RNA from chicks receiving only diethylstilbestrol (DES) to compete against labeled RNA from oviducts of
chicks treated either with DES alone or DES plus progesterone (DES
+ P). In these experiments, progesterone was administered six hours
prior to sacrifice of the chicks. Incomplete competition of the DES
+ P RNA by the unlabeled DES-RNA, indicated that certain species
present in the DES + P RNA were absent in the RNA from chicks
treated only with estrogen and suggested that progesterone was responsible for the presence of additional new specie(s) of RNA
molecules. In order to be certain that the differences were significant, we labeled the oviducts from animals given DES or DES +
P separately with different RNA precursor compounds (^{3}H-uridine
and ^{32}P-orthophosphoric acid); the oviducts were then combined,
homogenized and carried through the remainder of the purification
and hybridization procedures as a single unit. Since the RNA's
were handled simultaneously under a double-label protocol, technical error should have been eliminated. The results are shown in
Table 6. The competition curve, approaching that predictable on
a theoretical basis, was obtained when increasing amounts of unlabeled nuclear RNA from oviducts receiving DES alone was added

TABLE 6

EXTENT OF COMPETITION BY UNLABELED RNA
BEFORE AND AFTER PROGESTERONE

Unlabeled Competitor RNA (μg unlabeled RNA/μg labeled RNA)	Percent Hybridization* of Labeled RNA	
	DES alone	DES + Progesterone
I. DES alone		
0	100	100
1.5	55	66
3	40	50
6	24	35
9	10	22
12	4	19
II. DES + Progesterone (DES + P)		
0	100	100
1.5	67	67
3	41	42
6	20	19
9	11	11

*Chick oviduct DNA (40 μg) was incubated with labeled nuclear RNA (80 μg) from DES or DES + P treated oviducts for 17 hours at 67°C. Increasing amounts of unlabeled nuclear RNA from DES or DES + P treated oviducts were added to the initial reaction mixture to competitively hybridize to the DNA. The total labeled RNA hybridizing to DNA with an unlabeled competitor RNA present equals 100% hybridized. The specific activity of the labeled RNA ranged from 2000 to 8000 cpm/μg. The values are means of triplicates under a double-label protocol.

to the homologous ^{3}H-RNA. The ^{32}P-RNA from DES + P oviducts revealed certain RNA species which did not enter into competition with the unlabeled RNA (Table 6, I). However, when nuclear RNA from DES + P oviducts was used as the unlabeled competitor, the curves were virtually the same (Table 6, II). This would be expected if the unlabeled DES + P RNA contained the same species present in both ^{32}P-RNA (DES + P) and ^{3}H-RNA (DES alone). The hybridization competition results were also similar when the labels were reversed. Hahn et al. (19) using molecular hybridization, have also recently demonstrated the appearance of new species of oviduct RNA following progesterone administration.

The hybridization-competition studies suggest that progesterone induced the synthesis of a new specie(s) of nuclear RNA, during induction of avidin synthesis. These species of RNA were absent or present only in very small quantities prior to administration of the hormone. This evidence for new genome transcription was noted at both 6 and 16 hours following progesterone and occurred when either in vivo or in vitro labeling techniques were used. We have not detected avidin synthesis until 10 hours after progesterone administration, in vivo, to estrogen treated chicks. In such a specific model system for induction of a new protein as the chick oviduct, it is tempting to consider that this new species of RNA contains the messenger RNA for avidin. This interpretation is certainly complicated by reports of a heterogeneous high molecular weight, DNA-like class of RNA which, for the most part, may not even leave the nucleus (20,21). Therefore, we must await biologic testing of the material in a soluble chemically-defined system, demonstrating that a new RNA template for avidin synthesis has been created.

The precise mechanism of progesterone induction of avidin synthesis is not yet proven. We have recently reviewed numerous studies carried out in this laboratory over the last three years in an attempt to answer this question (22). Two major sites for hormonal regulation of protein synthesis now exist: at the transcriptional level in the nucleus or the translational level in the cytoplasm. The process does appear to be independent of new DNA synthesis. The inhibitory effect of actinomycin D when added to the incubation at zero time, the early changes in rapidly labeled nuclear RNA, and the early effect on nuclear RNA polymerase and a qualitative change in the RNA transcribed from DNA-chromatin template after progesterone would suggest a mechanism of action for this steroid hormone at the nuclear level of protein synthesis, resulting in new gene transcriptions (RNA) and the eventual de novo synthesis of avidin molecules. This unique model system should permit further biochemical studies on the mechanism of progesterone-mediated alteration of gene function.

REFERENCES

1. Corner, G.W.: The Hormones in Human Reproduction.
Princeton University Press, Princeton, p. 281 (1947).

2. Reynolds, S.R.M.: Physiology of the Uterus. P.B.
Hoeber, Inc., New York p.611 (1949).

3. Csapo, A. Brook Lodge Symposium of Progesterone, Brook
Lodge Press, Augusta, Michigan, p. 7 (1961).

4. Goto, M. and Csapo, A.: Biol. Bull. 115:335 (1958).

5. Marshall, J. and Csapo, A.: Biol. Bull. 117:419 (1959).

6. Mueller, G.C.: J. Biol. Chem. 204:77 (1953).

7. Wagatsuma, T., Sullivan, W.J. and Kumar, D.: Amer. J.
Obstet. Gynecol. 98:1050 (1967).

8. Varricchio, F.: Arch. Biophys. 121:187 (1967).

9. Brant, J.W.A. and A.V. Nalbandov: Poultry Sci. 35:692
(1956).

10. O'Malley, B.W., McGuire, W.L. and Korenman, S.G.:
Biochem. Biophys. Acta. 145:204 (1967).

11. Hertz, R., Fraps, R.M. and Sebrell, W.E.: Proc. Soc.
Exptl. Biol. Med. 52:142 (1943).

12. Korenman, S.G. and O'Malley, B.W.: Endocrinology 83:11
(1968).

13. Korenman, S.G. and O'Malley, B.W.: Biochem. Biophys.
Acta 140:174 (1967).

14. O'Malley, B.W. and Korenman, S.G.: Life Sciences 6:1953
(1967).

15. O'Malley, B.W.: Biochemistry 6:2546 (1967).

16. McGuire, W.L. and O'Malley, B.W.: Biochem. Biophys.
Acta 157:187 (1968).

17. Barker, K.L. and Warren, J.C.: Proc. Natl. Acad. Sci.
56:1298 (1966).

18.   O'Malley, B. W. and McGuire, W. L.:   Proc. Natl. Acad.
Sci. 60: 1527 (1968).

19.   Hahn, W.E., Church, R.B., Gorbman, A. and Willmot, L.:
Gen. Comp. Endocrinology (in press).

20.   Soeira, R., Birnboim, H. C., and Darnell, J. E.:   J.Mol.
Biol. 19: 362 (1966).

21.   Shearer, R. W., and McCarthy, B. J.:   Biochemistry 6:
283 (1967).

22.   O'Malley, B. W., McGuire, W. L., Kohler, P. O., and
Korenman, S. G.:   Recent Progress in Hormone Research, Vol. 29
(1969), in press.

THE EFFECTS OF GONADAL HORMONES AND CONTRACEPTIVE STEROIDS ON TRYPTOPHAN METABOLISM

D. P. Rose

University Department of Chemical Pathology,
The Royal Infirmary, Sheffield S6 3DA, England

The pathway by which tryptophan is metabolized to yield nicotinic acid ribonucleotide has been the subject of considerable interest in recent years. Abnormal urinary excretion of metabolites of this pathway in vitamin B_6 deficiency has led to the extensive use of a tryptophan load test for the study of pyridoxine requirements in man (1-3).

The metabolic reactions involved in the tryptophan-nicotinic acid ribonucleotide pathway are summarized in Figure 1. Vitamin B_6 deficiency causes the metabolites kynurenine, 3-hydroxykynurenine, xanthurenic acid, and to a lesser extent kynurenic acid to be excreted in abnormally large amounts after an oral dose of tryptophan (3). A lack of pyridoxal 5-phosphate coenzyme appears to affect kynureninase more severely than kynurenine aminotransferase, with the result that although there is a reduction in the rate of conversion of 3-hydroxykynurenine to 3-hydroxyanthranilic acid the production of xanthurenic and kynurenic acids proceeds at an increased rate. The excretion of xanthurenic acid in urine exceeds that of kynurenic acid, although both are formed by a similar transamination reaction. In vitro studies indicate that this is because the mitochondrial fraction of the aminotransferase, which yields xanthurenic acid, is less affected by a deficiency of pyridoxal 5-phosphate than is the supernatant fraction concerned in the formation of kynurenic acid (4).

Several studies have demonstrated a disturbance of tryptophan metabolism during normal pregnancy (5-7). Brown, Thornton, and Price found elevated outputs of xanthurenic acid, 3-hydroxykynurenine, kynurenine, and N-methyl-2-pyridone-5-carboxamide (2-pyridone)

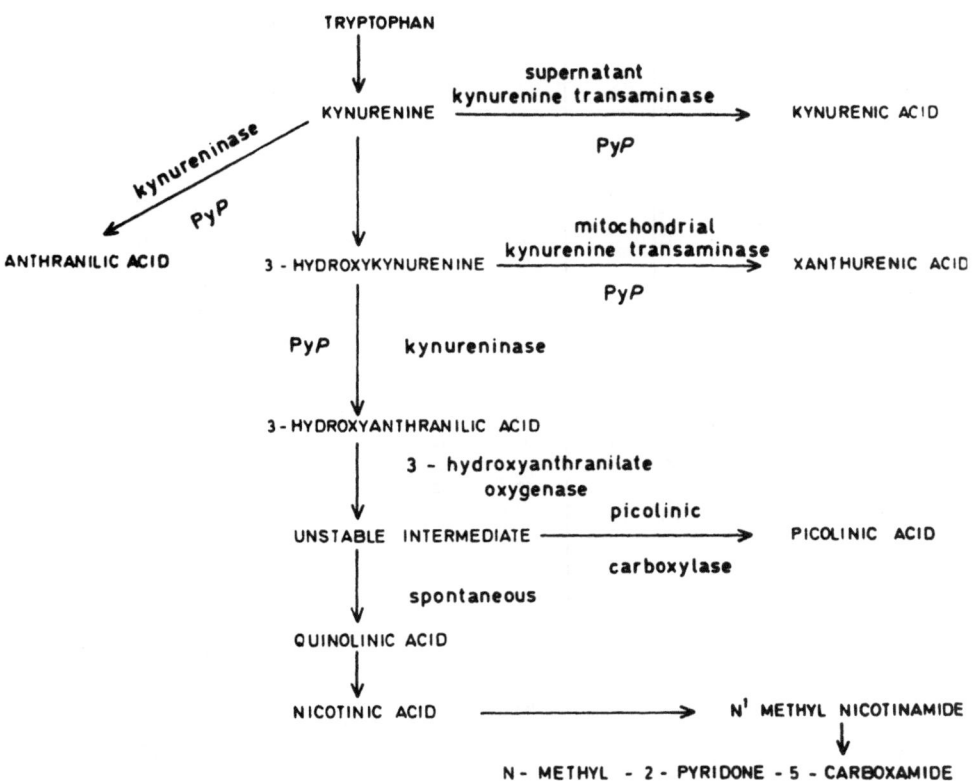

Fig. 1. THE METABOLIC PATHWAY OF TRYPTOPHAN CONVERSION TO
NICOTINIC ACID RIBONUCLEOTIDE. Enzymes concerned in reaction are
given in lower case. PyP = pyridoxal 5-phosphate.

TABLE 1

TRYPTOPHAN METABOLITE EXCRETION: CONTROL GROUP

Group	Mean Age (yr)	Excretion (μmoles in 8 hr) Mean ± S.E.			
		HK	XA	HA
Females 21 - 35 yrs. (11)	25.5	387 ± 34	186 ± 25	189 ± 24
Females 42 - 74 yrs. (10)	61.2	209 ± 32	141 ± 15	129 ± 23
Males 24 - 74 yrs.	46.8	189 ± 26	114 ± 14	114 ± 8

Number of subjects in each group is given in brackets.

Urine was collected for eight hours after a 5 g dose of L-tryptophan.

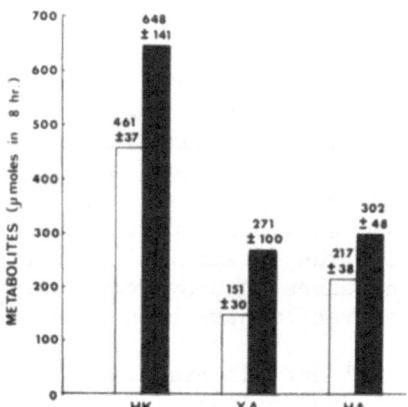

Fig. 2. VARIATION IN THE URINARY EXCRETION OF TRYPTOPHAN
METABOLITES WITH THE MENSTRUAL CYCLE. 3-Hydroxykynurenine (HK),
xanthurenic acid (XA), and 3-hydroxyanthranilic acid (HA) were
determined in urine collected for 8 hours after a 5 g dose of
L-tryptophan. The average values (±S.E.) are given for 5 subjects
studied on the first day after a menstrual period (open blocks)
and again on the 13th day of the cycle (solid black blocks).

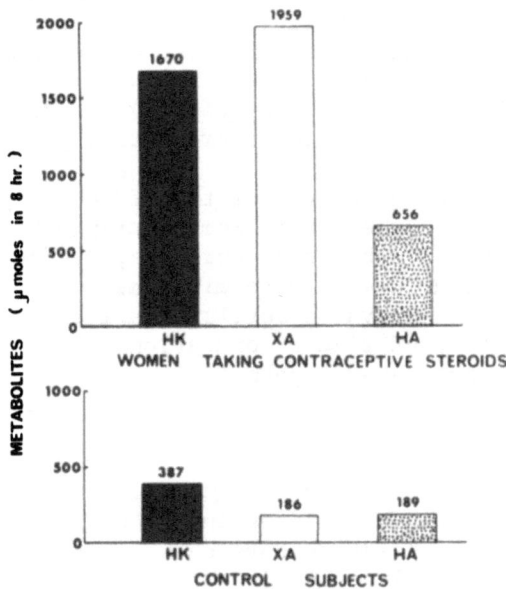

Fig. 3. THE EFFECT OF CONTRACEPTIVE STEROIDS ON THE URINARY
EXCRETION OF TRYPTOPHAN METABOLITES. The average excretions of
3-hydroxykynurenine (HK), xanthurenic acid (XA), and 3-hydroxy-
anthranilic acid (HA) by 10 women using contraceptive steroids
are compared with those of a control group of young adult females.
(5 g tryptophan load).

in urine collected after a 2 g tryptophan load. 2-Pyridone is the
major urinary excretion product of nicotinamide in man. When
supplements of pyridoxine were given, the excretion of these metabolites was lowered, but it still remained significantly higher
than the levels excreted by the non-pregnant controls. On the
basis of this observation it was suggested that the hormonal changes
associated with pregnancy might play a part in the disturbance of
tryptophan metabolism, as well as pyridoxine deficiency resulting
from fetal demands for the vitamin. In addition to the abnormalities noted above, increases in 3-hydroxyanthranilic acid and N^1-
methylnicotinamide excretion have been reported in pregnancy (8).

Studies by Michael and his associates suggested that gonadal
hormones influence the metabolism of tryptophan in the non-pregnant woman (9). They found a sex difference in the urinary excretion of metabolites, with higher levels occurring in women
than men. Table 1 shows the results of a study of tryptophan
metabolite excretions in urine collected for 8 hours after the
administration of a 5 g oral dose of L-tryptophan (10). Young
women (21-36 years of age) excreted 3-hydroxykynurenine (p =
< 0.001), xanthurenic acid (p = < 0.01) and 3-hydroxyanthranilic
acid (p = < 0.02) in significantly larger amounts than did men,
and 3-hydroxykynurenine in greater quantity than did a group of
older women who were post-menopausal or approaching the menopause
(p = < 0.001). There were no significant differences in the
excretions of the older women as compared with the men. These
results confirm those of Michael et al (9) and also relate the
higher excretions by women to the reproductive years of life.

In order to investigate further the effect of physiological
levels of hormones upon the metabolism of tryptophan by normal
women the excretions of 3-hydroxykynurenine, xanthurenic acid and
3-hydroxyanthranilic acid were determined at two stages of the
menstrual cycle (10). Elevated levels of all three metabolites
occurred at the estimated time of ovulation, when the urinary
excretion of estrogens is at a peak (11), as compared with the
levels on the first day after the menstrual period (Fig. 2).

The metabolic effects of estrogens and progestogens have
features in common with those of pregnancy. Studies of the
excretion of tryptophan metabolites in the urine of women taking
a combination of these hormones have shown that these similarities include an abnormal metabolism of the aminoacid (12,13).
Figure 3 compares the excretion of 3-hydroxykynurenine, xanthurenic
acid and 3-hydroxyanthranilic acid by ten women who were taking
an estrogen-progestogen preparation for the control of ovulation
with a control group of young women who were not taking hormones.
The levels of all three metabolites were markedly elevated by
hormone administration. Price, Thornton, and Mueller (13) have

TABLE 2

THE EFFECT OF ESTROGENS ON TRYPTOPHAN METABOLISM

Subject No.	Sex	Age (yr)	Hormone dosage	Duration of Therapy	Excretion (μmoles in 8 hr)			
					K	HK	XA	HA
1	M	68	Ethinyl estradiol 0.25 mg daily and methyl testosterone 5 mg daily	4 years	–	1120	1099	1612
2	M	59	Ethinyl estradiol 0.25 mg alternate days and methyl testosterone 5 mg alternate days	3 months	–	423	622	136
3	F	72	Ethinyl estradiol 0.05 mg every ten days	5 years	–	909	1589	474
4	F	70	Ethinyl estradiol 0.25 mg every three days	10 years	–	594	1186	305
5	F	24	(a) before starting estrogen	0	533	257	211	198
			(b) ethinyl estradiol 0.1 mg. daily {	2 weeks	470	338	806	332
				3 weeks	864	455	1320	436

Urine was collected for eight hours after a 5 g dose of L-tryptophan

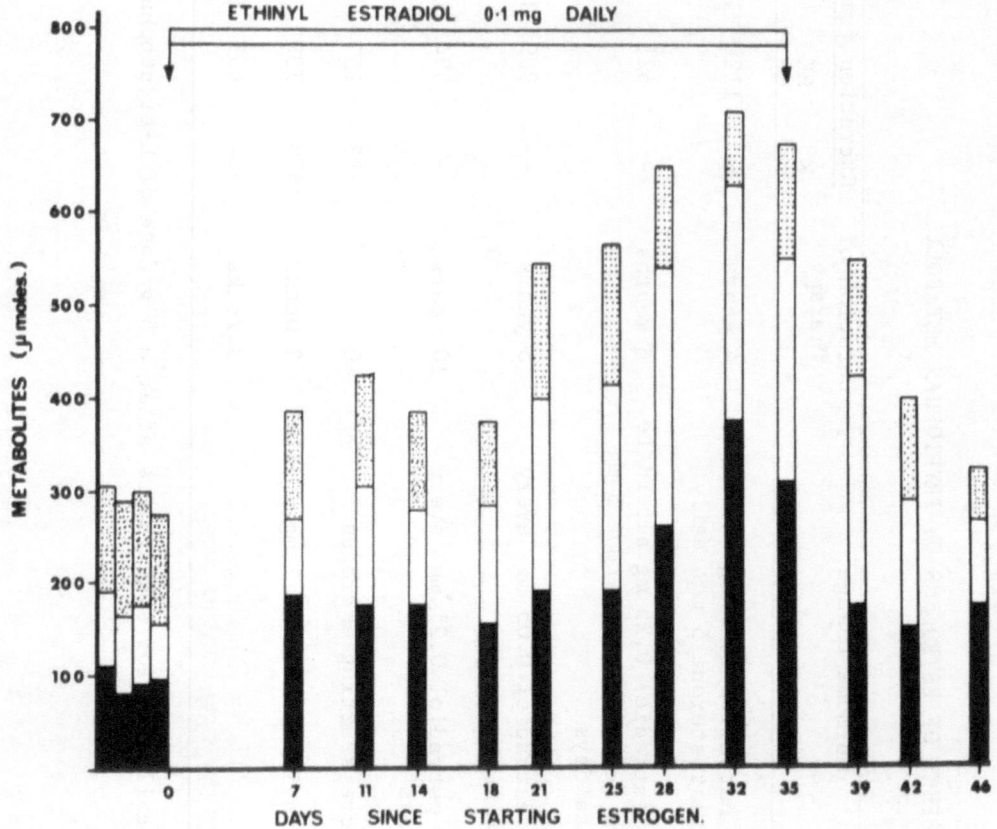

Fig. 4.   THE EFFECT OF ETHINYL ESTRADIOL ADMINISTRATION ON THE URINARY EXCRETION OF TRYPTOPHAN METABOLITES IN A NORMAL MALE SUBJECT.   Stippled part of column -- 3-hydroxyanthranilic acid; open part -- xanthurenic acid; solid black part -- 3-hydroxy-kynurenine.

shown that the excretion of kynurenine, acetylkynurenine and kynurenic acid are also raised abnormally following the administration of a tryptophan load to women taking Enovid-E (mestranol
0.1 mg and norethynodrel 2.5 mg) for contraceptive purposes.

The effect of contraceptive steroid preparations on tryptophan metabolism is also produced by treatment with estrogens alone.
Subjects Nos. 1 to 4 in Table 2 were receiving estrogen therapy
for hemorrhagic disorders due to capillary defects, and subject
No. 5 was a healthy volunteer. All of the metabolite levels were
elevated, including kynurenine which was determined in the urine
of subject No. 5. The time required for changes to appear in
the urinary excretion of tryptophan metabolites after starting
estrogen administration was studied in a healthy male volunteer
aged 30 years (12). Basal levels of 3-hydroxykynurenine, xanthurenic acid and 3-hydroxyanthranilic acid were determined on
four occasions, with at least 5 days between each of the 5 g
tryptophan loads. Ethinyl estradiol, 0.1 mg daily, was then taken
for 5 weeks during which period tryptophan metabolite excretions
were determined twice weekly. Figure 4 shows that the xanthurenic
acid and 3-hydroxykynurenine excretions began to rise at about
the seventh day, and continued to do so throughout the period of
hormone administration. The excretion of 3-hydroxyanthranilic
acid was unaltered in this particular instance.

When subjects receiving contraceptive steroids or estrogens
are treated with large doses of pyridoxine the excretion of
tryptophan metabolites is restored to normal levels (12,13)
(Table 3).

One divergence from the general similarity in the metabolism
of tryptophan by pregnant women and those taking contraceptive
steroids is that whereas the excretion of 2-pyridone is elevated
in pregnancy (7), normal levels were obtained in women taking
Enovid-E (13). However, a study of the excretion of N^1-methyl-
nicotinamide, the immediate precursor of 2-pyridone, has shown
that Enovid-treated women excrete an increased quantity of this
metabolite, both in urine collected without prior tryptophan
loading ('spontaneous') and following a 2 g dose of L-tryptophan
(Table 4) (14). The total yield of N^1-methylnicotinamide plus
2-pyridone is about 60 % greater in women taking Enovid-E than
it is in normal control subjects. Inhibition of N^1-methylnico-
tinamide oxidase activity would explain the elevated N^1-methyl-
nicotinamide excretion without a corresponding increase in
2-pyridone and such an effect of estrogens on this enzyme has been
described in the livers of mice (15).

TABLE 3

EFFECT OF PYRIDOXINE ADMINISTRATION ON EXCRETION OF

TRYPTOPHAN METABOLITES IN ESTROGEN-TREATED SUBJECTS

Estrogen Therapy	Pyridoxine	Excretion (μmoles in 8 hr)		
		HA	XA	HA
Enovid	(i) Pretreatment	2101	3551	578
	(ii) 1 mg daily for 1 month	1813	2630	383
	(iii) 20 mg night before load; 20 mg with load	121	538	234
Ethinyl estradiol	(i) Pretreatment	1120	1099	1612
	(ii) 40 mg night before load; 40 mg with load	67	78	71
Ethinyl estradiol	(i) Pretreatment	423	662	136
	(ii) 20 mg with load	54	87	45

Urine was collected for eight hours after a 5 g dose of L-tryptophan

TABLE 4

EFFECT OF ENOVID-E ADMINISTRATION ON THE EXCRETION OF

N^1-METHYLNICOTINAMIDE (N^1Me) AND 2-PYRIDONE (pyr) (μmoles/24 hr)

	Spontaneous excretion		Post-tryptophan excretion		Yield (post-tryptophan less spontaneous)	
	N^1Me	pyr	N^1Me	pyr	N^1Me	pyr
Enovid-E Group	60.0±8.2 *	63.5±8.4	148.3±16.9 *	136.4±13.7	88.3±15.3	72.9±9.3
ratio pyr/N^1Me	1.05		0.91			
Control Group	32.2±2.9	85.6±7.8	75.4±18.2	139.9±14.8	43.9±16.2	54.2±11.0
ratio pyr/N^1Me	2.65		1.85			

The control group consists of 13 subjects with results for N^1Me excretion and 24 subjects with pyr results. The results are expressed as mean ± S.E.. Those for the Enovid-E group marked * differ significantly from those of the control group; p < 0.05 (Student's t-test). In all cases urine was collected for 24 hours after a 2 g dose of L-tryptophan.

DISCUSSION

The very high excretions of xanthurenic acid, 3-hydroxy-
kynurenine and kynurenine in the urine of women taking estrogen or
estrogen-progestogen preparations, together with the correction of
these abnormalities by pyridoxine administration, suggest the
presence of vitamin B_6 deficiency. However, there is no direct
evidence that pyridoxal 5-phosphate has a role in the metabolism of
tryptophan to nicotinic acid ribonucleotide at a later stage than
the activity of kynureninase, and yet the excretion of 3-hydroxy-
anthranilic acid is elevated by estrogen administration (10), as it
is in pregnancy (8), and it returns to normal when pyridoxine is
given. As a possible explanation it has been suggested that
pyridoxal 5-phosphate may have an unrecognized role in tryptophan
metabolism beyond the step of 3-hydroxyanthranilic acid production
(16). Additional evidence for this is provided by the report that
the excretion of quinolinic acid is elevated when vitamin B_6
depletion is produced in man, and returns to normal following the
administration of large doses of pyridoxine (17).

It must be emphasized that increased excretions of tryptophan
metabolites in the urine of women using contraceptive steroids
have been demonstrated only following the administration of a
tryptophan load. Women taking Enovid-E appeared to excrete normal
quantities of these metabolites in urine collected without a prior
dose of L-tryptophan (13), although as only the unconjugated
urinary metabolites were determined it is possible that preliminary hydrolysis would reveal an increase in those derivatives,
incuding kynurenine, 3-hydroxykynurenine and xanthurenic acid,
which are also excreted as glucuronides and sulfate esters.

The excretion of N^1-methylnicotinamide is elevated in women
who are taking Enovid-E whether or not the urine is collected
after a dose of tryptophan (14). In view of this it has been
suggested that estrogens cause an increase in activity of one or
more enzymes concerned in the metabolism of tryptophan such that
there is an enhanced capacity to synthesize nicotinic acid ribonucleotide. When a tryptophan load is given, there may be insufficient pyridoxal 5-phosphate available to allow for the complete
metabolism of all of the amino acid entering the tryptophan-nicotinic acid ribonucleotide pathway, and so there is an increase
in the urinary excretion of xanthurenic acid, and those other
metabolites high levels of which are associated with vitamin B_6
deficiency (12,14).

A hormonal influence on tryptophan metabolism is well known
in the case of cortisol, which increases the activity of tryptophan
oxygenase by a process of induction (18). This same response has
been demonstrated in man and is accompanied by an increase in the

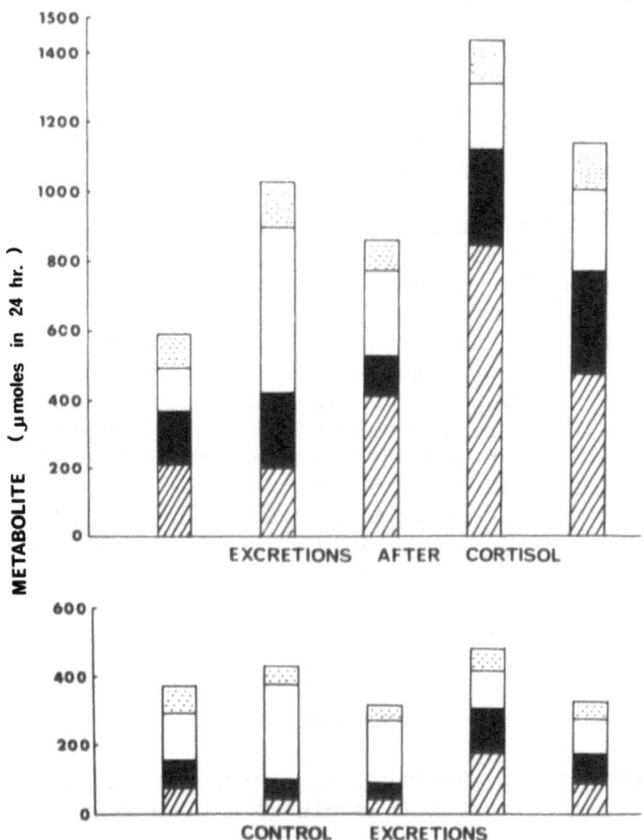

Fig. 5.   THE EFFECT OF CORTISOL ADMINISTRATION ON THE EX-
CRETION OF TRYPTOPHAN METABOLITES BY FIVE NORMAL SUBJECTS.
The excretions of kynurenine (crosshatched), 3-hydroxykynurenine
(solid black), xanthurenic acid' (open) and 3-hydroxyanthranilic
acid (stippled) were determined in urine collected for 24 hours
after a 5 g tryptophan load.   A week later hydrocortisone sodium
succinate, 250 mg, was injected intramuscularly and 5 hours later
a second study of tryptophan metabolite excretions was commenced.

urinary excretion of kynurenine (19), and other metabolites (20), in response to a tryptophan load. Figure 5 shows the elevated levels of kynurenine, 3-hydroxykynurenine, xanthurenic acid and 3-hydroxyanthranilic acid which occur when tryptophan is given after an injection of hydrocortisone. Treatment with pyridoxine causes a fall in the amounts of all four metabolites excreted after cortisol to levels which are as low as or lower than those excreted without cortisol administration (20). This would appear to indicate that a temporary lack of pyridoxal 5-phosphate develops similar to that which we have postulated to occur when a tryptophan load is given to an estrogen-treated subject.

If estrogens influence the metabolism of tryptophan to nico-tinic acid ribonucleotide by increasing the activity of a single enzyme, then tryptophan oxygenase would seem the most likely to be involved as it catalyses the first irreversible step in the sequence of metabolic reactions. However, although the activity of this enzyme is elevated in pregnant rats (21), the administra-tion of estrone and progesterone in combination (21), or estradiol alone (22) are without effect in the non-pregnant animal. The interpretation of these data is made difficult be-cause the changes in tryptophan metabolism seen in the pregnant rat differ from those seen in human pregnancy, for although kynurenine excretion is increased the levels of xanthurenic acid are normal (23). Further investigation of the effect of estro-gens on the enzymes involved in tryptophan metabolism, both in the rat and other species, is necessary before any firm conclusions may be drawn.

SUMMARY

Women using estrogen-progestogen preparations for the control of ovulation excrete elevated levels of a number of tryptophan metabolites in urine collected following a tryptophan load. The estrogenic component appears responsible for this abnormality as both men and women receiving an estrogen alone show a similar disturbance of tryptophan metabolism.

The excretions of kynurenine, 3-hydroxykynurenine, xanthurenic acid, and 3-hydroxyanthranilic acid are all increased in estrogen-treated subjects, but return to normal levels following the ad-ministration of pyridoxine.

The urinary excretion of N^1-methylnicotinamide is elevated in women using a contraceptive steroid preparation, although the output of N-methyl-2-pyridone-5-carboxamide remains at a normal level.

It is concluded that estrogens enhance the capacity for

conversion of tryptophan to nicotinic acid ribonucleotide, but
that they inhibit the oxidation of N^1-methylnicotinamide to yield
N-methyl-2-pyridone-5-carboxamide. A temporary depletion in
available pyridoxal 5-phosphate may be an additional factor
producing an abnormal excretion of metabolites in estrogen-
treated subjects given a tryptophan load.

REFERENCES

1. Greenberg, L.D., Bohr, D.F., McGrath, H., and Rinehart,
J.F.: Xanthurenic acid excretion in the human subject on a py-
ridoxine-deficient diet. Arch. Biochem. 21:237-239 (1949).

2. O'Brien, D. and Jensen, C.B.: Pyridoxine dependency in
two mentally retarded subjects. Clin. Sci. 24:179-186 (1963).

3. Yess, N., Price, J.M., Brown, R.R., Swan, P.B., and
Linkswiler, H.: Vitamin B_6 depletion in man: Urinary excretion
of tryptophan metabolites. J. Nutr. 84:229-236 (1964).

4. Ogasawara, N., Hagino, Y., and Kotake, Y.: Kynurenine
transaminase, kynureninase, and the increase of xanthurenic acid
excretion. J. Biochem. (Tokyo) 52:162-166 (1962).

5. Sprince, H., Lowy, R.S., Folsome, C.E., and Behrman,
J.S.: Studies on the urinary excretion of 'xanthurenic acid'
during normal and abnormal pregnancy; a survey of the excretion
of 'xanthurenic acid' in normal non-pregnant, normal pregnant,
pre-eclamptic, and eclamptic women. Am. J. Obstet. Gynec. 62:
84-92 (1951).

6. Wachstein, M. and Lobel, S.: Abnormal tryptophan
metabolites in human pregnancy and their relation to deranged
vitamin B_6 metabolism. Proc. Soc. Exptl. Biol. Med. 86:624-
627 (1954).

7. Brown, R.R., Thornton, M.J., and Price, J.M.: The effect
of vitamin supplementation on the urinary excretion of tryptophan
metabolites by pregnant women. J. Clin. Invest. 40:617-623
(1961).

8. Hernandez, T.: Tryptophan metabolite excretion in
pregnancy after a tryptophan load. Fed. Proc. 23:136 (1964).

9. Michael, A.F., Drummond, K.N., Doeden, D., Anderson,
J.A., and Good, R.A.: Tryptophan metabolism in man. J. Clin.
Invest. 43:1730-1746 (1964).

10. Rose, D.P.: The influence of sex, age and breast cancer
on tryptophan metabolism. Clin. Chim. Acta 18:221-225 (1967).

11. Brown, J.B.: Urinary excretion of oestrogens during the menstrual cycle. Lancet i:320-323 (1955).

12. Rose, D.P.: The influence of oestrogens on tryptophan metabolism in man. Clin. Sci. 31:265-272 (1966).

13. Price, J.M., Thornton, M.J., and Mueller, L.M.: Tryptophan metabolism in women using steroid hormones for ovulation control. Am. J. Clin. Nutr. 20:452-456 (1967).

14. Rose, D.P., Brown, R.R., and Price, J.M.: Metabolism of tryptophan to nicotinic acid derivatives by women taking oestrogen-progestogen preparations. Nature 219:1259-1260 (1968).

15. Gluecksohn-Waelsch, S., Greengard, P., Quinn, G.P., and Teicher, L.S.: Genetic variations of an oxidase in mammals. J. Biol. Chem. 242:1271-1273 (1967).

16. Rose, D.P.: Penicillamine and pyridoxine in man. Lancet i:489-490 (1966).

17. Brown, R.R., Yess, N., Price, J.M., Linkswiller, H., Swan, P., and Hankes, L.V.: Vitamin B_6 depletion in man: urinary excretion of quinolinic acid and niacin metabolites. J. Nutr. 87:419-423 (1965).

18. Civen, M. and Knox, W.E.: The independence of hydro-cortisone and tryptophan inductions of tryptophan pyrrolase. J. Biol. Chem. 234:1787-1790 (1959).

19. Altman, K. and Greengard, O.: Correlation of kynure-nine excretion with liver tryptophan pyrrolase levels in disease and after hydrocortisone induction. J. Clin. Invest. 45:1527-1534 (1966).

20. Rose, D.P. and McGinty, F.: The influence of adreno-cortical hormones and vitamins upon tryptophan metabolism in man. Clin. Sci. 35:1-9 (1968).

21. Greengard, P., Kalinsky, H.J., and Manning, T.J.: Tryptophan pyrrolase activity during pregnancy. Biochim. Biophys. Acta 156:198-199 (1968).

22. Rose, D.P. and Brown, R.R.: In preparation.

23. Mainardi, L.: Aspetti de metabolismo del triptofano nella gravidanza di animali di specie diversa. Acta Vitaminol. (Milan) 3:110-116 (1957).

CERTAIN METABOLIC EFFECTS OF ESTROGENS

A. A. Sandberg, H. E. Rosenthal and W. R. Slaunwhite, Jr.

Roswell Park Memorial Institute and the Medical
Foundation of Buffalo, Buffalo, New York

This presentation will concern itself with the effects of estrogenic hormones, either administered or through increased production during pregnancy, on two protein systems: 1. liver enzymes
involved in the metabolism of cortisol and 2. the elevation in
plasma transcortin concentration and its relation to progesterone-
cortisol interplay. Both of these parameters have been the subjects
of separate reports from our laboratory (Sandberg, Rosenthal and
Slaunwhite, 1966; Rosenthal, Slaunwhite and Sandberg, 1969) and
this paper will endeavor to stress the salient points of these effects.

A realistic evaluation of the parameters to be discussed requires accurate measurement of unbound cortisol (I) and albumin-
bound cortisol (I_A); in addition, other values which are of importance for a fuller interpretation of the observed phenomena are
necessary, i.e., total cortisol concentration in plasma, the plasma
transcortin concentration, and the amount of cortisol bound to
transcortin. Similar data are necessary for progesterone, if the
total picture in plasma is to be appreciated. Recently developed
techniques and mathematical computations (Rosenthal, Slaunwhite
and Sandberg, 1969) make it possible to measure accurately the
various levels mentioned above and allow an appraisal of the two
parameters listed (Table 1).

It appears that elevated estrogen levels in the body pro-
foundly affect the enzyme systems dealing with cortisol metabolism,
resulting in a markedly decreased ability of the liver to extract

This study has been supported in part by grant AM-01240 from
the National Institutes of Health.

Table 1

MEAN VALUES FOR CONCENTRATIONS OF CORTISOL IN VARIOUS

PLASMA COMPARTMENTS AND OF SOME METABOLIC PARAMETERS

OF CORTISOL

	Normal	Pregnancy (3rd trimester)	Estrogen Therapy
Plasma cortisol	12-14 µg%	35 µg%	40 µg%
(I)	1.1-1.25 µg%	2.2 µg%	3.2 µg%
(I_A)	1.4-1.6 µg%	2.9 µg%	4.2 µg%
(I_T)	9 µg%	30 µg%	33 µg%
Transcortin (T)*	17-25 µg	45-55 µg	40-60 µg
T-1/2	70-90 min.	120-150 min.	>240 min.
Daily secretion	16-28 mg	11-14.5 mg	8-16 mg

    *   Measured as mg of cortisol per 100 ml plasma
(I)   = unbound cortisol.
(I_A) = albumin-bound cortisol.
(I_T) = transcortin-bound cortisol.
T-1/2   = half-life of total plasma cortisol.
Data taken from Sandberg et al (1966).

from the blood and/or reduce enzymatically circulating cortisol.
Figures 1-3 and the following discussion will attempt to show that
under normal circumstances the liver metabolizes the unbound-cortisol
fraction (I) and possibly some of the albumin-bound cortisol (I_A)
and that following estrogen administration (or during pregnancy)
the enzymatic systems in the liver are incapable of effectively
metabolizing either one of these fractions. The legends to Figures
1 to 3 fully explain the conditions prevailing under various circumstances.

      Tait and Burstein (1964) in their evaluation of the metabolism
of cortisol in relation to transcortin-binding came to the conclusion, in support of the hypothesis first advanced by us some years
ago (Slaunwhite and Sandberg, 1959; Sandberg and Slaunwhite, 1959),
that the transcortin-cortisol complex is dissociated or metabolized
to only a small extent, if at all, during passage of the blood
through the liver. On the other hand, the cortisol moiety which
is unbound (I) and that which is bound to albumin (I_A) are almost
totally extracted from the plasma by the liver. If a realistic
secretion rate of cortisol per day is somewhere between 25-30 mg
and the mean unbound cortisol concentration in the plasma is 1.1-
1.25 µg % and the mean total cortisol concentration is 12-14 µg %,
an estimation can be made of the plasma cortisol compartment being

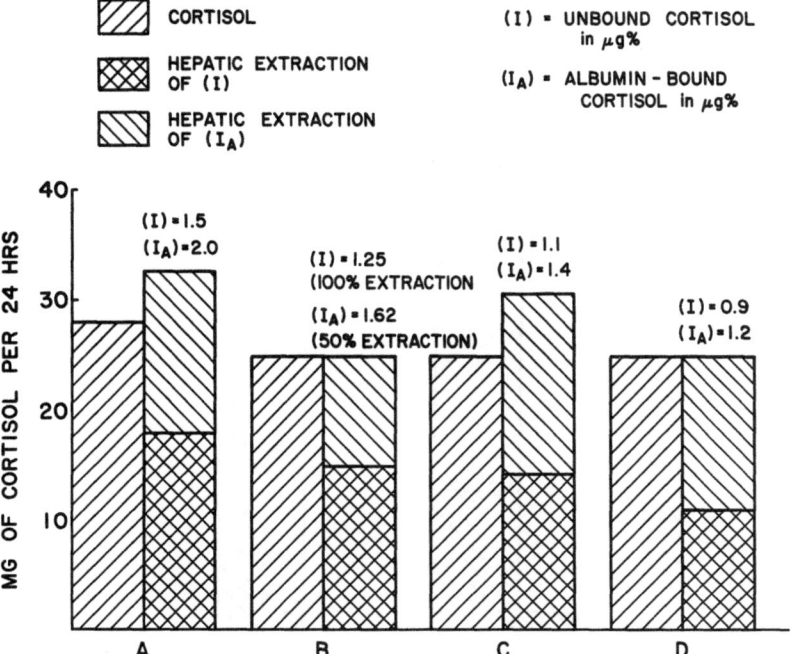

Fig. 1.   Cortisol secretion and hepatic extraction in 24 hours
in normal subjects. A represents the conditions presented for
normal subjects by Tait and Burstein (1964) from the data of
Peterson et al (1960). It is apparent that were extraction of
the total unbound and albumin-bound cortisol to occur, the hepatic
clearance would account for considerably more cortisol than is
secreted per day. In B are shown the secretion data for cortisol
in male subjects obtained by Plager, Schmidt and Staubitz (1964)
and the hepatic extraction has been calculated by us on the basis
of (I) found by these authors. If extraction of the total (I)
fraction and only 50% of the (I_A) fraction occurred, the results
would account for the daily secretory rate. It should be pointed
out that this is an assumption, based on the theory that extraction
of the albumin-bound moiety of cortisol may not be complete in the
liver due to the association involved between the steroid and
protein. In C, the cortisol secretion rate is shown to be only
slightly smaller than can be accounted for by the hepatic extraction
of the total (I) and (I_A) compartments, based on binding data obtained in our laboratory. In D, the hepatic extraction data have
been adjusted to match the cortisol secretory rate. The values
indicate that total hepatic extraction of (I) + (I_A) could easily
account for the 25 mg of cortisol secreted daily if the (I) and
(I_A) were to be slightly overestimated due to technical factors.

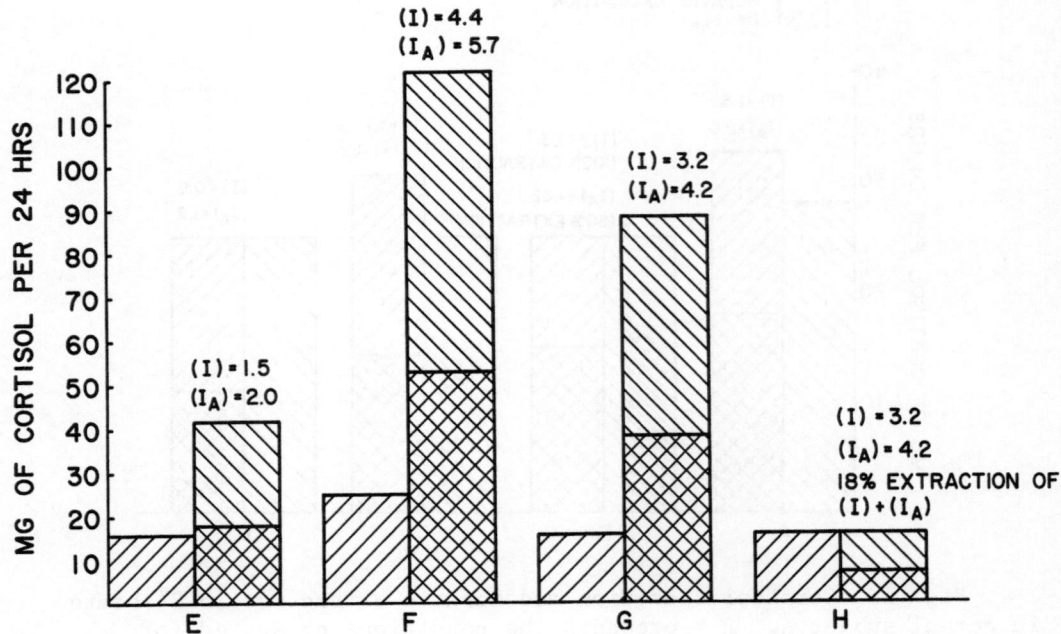

Fig. 2.　Cortisol secretion and hepatic extraction in 24 hours in estrogen-treated subjects.　In E are presented the derivations of Tait and Burstein (1964) based on the data of Peterson et al. (1960) for an estrogen-treated subject.　The calculation of Tait and Burstein (1964) arrived at (I) and (I$_A$) values in the estrogen-treated subject identical to those of normals.　Were (I) + (I$_A$) to be totally cleared in the liver, the amount of cortisol so cleared would greatly exceed the reduced cortisol secretion in this patient. In F, the data of Plager et al (1964) are similarly shown and here, too, the hepatic clearance would greatly exceed the cortisol secretion rate of 25 mg.　The latter value is rather high for estrogen-treated subjects.　The (I) and (I$_A$) values were obtained in our laboratory on a group of estrogen-treated subjects.　In G, it is shown that total extraction of even the (I) fraction would exceed the cortisol secretory rate.　Our adjusted values in H, based on 18% extraction (I) + (I$_A$) are compatible with the reduced clearance rate of cortisol by a factor of 4.5 (Tait and Burstein, 1964).

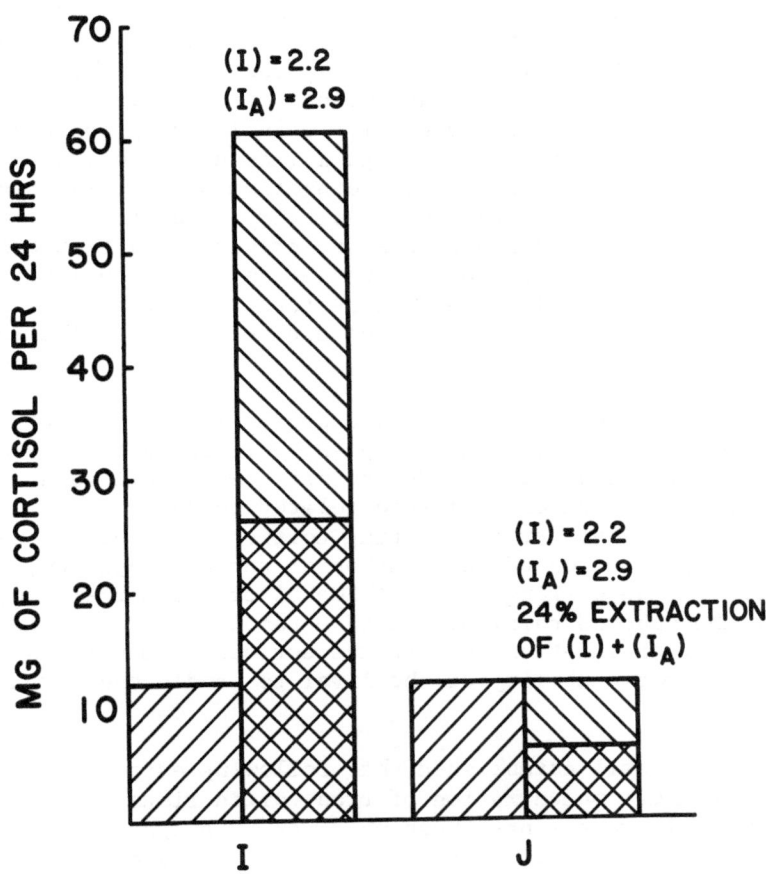

Fig. 3. Cortisol secretion and hepatic extraction in pregnancy
(third trimester). The secretory values are those of Migeon et al
(1963). The (I) and (I$_A$) values were obtained in our laboratory
(see Table 1). In I, it is shown, again, that total extraction of
the (I) + (I$_A$) compartments would greatly exceed the cortisol
secretory level. To match the latter only 24% extraction and
metabolism of (I) + (I$_A$) need occur. This and the preceding two
figures are adapted from Sandberg, Rosenthal and Slaunwhite (1966).

metabolized. It has been demonstrated that from 175 to 180 liters
of plasma are cleared of cortisol per day (Peterson, Nokes, Chen
and Black, 1960). Since the transcortin-cortisol complex cannot be
metabolized, it is apparent that the above figure for clearance is
artificial and we must look for more factual expression of the plasma clearance. It appears that 1200 liters of plasma pass through
the liver every 24 hours (for references, see Tait, Little, Tait
and Flood, 1962). Were all of the unbound cortisol to be cleared
from the plasma, this would account for only 13-18 mg of cortisol
metabolized by the liver per day (Fig. 1), assuming no extra-
hepatic metabolism of the steroid. Metabolism of the albumin-bound
cortisol would result in a cortisol secretory rate exceeding that
described. The various permutations are presented in Figure 1 and
the most likely explanation for the manner in which the liver
metabolizes cortisol would appear to be total extraction and metabolism of the unbound cortisol fraction and some of the albumin-
bound fraction.

The possibilities and the picture prevailing in subjects who
had received estrogens or during pregnancy are shown in Figures 2
and 3 and the accompanying legends go into some detail regarding
the most plausible metabolic picture related to the extraction and
metabolism by the liver or circulating cortisol. In either case,
i.e., following estrogen administration or during pregnancy, the
liver appears to be working at about 20-25% of its normal capacity
to extract the unbound cortisol and to metabolize the steroid. Thus,
the most likely explanation is that the estrogenic materials decrease the enzymatic ability of the liver to handle the circulating
cortisol.

It has been well established that following estrogen administration the plasma concentration of transcortin rises three to four
fold. Similar increases have been observed in pregnancy, though,
in general, the transcortin levels do not reach the height observed
following estrogen therapy. Recently, it has been demonstrated
that transcortin has a high affinity for progesterone and that this
steroid does, in fact, bind to transcortin to a significant extent
(Seal and Doe, 1966; Sandberg, Rosenthal, Schneider and Slaunwhite,
1966). The distribution of progesterone and cortisol among the
various circulating proteins are shown in Figures 4 to 9. Thus, it
is readily apparent that during pregnancy even though the levels
of transcortin rise considerably, resulting in increased binding of
cortisol and, thus, in an increased concentration of plasma cortisol,
and increased binding of progesterone as well, the proportion of each
steroid bound by the various protein fractions remains about the
same as in normal subjects. This maintenance of regularity in the
proportion of steroid bound to various protein indicates that the
elevated levels of transcortin are more than sufficient to accom-
modate the circulating cortisol and progesterone in pregnancy. Even

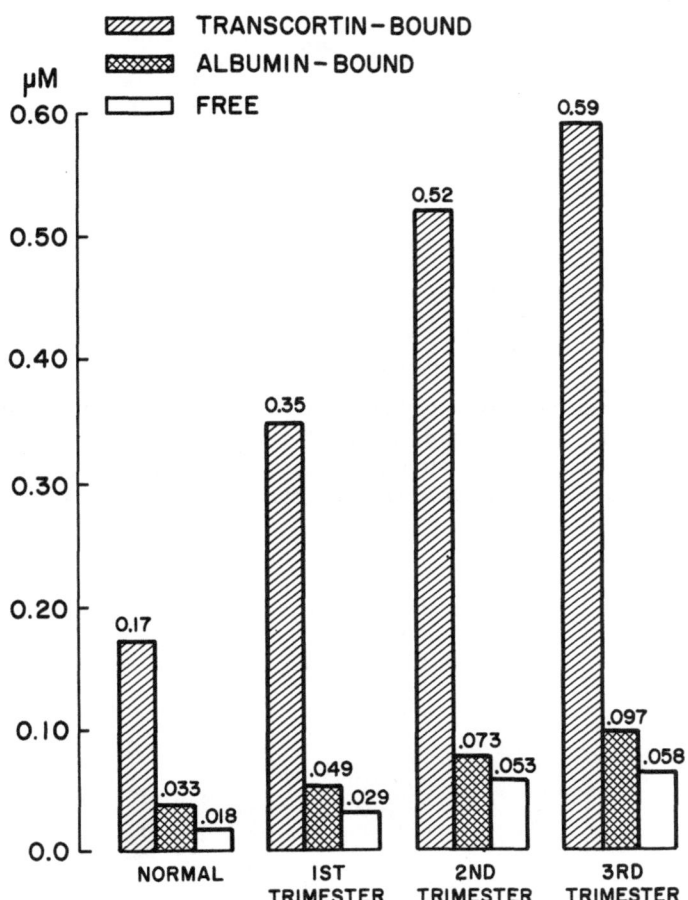

Fig. 4.   The distribution of cortisol in normal and pregnancy plasma. In normal women the preponderant amount of cortisol is transcortin-bound, with only a minor fraction being bound to albumin. About 10% of the total cortisol is unbound. The plasma cortisol concentration rises with progression of the pregnancy, reaching the highest level during the third trimester. With this rise, the amounts bound to transcortin increase, as do the albumin-bound and unbound fractions. This and the following five figures are from Rosenthal, Slaunwhite and Sandberg (1969).

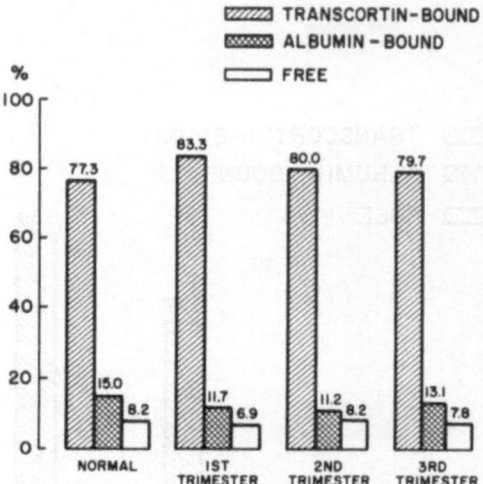

Fig. 5. Percentage of cortisol distribution among transcortin, human serum albumin (HSA), and unbound fractions in the plasma of normal women and during the three trimesters of pregnancy. In general, the ratio of cortisol found among these fractions appears to remain unchanged.

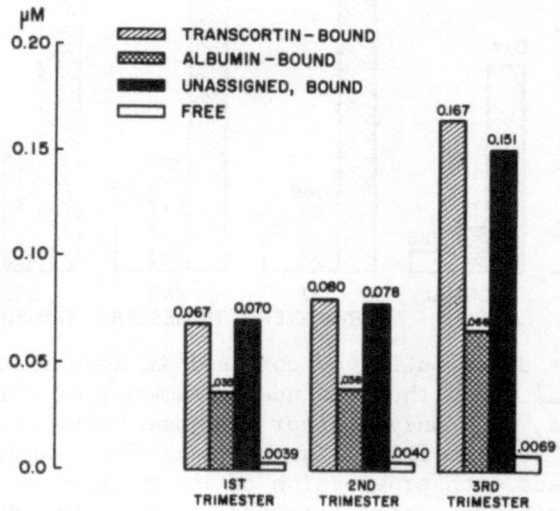

Fig. 6. The distribution of progesterone plasma during the three trimesters of pregnancy. Most of the progesterone is bound to transcortin and to a protein fraction whose nature is still unknown (called "unassigned" in the figures). Note that the amount of progesterone bound to albumin is much less than that to the two previously mentioned fractions. The unbound progesterone constitutes a very small part of the total progesterone, even in the third trimester of pregnancy.

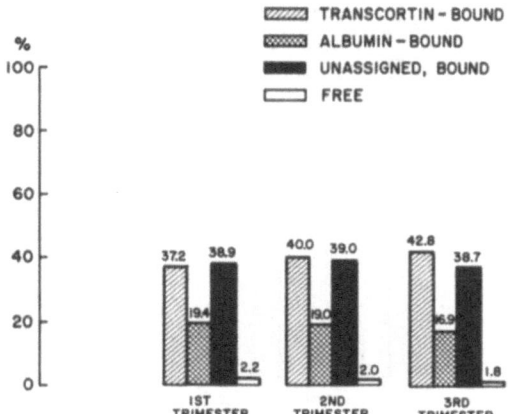

Fig. 7. The percentage of progesterone distributed among the various fractions in the plasma of pregnant women. Note that the percentage of progesterone bound by the various fractions remains essentially unchanged, even though the levels of progesterone increase with the advance of pregnancy. The percentage of progesterone unbound is much lower than that of cortisol.

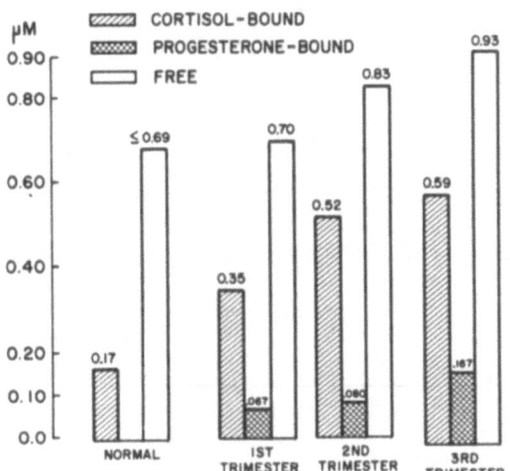

Fig. 8. The concentration of transcortin in the plasma of normal women and in the three trimesters of pregnancy. The total level of transcortin is markedly increased in the last trimester. Even though a substantial amount of transcortin is associated with cortisol, and to a lesser degree with progesterone, it can be seen that most of the transcortin appears to be available for binding (shown as "unbound") and explains why the ratio of distribution of cortisol and progesterone among various proteins remains essentially unchanged.

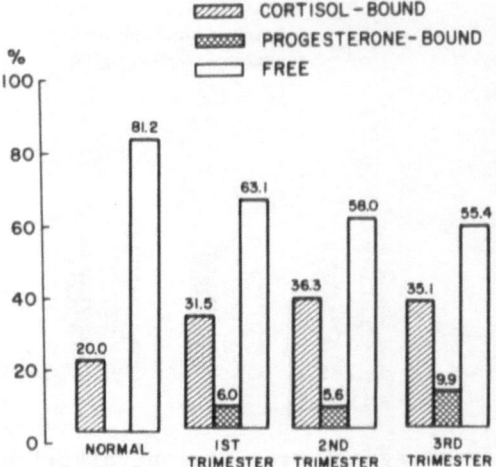

Fig. 9. The percentage of transcortin occupied by cortisol and progesterone and that "unbound" in normal women and in the three trimesters of pregnancy. Even though a higher percentage of the protein is occupied by cortisol and progesterone, resulting in lesser amounts of transcortin being available for binding with other substances, a substantial percentage of transcortin is still available for further binding.

Table 2

THE EFFECT OF PROGESTERONE ON THE VALUES OBTAINED BY

EQUILIBRIUM DIALYSIS FOR ENDOGENOUS CORTISOL LEVELS

Additions	Apparent µg% Cortisol found	Δ*
None	13	--
33.3 µg% cortisol	47	34
50 µg% progesterone	23	10
100 µg% progesterone	33	20
150 µg% progesterone	42	29
33.3 µg% cortisol 100 µg% progesterone } combined	70	57

*Increase in apparent µg% cortisol found over the value for endogenous cortisol.

Data taken from Rosenthal et al (1969).

though progesterone readily displaces cortisol from transcortin when
the protein is studied in the isolated state, the picture in the
plasma is more complicated (Table 2). It requires at least four to
five times as much progesterone in plasma to displace cortisol from
transcortin, this being due to the fact that the association constants of serum albumin and other proteins for progesterone are
relatively high and the binding systems have a high capacity for
this steroid. Thus, even in pregnancy it would appear that the
amount of cortisol displaced from transcortin by progesterone is
probably of a very small order of magnitude. Sight should not be
lost of the possibility, however, that some of the synthetic progestational agents may have a much higher affinity for transcortin than
progesterone, in which case they may play a more important role in
affecting the levels of unbound cortisol in the circulation than
does progesterone.

The administration of estrogenic compounds, including those
present in some of the contraceptive medications, results in elevated
levels of transcortin, leading to a definitely elevated level of unbound cortisol. In addition, progesterone and related compounds may
play some part in displacing cortisol from transcortin in plasma of
pregnant women and, thus, contribute to the elevation of the unbound
cortisol. The effects of elevated unbound cortisol levels on human
physiology, particularly when such levels are active over a very
prolonged period of time as may occur in patients receiving contraceptive therapy, is at present totally unknown. The question of the
effects of the elevated unbound cortisol levels on pituitary function and on other metabolic parameters remains at present unanswered.
When this is combined with the indications that estrogens definitely
decrease the ability of the liver to metabolize unbound cortisol,
the problem is compounded in our understanding of the significance
and the ultimate effects elevated unbound cortisol levels may have
in human subjects over prolonged periods of time.

REFERENCES

1. Peterson, R.E., Nokes, G., Chen, P.S., Jr. and Black, R.L.:
Estrogens and adrenocortical function in man. J. Clin. Endocr.
20: 495 (1960).

2. Plager, J.E., Schmidt, K.G. and Staubitz, W.J.: Increased
unbound cortisol in the plasma of estrogen-treated subjects. J.
Clin. Invest. 43: 1066 (1964).

3. Rosenthal, H.E., Slaunwhite, Jr., W.R. and Sandberg, A.A.:
Transcortin: A corticosteroid-binding protein of plasma. X. Cortisol and progesterone interplay and unbound levels of these steroids
in pregnancy. J. Clin. Endocr. (in press 1969).

4. Sandberg, A.A. and Slaunwhite, W.R., Jr.: Transcortin: A conticosteroid-binding protein of plasma. II. Levels in various conditions and the effects of estrogens. J. Clin. Invest. 38: 1290 (1959).

5. Sandberg, A.A., Rosenthal, H., Schneider, S.L. and Slaunwhite, W.R., Jr.: In Steroid Dynamics, (eds.) Pincus, G., Nakao, T. and Tait, J.F. Academic Press, New York. p. 9 (1966).

6. Seal, U.S. and Doe, R.P.: In Steroid Dynamics, (eds.) Pincus, G., Nakao, T. and Tait, J.F. Academic Press, New York. p. 63 (1966).

7. Slaunwhite, W.R., Jr. and Sandberg, A.A.: Transcortin: A corticosteroid-binding protein of plasma. J. Clin. Invest. 38: 384 (1959).

8. Tait, J.F. and Burstein, S.: In vivo studies of steroid dynamics in man. The Hormones, Academic Press, New York. Vol. 5 p. 441 (1964).

9. Tait, J.F., Little, B., Tait, S.A.S. and Flood, C.: The metabolic clearance rate of aldosterone in pregnant and nonpregnant subjects estimated by both single-injection and constant-infusion methods. J. Clin. Invest. 41: 2093 (1962).

RESPIRATION

RESPIRATION

EFFECTS OF GONADAL HORMONES AND CONTRACEPTIVE STEROIDS ON

RESPIRATION

M. Stein, A. Tarabeih, T. Yasutake and T. Hirose

Department of Biology and Medical Sciences, Brown
University and the Department of Medicine, Rhode Island
Hospital, Providence, Rhode Island

When the editors assigned me the task of reviewing the effects
of gonadal hormones and contraceptive steroids on the pulmonary
system, I replied that I was in somewhat of a quandry as to where
to begin. Their suggestion was merely that all biological literature be reviewed and any appropriate data pertaining to these
steroids and respiration be presented. Thus, my first reference
was found in Genesis (1) and describes a most dramatic effect of
estrogens on a portion of the pulmonary system of man (Fig. 1).
Thus far, no one has been able to reproduce that experiment.

Actually, a review of the effects of these steroids on the
pulmonary system is fairly simple as there have not been many
presentations in the literature. This report will be divided into
considerations of the effects of these chemicals (1) on the control of respiration, (2) on lung mechanics, (3) on gas transfer
(diffusion), and (4) on the lung parenchyma.

EFFECTS ON CONTROL OF RESPIRATION

Observations were made many years ago of an increase in ventilation during pregnancy (2) and the luteal phase of the menstrual
cycle (3-5). With both of these conditions the increase in alveolar

*Supported in part by United States Public Health Service
Research Grant HE 10017, a grant from the Rhode Island Heart
Association, and also supported by United States Public Health
Service Training Grant #1 T12 HE 5862-01. Figures 10-13 were made
available through the kindness of Dr. El-Heneidy, Department of
Medicine, University of Alexandria, Egypt.

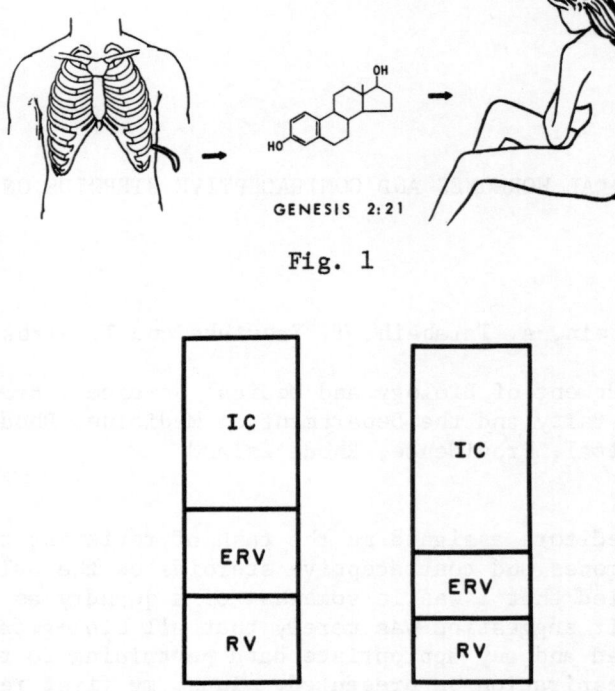

Fig. 1

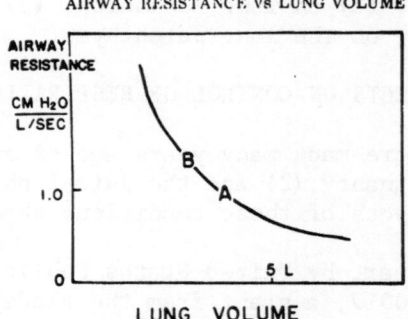

Fig. 2. Lung volumes in pregnant and non-pregnant women.
IC = inspiratory capacity, ERV = expiratory reserve volume, RV =
residual volume. ERV + RV = functional residual capacity (FRC).
IC + ERV + RV = total lung capacity (TLC). IC + ERV = vital
capacity. In pregnancy, FRC is decreased by approximately 25%,
although TLC remains near non-pregnant levels (9,10).

AIRWAY RESISTANCE vs LUNG VOLUME

AIRWAY
RESISTANCE

$\dfrac{CM\ H_2O}{L/SEC}$

1.0

B

A

5 L

0

LUNG VOLUME
PLEURAL PRESSURE

Fig. 3. Relationship among lung volume, pleural pressure
and lung flow resistance. A, lung volume and flow resistance
at higher lung volume. B, lung volume and flow resistance at
decreased lung volume.

ventilation is sufficient to produce considerable decreases in arterial PCO_2. More recently, enhanced alveolar ventilation has been described in male and female subjects following progesterone but not estrogens (6,7). The following paper in this volume by Dr. Lyons (8) considers in detail the effects of progesterone on ventilation.

EFFECTS ON LUNG MECHANICS

In physical terms, mechanics describes the effects of forces on a solid, liquid, or gaseous body at equilibrium or during motion of the body. The resistance to movement of gas during laminar flow in the airways can be described according to the Poiseuille Formulation*:

$$R_L = \frac{Pressure}{Flow} \qquad \frac{8 \ln}{\pi \, r^4}$$

where R = resistance of lung to air flow, pressure is the driving pressure utilized to overcome frictional forces in the airway, flow is the gas flow, I = length of tube, n = viscosity of gas and r = radius of the tube or airway.

Lung compliance describes the elastic characteristics of the lungs and is given by the slope C_L = dV/dP, C_L = lung compliance, dV = change in volume from the point of one equilibrium to another (e.g., the tidal volume) and dP = the concomitant pressure utilized to overcome elastic recoil properties of the lung. Lung compliance is affected by numerous factors including the lung volume at which it is measured, the number of functioning alveolar units, surface forces and the nature of the air-liquid interface.

A possible effect of gonadal hormones on lung mechanics has been indicated by observations made during pregnancy. It has been known for some time that the functional residual capacity (FRC) decreases during the latter half of pregnancy (Fig. 2) (9,10). When FRC decreases, the expected response is an increase in lung flow resistance (R_L). As shown in Figure 3, at smaller lung volumes, the recoil pressure which tends to distend intrapulmonary airways is less, the airway caliber decreases, and R_L increases. However, in the pregnant female, R_L decreases in the presence of a reduced FRC (11,12). Thus, near term R_L was reported as 0.9 cm. H_2O/L/sec. and shortly after delivery, values rose to 1.8 cm.H_2O/L/sec. (12).

However, evidence to attribute the reduction in R_L during pregnancy directly to sex hormones is lacking. Recently, Winter

_____

*The Poiseuille law applies to laminar flow in a rigid tube. Although the pulmonary airways are not rigid, the formulation can still be used.

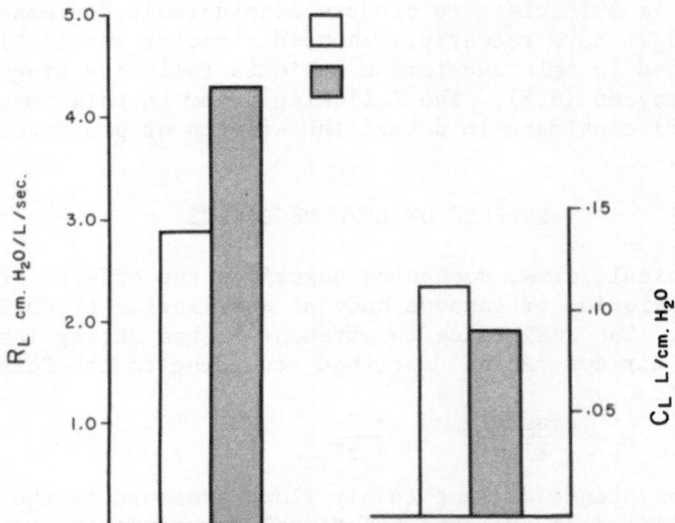

Fig. 4. R_L and C_L in animals treated with diethylstilbesterol, 1 mg/day for 25 days and in non-treated animals.

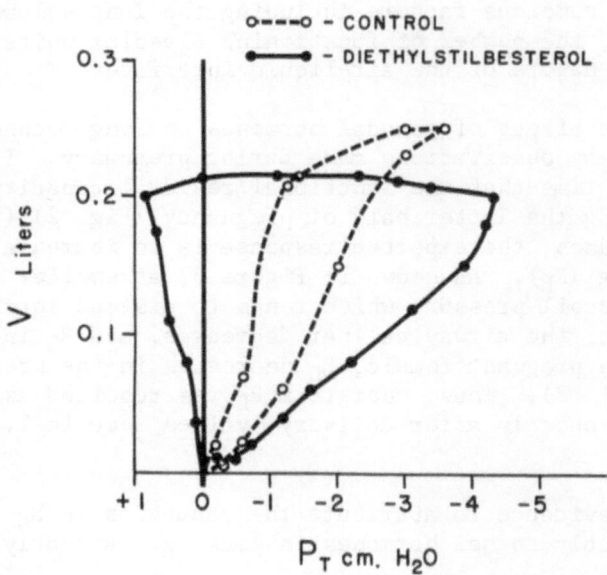

Fig. 5. Pressure-volume curves in control animal and animal treated with diethylstilbesterol for 25 days. Pressures are in reference to atmosphere.

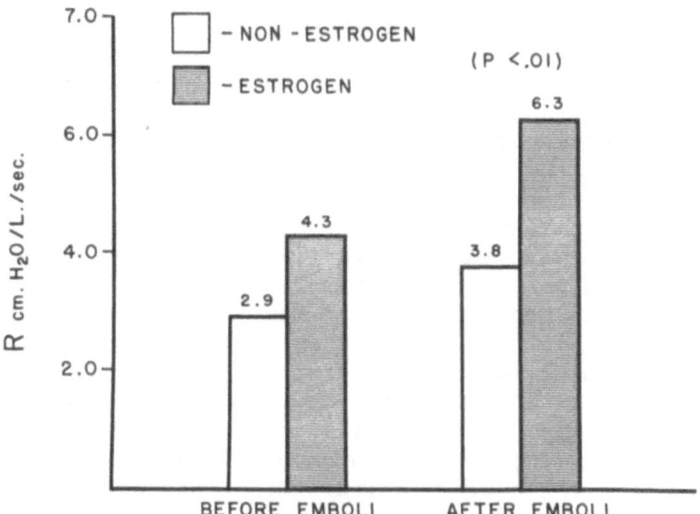

Fig. 6. Lung flow resistance before and after autologous
pulmonary thromboemboli in estrogen and non-estrogen treated dogs.
In both the treated and non-treated animals, there were significant
increases in flow resistance. However, following emboli the increments in the estrogen-treated animals were significantly larger.

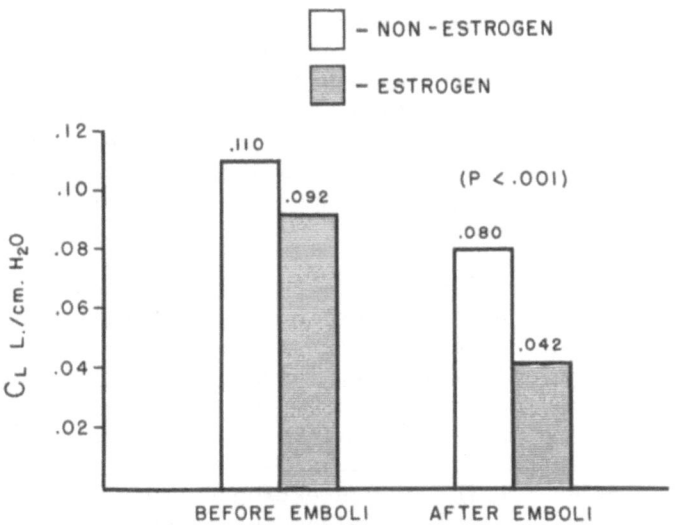

Fig. 7. Lung compliance changes before and after autologous
pulmonary thromboemboli in estrogen-treated and non-treated animals.
The post-embolic fall in C_L was greater in the treated animals.

and Sullivan (13), showed that a progestin (250 mg Delalutin), an estrogen (1 mg diethylstilbesterol) or a sequential combination (C-Quens) changes neither lung volume nor flow resistance in the non-pregnant female. However, the possibility exists that the changes in pregnancy were related to higher quantities of hormone during pregnancy, other hormones or metabolites.

Evidence can also be found to suggest that contraceptive steroids can produce an increase in flow resistance. Trethewie and Gaffney (14) demonstrated that animals treated with gonadal hormones (estrogen, progesterone and testosterone) had higher histamine contents in their lungs than controls. Histamine, of course, is a potent bronchoconstrictor. Possible data to support this latter concept has been obtained in our laboratory. Utilizing a model described by Wessler (15,16), we have studied the pulmonary physiologic responses to thromboembolism in the dog (17). Recently, we have explored the alterations induced by giving the animals estrogen prior to pulmonary embolism. A single intravenous dose of estrogen produced neither acute changes in lung mechanics nor differences in the ventilatory responses to embolism when compared to untreated animals. However, when male and female animals were given diethylstilbesterol, 1 mg/day for 25 days, the values of R_L were significantly higher than in untreated animals (Fig. 4). Since lung compliance in the two groups of animals were similar, bronchoconstriction in relatively large airways (proximal to the terminal bronchioles) was indicated. Figure 5 compares a pressure-volume curve of an animal treated with diethylstilbesterol to an untreated animal. In both examples, inspiration begins at resting lung volumes (zero volume and zero pressure) and proceeds counter clockwise. In the untreated animal, the pleural pressure is always negative becoming zero only at end expiration. However, in the animal treated with diethylstilbesterol, the pleural pressure became positive during expiration. Thus, the energy of elastic recoil of the lungs was not sufficient to empty the lungs during expiration and it was necessary for expiratory muscles to produce positive pleural pressure to overcome increased frictional forces following estrogen therapy.

When emboli were released from peripheral veins of the estrogen treated animals, the responses in lung mechanics were of some interest. Although the increases in respiratory rate were similar in the untreated animals following thromboemboli, the increases in flow resistance and decreases in lung compliance were significantly different (Figures 6 and 7). There is no clear explanation of these increased responses. Previously, we suggested that alterations in lung mechanics in the non-estrogen treated animal following thromboembolism are related to release of amines from platelets aggregated on the surface of the thromboembolism (Fig. 8) (18,19). Whether the enhanced response to pulmonary thromboembolism in estrogen treated animals is mediated through increased plaetlet

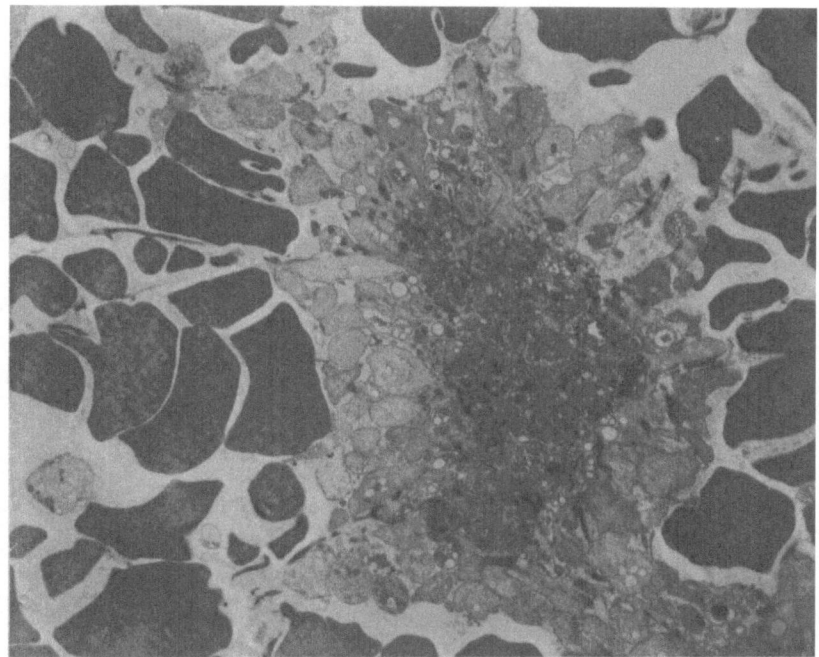

Fig. 8. Aggregation of platelets on surface of a thrombo-embolus removed from vena cava of dog. Many platelets have lost their dense osmiophilic staining granules believed to contain serotonin. (Reproduced with permission of Charles C. Thomas and Grune and Stratton).

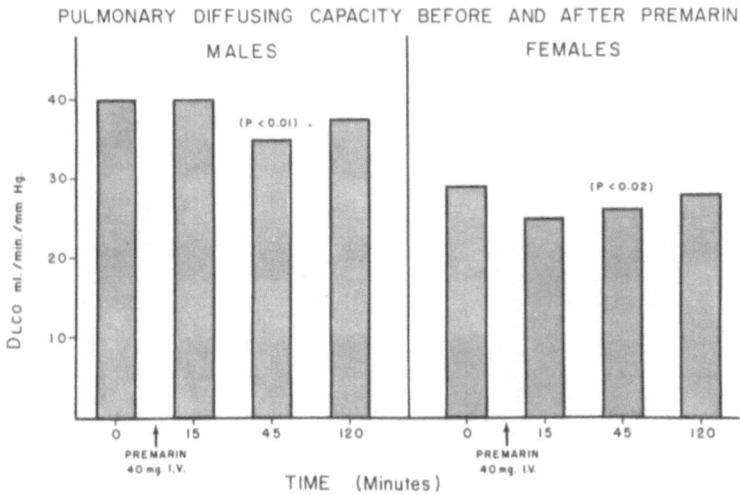

Fig. 9. Changes in $D_L CO$ after intravenous Premarin in male and female subjects.

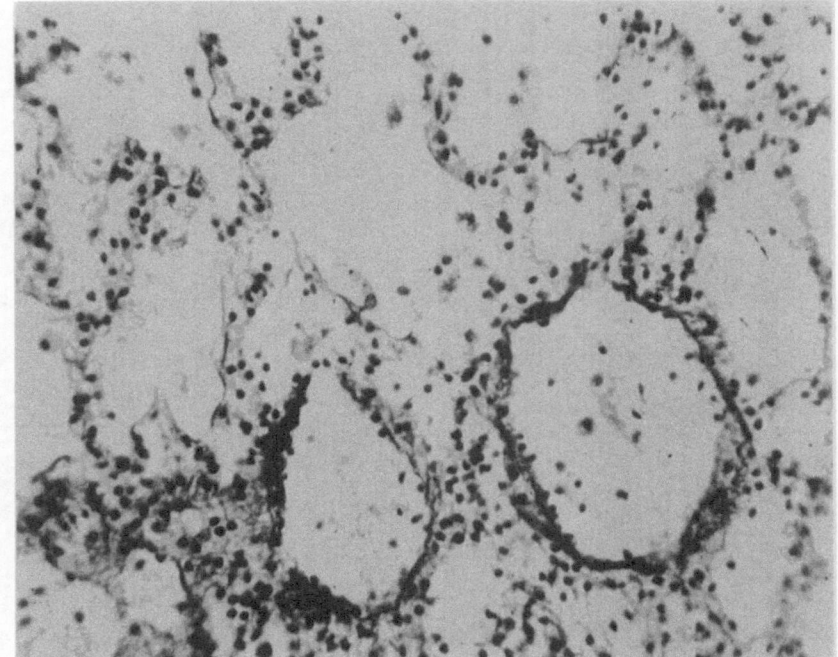

Fig. 10

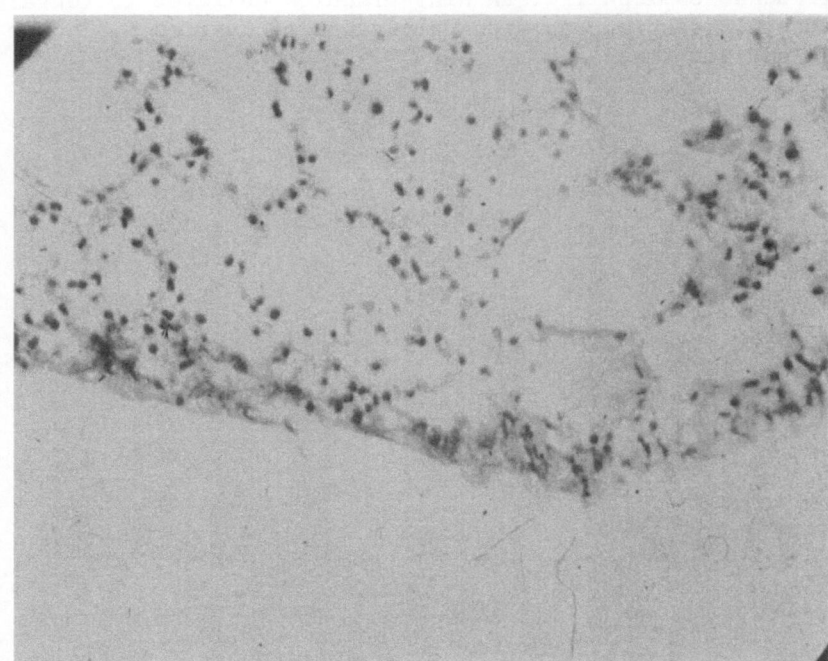

Fig. 11

aggregation, release of increased amounts of serotonin from dog platelets, sensitization of the airway or other mechanisms is unknown at the present time.

Further, although not well documented, observations of sensitization of the airway following gonadal hormones and/or contraceptive steroids and a possible role in asthma can be found in the literature (20-22).

EFFECTS ON GAS TRANSFER

The vital gases, oxygen and carbon dioxide, diffuse passively across the alveolar capillary membranes. Physiologically, carbon dioxide has such a high solubility and diffusivity that its transfer is rarely a matter of clinical concern. Measurement of the pulmonary diffusing capacity for oxygen is indirect and difficult to perform. The assay of pulmonary diffusing capacity is usually made using small concentrations of carbon monoxide. Forster et al (23) have devised a relatively simple single breath test using carbon monoxide to quantitate pulmonary diffusing capacity (D_LCO). Pecora, Putnam, and Baum (24) gave intravenous estrogens and diluent placebo to five female and eleven male volunteers. They then measured the single breath D_LCO at 15, 45, and 120 minutes after the estrogen infusion (Fig. 9). Small but significant decreases in D_LCO were observed in male and female subjects 45 minutes after intravenous premarin. At 120 minutes, the decreases were smaller and no longer significant. Although they had neither histological nor biochemical observations to explain their data, they speculated that the estrogens induced increases in mucopolysaccharides and the length of polymers around small blood vessels (25,26), thereby increasing the path length of diffusion.

EFFECT ON LUNG PARENCHYMA

Dr. El-Heneidy, the Faculty of Medicine, Alexandria Medical School, has kindly supplied his observations and slides of changes induced by estrogenic drugs on the lungs of animals. El-Heneidy, Helmy, and Michael (27) gave stilbesterol (1-5 mg) or ethinyl estradiol (10-125 mg) to guinea pigs. They observed progressive pulmonary lesions beginning with (a) an accumulation of macrophages in pulmonary capillaries, (b) migration of macrophages to the alveolar interstitium and alveolar spaces with pleural and interstitial reaction, and (c) diffuse interstitial pneumonitis. In Figure 10, after two weeks of therapy, mononuclear phagocytes have invaded the interstitial spaces especially around blood vessels. Alveolar walls appear to be thickened and some mononuclear cells have penetrated the alveolar spaces. Figure 11 shows the lung periphery four to six weeks after estrogen therapy. The

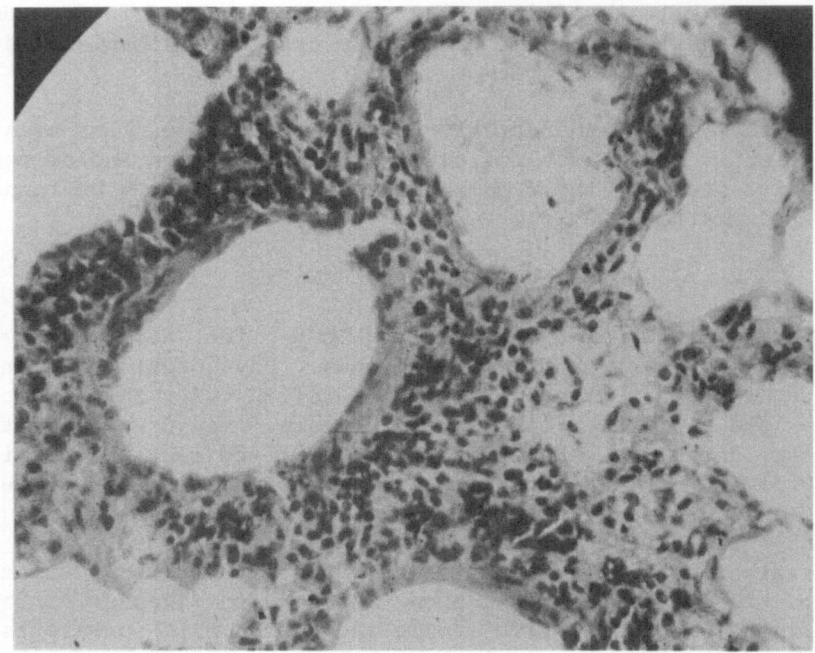

Fig. 12

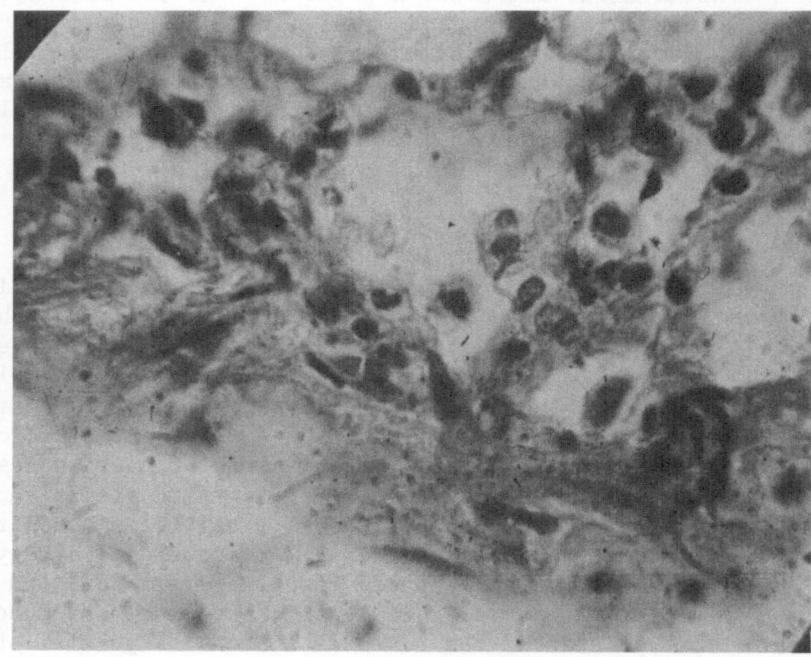

Fig. 13

pleura is hypertrophic and there is fibrosis. After two months (Fig. 12), there is definite fibrosis of the pleura and interstitial lung tissues. Figure 13 reveals observations made in an animal treated with 5 mg stilbesterol daily for three months. There are empty cystic air spaces and diffuse interstitial fibrosis.

An effect on the airways was also demonstrated in their experiments. Guinea pigs treated with stilbesterol, 5 mg/day, for three months showed goblet cell hypertrophy of the bronchi. This could account for the increases in flow resistance that we observed if similar changes occurred in the estrogen treated dog.

SUMMARY

Most of the data presented here, including those from our own laboratory, are unconfirmed. Investigations concerning the effects of gonadal hormones and contraceptive steroids on lung structure and function have been few in number. Nevertheless, it is apparent that certain progestins can alter the systems that control the minute volume of gas moving in and out of the alveoli. Estrogens given to animals in large dosage can produce histologic alterations in lung airways and parenchyma as well as functional changes. Additional data are required to determine the role of these substances in various pulmonary diseases (e.g., chronic bronchitis, emphysema, pulmonary fibrosis) and their relationships to the pulmonary responses to diseases such as asthma and pulmonary embolism.

REFERENCES

1. Genesis: 2: 21

2. Hasselbalch, K.A., and Gammeltoft, S.A.: Die Neutralitaetregulation des graviden Organisms. Biochem. Ztchr. 68: 206 (1915).

3. Heerharber, I., Loeschcke, H.H., and Westphal, U.: Eine Wirkung des Progesterons auf die Atmung. Arch. f. d. ges. Physiol. 250:42-55 (1948).

4. Bokelmann, O., u. I Rother: Z. Geburtsh. Gynak. 87: 584 (1924).

5. Wilbrand, U., Porath, C.H., Matthies, P., and Jaster, R.: Der Einfluss der Ovarialsteroid auf die Funktion des Atemzentrum. Arch. fur gynkologie. 191:507-531 (1959).

6. Tyler, J.M.: The effect of progesterone on the respiration of patients with emphysema and hypercarbia. J. Clin. Invest. 39:34-41 (1960).

7. Lyons, H.A., and Huang, C.T.: Therapeutic use of pro-gesterone in alveolar hypoventilation associated with obesity. Am. J. Med. 44:881-888 (1968).

8. Lyons, H.A.: Ventilatory responses to progesterone. (this volume)

9. Cugell, W.D., Frank, N.R., Gaensler, E.A., and Badger, T.L.: Pulmonary function in pregnancy. Am. Rev. Tuberc. 67: 568-597 (1953).

10. Novy, M.J., and Edwards, M.J.: Respiratory problems in pregnancy. Am. J. Obs. and Gyn. 99:1024-1045 (1967).

11. Rubin, A.M.D., Russo, N., and Gaucher, D.: The effect of pregnancy on pulmonary functions in normal women. Am. J. Obs. and Gyn. 72:963-969 (1956).

12. Gee, J.B.L., Packer, B.S., Miller, J.E. and Robin, E.D.: Pulmonary mechanics during pregnancy. J. Clin. Invest. 16:945-952 (1967).

13. Winter, L.W., and Sullivan, K.N.: The role of the dia-phragm and hormones in changing pulmonary functions during preg-nancy. Clin. Res. 16:474 (1964).

14. Trethewie, E.R., and Gaffney, F.M.: Influence of gonado-trophic hormones on the histamine content of and ease of release of histamine by trypsin from guinea pig lung. Austral. J. Exp. Biol. and M. Sc. 27:867-868 (1949).

15. Wessler, S., Freiman, D.G., Ballon, J.D., Katz, J.H., Wolff, R., and Wolf, E.: Experimental pulmonary embolism with serum-induced thrombi. Am. J. Pathol. 38:89-100 (1961).

16. Wessler, S. and Thye Yin, E.: Hypercoagulability. (this volume).

17. Stein, M. and Thomas, D.P.: Role of platelets in the acute pulmonary responses to endotoxin. J. Appl. Physiol. 23: 47-51 (1967).

18. Thomas, D.P., Gurewich, V., and Ashford, T.P.: Platelet adherence to thromboemboli in relation to the pathogenesis and treatment of pulmonary embolism. New Eng. J. Med. 274:953-956 (1966).

19. Stein, M., Hirose, T., Yasutake, T., and Khan, M.A.: The effects of platelet amines on airway function. in Conference on Airway Dynamics, A. Bouhuys, editor, Charles C. Thomas, Chicago, Illinois, In Press.

20. Horan, J.D. and Ledeman, J.J.: Possible asthmogenic effect of oral contraceptives. Correspondence. Canad. Med. Ass. J. 99:130-131 (1968).

21. Mears, E.: Letter to the editor. Lancet i:981 (1964).

22. Chen, C.Y.: Clinical studies in bronchial asthma. The influence of the gonadal hormones on asthma in the female. J. Formosa Med. Ass. 61:766-773 (1962).

23. Ogilvie, C.M., Forster, R.E., Blakemore, W.S., and Morton, J.W.: A standardized breath holding technique for the clinical measurement of the diffusing capacity of the lung for carbon monoxide. J. Clin. Invest. 36:1-17 (1957).

24. Pecora, L.J., Putnam, L.R., and Baum, G.L.: Effects of intravenous estrogens on pulmonary diffusing capacity. Am. J. Med. Sci. 246:48-52 (1963).

25. Wayne, L., Coots, M., Glueck, H.I., Baum, G., Pecora, L., and Putnam, L.: The effect of intravenous estrogen on tissues and capillaries as measured by coagulation tests, intradermal hyaluronidase, hyaluronidase serum inhibitor and pulmonary diffusion studies. J. Lab. and Clin. Invest. 58:970 (1961).

26. Schiff, M. and Burn, H.F.: The effect of intravenous estrogen on ground substance. Arch. Otolaryng. 73:43-51 (1961).

27. El-Heneidy, A.R., Helmy, I.D., and Michael, M.A.: Experimental diffuse interstitial fibrosis of the lungs and capillary cellular trapping. Alex. Med. J. 12:275-307 (1966).

RESPIRATORY EFFECTS OF GONADAL HORMONES

H. A. Lyons

Cardiopulmonary Section, Department of Medicine, State
University of New York Downstate Medical Center

Most knowledge of respiratory changes due to hormones has been
gained from studies which were made years ago. Even that knowledge
is limited and incomplete. In fact, modern models of the control
of respiration do not include or consider the role of hormones (1,
2).

This review will attempt to discuss previous observations and
present our own studies made with progesterone. The review will
be restricted to the gonadal hormones.

OVARIAN HORMONES

The observation of hyperventilation occurring during pregnancy
suggested a hormonal factor. This hyperventilation was observed
by Hasselbalch and Gammeltoft to be associated with a decrease in
alveolar carbon dioxide tension (P_ACO_2) (3). A lowered P_ACO_2 was
observed not only during pregnancy but also during the luteal phase
of the menstrual cycle (3,4). The fall of P_ACO_2 during the luteal
phase observed among women in our studies average 8.2 mm. Hg (5,7).
Griffith and his associates (6), and Bokelmann with Rother (7)
showed that the cyclic variation of the P_ACO_2 disappeared with the
menopause. These several observations suggested a relation between
the endocrine changes of pregnancy and menstruation. Subsequent
workers attempted to associate these respiratory changes with
specific hormones (8-14).

Supported by United States Public Health Service Training
Grant # 1 T12 HE 5862-01.

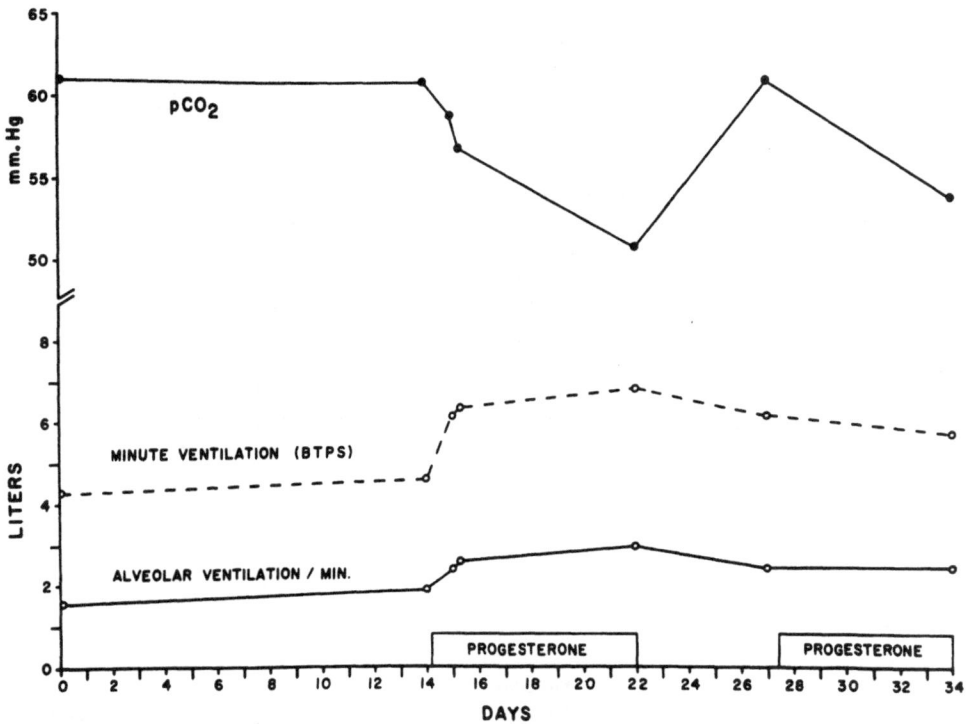

Fig. 1. The change in minute and alveolar ventilation and lowering of alveolar carbon dioxide tension resulting from the administration of progesterone is shown.

The common factor considered was the secretion from the corpora lutea of pregnancy and from the corpora lutea of the menstrual cycle for producing the changes of the alveolar carbon dioxide tension; progesterone seemed to be the responsible agent.

The effect of progesterone on respiration has been extensively studied. That progesterone is a respiratory stimulant has been generally accepted. The effects of progesterone on respiration has been studied in women during pregnancy, in postmenopausal women and in normal men (8-10, 13, 17) (Fig. 1). The maximal response after the administration of progesterone follows within three to twenty-four hours (7, 14). Stimulation to respiration after the administration of progesterone has been observed in emphysematous patients and patients with carbon dioxide retention (16, 17, 20). Lyons and Antonio demonstrated an increased response of ventilation to inhalation of carbon dioxide in pregnant women and in normal men, the latter after the administration of progesterone (15) (Fig. 2). Doring, Loeschke and Ochwaldt observed the response was enhanced and prolonged by the simultaneous administration of estrogen with progesterone (9). Willbrand considered that this

altered response indicated that the threshold to carbon dioxide
was reduced by progesterone and that the sensitivity of the respiratory center was increased by estrogen (19). The response
of ventilation appears to be additive when these two female
hormones are administered.

     Estrogens have a catabolic action and raise the metabolic rate
and so may directly affect ventilation in this way (12). Although
no strong evidence has been advanced to show that progesterone
produces any effect on metabolism, Goodland and his associates
thought that progesterone raises the metabolic rate (10). If this
were confirmed, then the respiratory effect due to progesterone
could be explained on this basis. On the other hand, the similarity of the observations of ventilation during the luteal phase of
the menstrual cycle, during pregnancy and after the administration
of progesterone strongly suggests that progesterone is the responsible agent in producing these responses.

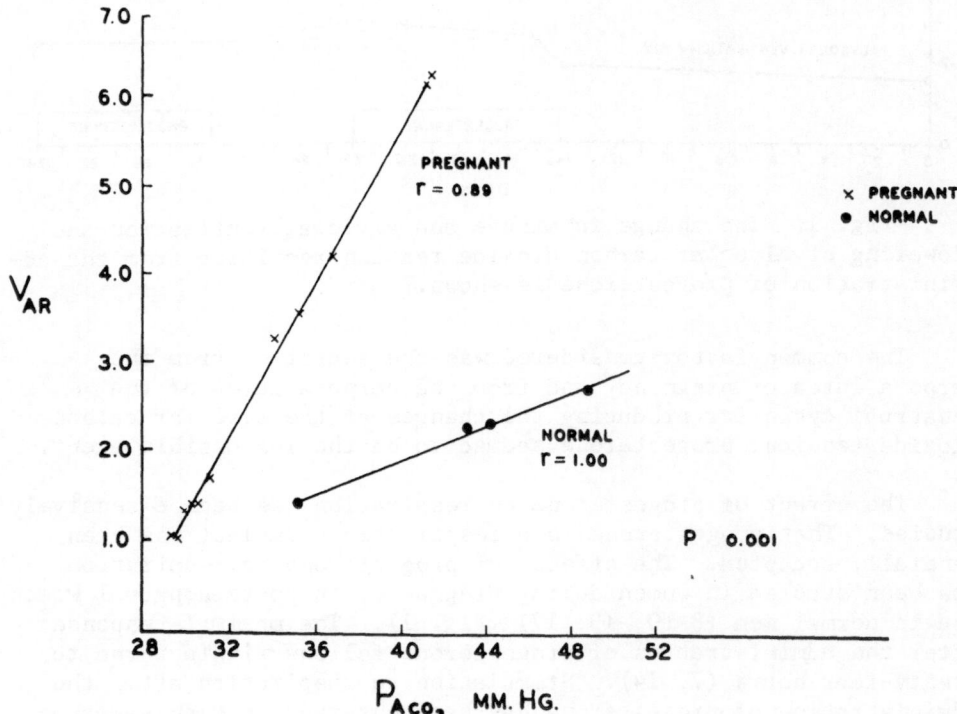

Fig. 2. The stimulus response to carbon dioxide expressed as
the alveolar ventilation ratio related to the alveolar carbon
dioxide tension for normal and pregnant subjects. The slope of the
curve determines the sensitivity of the respiratory center to the
stimulus. A similar response was observed in normal men after the
administration of progesterone (not shown) (after Lyons and Antonio
(15))--reproduced with permission.

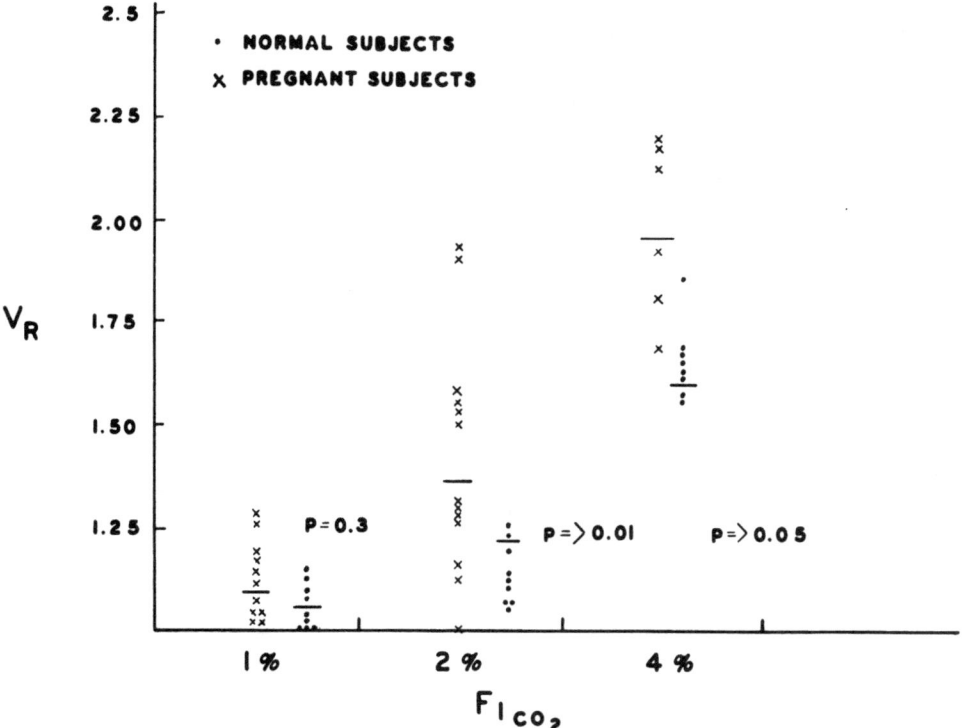

Fig. 3. Scattergram of the ventilatory response related to the concentration of inspired carbon dioxide for normal and pregnant subjects. The horizontal lines represent the mean values.

The alteration of the carbon dioxide sensitivity resulting from the administration of progesterone and pregnancy is shown by the shift of the response curves to the left and a steeper slope. The changes in alveolar carbon dioxide tensions found during the luteal phase of the menstrual cycle also are associated with an increase in the sensitivity to the breathing of carbon dioxide (8). The threshold of the respiratory center is lowered and the ventilatory response exhibits an increased steepness of the slope just as in pregnancy. Normally, minute ventilation increases 1.5 to 2.0 liters per minute per mm. mercury rise of alveolar carbon dioxide tension. Lyons and Antonio observed a 6 liter increase in ventilation for each mm. mercury rise in alveolar carbon dioxide tension for pregnancy (15) (Fig. 3). When progesterone is administered to nonpregnant women and men, an increased respiratory response to the inhalation of carbon dioxide is observed, similar to that of pregnancy (8, 9, 15, 19). The threshold to the stimulation of ventilation occurs at lower alveolar levels (25.7 to 32.5 mm. Hg) (Table 1).

TABLE 1

RELATION OF VE/M^2 AND PaCO$_2$ ON SIX PATIENTS

AFTER PROGESTERONE AND BICARBONATE

Direction of Changes	VE/M^2						PaCO$_2$ mm. Hg.					
	Before NaHCO$_3$			After NaHCO$_3$			Before NaHCO$_3$			After NaHCO$_3$		
	Rm.Air	4%CO$_2$	6%	Rm.Air	4%CO$_2$	6%	Rm.Air	4%CO$_2$	6%	Rm.Air	4%CO$_2$	6%
Mean Value Before Progesterone	5.31	10.32	17.94	4.41	9.47	16.25	40.80	44.48	52.17	42.40	47.18	53.72
Mean Value After Progesterone	7.28	13.39	23.39	7.79	11.98	21.14	29.88	37.40	47.47	33.65	43.08	47.75
Average increase L/min/m^2	1.97	3.07	5.45	3.38	2.51	4.89	10.92	7.08	4.70	8.75	4.10	5.97

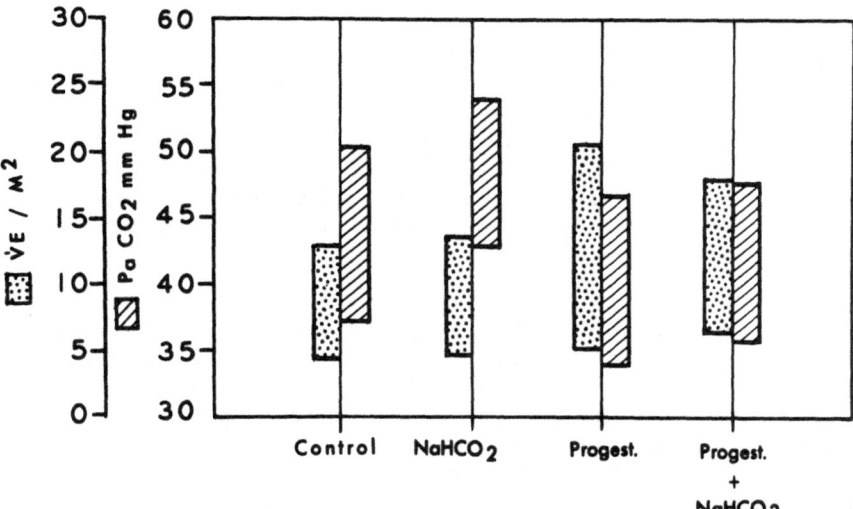

Fig. 4. The changes in ventilation and arterial carbon dioxide tension in four subjects following the administration of bicarbonate, progesterone or progesterone and bicarbonate together.

Progesterone is able to overcome the depressed ventilatory response produced by induced metabolic alkalosis both in humans and in experimental dogs (Fig. 4). Progesterone has been found useful in the obesity hypoventilation syndrome and emphysema by restoring alveolar hypoventilation to normal (16, 17).

Attempts to explain the mode of action of progesterone have been made. No demonstrable increase in the basal metabolic rate has been observed as a result of administration of progesterone. This lack of metabolic change was not present with hormones testosterone, corticosteroids, estradiol, or gonadotrophic hormones (8). A slight elevation of temperature has been observed after the administration of progesterone, but this elevation of temperature has never exceeded 0.5° F. in our studies (17) and failed to explain the level of respiratory response. Doring and his associates were unable to register hyperventilation to any febrile response after using pyrogens (9).

The way progesterone acts upon the respiratory center remains unexplained. Perkins stated: "progesterone and estrogens are involved in some mysterious way, possibly by modifying the permeability of the membrane of the chemoreceptor cell" (17). The most reasonable explanation is that the hormonal stimulation of respiration causes a drop in alveolar pCO_2 with a transient alkalosis. Then compensation takes place by a lowering of the plasma bicarbonate level and restoring pH to normal level. The observation

of Plass and Oberst that in pregnancy the total acid and the total
base are lowered approximately 5.0 mEq./l is consistent with this
probability (14).   Tyler observed that synthetic progestional compounds, ethinyl-testosterone, 19-norethinyl-testosterone, and
1,2-dehydroprogesterone failed to produce the lowering of alveolar
carbon dioxide tension (20) (Fig. 5). He suggested that the
ethinyl group prevents the respiratory action, even though these
compounds have strong progestional activity on the uterine endometrium.

The probability exists that progesterone acts at the cellular
level of the respiratory center. Doring suggested a central action,
but offered no proof. In studies made in our laboratory, we were
unable to demonstrate any changes of the cerebrospinal fluid to
indicate a site of action (21). Whatever the mode of action of
these hormones, the effects on respiration in the latter half of the
menstrual cycle, in pregnancy and after progesterone administration
are the same.

EFFECT OF PROGESTERONE ON RESPIRATION IN EMPHYSEMA

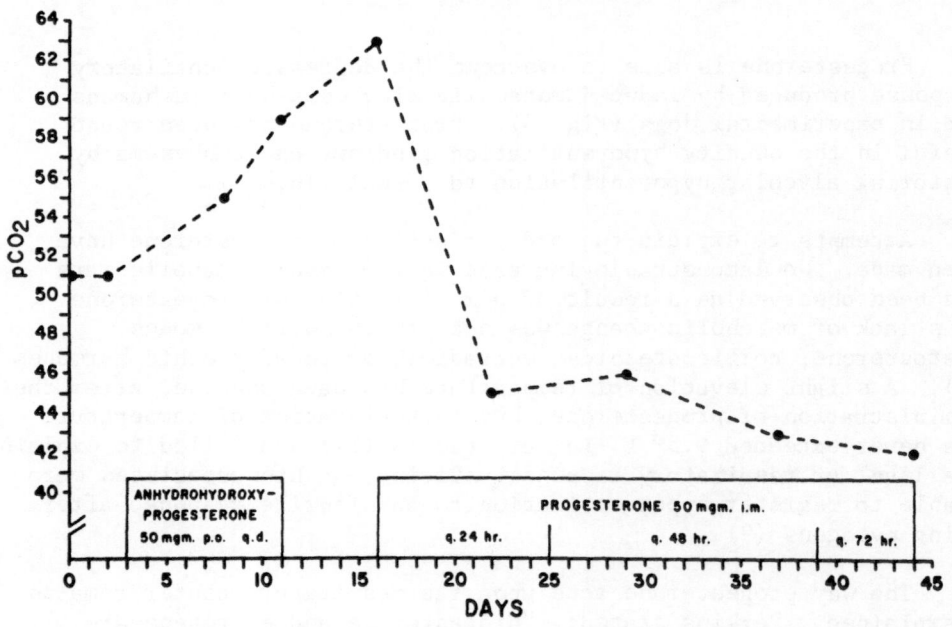

Fig. 5. The change in carbon dioxide tension after the administration of a synthetic progestional compound (ethinyl-testosterone) is elevated unlike the marked decrease following the
administration of progesterone. The presence of the ethinyl group
has been considered responsible for the lack of the respiratory
response. (After Tyler, J.M. (20))--reproduced with permission of
the Journal of Clinical Investigation.

SUMMARY

The administration of progesterone lowers alveolar carbon dioxide tensions and is probably responsible for the same effect during pregnancy and the luteal phase of the menstrual cycle. The hormone increases minute ventilation and increases the sensitivity of the respiratory center to carbon dioxide.

Progestional agents which have an ethinyl group fail to show a similar effect on respiration. It appears that the presence of the ethinyl group in the molecule prevents the respiratory effect.

The mode of action of progesterone on ventilation remains unexplained.

Estrogens affect ventilation by raising the metabolic rate and, when given simultaneously with progesterone, increase the ventilatory response to carbon dioxide.

REFERENCES

1. Grodins, F.S.: Control Theory and Biological Systems. Columbia University Press, New York, New York, 1963.

2. Milhorn, H.T.: The Application of Control Theory to Physiological Systems. W. B. Saunders Co., Philadelphia, Pa., 1966.

3. Hasselbalch, K.A.: Ein Beitrag zur Respirationsphysiologia der Graviditat. Scandanav. Arch. Physiol. 22: 1, 1912.

4. Hasselbalch, K.A. and Gammeltoft, S.A.: Die Neuralitatsiegulatren des gravidesn organismus. Biochem. Z. 68: 206, 1915.

5. Lyons, H.A. and Robeson, A. Unpublished observations.

6. Griffith, F.R., Jr., Pacher, G.W., Brownele, K.A., Klein, J. and Cainer, M.E.: Studies in human physiology, alveolar air and blood gas capacity. Amer. J. Physiol. 89: 449, 1929.

7. Bohelmann, O. and Rother, J.: Problem der extragenitalen Wellenbervegung im Leben des Weibes. Z. geburtsh gynak 87: 584, 1924.

8. Heerhaber, I., Loeschcke, H.H. and Westphal, V.: Eine Wirkung des Progesterons auf die atmung. Arch. ges Physiol. 250: 42, 1948.

9. Doring, G.K., Loeschcke, H.H. and Ochwaldt, B.: Weitere Untersuchungen uber die Wirkung der Sexual hormone auf die Atmung. Arch. ges Physiol. 252: 216, 1950.

10. Goodland, R.L., Reynolds, J.G., McCoord, A.B. and Pommerenke, W.J.: Respiratory and electrolyte effects induced by estrogen and progesterone. Fertil. Steril. 4: 300, 1953.

11. Landau, R.L., Bergenstal, D.M., Lugibihl, K. and Kascht, M.E.: The metabolic effects of progesterone in man. J. Clin. Endocr. 15: 1194, 1955.

12. Hagerman, D.D. and Villee, C.A.: Metabolic studies of the mechanism of action of estrogens. Recent Progress in the Endocrinology of Reproduction, edited by C. W. Lloyd, New York, Academic Press, p. 317, 1959.

13. Kydd, D.M.: Hydrogen ion concentration and acid-base equilibrium in normal pregnancy. J. Biol. Chem. 91: 63, 1931.

14. Plass, E.D. and Oberst, F.W.: Respiration and pulmonary ventilation in normal non-pregnant, pregnant and puerperal women (With interpretation of the acid base balance). Amer. J. Obstet. Gynec. 35: 44, 1938.

15. Lyons, H.A., and Antonio, R.: The sensitivity of the respiratory center in pregnancy and after the administration of progesterone. Trans. Ass. Amer. Phys. 72: 173, 1959.

16. Cullen, J.H., Brum, V.C. and Reidt, W.V.: The respiratory effects of progesterone in severe pulmonary emphysema. Amer. J. Med. 27: 551, 1959.

17. Lyons, H.A. and Huang, C.T.: Therapeutic use of progesterone in alveolar hypoventilation associated with obesity. Amer. J. Med. 44:881-888, 1968.

18. Perkins, J.F.: Arterial CO_2 and hydrogen ion as independent additive respiratory stimuli: Support for one portion of the Gray Multiple Factor Theory. In the Regulation of Human Respiration, edited by Cummingham, O.J.C. and Lloyd, B.B., Blackwell Scientific Publications, Oxford, England, 1963.

19. Wilbrand, V., Porath, C.H., Matthaes, P. and Jaster, R.: Der Einfluss der Ovarialsteroide auf die Funktion des Atemuzentrum. Arch. Gynek 191: 507, 1959.

20. Tyler, J.M.: The effects of progesterone on patients with emphysema and hypercapnia. J. Clin. Invest. 38: 38, 1960.

21. Huang, C.T. and Lyons, H.A.: Ventilatory effects of progesterone in acute metabolic acidosis and alkalosis with reference to the changes in CSF. The Physiologist 9: 207, 1966.

HYPERTENSION AND ELECTROLYTES

ORAL CONTRACEPTIVES AND HIGH BLOOD PRESSURE: CHANGES IN PLASMA

RENIN, RENIN SUBSTRATE AND ALDOSTERONE EXCRETION

J.H. Laragh, M.A. Newton, J.E. Sealey and
J.G.G. Ledingham

Department of Medicine, Columbia University, College of
Physicians and Surgeons, and the Presbyterian Hospital
in the City of New York

In this communication I will review for you studies, stimulated
by clinical observations in certain of our hypertensive patients,
which first suggested the possibility of a cause and effect relationship between the use of oral contraceptives and either the
development or enhancement of high blood pressure.

At the outset, it should be emphasized that because of the
widespread use of these medications, we believe that in the large
majority of women who take them, they do not induce hypertension.
However, observations that we have made in 11 selected hypertensive
patients suggest that in special circumstances these hormonal
agents may become critically involved in the production of hypertensive disease. A preliminary report of these findings has been
published (1).

When our clinical observations first suggested this relationship, it was decided to investigate concurrently the effects of
these female hormonal substances on electrolyte metabolism and on
the behavior of the renin-angiotensin-aldosterone hormonal interaction. This seemed appropriate because of the known relationship
of this hormonal system to other forms of hypertensive disease and
because previous work (Table 1) had indicated that estrogens and
progestogens can significantly affect various components of this
renal-adrenal hormonal system (1-9).

This work was supported by grants HE-01275 and HE-05741 from
the National Institutes of Health, U.S. Public Health Service.

TABLE 1

ORAL CONTRACEPTIVES, HYPERTENSION AND ABNORMALITIES
IN THE RENIN ANGIOTENSIN ALDOSTERONE HORMONAL INTERACTION

Elevated Levels	Agent	Authors
1. Plasma Angiotensinogen	Estrogen	Helmer and Griffith, 1952[2]
2. Aldosterone Secretion	Progestogen, Estrogen	Layne et al, 1962[3]
3. Plasma Renin	Pregnancy	Brown et al, 1963[5] Winer 1965[6] Genest et al, 1965[7]
4. Plasma Renin	Estrogen (large doses)	Crane et al, 1966[8]
5. Blood Pressure	Oral Contraceptives	Laragh et al, 1967[1] Woods 1967
6. Plasma Reactivity to Renin	Oral Contraceptives	Laragh et al, 1967[1]

TABLE 2

ORAL CONTRACEPTIVES AND HIGH BLOOD PRESSURE

Eleven Patients Presenting with Hypertension

1. Six normotensive prior to medication

2. Five hypertensive known prior to medication
    2, - hypertension augmented
    3, - hypertension unchanged

3. Nine medication withdrawn
    3, - normalized blood pressure
    3, - improved
    3, - unchanged

4. Reappearance of hypertension with restoration of
    treatment in each of two.

5. Marked consistent elevation of angiotensinogen with
    increased plasma reactivity to renin.

6. Less consistent or persistent increases in plasma
    renin levels and aldosterone secretion.

METHODS AND MATERIALS

Eleven women with high blood pressure have been studied.
Using previously defined criteria (10), we classified eight as
having uncomplicated benign "essential" hypertension, two as renal
hypertension and one as advanced hypertension. Most of the
patients were observed in the out-patient department, but three
were admitted to the metabolism ward and studied under conditions
of controlled electrolyte balance. In addition, the effects of
oral contraceptives were evaluated further in metabolism ward
studies of two normal volunteers and a male subject with uncomplicated essential hypertension.

Aldosterone secretion and excretion rates were measured by a
double isotope dilution technic previously described (10,11).
Blood samples for estimation of renin were taken at noon, when the
patients had been ambulatory for about four hours. Renin activity,
renin substrate concentration and the rate of angiotensin formation
in response to a fixed amount of exogenous renin were all measured
by a modification of the method of Pickens et al (12). In our
modification each incubation is carried out for 16 and 24 hours in
isotonic salt in the presence of EDTA and DFP. For studies designed to evaluate the capacity for angiotensin formation in a
given plasma, a fixed amount of exogenous renin was added to the
sample. In the earlier studies, a final concentration of .0034
Goldblatt units/ml. of renin was employed in a four-hour aqueous
incubation (1). In more recent studies (Fig. 6), .0017 Goldblatt
units/ml was employed with a one-hour incubation in saline.
Highly purified angiotensinase-free renin was prepared from human
kidneys according to the method of Haas et al (13).

RESULTS

A summary, in grosso modo, of our previously reported observations (1) associating oral contraceptive therapy with changes in
arterial blood pressure and with changes in the renin-angiotensin-
aldosterone system is presented in Table 2.

Effects on Arterial Blood Pressure

Because of the frequent usage of oral contraceptives and the
high incidence of hypertensive disease in the population at large,
the fact that hypertensive disease was first discovered in six of
our patients receiving this treatment, does not in itself imply any
specific interrelationship (Table 2). Furthermore, even the augmentation of pre-existing hypertension observed in two of five
previously hypertensive patients could be a chance occurrence.

However, the complete reversal of documented hypertension

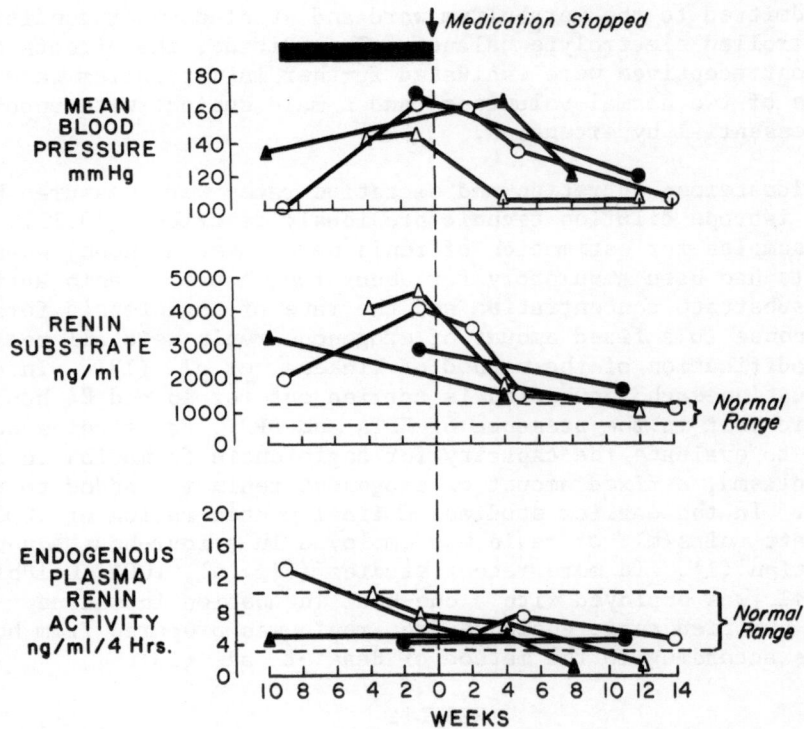

Fig. 1. Effects of withdrawal of oral contraceptives in four patients. After withdrawal of medication elevated blood pressure was improved in two and completely corrected in two others. At the same time elevated renin substrate levels returned to normal, and plasma renin levels, though not abnormal, tended to decline. It is of note that plasma renin levels were at times elevated earlier in treatment, but tended to decline as therapy was continued. (From Newton et al: Am. J. Obstet. and Gynec. 101:1037, 1968.)

after drug withdrawal in three of nine and the improvement of
hypertension in another three of the nine raises the possibility
of a more specific relationship. In Figure 1, the time course for
blood pressure improvement and for correction of associated abnormalities in the renin-angiotensin system is presented for four of
these patients.

In two patients, in each of whom correction or considerable
improvement in blood pressure was observed after drug withdrawal,
the oral contraceptives were re-administered. In both, hypertension
returned, and concurrently characteristic abnormalities in the
renin-angiotensin-aldosterone system reappeared. Such sequential
observations (Fig. 2), demonstrating reappearance and redisappear-
ance of hypertension perhaps provide the most convincing evidence
to suggest a specific connection between the administration of oral
estrogen-progestogen and the development of high blood pressure.

One patient (Table 2) who had hypertension prior to the use
of contraceptives also seems to have been cured of the condition
by drug withdrawal (1). She first developed hypertension during
pregnancy and subsequently underwent nephrectomy for unilateral
renal infection. Pre-existing hypertension in the region of
180/110 persisted during 20 months of oral contraceptive therapy.
However, she had been normotensive for over a year since stopping
medication.

Effects on Renin Substrate

The most consistant attendant biochemical abnormality was the
appearance of marked and persistent increases in the concentration
of plasma angiotensinogen, observed in all but one of the hypertensive women studied (Figs. 1-4). The elevated values ranged from
1980 to 8650 ng of angiotensin generated per ml of plasma or to
as much as eight times the normal concentration. In two normal
male subjects and in one male hypertensive patient, entirely similar changes were produced by treatment with these agents (Fig. 5,6).

The maximum effect on renin substrate with the use of combined
estrogen-progestogen treatment was observed to develop from as soon
as four days to as long as two weeks after starting treatment
(Figs. 2,3). The time required for the return of substrate levels
to the normal range after drug withdrawal exhibited even more variation. Two to four weeks or even longer often was required for
the return of substrate levels to a normal range (Fig. 1).

An attempt was made to determine which component of an oral
contraceptive preparation was responsible for this biochemical
effect (Fig. 5). The administration of norethynodrel produced
significant increases in renin substrate but less than that observed

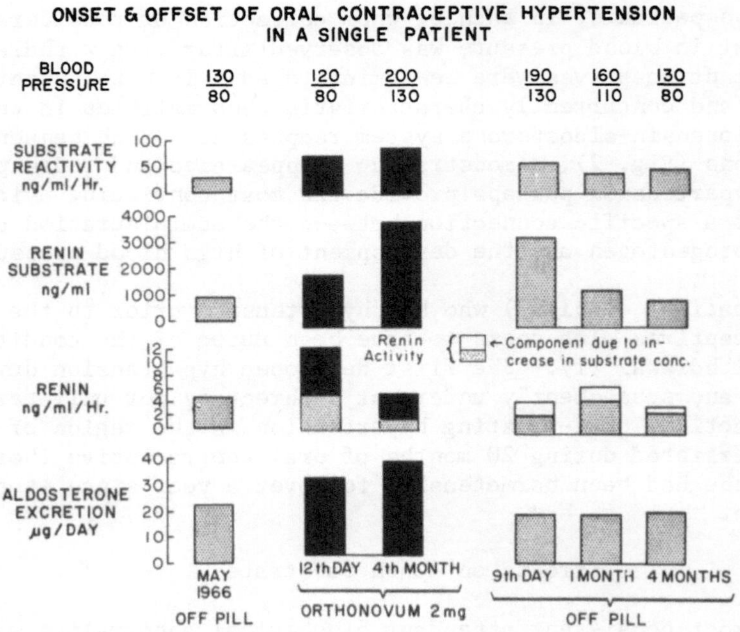

Fig. 2. A 32 year old woman in whom hypertension was first discovered after three years of oral contraceptive therapy with Enovid 5 mg. Hypertension disappeared after drug withdrawal. It reappeared, as shown here, when treatment was renewed, and then disappeared again after drug withdrawal. The onset and disappearance of hypertension was associated with concomitant increases and decreases in renin, aldosterone, renin substrate and renin activity. The data illustrate that, in this patient, the observed increase in renin activity was largely due to an increased substrate concentration. (From Newton et al: Am. J. Obstet. and Gynec. 101:1037, 1968.)

with the use of either ethynyl estradiol or the combination pill.
Such results in two male subjects suggest that both components of
the oral contraceptives can stimulate substrate formation with the
predominant effect being referable to the estrogen. The stimulating
effect of norethynodrel may be derived from its estrogenic properties since progesterone was found not to increase renin substrate
in a previous report (2).

Effects on the Plasma Reactivity to Exogenous Renin

Because of the striking increases observed in renin substrate
levels, a study was made to determine whether this abnormality
might produce a change in the character or magnitude of the response to renin (Figs. 2-6). This question was approached by
employing an _in vitro_ system in which the capacity to form angiotensin was measured after the addition of a fixed amount of renin
to the individual plasma.

Significant increases in substrate reactivity were consistently
observed. These increases were directly related to the corresponding induced rise in renin substrate concentration. Increased
reactivity was produced as the substrate concentration increased
to the region of 2000 ng/ml. Above this concentration further
increases in substrate induced lesser increments in reactivity.
In the one patient in whom substrate failed to increase significantly, no increase in reactivity to renin was produced (1).
These results suggest that it is the change in concentration of
substrate which accounts for the increased reactivity. Other _in
vitro_ studies in which reactivity was measured after addition of
estrogen to normal plasma indicated that the presence of the estrogen does not _per se_ modify the rate of reaction between renin and
its substrate.

Previous studies have suggested that under normal conditions
substrate concentration is not rate limiting so the reaction
velocity for a given amount of renin is near maximum (12,14,15).
Because of these reports the possibility may be raised that the
consistent increases in reactivity to renin produced by the contraceptives might have resulted from modification of the plasma
concentration of either an activator or an inhibitor. To test
this possibility, a plasma sample with a substrate concentration
of 3000 ng/ml angiotensinogen, drawn at the time of maximum effect
on substrate concentration, was diluted, and the reactivity of
various dilutions of this sample was compared with that of other
samples drawn from the same patient as his substrate concentration
was rising (Fig. 6). The two curves of reactivity as related to
substrate concentration were superimposable. This result does not
fully exclude but neither does it provide positive evidence for an
activator or inhibitor; instead, it suggests that the increased

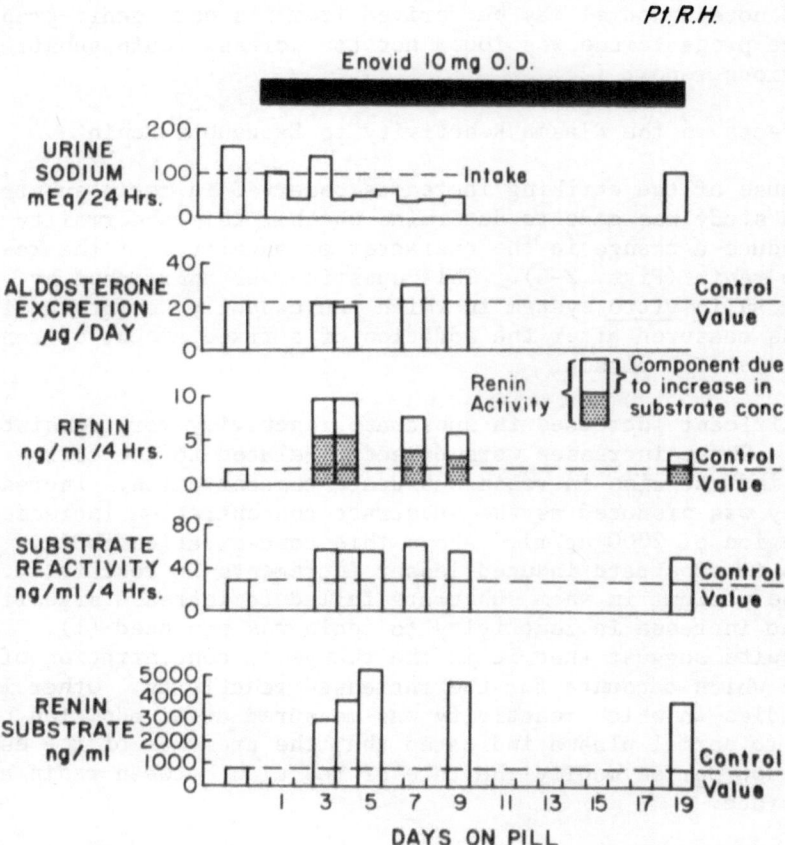

Fig. 3. Effects of administration of an oral contraceptive for 19 days to a 41 year old woman with essential hypertension. In this patient, the drug produced a slightly positive sodium balance. At the same time, aldosterone excretion exhibited a significant rise which seemed slightly out of phase with the increased renin. The prompt rise in plasma renin activity appeared to be due to both an increase in endogenous renin and to an increased reactivity from increased substrate concentration. With continued treatment, elevated renin activity tended to fall back to the normal range even though the increased renin substrate persisted. (From Newton et al: Am. J. Obstet. and Gynec. 101:1037, 1968.)

reactivity to renin merely results from an increased substrate concentration. Whether the substrate is qualitatively as well as quantitatively changed by the sex hormones also remains a subject for further studies involving both dilution and concentration and determination of Km values.

Effects on Endogenous Plasma Renin Activity

Because of the consistently produced enhancement of plasma reactivity to renin, proper evaluation of the influence of oral contraceptive therapy on the true renin concentration requires that each measurement of endogenous renin activity be corrected by taking into account the contribution of these alterations in reactivity (Figs. 1-5). Such data indicate that the observed apparent increases in endogenous renin activity resulted from either an increase in plasma reactivity or an increase in the true renin concentration or both (Fig. 3).

With long-term administration of oral contraceptives, endogenous renin activity remained elevated in four patients, but in five others the values were normal (1). The return of the endogenous renin to normal levels in this situation suggests that the true renin concentration actually may have been depressed below normal.

An example of a patient with persistently increased plasma renin levels is presented in Figure 4. The data illustrate that the abnormality persists at all levels of sodium intake. The second pattern, i.e., the tendency for endogenous renin activity to return to normal after an initial rise, is illustrated by studies of two other hypertensive patients (Figs. 2,3) and of two normotensive males (Fig. 5).

Effects on Aldosterone Secretion or Excretion

Abnormalities in aldosterone tended to be transient, and they were observed less consistently than the renin abnormalities. In four of eight hypertensive patients studied, the levels remained elevated. However, in one, the increase seemed referable to severe pre-existing hypertensive disease. In the other three, the values were restored to normal by cessation of therapy (Figs. 2-4). In two normal male subjects only transient increases in aldosterone excretion were induced in association with the transiently increased endogenous renin activity.

DISCUSSION

Because both hypertensive disease and the use of oral contraceptives are such common phenomena in the adult female premenopausal

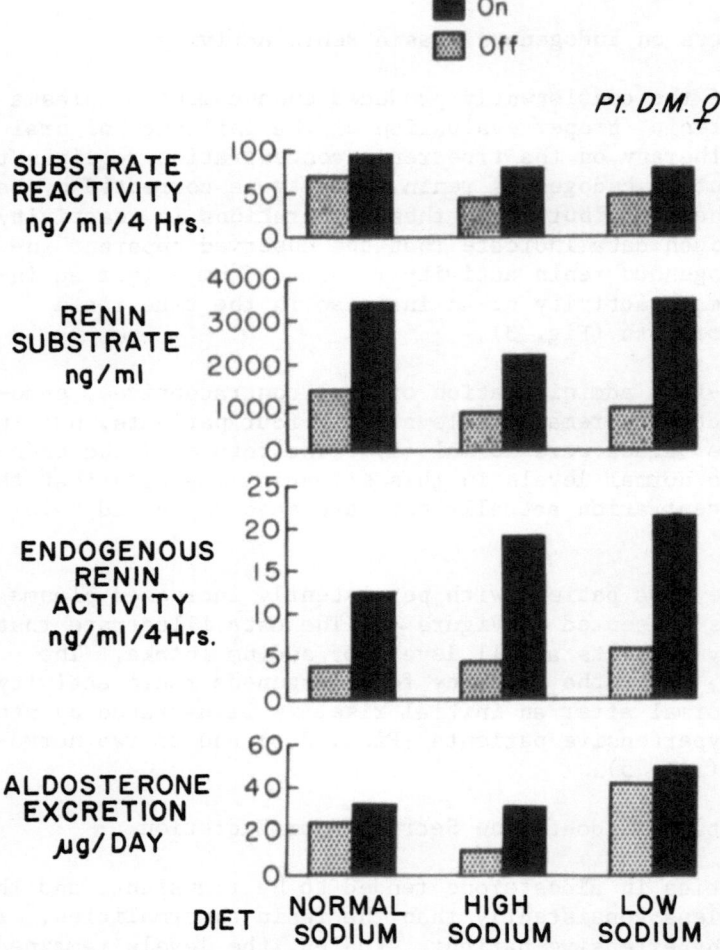

Fig. 4. The influence of changes in dietary salt intake on oral contraceptive induced abnormalities in the renin-angiotensin-aldosterone system. Data taken from a metabolism balance study of a 30 year old woman who had been maintained on Enovid-E, 2.5 mg, for 17 months and whose hypertension in the region of 160/110 was discovered shortly after starting treatment. This patient exhibited persistent and significant increases in all of the measured components of the renin-angiotensin system. The abnormalities were apparent at all levels of sodium intake. The fluctuations of plasma renin levels with various regimens did not appear altogether appropriate. (From Newton et al: Am. J. Obstet. and Gynec. 101:1037, 1968.)

population, the development or enhancement of hypertension in subjects taking this medication could be mere coincidence. Nevertheless, in the present study, considerable evidence has been advanced to suggest a cause and effect relationship between the use of this type of medication and the development or aggravation of high blood pressure in certain individuals who seem especially sensitive in this regard. Furthermore, these clinical observations are now supported by findings from other clinics (9,16,17).

The most impressive and consistent abnormality observed in the present investigation was the striking increase in the concentration of plasma angiotensinogen. In every instance, it was possible to demonstrate that this observed increase in renin substrate concentration was associated with a marked enhancement in the rate of angiotensin formation upon addition of a fixed amount of endogenous renin to the plasma. These increased responses suggest that increases in the concentration of substrate above normal levels can exert an important accelerating influence on the rate of production of angiotensin, so that the rate of angiotensin formation can be increased by as much as the factor of two. The finding is somewhat surprising since it has previously been thought that substrate is normally present in amounts which are sufficient to provide nearly maximum enzyme velocity (12,14,15). The possibility exists that oral contraceptives also produce a qualitative change in renin substrate which shifts the concentration at which near maximum velocity is reached and which, per se, might also alter its reactivity to renin. Whatever the case in this regard, it is clear that the net result of these pills is an increased substrate reactivity to a fixed amount of renin. Thus, the findings in the study strongly suggest that normal concentration of renin substrate is insufficient to produce a maximum rate of reaction with renin and they also imply that, from a physiological standpoint, the suboptimum substrate concentrations of normal subjects are probably not rate-limiting for angiotensin production. This possibility is supported by the observation that when substrate concentrations are elevated by the drugs, there is often a tendency for the renin concentration to fall so that the rate of formation of angiotensin tends to remain unchanged. Thus, there is a tendency to autoregulate the formation of the final product, angiotensin.

In addition to their effects on substrate concentration, these hormonal substances appear to act by another means to produce true increases in levels of plasma renin. Thus, in some patients, increased endogenous plasma renin activity could be accounted for by increases in the plasma angiotensinogen concentration. However, in others, either transient or sustained increases in renin activity were of greater magnitude than could be accounted for by the aforementioned mechanism. Therefore, it seems likely that these female hormonal substances can act by other, possibly more

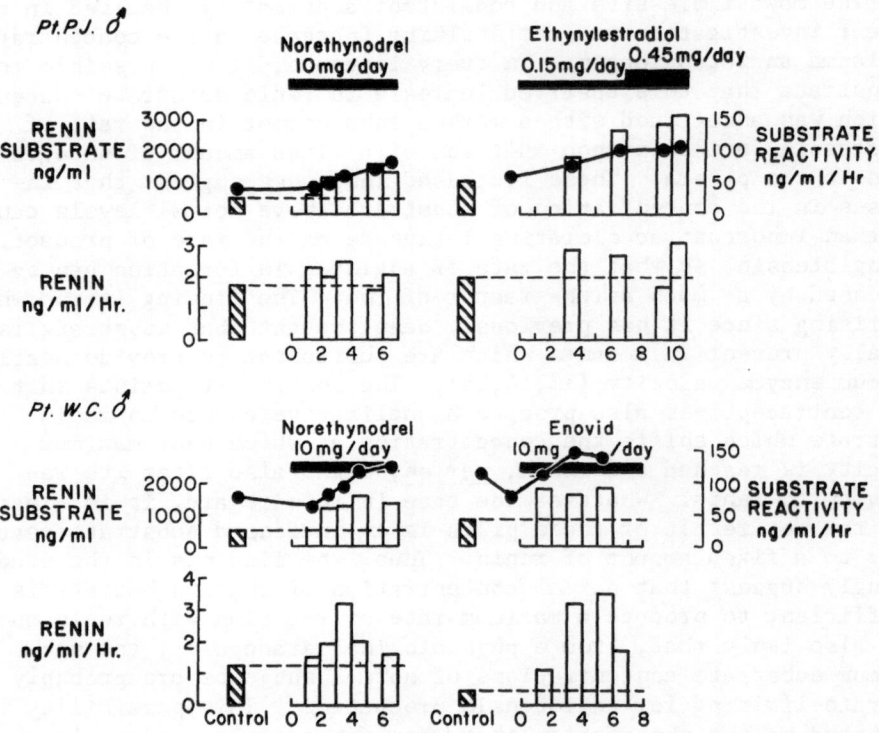

**EFFECT OF NORETHYNODREL, ENOVID, OR ETHYNYLESTRADIOL
ON RENIN, RENIN SUBSTRATE, & SUBSTRATE REACTIVITY**

Fig. 5. Relative effects of progestogen and estrogen in renin, renin substrate and plasma reactivity to renin. Studies were made in two normal male volunteers receiving a constant regimen. In both subjects, renin substrate and plasma reactivity to renin were increased to a greater extent by either estrogen or an estrogen combination. The progestogen exhibited similar but smaller effects. (From Newton et al: Am. J. Obstet. and Gynec. 101:1037, 1968.)

direct, means to increase plasma renin concentration. Clearly, the
increases in plasma renin were not due to induced sodium depletion
since oral contraceptives or their components generally tend to
promote fluid retention.

The relevance of the observed derangements in the renin-
angiotensin-aldosterone system to the associated production or augmentation of hypertensive disease remains obscure. We have
repeatedly observed the same abnormalities in patients receiving
the same medications, who at the same time exhibited no change
whatever in their blood pressure. However, one may speculate about
the possibility that in certain susceptible individuals the induced
increased reactivity towards endogenous renin may reduce the buffer
capacity of this hormonal interaction. In this way, the increased
responsiveness to renin, perhaps aided by the second direct stimulating effect on renin secretion, might create a situation leading
to an exaggerated pressor response to the usual physiologic stimuli
for renin release. This idea that, in certain subjects, feedback
compensation for the angiotensinogenemia produced by these drugs
may be incomplete, is perhaps supported by our observations illustrating that only some patients fully compensated for the induced
angiotensinogenemia by suppressing their renin secretion.

One can only speculate about the factors which might act to
sensitize certain individuals to the pressor action of these contraceptive agents. Pre-existing occult renal disease with reduced
buffer capacity of the renin angiotensin system may be one factor
as evidenced in two such patients included in our series and in one
other patient now under study. Another sensitizing factor may be
related to the tendency for sodium and water retention produced by
these drugs in certain individuals. In future studies, serial measurements of sodium balance or of sodium spaces or weight fluctuations (18) in out-patients may be especially illuminating. The
often repeated proposal (3) that the aldosteronism of progestational
compounds is secondary to a natriuresis seems quite unlikely in
these patients, who often exhibit a weight gain on these drugs.

Renin substrate is made by the liver (19). Estrogens appear
to increase or decrease the synthesis of various other proteins (1),
including a cortisol binding globulin and an aldosterone binding
protein (20). It therefore seems possible that the estrogens raise
the serum renin substrate by stimulating hepatic biosynthesis.
Renin substrate levels may be sharply reduced in patients with
cirrhosis (21). However, in one such patient, we produced a
striking rise in angiotensinogen with oral contraceptives, possibly
indicating a potentially adequate hepatic biosynthetic capacity.
An alternate possibility to explain the angiotensinogenemia would
be an effect of estrogens and progestogens on the kidney, since
renal insufficiency and nephrectomy often produce sharp rises in
renin substrate concentration.

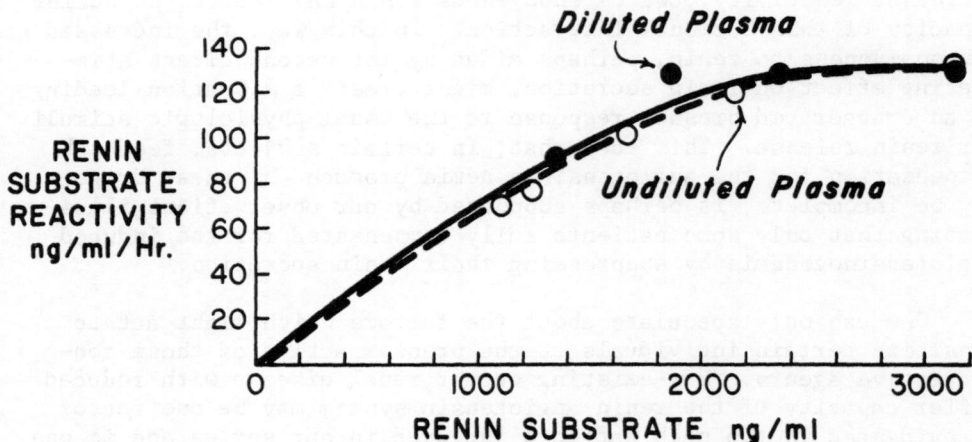

Fig. 6. Effect of dilution of renin substrate on substrate reactivity compared with undiluted samples exhibiting various concentrations. These samples were obtained at other times in the course of oral contraceptive administration. The data strongly suggest that observed changes in the substrate capacity to release angiotensin are directly related to changes in the substrate concentration rather than the result of variation in concentration of an activator or inhibitor. (From Newton et al: Am. J. Obstet. and Gynec. 101:1037, 1968.)

Full understanding of the role of estrogenic and progestogenic steroids in the pathogenesis of various forms of hypertensive disease, especially the forms observed during pregnancy, will require further study. The observations reported here may be applicable to the study of hypertension in experimental models. Furthermore, they may be relevant to the use of female hormones in other clinical situations. Of note in this regard are the reports of strokes in young women using oral contraceptives (22) and of a significant incidence of cerebral vascular accidents in a large group of males (23) receiving estrogen treatment for prostatic carcinoma.

SUMMARY

A group of patients have been described in whom the development or augmentation of hypertensive disease was associated with the use of oral contraceptives. The experience suggests a causal role for these hormonal substances in certain susceptible individuals. Factors which might sensitize to the pressor effect of these drugs remain undefined. However, the effect may be related to marked associated changes observed in certain components of the renin-angiotensin-aldosterone hormonal interaction. The contraceptive medications consistently produced large, sustained increases in plasma renin and in aldosterone were also observed. Parallel in vitro studies demonstrated that renin substrate is normally not present in excess because the contraceptive-induced increased substrate concentration was always accompanied by a significantly increased capacity for angiotensin formation when renin was added to the plasma. It seems possible to us that, in certain susceptible subjects, these induced hormonal changes, together with associated changes in sodium metabolism, could compromise the buffer capacity of the renin-angiotensin-aldosterone hormonal system, permitting exaggerated (pressor) responses to circulating renin when it is released by the normal physiologic stimuli. These observations also may be relevant to the use of female hormones in other clinical situations, and they may be applicable to the study of hypertension in experimental models.

REFERENCES

1. Laragh, J.H., Sealey, J.E., Ledingham, J.G.G. and Newton, M.A.: Oral contraceptives. Renin, aldosterone and high blood pressure. J.A.M.A. 201:918 (1967).

2. Helmer, O.M. and Griffith, R.S.: The effect of the administration of estrogens on the renin-substrate (hypertensinogen) content of rat plasma. Endocrinology 51:421 (1952).

3. Layne, D.S., Meyer, C.J., Vaishwanar, P.S. and Pincus, G.: The secretion and metabolism of cortisol and aldosterone in normal and in steroid-treated women. J. Clin. Endocr. 22:107 (1962).

4. Laidlaw, J.C., Ruse, J.L. and Gornall, A.G.: The influence of estrogen and progesterone on aldosterone excretion. J. Clin. Endocr. 22:161 (1962).

5. Brown, J.J., Davies, D.L., Doak, P.B., Lever, A.F. and Robertson, J.I.S.: Plasma renin in normal pregnancy. Lancet ii:900 (1963).

6. Winer, B.M.: Renin in pregnancy and the menstrual cycle. J. Clin. Invest. 44:112 (1965).

7. Genest, J., deChamplain, J. Veyrat, R., Boucher, R., Tremblay, G.Y., Strong, C.G., Koiw, E. and Marc-Aurèle, J.: Role of the renin-angiotensin system in various physiological and pathological states in Proc. Council for High Blood Pressure Research 13:97 (1964).

8. Crane, M.G., Heitsch, J., Harris, J. and Johns, V.J.,Jr.: Effect of ethinyl estradiol (estinyl) on plasma renin activity. J. Clin. Endocr. 26:1403 (1966).

9. Woods, J.W.: Oral contraceptives and hypertension. Lancet ii:653 (1967).

10. Laragh, J.H., Sealey, J.E. and Sommers, S.C.: Patterns of adrenal secretion and urinary excretion of aldosterone and plasma renin activity in normal and hypertensive subjects. Circ. Res. Suppl. I, 18 & 19: 1-158, 1966.

11. Laragh, J.H., Sealey, J.E. and Klein, P.D.: The presence and effect of isotope fractionation in isotope dilution analysis: A factor in the measurement of aldosterone secretory rates in man, in Radiochemical Methods of Analysis, Vienna: International Atomic Energy Agency, 2:353 (1965).

12. Pickens, P.T., Bumpus, F.M., Lloyd, A.M., Smeby, R.R. and Page, I.H.: Measurement of renin activity in human plasma. Circ. Res. 17:438 (1965).

13. Haas, E., Goldblatt, H. and Gipson, E.C.: Extraction, purification and acetylation of human renin and the production of anti-renin to human renin. Arch. Biochem. 110:438 (1965).

14. Haas, E. and Goldblatt, H.: Kinetic constants of the human renin and human angiotensinogen reaction. Circ. Res. 20:45 (1967).

15. Skinner, S.L.: Improved assay methods for renin "concentration" and "activity" in human plasma. Circ. Res. 20:391 (1967).

16. Swaab, L.I.: Blood pressure and oral contraception in Proceedings of Second International Congress on Hormonal Steroids, Milan, Italy, Amsterdam, Excerpta Medica Foundation, 1966, p. 198.

17. Shapiro, A.P.: Personal communication.

18. Thomas, C.B.: Some observations on the relationship between weight changes following sodium restriction and those associated with the menstrual cycle in normal young women. Ann. Int. Med. 39:289 (1953).

19. Braun-Menendez, E., Fasciola, J.C., Leloir, L.F., Munoz, J.M. and Taquini, A.C.: Renal Hypertension, Springfield, Ill. Charles C. Thomas, Publisher, p. 130, (1946).

20. Meyer, C.J., Layne, D.S., Tait, J.F. and Pincus, G.: The binding of aldosterone to plasma proteins in normal, pregnant and steroid-treated women. J. Clin. Invest. 40:1663 (1961).

21. Ayers, C.R.: Plasma renin activity and renin-substrate concentration in patients with liver disease. Circ. Res. 20:594 (1967).

22. Cole, M.: Strokes in young women using oral contraceptives. Arch. Int. Med. 120:551 (1967).

23. The Veterans Administration Co-operative Urological Research Group: Treatment and survival of patients with cancer of the prostrate. Surg. Gyn. & Ob. 124:1011 (1967).

THE EFFECTS OF GONADAL HORMONES ON WATER AND ELECTROLYTE METABOLISM IN THE HUMAN

J. R. K. Preedy

Department of Medicine, Emory University,
Atlanta, Georgia

For many years, physicians have had the impression that the administration of gonadal hormones could under certain circumstances cause fluid retention in the human subject. The impression was strengthened by experiments in the late nineteen-thirties showing that gonadal hormones could cause marked fluid retention in animals (1,2). These experiments led in turn to the proposal that gonadal hormones were responsible for the cyclical fluid retention frequently seen in women before the menses (3).

Subsequent reports have documented changes in water and electrolyte metabolism following the administration to the human of the gonadal hormones, testosterone, progesterone and certain estrogens, using the overall balance technique. These studies have confirmed that each of these hormones can alter water and electrolyte metabolism, but not necessarily in the same direction.

The effects of these hormones tend to be complex. Water can be retained or lost in association with K, PO_4 and nitrogen as part of an anabolic or catabolic action. Water can also be retained or lost in association with Na and Cl and expansion or contraction of extracellular fluid volume. These effects are apparently separate. Furthermore, the effects of the various hormones on sodium and chloride excretion may be biphasic, or even triphasic, during the period of hormone administration, particularly in the normal subject, and particularly with lower doses. Consequently, it is a gross over-simplification to describe any of these hormones solely as "fluid-retaining" or "diuretic."

Interpretation of some of the published balance studies in

terms of normal physiology is rendered difficult by certain features of the experiments, of which the following are examples:-
1) hormones may be administered in unphysiologically large amounts,
2) subjects may not be normal, 3) study periods may be too short, and may include only one phase of the effect. Finally, of course, observed changes in the intact subject may not be due to a direct action of the administered hormone on some target tissue, but to some complex readjustment in the secretion, metabolism, excretion, or in the action, of one or more endogenous hormones.

In this brief review I shall deal principally with the effects of testosterone, progesterone and estrogens on sodium chloride and water metabolism, and to a less extent on potassium and phosphate metabolism. I shall not deal with possible mechanisms, since this is to be covered by the next speaker, Dr. Katz.

TESTOSTERONE

Testosterone has been least well studied of the three. The best studies are still those of Knowlton and co-workers (4) of 30 years ago. In Figure 1, taken from the publications of the above workers, is shown the typical effect of testosterone in a normal male. There is a sustained decrease in the urinary output of nitrogen, potassium and phosphate, in urinary sodium and chloride output, and in urinary volume, accompanied by an increase in weight. This appears to continue for so long as treatment is given. Following cessation of treatment there is a diuresis of all substances, followed by a return to control levels. The daily dose of testosterone given in these experiments was approximately three times the normal production rate per day for males.

In a "hypogonad" woman, exactly similar results were obtained (4). In this case, the daily dose of testosterone was about 50 times the normal production rate per day for females.

It would appear therefore that testosterone can cause salt and water retention in males and females, at least in the unphysiologically high dosage used. However, we need considerably more information, using a larger number of subjects and varying dose levels.

The effect of testosterone on salt and water metabolism can be abolished on a low sodium diet, leaving the effects on urinary potassium, phosphate and nitrogen unchanged (5). This may be of some theoretical interest.

PROGESTERONE

The effects of progesterone have been studied in recent years

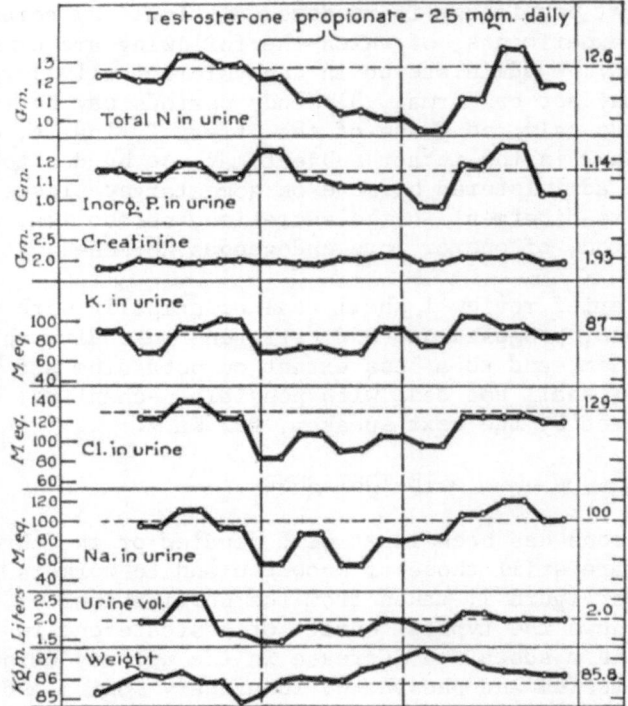

Figure 1.   The effect of testosterone propionate on nitrogen,
electrolyte and water balances in a normal male subject (4).

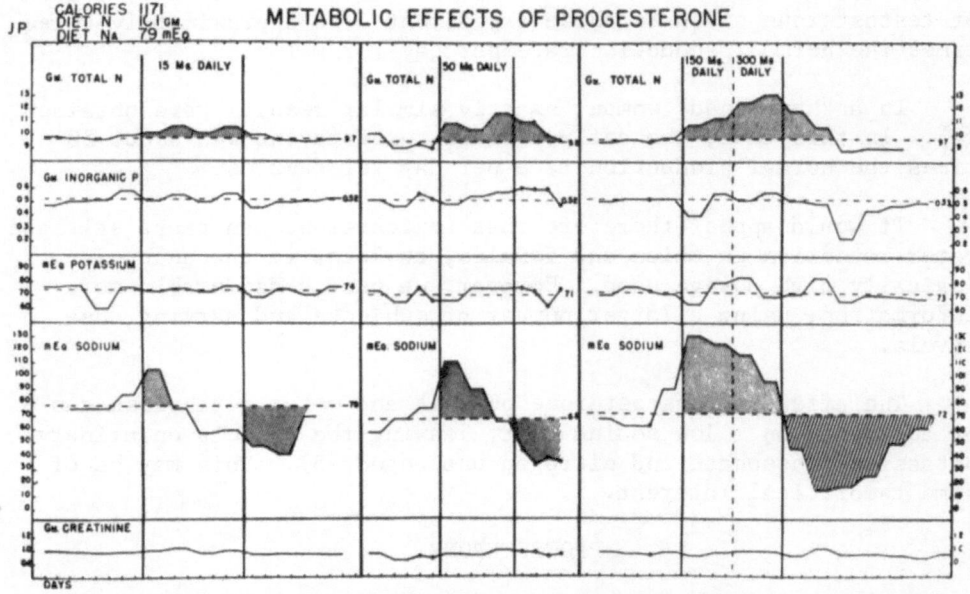

Figure 2.   The effect of progesterone on nitrogen, electrolyte
and water balances in a female subject with diabetes (6).

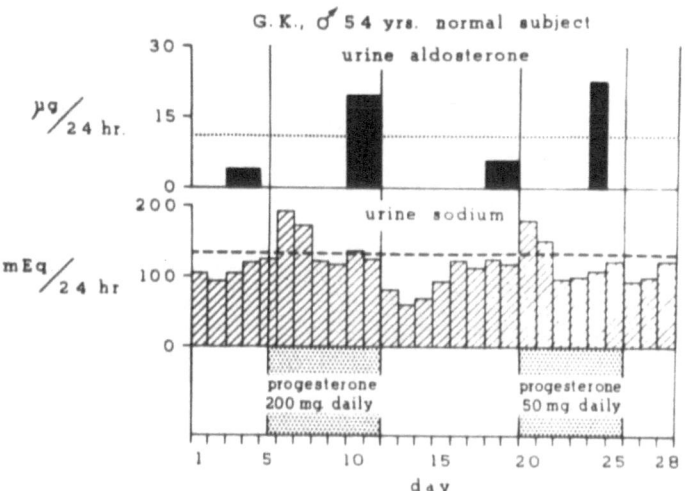

Figure 3.   The effect of progesterone on urinary sodium and urinary aldosterone excretion in a normal male (7).

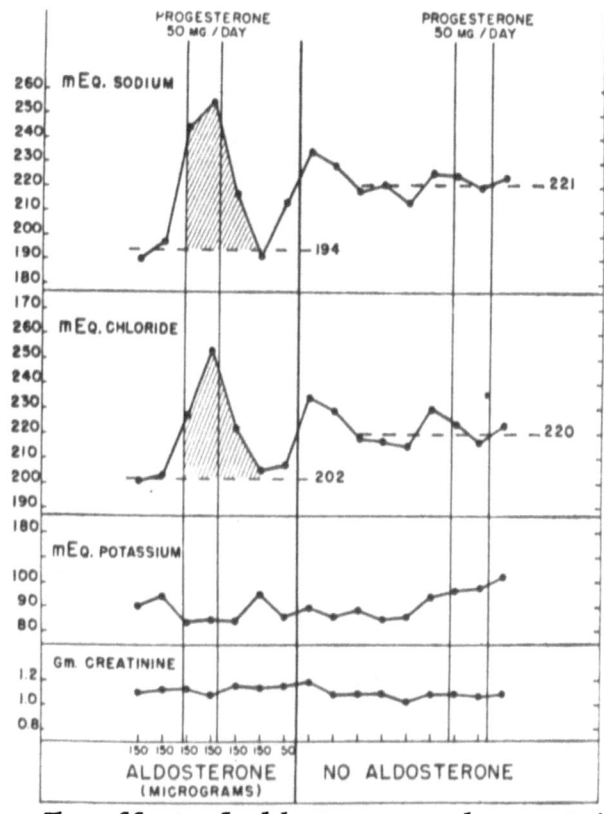

Figure 4.   The effect of aldosterone replacement in the progesterone-induced sodium chloride diuresis in a subject with Addison's disease (6).

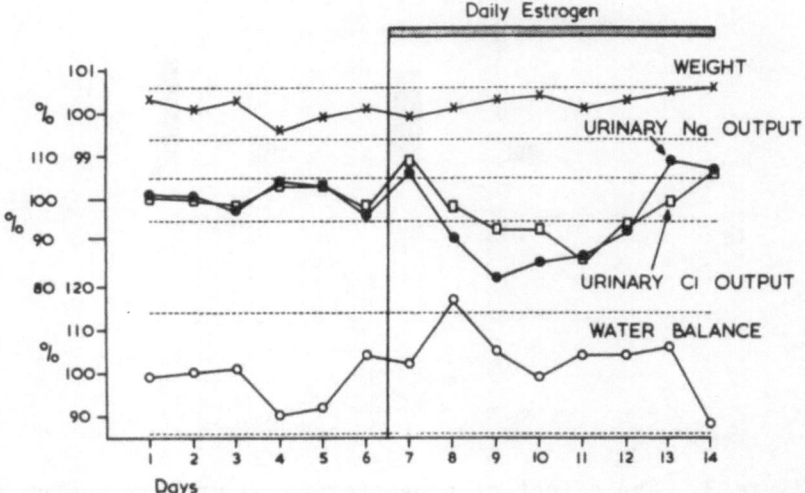

Figure 5. The effect of estradiol-17β on sodium, chloride and water balances in a group of normal subjects (9).

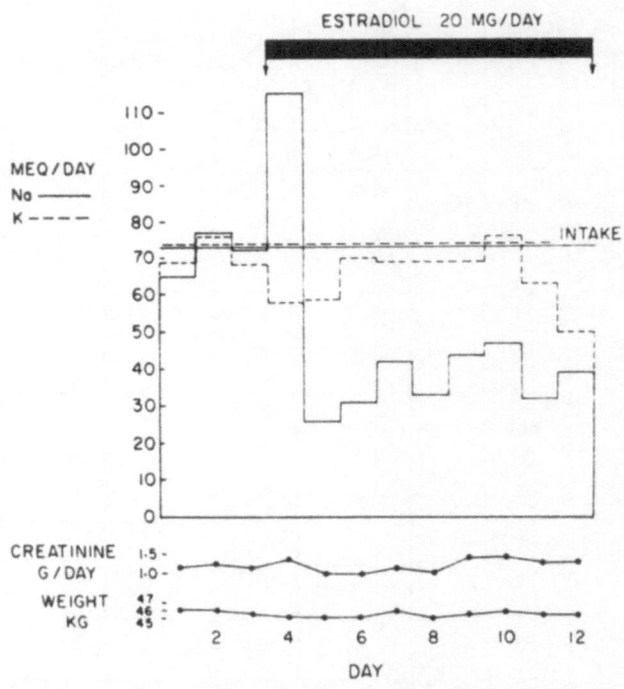

Figure 6. The effect of a large dose of estradiol-17β on urinary sodium and potassium excretion in a male with emphysema (12).

by Landau (6), Laidlaw (7), Bartter (8) and their respective co-workers.

Figure 2, taken from Landau's studies, shows the effect of increasing doses of progesterone in a woman (who happened to have diabetes). The dose range is from 15-300 mg /day. This is equivalent to the normal production rate in women during the latter half of the menstrual cycle (lower dose range), and to the production rate in late pregnancy (upper dose range). These levels could therefore be regarded perhaps as physiological.

The results obtained are typical of those seen in both sexes. There is a catabolic effect (increase of nitrogen in the urine), but no consistent effect on urinary potassium or phosphate. There is however a definite effect on urinary sodium. In the lower dose the effect is clearly biphasic. There is a diuresis followed by retention during the continued administration of the hormone. In the middle and higher doses, there is diuresis, and although no actual retention occurs during the period of hormone administration the biphasic nature of the curve is still quite obvious. Perhaps if administration of the hormone were continued for a long period, actual retention would have been observed.

The same effects were noted by Laidlaw (Fig. 3), that is, a diuresis of sodium followed by retention while the progesterone was still being given. As in the previous Figure 2, the biphasic nature of the effect was more obvious at the lower dose level (7).

Similar results were also reported by Bartter and co-workers (8), but the periods were shorter and only the natriuretic phase of the effect was observed.

The effect of progesterone on water and salt metabolism appears to be dependent on the presence of a mineralocorticoid. In Figure 4, taken from Landau's work (6), progesterone was administered to a woman with Addison's disease with and without aldosterone. With aldosterone the typical diuresis of Na and Cl was obtained (with no alteration in K). In the absence of aldosterone, however, progesterone appeared to have no effect at all on urinary electrolyte excretion. Bartter and co-workers obtained similar results in Addisonian patients with and without the administration of desoxycorticosterone (DOC) (8).

ESTROGENS

We ourselves have carried out extensive studies of the effect of the administration of one of the estrogens, estradiol-17β, in human subjects both in health and in disease states (8-10).

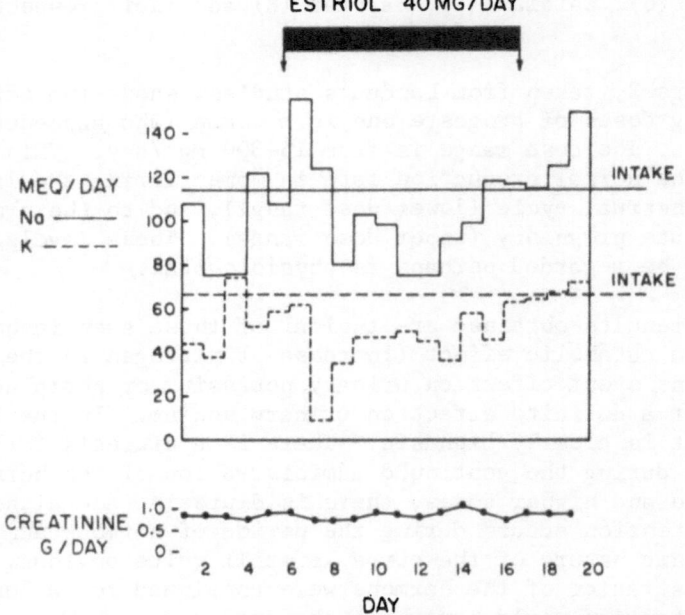

Figure 7. The effect of estriol on urinary sodium and potassium excretion in a subject with duodenal ulcer (12).

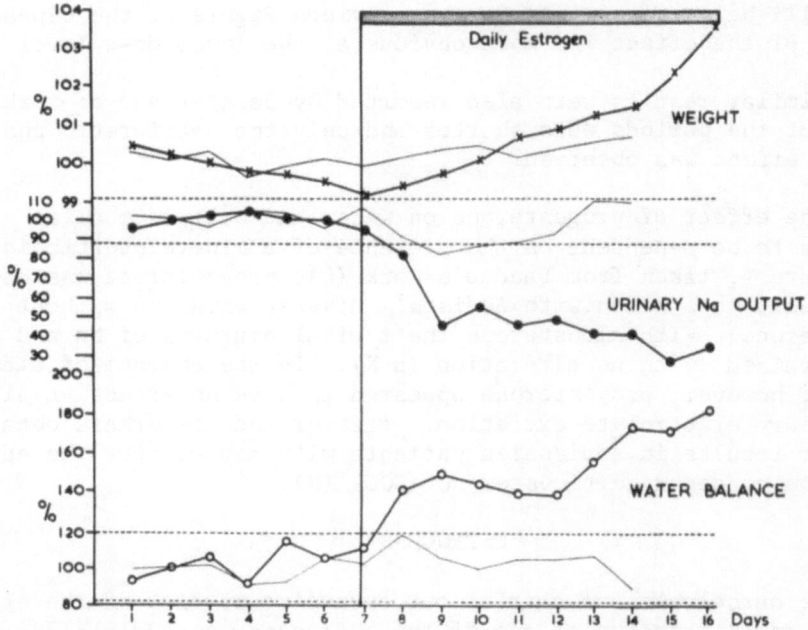

Figure 8. The effect of estradiol-17β on sodium and water balances in a group of subjects with hepatic cirrhosis and ascites (10).

Figure 5 is a composite graph showing the effect of estradiol-17β in 12 normal subjects (males and females). The time intervals on the graph are divided into control and estrogen periods. The daily amount of the estrogen given was 7 mg , which is 60 to 100 times the daily production rate in females during reproductive life, but corresponds with the daily production in late pregnancy.

Each value for weight, urinary sodium and chloride output and "water balance" is the average for the group expressed as a percentage of the mean control value. The horizontal lines represent 2 SDs above and 2 SDs below this mean. Consequently, any values above or below these lines are significantly different from control values. "Water balance" is total water intake less urine output. Therefore, a <u>rise</u> in this value is consistent with water retention.

It will be seen that there are elements of a triphasic response for sodium and chloride, that is, a diuresis on the first day, followed by retention for several days, followed again by a diuresis, all occurring while the hormone is still being given. However, it should be emphasized that with this dose the effects are minor as well as transient, and can only be clearly established when results from a number of cases are analyzed. There was apparently a slight tendency to gain weight in these normal subjects and a slight rise in water balance, but these changes were too small to achieve significance. There was no change in urinary K, PO$_4$ or nitrogen output.

At a higher dose level, the effect appears to be exaggerated (Fig. 6). This figure is taken from recent work of Katz and Kappas (12) with Dr. Katz' permission. Here, estradiol-17β in three times the amount used by ourselves was given to one male. There is a marked diuresis on the first day, followed by sustained retention with no subsequent diuresis of sodium during the period of observation.

Figure 7, taken from the same authors' work (12) shows the effect of estriol. This is of particular interest, since estriol has comparatively weak estrogenic potency in most bioassays, and is usually thought to be a relatively inactive product of the highly active estrogens estradiol-17β and estrone, at least in the non-pregnant subject. In spite of this, a typical triphasic effect on urinary sodium output was observed, similar to that seen in our own cases with estradiol-17β.

We have shown above (Fig. 5) that estradiol-17β in doses of 7 mg daily causes only slight and transient changes in water and salt metabolism in the normal human. In certain disease conditions, however, such as cirrhosis with ascites and congestive heart failure, the effect of estradiol-17β in the same dose is neither slight nor transient. In fact, a marked and sustained retention

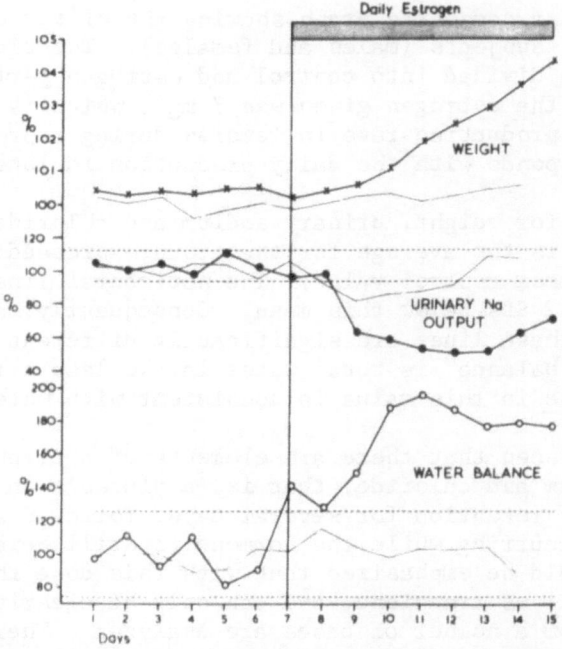

Figure 9.   The effect of estradiol-17β on sodium and water balances in a group of subjects with constrictive pericarditis (11).

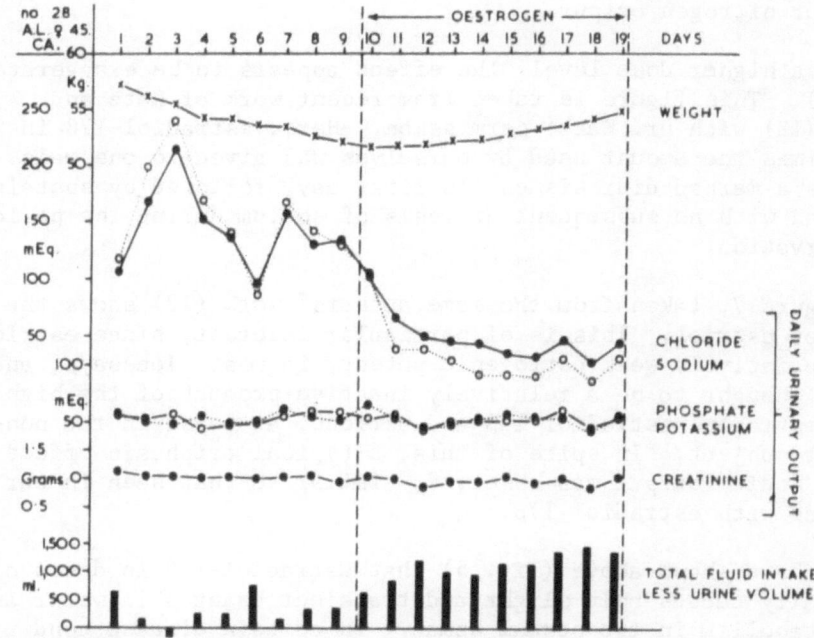

Figure 10. The effect of estradiol-17β on sodium, chloride, phosphate, potassium and water balances in a subject with hepatic cirrhosis and ascites (10).

of sodium and water usually occurs.

Figure 8 shows a composite graph taken from our own publications (9) of the results in 8 cases of cirrhosis with ascites. The format is the same as in Figure 5 (normal series) and the corresponding values for the normal are reproduced as faint lines for comparison. As you see, estradiol-17β causes marked and sustained retention of sodium and water, accompanied by a gain in weight. Note that during the control period weight was lost steadily due to spontaneous diuresis. This weight loss is actually converted into weight gain by the estrogen administration.

The same results are seen in congestive heart failure, and particularly in constrictive pericarditis (Fig. 9). Here, the retention of sodium and water is again very marked.

The record of an individual case of cirrhosis with ascites is shown in Figure 10. This shows that the marked retention of sodium, chloride and water which occurs in these cases is not accompanied by any significant change in the output of potassium or phosphate.

SUMMARY

We have provided evidence obtained from the literature that testosterone (in daily doses three times the production rate in males and 30 times that in females) causes salt and water retention, as well as retention of nitrogen, potassium and phosphate. However, more information regarding this effect is needed.

Progesterone, in roughly physiological doses, causes a diuresis of sodium followed by retention while the hormone is still being given. The diuretic effect seems to predominate at higher dosage levels. Whether the retention phase is completely obliterated at these high levels or merely delayed is not yet clear. To determine this would require a longer period of progesterone administration. Thus, we cannot be certain at this time whether long-term progesterone administration causes sodium diuresis or sodium retention.

Estradiol-17β administration in daily doses equivalent to the production rate in late pregnancy, but 60 to 100 times that during the menstrual cycle, causes only transient changes in urinary sodium and chloride output in the normal. (At higher doses, retention of sodium seems to predominate). However, the same doses of estradiol-17β causes massive and prolonged retention of sodium chloride and water (but not of potassium or phosphate) in cases of cirrhosis with ascites and congestive heart failure (and particularly in constrictive pericarditis).

Although as mentioned above we cannot yet be certain that progesterone has a natriuretic effect in the <u>long term</u>, it certainly appears to be natriuretic in the short term. If this hormone is in fact predominantly natriuretic, then it has an opposite effect to that of estradiol-17β which is predominantly sodium-retaining. Such a relationship would be of some interest and importance. For instance, in late pregnancy when both hormones are produced in large quantity, progesterone could exert a protective effect by minimizing salt and water retention which might otherwise occur due to the effect of estradiol-17β and perhaps other estrogens. The same protective effect might be present to a lesser extent in the latter part of the menstrual cycle. An imbalance in the pregesterone-estrogen ratio might be responsible in part for objective fluid retention at this time. Finally, a protective effect could conceivably be present when progestogens and estrogens are administered together, as in oral contraceptive medication.

REFERENCES

1. Thorn, G.W. and Harrop, G.A.: Sodium retaining effect of sex hormones. Science 86:40-41 (1937).

2. Thorn, G.W. and Engel, L.L.: Effect of sex hormones on renal excretion of electrolytes. J. Exper. Med. 68:299-312 (1938).

3. Thorn, G.W. and Emerson, K., Jr.: Role of gonadal and adrenal cortical hormones in production of edema. Ann. Int. Med. 14:757-769 (1940).

4. Knowlton, K., Kenyon, A.T., Sandiford, I., Lotwin, G. and Fricker, R.: Comparative study of metabolic effects of estradiol benzoate and testosterone propionate in man. J. Clin. Endocr. 2:671-684 (1942).

5. Borun, E.R. and Geiger, E.: Interrelationships of some metabolic effects of testosterone propionate in normal males during restricted sodium intake. J. Clin. Invest. 35:1109-1118 (1956).

6. Landau, R.L. and Lugibuhl, K.: The catabolic and natriuretic effects of progesterone in man. Recent Progr. Hormone Res. 17:249-292 (1961).

7. Laidlaw, J.C., Ruse, J.L. and Gornall, A.G.: The influence of estrogen and progesterone on aldosterone excretion. J. Clin. Endocr. 22:161-171 (1962).

8. George, J.M., Saucier, G. and Bartter, F.C.: Is there a potent naturally occurring sodium-losing steroid hormone? J. Clin. Endocr. 25:621-627 (1965).

9. Preedy, J.R.K. and Aitken, E.H.: Effect of estrogen on water and electrolyte metabolism; normal. J. Clin. Invest. 35:423-429 (1956).

10. Preedy, J.R.K. and Aitken, E.H.: Effect of estrogen on water and electrolyte metabolism; hepatic disease. J. Clin. Invest. 35:430-442 (1956).

11. Preedy, J.R.K. and Aitken, E.H.: Effect of estrogen on water and electrolyte metabolism; cardiac and renal disease. J. Clin. Invest. 35:443-451 (1956).

12. Katz, F.H. and Kappas, A.: The effects of estradiol and estriol on plasma levels of cortisol and thyroid hormone-binding globulins and on aldosterone and cortisol secretion rates. J. Clin. Invest. 46:1768-1776 (1967).

EFFECT OF GONADAL HORMONES ON ADRENOCORTICAL SECRETION
AND ITS SIGNIFICANCE

F. H. Katz

Section of Endocrinology, Department of Medicine,
Loyola University, Stritch School of Medicine, Hines,
Illinois

Alterations of adrenocortical secretion during pregnancy and
differences between males and females of various species have been
extensively studied for many years and it would be beyond the limitation of this brief survey to attempt to cover this entire field.
We will therefore review the highlights of work done in this area
especially as it affects our understanding of normal human physiology and alterations that occur with hormone treatment in man.
In addition, work from our laboratory will be discussed.

ESTROGENS

Glucocorticoids

The considerable increase in plasma corticosteroid concentration during the third trimester of normal pregnancy (1) has long
been known to be easily reproducible by a short course of treatment
with estrogens (2,3). It was found that estrogens increase the
production of the specific corticosteroid binding globulin (CBG)(4)
and that most of the increased plasma corticosteroid is protein-
bound. Figure 1 shows that although estradiol will increase plasma
CBG capacity for cortisol, estriol, which, like the estradiol, was
administered in amounts similar to those present in the third

The clinical studies described were carried out at the Argonne
Cancer Research Hospital, operated for the United States Atomic
Energy Commission by the University of Chicago, and at the Veterans
Administration Hospital, Hines, Illinois. Additional support was
provided by U.S. Air Force Contracts 41(609)-2786 and 41609-67-
C0008. Technical assistance was rendered by Miss Janet Marie Cobb.
Miss Synetra Williams rendered secretarial assistance.

434

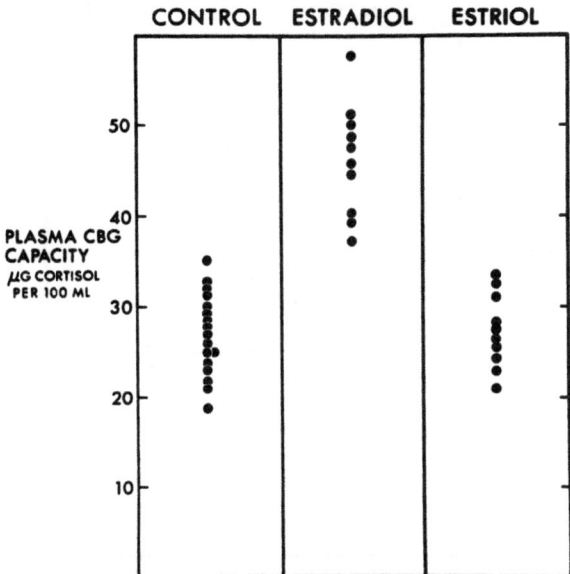

Figure 1. Estrogen effects on cortisol-binding-globulin
(CBG). Subjects receiving estradiol had an increase in CBG
capacity while those given estriol had no change. From Katz and
Kappas (5).

TABLE 1*

		Plasma Total Cortisol		Plasma Free Cortisol	
			μg per 100 ml		
	N	Mean	S.D.	Mean	S.D.
Control	34	8.55	0.82	0.53	0.06
Estrogen	9	39.44	4.00	1.21	0.13

*Plasma total cortisol was measured by a double isotope derivative
method or by competitive protein binding analysis (8). Free
cortisol is that fraction of the total dialyzable at 37°. The
subjects were young men who were given 5 mg diethylstilbestrol
daily for seven days.

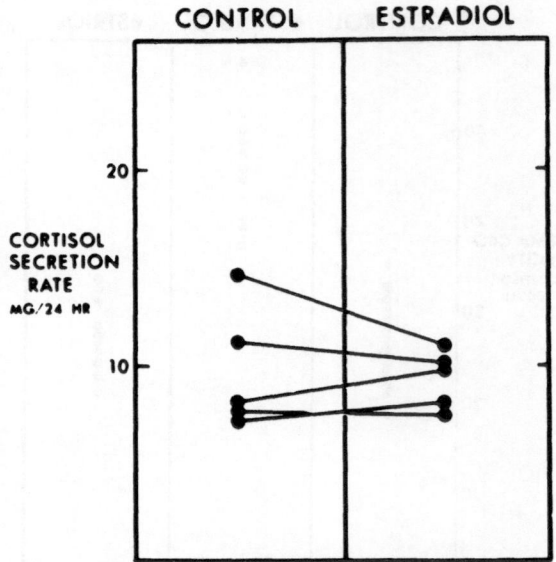

Figure 2.   Estradiol effects on cortisol secretion rate.
Doses of estradiol approximating amounts produced in the third
trimester of pregnancy had no significant effect on cortisol
secretion.

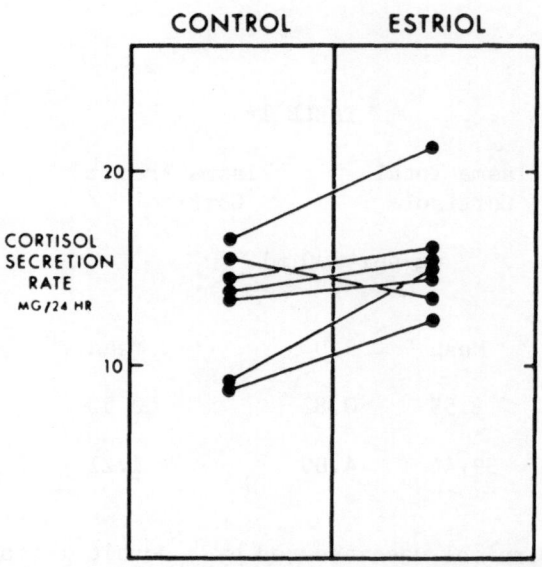

Figure 3.   Estriol effects on cortisol secretion rate. Doses
of estriol approximating amounts produced in the third trimester
of pregnancy produced a small but significant increase in cortisol
secretion.

trimester, did not have this effect on CBG (5). Although much of
the hormone present in pregnancy plasma is bound to transcortin
(CBG), most workers in the field have found increased absolute
levels of non-protein-bound cortisol in pregnancy and after estrogen treatment (6,7). Our own data are shown in Table 1. Control
levels of plasma cortisol of 8.5 µg per 100 ml. rose to near 40
after one week of diethylstilbestrol 5 mg. daily administered to
normal men. Non-protein-bound cortisol rose from 0.5 to 1.2 (8).

As would be expected under such circumstances, the half life
of cortisol in the plasma after estrogen is considerably increased
(3) and consequently urinary excretion and adrenocortical secretion
are diminished (9). Our studies with third trimester quantities
of estradiol (5) are shown in Figure 2. Although two of our subjects had small diminutions in cortisol secretion, values for the
group as a whole did not change after estradiol. Figure 3 shows
that there was a small but statistically significant increase in
cortisol secretion following a week or more of estriol administration. It is possible that this effect of estriol may be responsible for the increased cortisol secretion observed in pregnant subjects by Cope and Black (10), although more recently it has been
claimed (11) that there is a small reduction in cortisol secretion
in pregnancy, with an increase at the time of the onset of labor.
Our failure to observe a decrease in cortisol secretion after estradiol may be related to its metabolism to estriol.

Insofar as the estrogens present in oral contraceptives are
concerned, these dosages have been shown to cause statistically
significant but relatively small reductions in cortisol secretion
rate after the administration of the antiovulatory agents (12).
Norethynodrel also was able to effect a significant reduction in
cortisol secretion. Since norethynodrel also increased cortisol
concentration and cortisol binding it would appear that these
effects of norethynodrel are related to its estrogenic activity.
Progesterone is unable to effect these changes.

Mineralocorticoids

During the normal menstrual cycle, aldosterone secretion is
significantly increased during the luteal as compared to the
follicular phase (13). This could be due to the increased progesterone or the increased estrogen during the latter part of the
cycle.

It is now well established that aldosterone production is increased during the course of normal pregnancy. The most extensive
study (14) indicated that this increase in aldosterone secretion
begins as early as the fifteenth week and continues as pregnancy
proceeds. In addition, it can be partially suppressed by adding
salt to the diet and stimulated by sodium restriction.

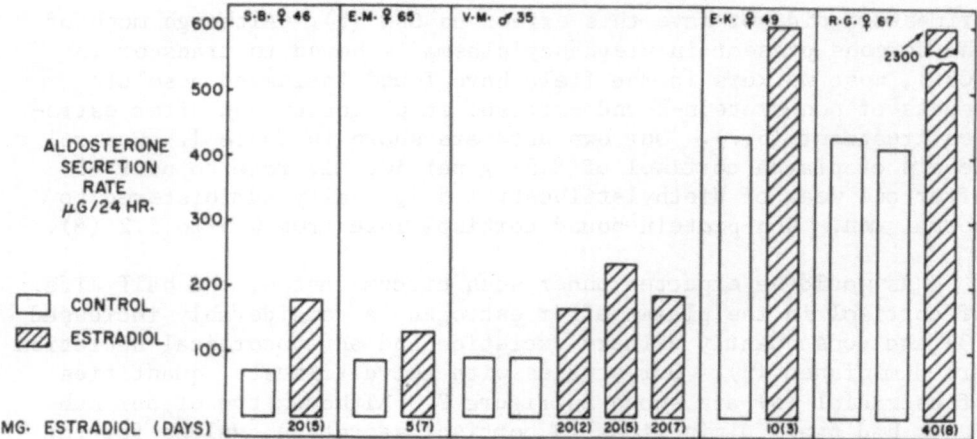

Figure 4.　Estradiol effect on aldosterone secretion.
Secretion of aldosterone was increased in individuals with normal
or elevated baseline excretion rates when estradiol was
administered.

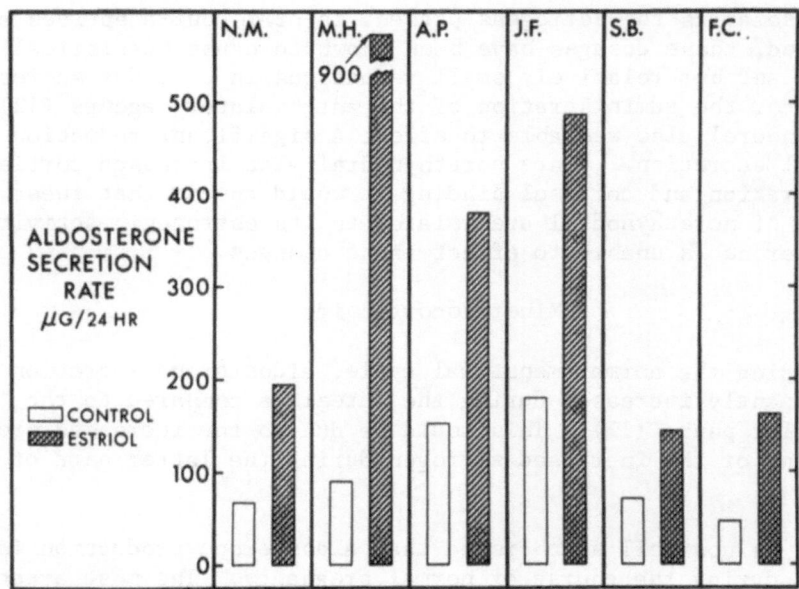

Figure 5.　Estriol effect on aldosterone secretion.　Estriol
consistently increased aldosterone secretion when given in excess
of 40 mg daily.

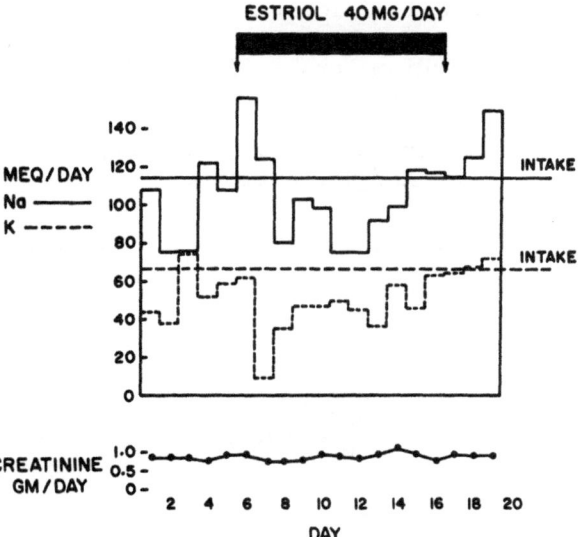

J·N· ♀ 42 DUOD· ULCER

Figure 6. Estrogen effect on sodium and potassium balance. Natriuresis followed by sodium retention and eventual escape were observed. From Katz and Kappas (5).

TABLE 2*

M.I. ♀ 65

Time	Urine Sodium mEq/hr	
10 a.m.	5.2	
11	5.4	
12	4.5	
1 p.m.	3.6	
2	2.0	← Estradiol
3	2.9	10 mg iv/6 hr
4	9.0	
5	19.2	
6	1.1	
7	1.4	
8	1.4	

*Hourly urinary sodium excretion was measured while the subject was receiving the solvent vehicle (10% N, N-dimethylacetamide in propylene glycol) alone and after estradiol was added.

TABLE 3*

Y.B. ♀ 37 Total Adrenalectomy

Sodium Intake 200 mEq/day
Cortisone 37.5 mg/day

Sodium Excretion - Urinary
mEq/gm Creatinine

Control	Estradiol 20 mg	Estriol 40 mg
193	239	229
238	230	157
158	255	175
222	279	229
206	205 ← D.C.	214
204	201	
186	235	
173	242	

*Daily values for sodium excretion are listed. The values during estradiol treatment differed significantly from the control values at the 5% level.

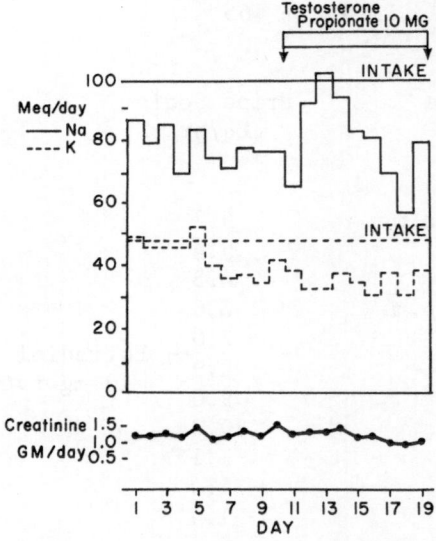

Figure 7. Effect of testosterone on sodium balance in an orchidectomized male. Natriuresis was observed during the first few days of hormone treatment.

Amounts of natural estrogens similar to those produced in the third trimester of normal pregnancy can increase aldosterone secretion (5). The effect of estradiol in five subjects is shown in Figure 4. Subject E.K. was suspected of having primary aldosteronism and her secretion rate was increased by the administration of estradiol. Subjects receiving diets containing less than 10 milliequivalents of sodium per day such as R.G. at the right of the figure also had an increase in aldosterone secretion following the administration of estradiol. Estradiol also increased the aldosterone secretion in a patient with bilateral adrenocortical hyperplasia with increased aldosterone secretion and suppression of plasma renin. Dosages of estrogen as low as those in oral contraceptives can also significantly increase the aldosterone secretion rate (12).

Estriol administered in amount similar to those present in the third trimester also increases aldosterone secretion (5), as shown in Figure 5.

Figure 6 illustrates what we believe to be a possible mechanism of the increased aldosterone production following estrogen administration. We have observed in a number of individuals now an early natriuresis, sometimes with a reciprocal potassium retention, immediately after the administration of the estrogen has begun. This is followed by a period of sodium retention with escape from the sodium retaining effect as occurs after the administration of mineralocorticoids. Eventual excretion of the excessively retained sodium occurs after the estrogen has been discontinued. Since it has been shown that plasma renin activity increases after estrogen administration (15) just as is true in pregnancy (16) we believe that estrogens, like progesterone (17), have antagonistic action to aldosterone at the renal tubular level and that the increase in renin and aldosterone after the administration of estrogen is a compensatory effect with some overcompensation. Table 2 demonstrates that a totally adrenalectomized woman had an increased mean sodium excretion while estradiol was being administered compared to a control period, although she was receiving the same diet with a constant sodium intake. A similar effect could not be shown after estriol. The effect of intravenous estriol on hourly sodium excretion in one subject is shown in Table 3.

PROGESTATIONAL AGENTS

As is detailed in Dr. Preedy's paper, the role of progesterone as a natriuretic agent in man has been well established by the elegant studies of Dr. Landau (18). The expected effect of this aldosterone antagonist in reducing aldosterone secretion was found by Laidlaw et al (19). The early natriuresis after the beginning of progesterone administration was followed by an increase in

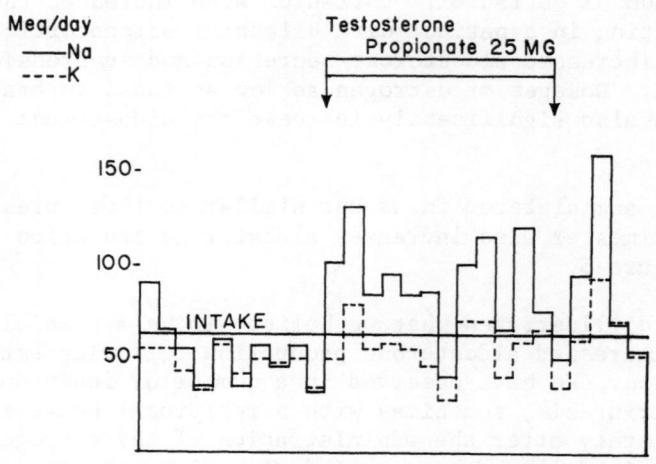

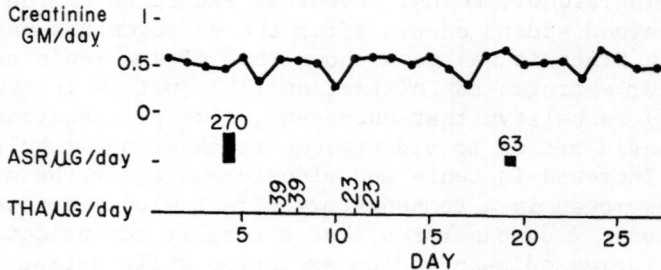

Figure 8.   Testosterone effects on aldosterone secretion.
Natriuresis and a reduction in aldosterone secretion rate (ASR)
and tetrahydroaldosterone (THA) excretion were observed.

aldosterone secretion. The increase in aldosterone secretion was slightly excessive, resulting in the net sodium retention also demonstrated previously by Landau. When progesterone injections were discontinued the aldosterone secretion returned to baseline values. Others have demonstrated that the dosages of progestational agents like the 10 mg norethynodrel in the early oral contraceptives could increase the aldosterone secretion rate significantly (12). The estrogenic effect of norethynodrel, demonstrated for cortisol binding capacity, could have been playing a role, however. The effect of smaller amounts of progestational agents present in the currently used oral contraceptives has not been reported.

ANDROGENS

Since a number of androgenic materials have been shown to be antagonistic to the action of aldosterone, both competitively (20) and noncompetitively (20,21), we have begun to study the effect of testosterone on the renin-angiotensin system in man. Figure 7 shows some evidence of natriuresis early during the course of administration of testosterone to an orchiectomized man. This is followed by slight sodium retention, as we would expect in the event that aldosterone production had been stimulated excessively by natriuresis. A second study in an elderly man, shown in Figure 8, demonstrated some natriuresis throughout the two-week period of testosterone administration. Aldosterone secretion, however, decreased from 270 to 63 µg/day and, as can be seen on the bottom of the graph, tetrahydroaldosterone excretion also diminished from 39 on each of two days prior to testosterone to 23 µg per day on the first and second days of testosterone injection. This would suggest that testosterone had some direction suppressive effect on the renin-angiotension mechanism or on the adrenal secretion of aldosterone. Two younger men have recently been given similar dosages of testosterone. They had only small diminutions of aldosterone secretory rate, of questionable significance, from 260 to 210 µg per day and from 400 to 375 µg per day. Further studies are proceeding.

CONCLUSIONS

There is evidence that all three classes of gonadal hormones have some antagonistic function to aldosterone at the renal tubular level. Both estrogens and progestational agents increase the aldosterone secretion rate and their natriuretic effect may well stimulate the renin-angiotensin system. Although, in animals, there is evidence also for renal antagonism to aldosterone by androgens, in man preliminary studies indicate a reduction of aldosterone secretion after testosterone treatment.

REFERENCES

1. Gemzell, C.A.: Blood levels of 17-hydroxycorticosteroids in normal pregnancy. J. Clin. Endocrin. Metab. 13:898 (1953).

2. Taliaferro, I., Cobey, F. and Leone, L.: Effect of diethylstilbestrol on plasma 17-hydroxycorticosteroid levels in humans. Proc. Soc. Exp. Biol. Med. 92:742 (1956).

3. Wallace, E.Z., Silberberg, H.I. and Carter, A.C.: Effect of ethinyl estradiol on plasma 17-hydroxycorticosteroids, ACTH responsiveness, and hydrocortisone clearance in man. Proc. Sci. Exp. Biol. Med. 95:805 (1957).

4. Sandberg, A.A., Woodruff, M., Rosenthal, H., Nienhouse, S. and Slaunwhite, W.R.: Transcortin: a corticosteroid-binding protein of plasma. VII. Half-life in normal and estrogen-treated subjects. J. Clin. Invest. 43:461 (1964).

5. Katz, F.H. and Kappas, A.: The effects of estradiol and estriol on plasma levels of cortisol and thyroid hormone-binding globulins and on aldosterone and cortisol secretion rates in man. J. Clin. Invest. 46:1768 (1967).

6. Plager, J.E., Schmidt, K.G. and Staubitz, W.J.: Increased unbound cortisol in the plasma of estrogen-treated subjects. J. Clin. Invest. 43:1066 (1964).

7. Doe, R.P., Dickinson, P.B., Swain, W.R., Zinneman, H.H. and Seal, U.S.: Nonprotein-bound 17-OHCS at 9 A.M. and 9 P.M. in normals, pregnancy, estrogen-treated females and males with cancer of the prostrate. Program, 49th meeting of the Endocrine Society, Abstract No. 80 (1967).

8. Katz, F.H. and Shannon, I.L.: Parotid fluid cortisol and cortisone. In preparation.

9. Peterson, R.E., Nokes , G., Chen, P.S. and Black, R.L.: Estrogens and adrenocortical function in man. J. Clin. Endocrin. Metab. 20:495 (1960).

10. Cope, C.L. and Black, E.: The hydrocortisone production in late pregnancy. J. Obstet. Gynec. Brit. Emp. 66:404 (1959).

11. Migeon, C.J., Kenny, F.M. and Taylor, F.H.: Cortisol production rate. VIII. Pregnancy. J. Clin. Endocrin. Metab. 28:661 (1968).

12. Layne, D.S., Meyer, C.J., Vaishwanar, P.S. and Pincus, G.:
The secretion and metabolism of cortisol and aldosterone in normal
and in steroid treated women. J. Clin. Endocr. Metab. 22:107 (1962).

13. Gray, M.J., Strausfeld, K.S., Watanabe, M., Sims, E.A.H.
and Solomon, S.: Aldosterone secretory rates in the normal menstrual cycle. J. Clin. Endocrin. Metab. 28:1269 (1968).

14. Watanabe, M., Meeker, I., Gray, M.J., Sims, E.A.H. and
Solomon, S.: Secretion rate of aldosterone in normal pregnancy.
J. Clin. Invest. 42:1619 (1963).

15. Crane, M.G., Heitsch, J., Harris, J.J. and Johns, V.J.:
Effect of ethinyl estradiol (Estinyl) on plasma renin activity.
J. Clin. Endocrin. Metab. 26:1403 (1966).

16. Brown, J.J., Davies, D.L., Doak, P.B., Lever, A.F. and
Robertson, J.I.S.: Serial estimation of plasma renin concentration
during pregnancy and after parturition. J. Endocrin. 35:373 (1966).

17. Landau, R.L. and Lugibihl, K.: Inhibition of the sodium-
retaining influence of aldosterone by progesterone. J. Clin.
Endocrin. Metab. 18:1237 (1958).

18. Landau, R.L. and Lugibihl, K.: The catabolic and natriuretic effects of progesterone in man. Recent Prog. Hormone Res.
17:249 (1961).

19. Laidlaw, J.C., Ruse, J.L. and Gornall, A.G.: The
influence of estrogen and progesterone on aldosterone excretion.
J. Clin. Endocrin. Metab. 22:161 (1962).

20. Kagawa, C.M. and Jacobs, R.S.: Action of testosterone in
blocking urinary electrolyte effects of desoxycorticosterone.
Proc. Soc. Exp. Biol. Med. 120:512 (1959).

21. Williamson, E.E.: Natriuretic action of certain
adrenocortical androgens. Steroids 6:365 (1965).

EFFECTS OF GONADAL HORMONES ON PLASMA RENIN ACTIVITY AND ALDOSTERONE EXCRETION RATE

M. G. Crane* and J. J. Harris

Department of Medicine, Loma Linda University
Loma Linda, California

We have reported elsewhere (1) that the administration of ethinyl estradiol increased plasma renin activity (PRA) and aldosterone excretion rate. We were led to make these observations because of the findings of a markedly increased PRA in a normal subject who was taking Orthonovum for contraceptive purposes. Her PRA decreased to normal after the oral contraceptive was discontinued.

In 1967 Helmer and Judson (2) observed elevated PRA in three of five subjects who had been given oral contraceptive pills (OCP). Laragh and associates (3) have also reported elevated PRA and renin substrate levels in hypertensive patients on oral contraceptives.

In this report, we present the effect of ethinyl estradiol (E.E.) and medroxyprogesterone acetate (M.P.A.) on PRA and aldosterone excretion rate in normal male and female subjects. We also describe the effect of three different oral contraceptives (Enovid-10, Orthonovum-10, or Provest) on PRA and aldosterone excretion rate in 15 normal female subjects.

METHODS AND MATERIALS

Observations of the effect of the drugs on PRA and aldosterone

---

These studies were supported by the following Grants in Aid from the National Institutes of Health of the USPHS: HE-11031, HE-04745, and FR-00276.

*Career Development Awardee K3-HE-7627 of the National Institutes of Health of the USPHS.

excretion rate were made under three different conditions as described below:

Condition (1) unrestricted sodium intake and supine overnight;
measurement of PRA and urinary aldosterone excretion rate.

Condition (2) after 72 hours of sodium restriction and supine
overnight; measurement of PRA and urinary aldosterone excretion
rate.

Condition (3) after 72 hours of sodium restriction and four
hours standing; measurement of PRA.

Plasma renin activity was quantitated by the method of Boucher
and associates (4) as modified by Cohen and associates (5). Urinary aldosterone excretion rate was measured by the double isotope
derivative method of Kliman and Peterson(6).

Ethinyl estradiol (Estinyl) was given in doses of 0.5 mg daily
for 21 days to 14 normal subjects (nine male and five female) without obvious endocrine disorders ranging in age from 23 to 38 years.
Seven subjects were given Estinyl that was six to seven years old
(older E.E.). Seven subjects were given Estinyl that had been
manufactured within the year of use (newer E.E.).

Five normal subjects (four male and one female) without known
endocrine disorders were given medroxyprogesterone acetate
(Provera). One subject received 10 mg daily and four received
20 mg daily in a single oral dose for 21 days.

A total of 15 normal normotensive female subjects ranging in
age from 21 to 44 years of age were given Enovid-10, Orthonovum-10,
or Provest for 21 days. Each medication was given to five different control subjects. Eight of the subjects had been taking oral
contraceptive pills for ten months or longer before the study.
Seven of the subjects had never taken oral contraceptives before.

The outline of study for the individual steroids was as follows:
When E.E. or M.P.A. was administered, the PRA and urinary aldosterone
excretion rate measurements were made under the three different
conditions mentioned above before and during the first and third
week of administration of the drug.

The outline of study for the oral contraceptives was as follows: The oral contraceptive pills were started on the fifth or
sixth day after the onset of menstruation. During the first and
third week of the administration of the oral contraceptive, PRA
and aldosterone excretion rate measurements were made under the
three conditions outlined above. The OCP was then discontinued;
and, during the time period three to seven days after the last
pill was taken, the third renin activity-aldosterone study was
made.

RESULTS

The results of PRA and aldosterone excretion rate under the condition of sodium restriction and supine overnight will not be presented in this report for the sake of brevity.

The average normal values for PRA in our laboratory for 36 normal subjects are as follows: With the subjects on a normal sodium intake and supine overnight, the mean value was 161 PRA units/100 ml plasma (±2 S.D. 30-310). After the subjects had been on sodium restriction for three days and standing for four hours, the mean was 810 PRA units/100 ml plasma (±2 S.D. 310-1310).

The average values for aldosterone excretion rate of 29 normal subjects on unrestricted sodium intake was 10.4 μg/24 hrs (±2 S.D. 3.8-55.0).

The effects of ethinyl estradiol on PRA and aldosterone excretion rate are presented in Figures 1 to 4.

The effects of medroxyprogesterone acetate on PRA and aldosterone excretion rate are presented in Figures 5 to 8.

The effects of oral contraceptives on PRA and aldosterone excretion rate are presented in Figures 9 to 12.

DISCUSSION

The following general conclusions can be made from the preceeding results. Oral contraceptive pills caused as much as a two-fold average increase in plasma renin activity and aldosterone excretion rate. Not all subjects responded with an increase in PRA and aldosterone excretion rate. The subjects who had in the past been using OCP for contraceptive purposes responded more promptly and to a slightly greater degree to the course of OCP than did those who were taking contraceptive pills for the first time. The effect of the pills persisted in some of the subjects for at least one week after the last dose was given.

The administration of recently manufactured E.E. (in much larger doses than used in OCP) resulted in an increase in PRA and aldosterone excretion rate to about the same extent as that produced by the OCP in both the male and female subjects. We have also observed in four normal subjects that mestranol in doses equivalent to that of E.E. caused approximately a two-fold increase in PRA.

Medroxyprogesterone acetate in contrast with the estrogenic

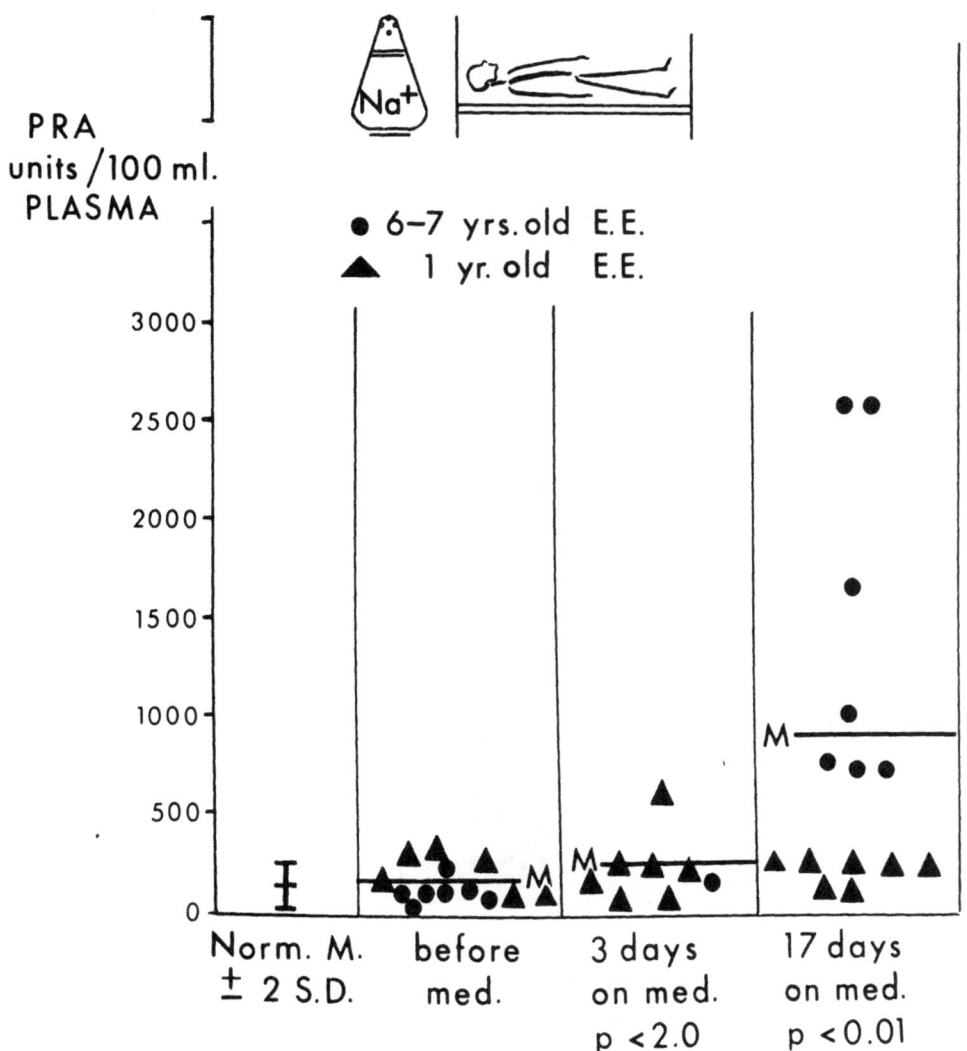

Figure 1 presents the results of the PRA studies in 14 subjects under the conditions of normal sodium intake and supine. (PRA measurements were not made in the first week on those subjects who were given the older E.E.) After three days on the medication, 1 out of 7 of the subjects had a PRA value greater than normal. After 18 days on the medication, none of those who were taking the newer E.E. had a PRA value above normal, however, all of those who were taking the older E.E. had values greater than normal. The average increase in PRA was significantly greater than that of normal subjects (p <0.01).

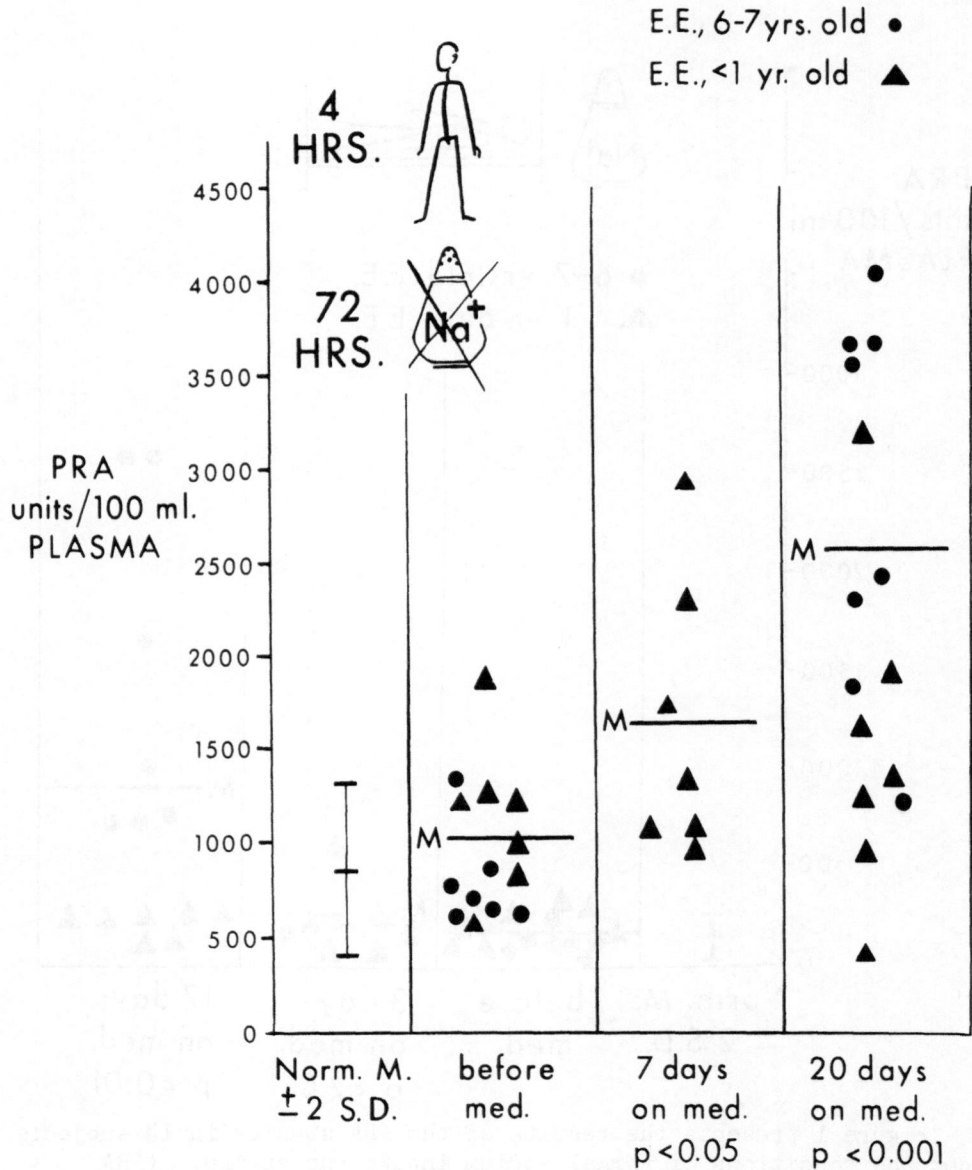

Figure 2 presents the results of PRA under the condition of sodium restriction and standing. After 7 days on the E.E., there was a 2-fold average increase in PRA under these conditions. The increase was significant only at $p < 0.05$ value when compared with the before E.E. value of the same individual, but was highly significant in comparison with the normal mean ($p < 0.001$). After 20 days on the E.E., there was a 2.9-fold average increase in PRA under these conditions. The increase was significant ($p < 0.001$) for those taking the newer as well as the older E.E. in comparison with the normal subjects.

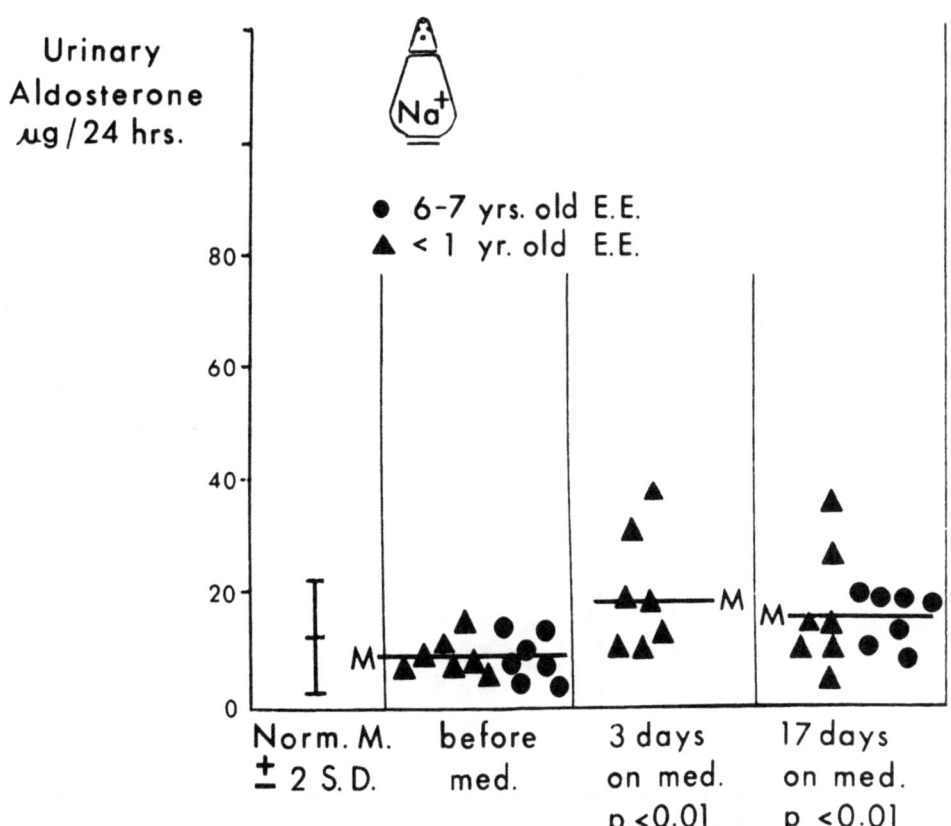

Figure 3 presents the results of E.E. on urinary aldosterone excretion rate under the conditions of unrestricted sodium intake. The average increase in aldosterone excretion rate in the first and third week of E.E. was 1.8 to 2.2-fold respectively. The mean increase on both occasions was significantly greater than the normal mean values (p <0.01).

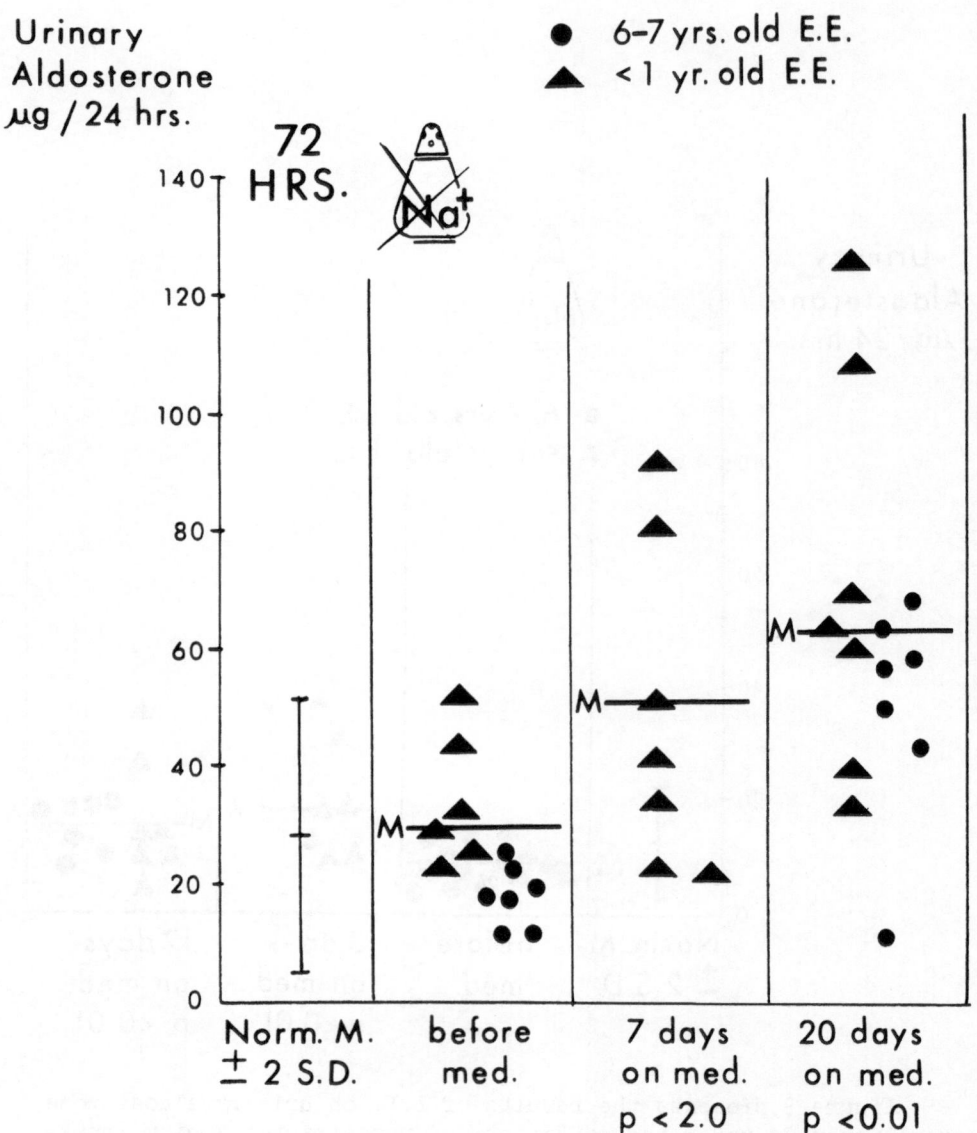

Figure 4 gives the results of the aldosterone excretion rate on Day-3 of sodium restriction before and during the first and third week of administration of E.E. The results show that the responsiveness to sodium restriction during the first week of E.E. administration was slightly increased, but not significantly greater than the values before medication. However, there was a significant, a 2-fold average, increase in aldosterone excretion rate in response to sodium restriction in the third week of administration of E.E. (p <.01).

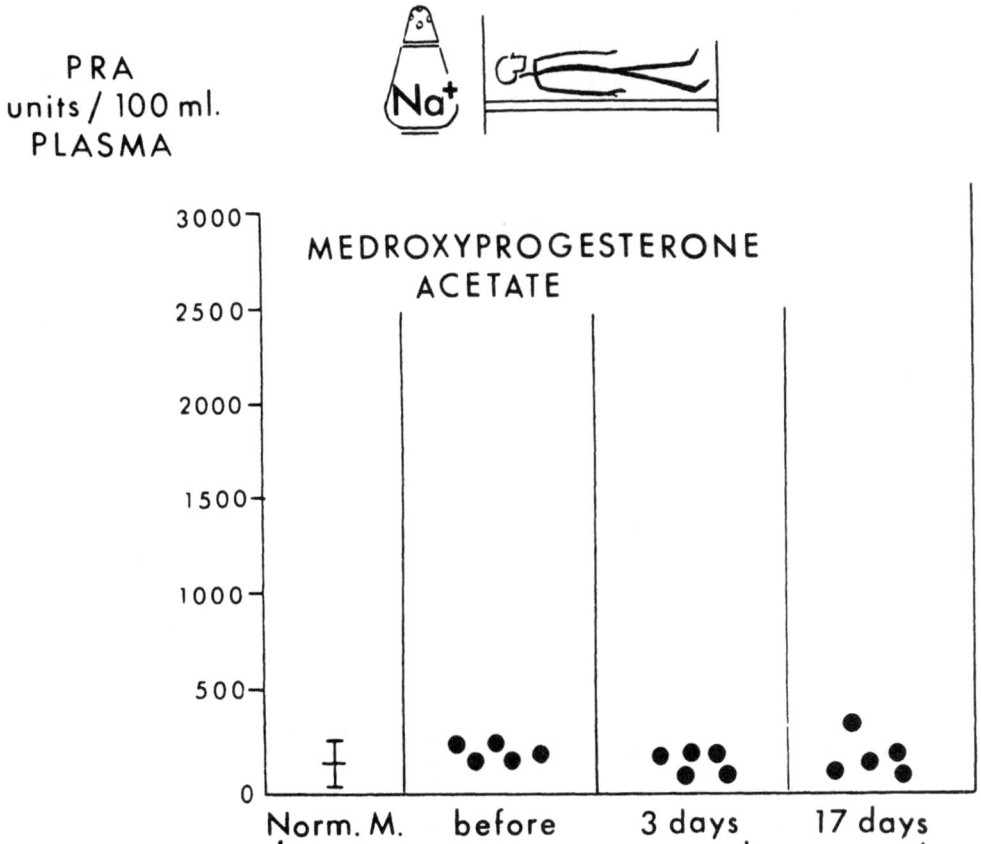

Figure 5 presents the results of the PRA obtained before and during the administration of M.P.A. with the subjects on a normal sodium intake and supine overnight. There was no essential difference in PRA under this condition during the first or third week of administration of the drug. All values were within 2 S.D. of the normal mean.

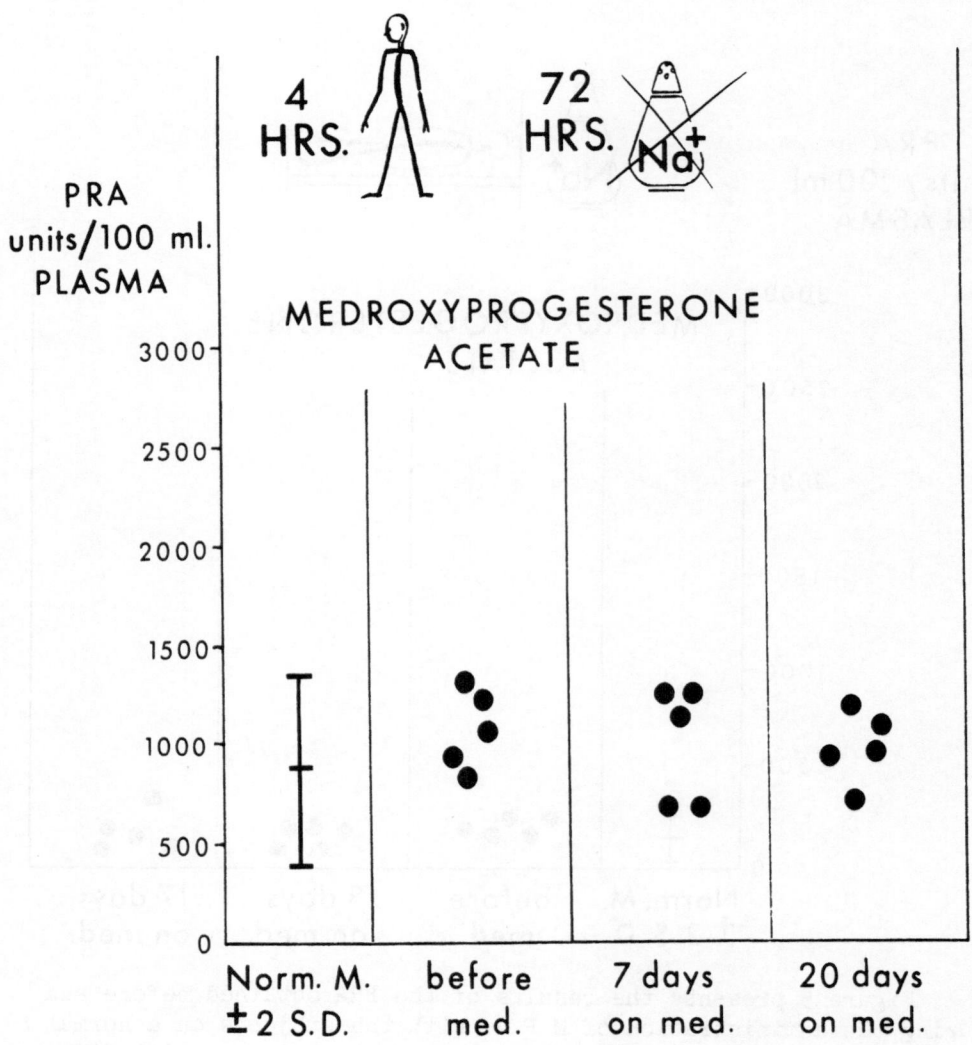

Figure 6 presents the results of PRA obtained before and during the administration of M.P.A. under the condition of sodium restriction and standing. The results show that there was no appreciable effect on PRA under this condition during the first and third week of administration of M.P.A.

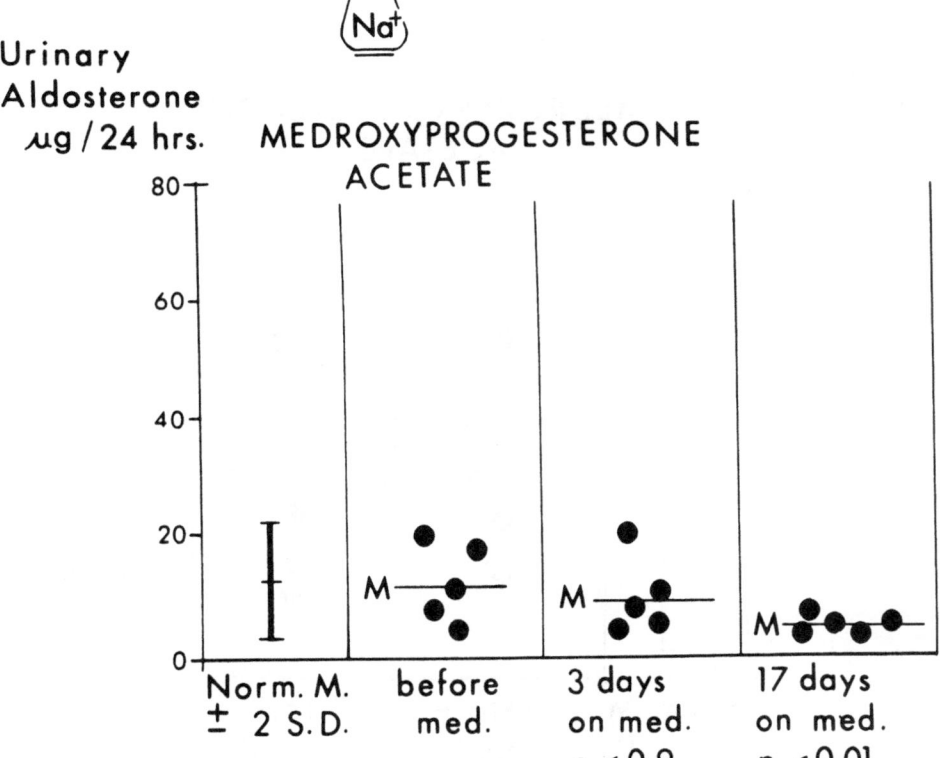

Figure 7 presents the results of the aldosterone excretion rate obtained when the subjects were on normal sodium intake before and during the administration of M.P.A. There was about a 50% decrease in aldosterone excretion rate in comparison with normal values in the third week of administration of medroxyprogesterone acetate. The average decrease was significant ($p < 0.01$).

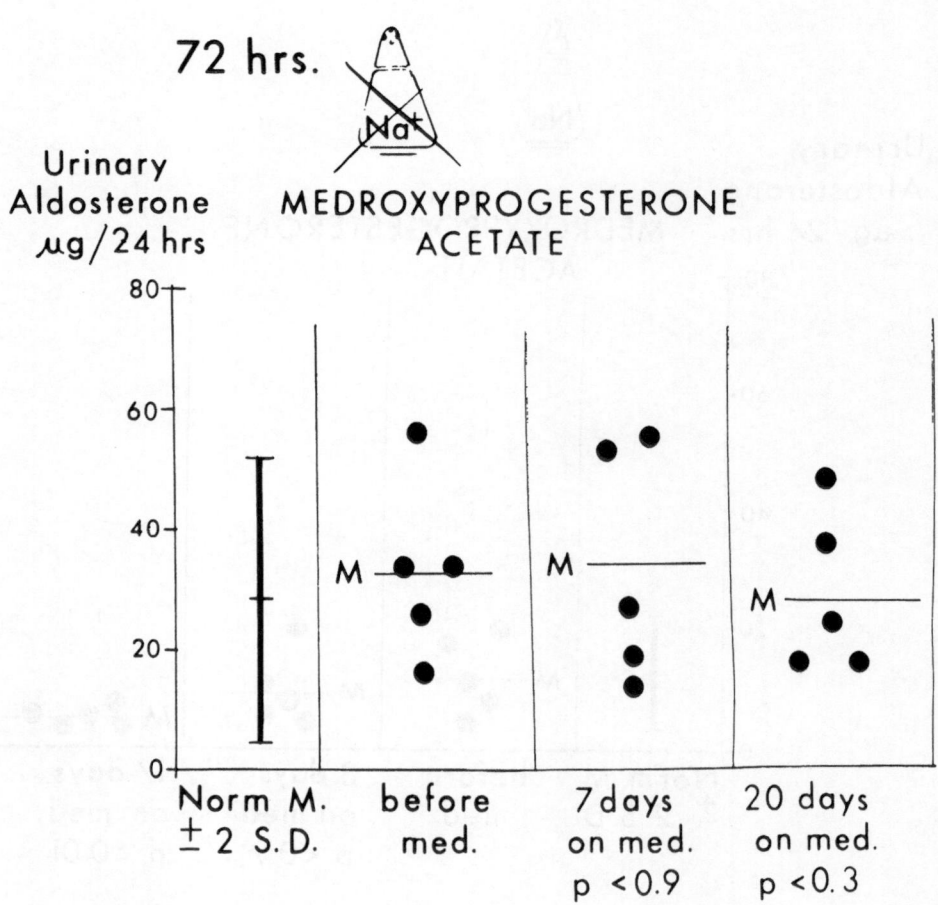

Figure 8 presents the results of the aldosterone excretion rates obtained on Day-3 of sodium restriction before and during the administration of M.P.A. There was essentially no difference in the aldosterone excretion rate in response to sodium restriction during the administration of M.P.A.

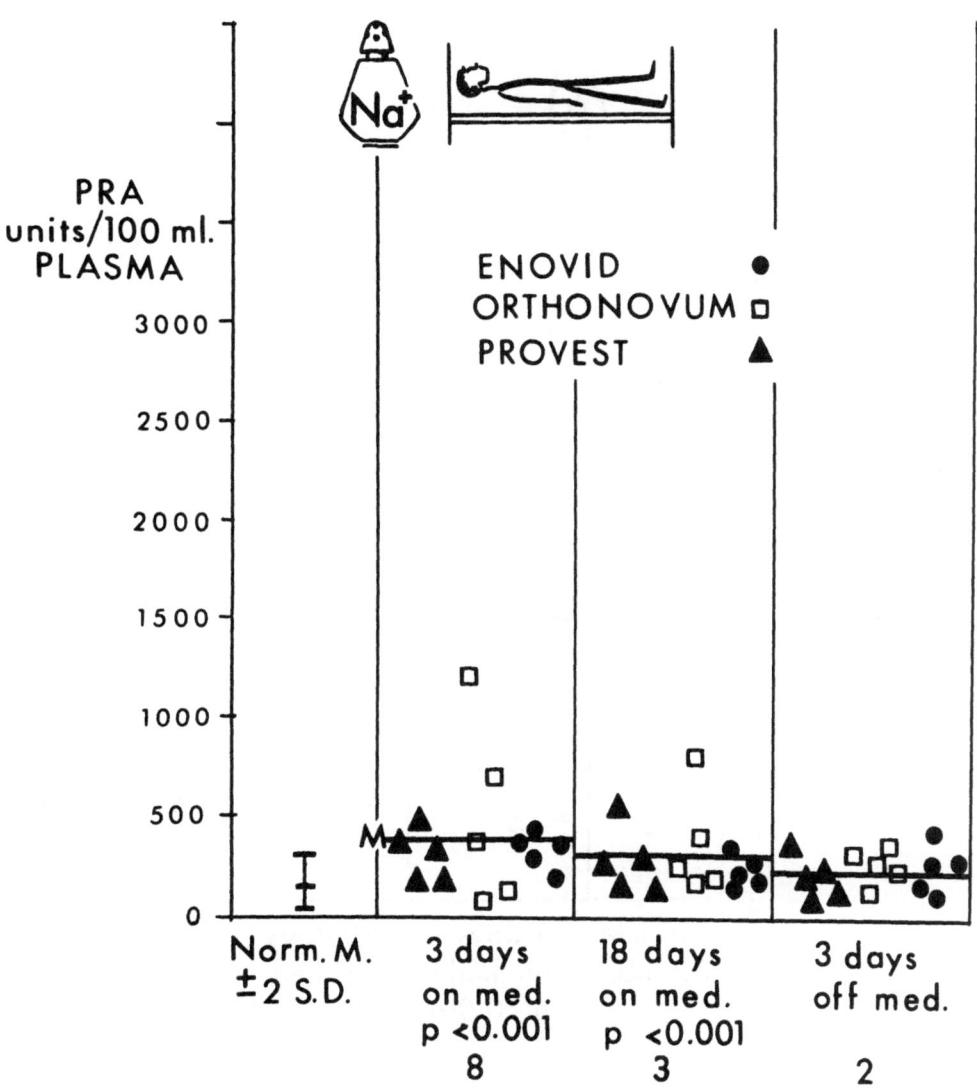

Figure 9 presents the values of PRA obtained during and after the administration of the three oral contraceptive pills with the subjects on normal sodium intake and supine overnight. Eight out of 15 values were greater than normal on the third day of administration of the oral contraceptive pill. There was an average increase in PRA of about 2.4-fold which was significant (p <0.001). After 18 days on the medication, 3 values were greater than normal. There was an average increase in PRA of 1.9-fold which was significant (p <0.001). During the three days off OCP, the PRA under this condition had returned to normal in all but 2 subjects.

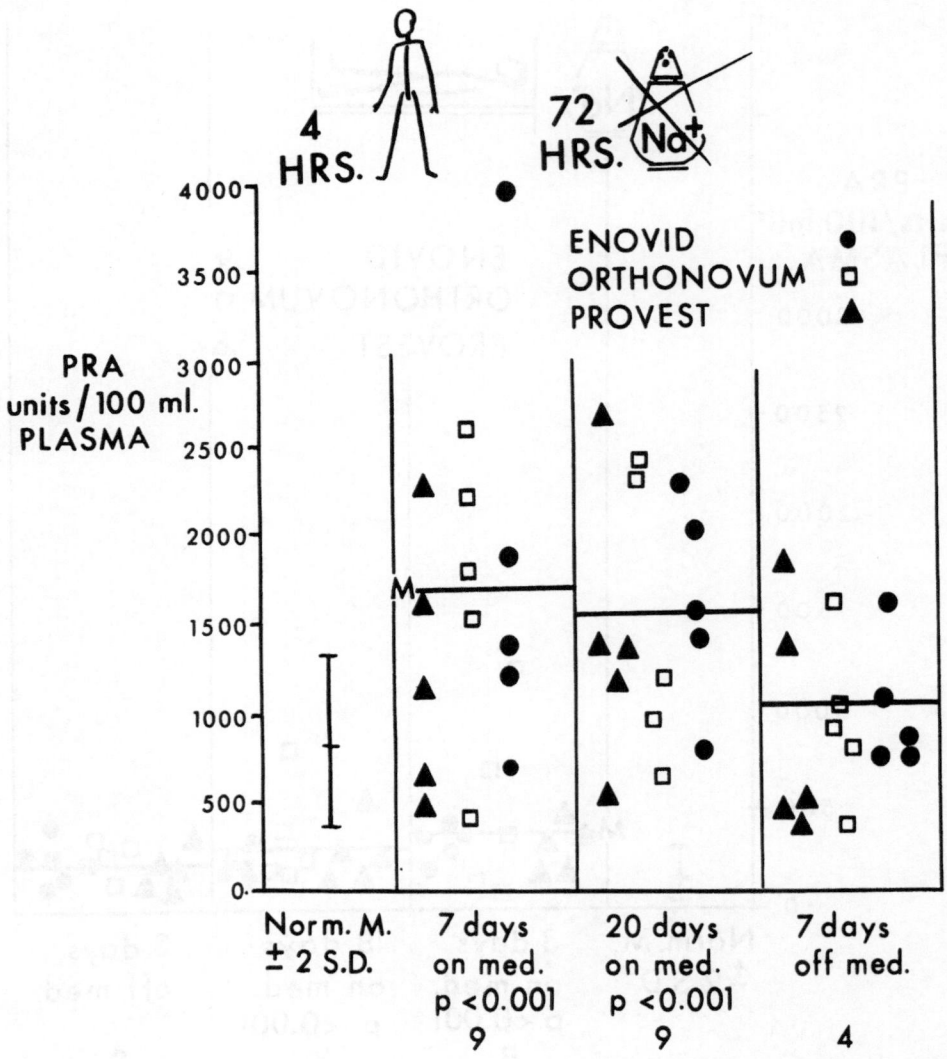

Figure 10 presents the values of PRA obtained during and after the administration of the OCP with the subjects under the condition of sodium restriction and standing. Nine of the 15 values on both the first and third week of administration of the oral contraceptives were greater than the normal range. On both occasions while on OCP, the PRA was significantly greater than normal and greater than the corresponding values obtained in the week after discontinuing the medication (p <0.001). Four of the subjects during the week off the OCP continued to have values which were above normal. One of these continued to have above normal PRA for 3 weeks after discontinuing the OCP. Three of these 4 were studied 3 to 6 months after discontinuing the medication, and all three were then found to be within normal limits.

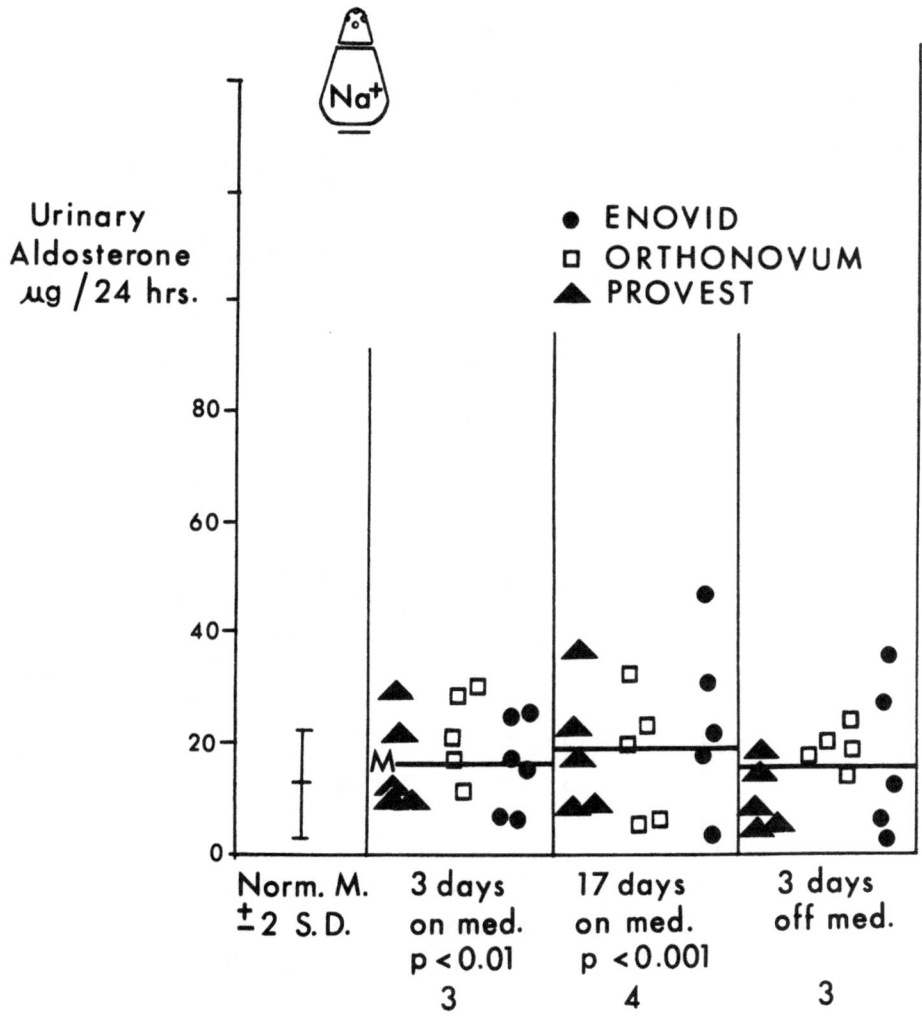

Figure 11 presents the results of the aldosterone excretion rate obtained during and after the OCP with the subjects on unrestricted sodium intake. After three days on the OCP, there was a 1.5-fold average increase in aldosterone excretion rate which was significant in comparison with the normal mean (p <0.01). After the subjects had been on the contraceptive for three weeks, there was a 1.9-fold average increase in the aldosterone excretion rate which was significant (p <0.001). After the medication was discontinued, the urinary aldosterone excretion rates were greater than normal in 3 of the 15 subjects. However, the average aldosterone value was not significantly elevated (p <0.05).

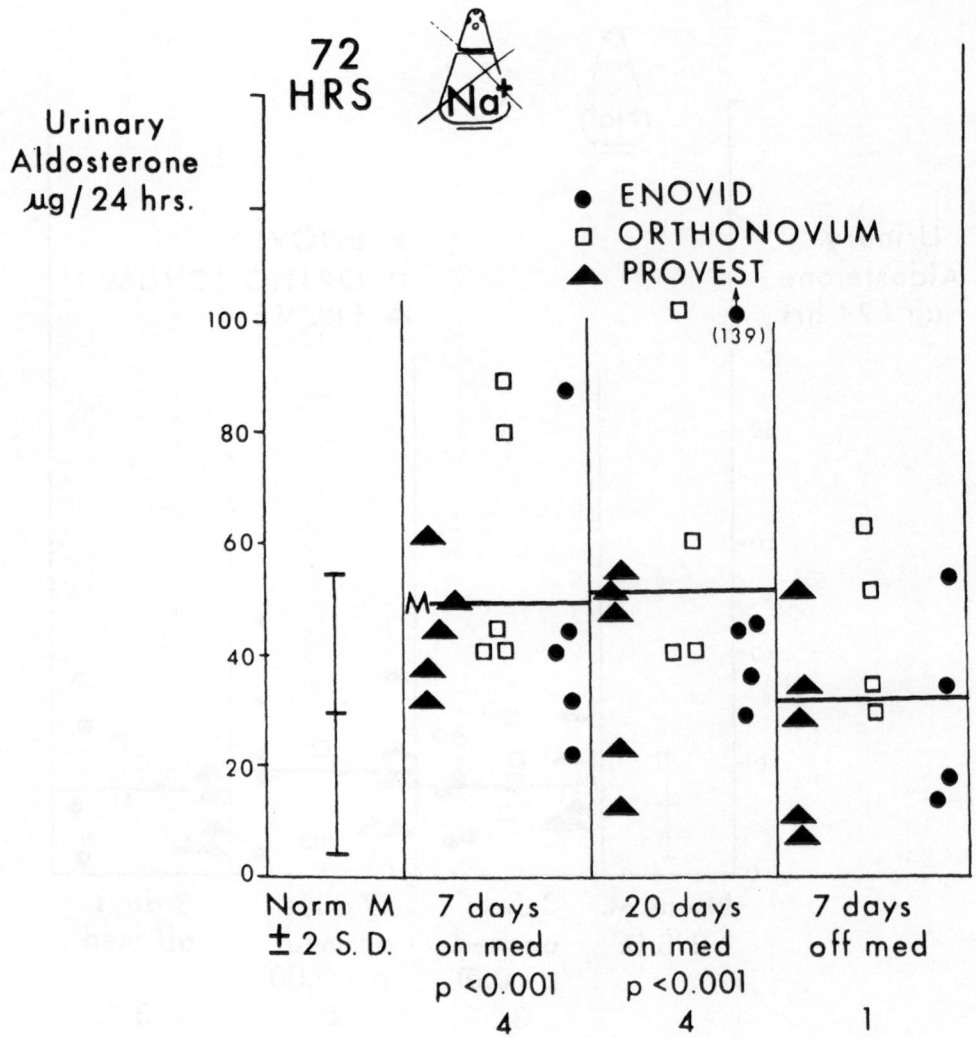

Figure 12 presents the effect of OCP on aldosterone excretion rate obtained in response to three days of sodium restriction. On both the 7th and 20th day of administration of the contraceptive pills, four values for aldosterone excretion rate were greater than the upper limits of normal. The average aldosterone excretion was significantly increased on both occasions in comparison with the aldosterone excretion rate of normal subjects (p <0.001) and with those observed in the same subjects on the 7th day after the OCP had been discontinued.

steroids caused a 50% decrease in aldosterone excretion rate but without causing a detectable effect on PRA under the conditions studied.

Laidlaw and associates (7) have reported that the administration of estrogens caused a slight increase in aldosterone excretion rate, but their values during estrogens were still within normal range. Layne and associates (8) found that OCP or estrogen alone increased both the secretion rate and excretion rate of aldosterone. They also observed that the amount of aldosterone excreted as a glucuronide was less during the adminstration of estrogens indicating that estrogens changed the metabolism of aldosterone.

Several authors (2,3,9) have found a two- to four-fold increase in renin substrate in response to estrogen administration. Time does not permit a presentation of data on renin substrate, but we have observed an increase in renin substrate in all subjects given OCP. There was a two and a half to three-fold average increase in renin substrate. The effect of the OCP on the substrate persisted into the week after they were discontinued. Helmer and Judson (2) have presented evidence indicating that an increase in substrate, such as that seen during OCP administration, could account for the increase in PRA without an increase in renin.

Progesterone has been found to cause sodium diuresis and an increase in aldosterone excretion rate, the so-called "anti-aldosterone" effect of progesterone. Our findings of a decrease in aldosterone excretion rate during medroxyprogesterone acetate administration would appear to contradict that. However, the work of Chagoya and associates (10) indicates that synthetic progestational compounds may not have anti-aldosterone properties. Landau and associates (11) stated in 1958 that progestational compounds with an α side chain at carbon-17 did not have anti-aldosterone effects, but instead caused sodium retention. We would interpret the decrease in aldosterone excretion rate that we observed during the administration of medroxyprogesterone acetate to indicate that there was sodium retention with expansion of extracellular volume. However, it remains to be determined whether or not this was the mechanism by which the aldosterone excretion rate was suppressed.

The most important issue to us seems to be this: Are these effects on PRA and aldosterone metabolism a major factor in the etiology of the hypertension that has been reported (3,12) to occur in some women on the pills? We have studied 18 women who developed hypertension after starting OCP. Eleven of these women have become normotensive since discontinuing the OCP. We hope to discuss this further, later on in the program.

REFERENCES

1. Crane, M.G., Heitsch, J., Harris, J., and Johns, V.J., Jr.: Effect of ethinyl estradiol (Estinyl) on plasma renin activity. J. Clin. Endocr. 26:1403 (1966).

2. Helmer, O.M., and Judson, W.E.: Influence of high renin substrate levels on renin-angiotensin system in pregnancy. Amer. J. Obstet. Gynec. 99:9-17 (1967).

3. Laragh, J.H., Sealey, J.E., Ledingham, J.G.G., and Newton, M.A.: Oral contraceptives, renin, aldosterone and high blood pressure. J.A.M.A. 201:918-922 (1967).

4. Boucher, R., Veyrat, R., de Champlain, J., and Genest, J.: New procedures for measurement of human plasma angiotensin renin activity levels. Canad. Med. Ass. J. 90:194 (1964).

5. Cohen, E.L., Conn, J.W., and Rovener, D.R.: Postural augmentation of plasma renin activity and aldosterone excretion in normal people. J. Clin. Invest. 46:418 (1967).

6. Kliman, B., and Peterson, R.E.: Double isotope derivative assay of aldosterone in biological extracts. J. Biol. Chem. 235:1639 (1960).

7. Laidlaw, J.C., Ruse, J.L., and Gornall, A.G.: The influence of estrogen and progesterone on aldosterone excretion. J. Clin. Endocr. 22:161 (1962).

8. Layne, D.S., Meyer, C.J., Vaishwanar, P.S., and Pincus, G.: The secretion and metabolism of cortisol and aldosterone in normal and in steroid treated women. J. Clin. Endocr. 22:107 (1962).

9. Helmer, O.M., and Griffith, R.S.: The effect of the administration of estrogens on the renin-substrate (hypertensinogen) content of rat plasma. Endocrinology 51:421 (1952).

10. Chagoya, L., Nurko, B., Santos, E., and A. Rivera: 6-chloro, 6-dehydro, 17 α-acetoxyprogesterone: its possible action as an aldosterone antagonist. J. Clin. Endocr. 21:1364 (1961).

11. Landau, R.L., Lugibihl, K., and Dimick, D.F.: Metabolic effects in man of steroids with progestational activity. Ann. New York Acad. Sc. 71:588 (1958).

12. Weinberger, M.H., Dowdy, A.J., Nokes, G.W., and Luetscher, J.A.: Reversible increases in plasma renin activity, aldosterone secretion, and blood pressure in women taking oral contraceptive preparations. Clin. Res. 16:150 (1968).

PROPERTIES AND ORIGIN OF UTERINE RENIN

P.J. Mulrow, T.F. Ferris, P. Gordon, R.C. Anderson and
P.N. Herbert

Department of Internal Medicine, Yale University School
of Medicine, New Haven, Connecticut

For many years, renin has been considered to be an enzyme
that is synthesized and stored in the juxtaglomerular apparatus of
the kidney. Recently, substantial quantities of renin have been
extracted from the salivary gland of the white mouse and from the
pregnant rabbit uterus and placenta (1-3). In view of the recent
reports of high concentrations of renin in the plasma and amniotic
fluid of pregnant women, this finding takes on special significance
(4,5). The present report summarizes some of our studies on rabbit
uterine renin that have been published in more detail elsewhere
(6-8).

The pressor substance isolated from rabbit uterus has several
characteristics of renin. It is acid stable, heat labile, non-
dialyzable and ammonium sulfate precipitable. It produces a renin-
like pressor curve when injected into the rat, rabbit or dog and
is inactivated by incubation with renin antibodies. On incubation
with renin-substrate, it produces a pressor material similar to
synthetic angiotensin II. Uterine and kidney renin have optimum
activity at approximately pH 6; the enzymes are identical with
respect to mobility on disc electrophoresis and molecular weights
determined by gel filtration are approximately the same, 45,000
(Figs. 1,2). Although a small reproducible difference between the
apparent Km values of the two enzymes can be demonstrated, most of
the evidence indicates the enzymes are very similar if not
identical.

The concentration of renin in the pregnant uterus of the
rabbit is greater than in the non-pregnant uterus and is equal to
that of the whole kidney, but because of the greater weight of the
pregnant uterus, it is a greater potential source of renin than

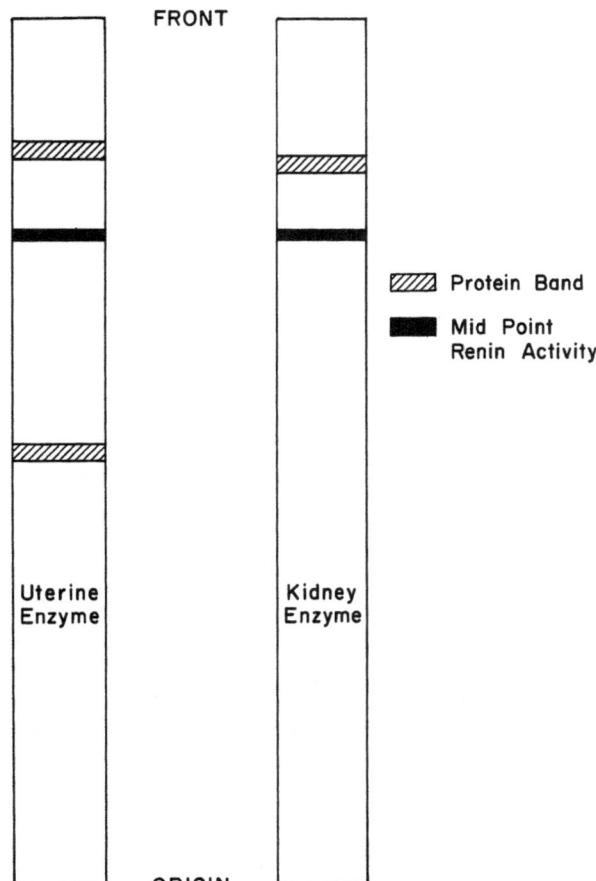

Figure 1. "Disc electrophoresis patterns. The drawing
indicates the position of the major protein bands and the location
of the renin enzymatic activity after electrophoresis of 0.1 ml.
enzyme preparation. Electrophoresis was conducted with Tris-
glycine buffer pH 8, at 5 ma/sample at room temperature".
(Anderson, R.C., Herbert, P.N. and Mulrow, P.J. Am. J. Physiol.
215:777, 1968.)

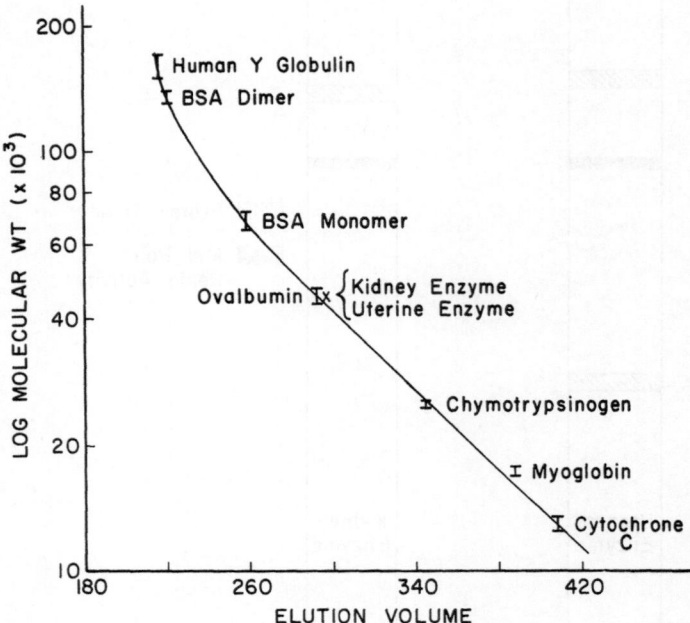

Figure 2. "Average elution volume as a function of log
molecular weight. Reference proteins and enzyme solutions were
applied to a 2.5 x 100 cm. column Sephadex G-100 in volume of 2 ml.
Sodium phosphate buffer (0.1 M, pH 6) was used for elution.
Reference proteins were located by OD measurements. Renin activity was located by incubation of aliquots of eluate with renin
substrate. Each point is an average of more than two determinations. The height of the bars represents the range of molecular
weights reported in the literature for the reference proteins.
The elution volume of the kidney and uterine enzyme is indicated
by X". (Anderson, R.C., Herbert, P.N. and Mulrow, P.J. Am. J.
Physiol. 215:777, 1968.)

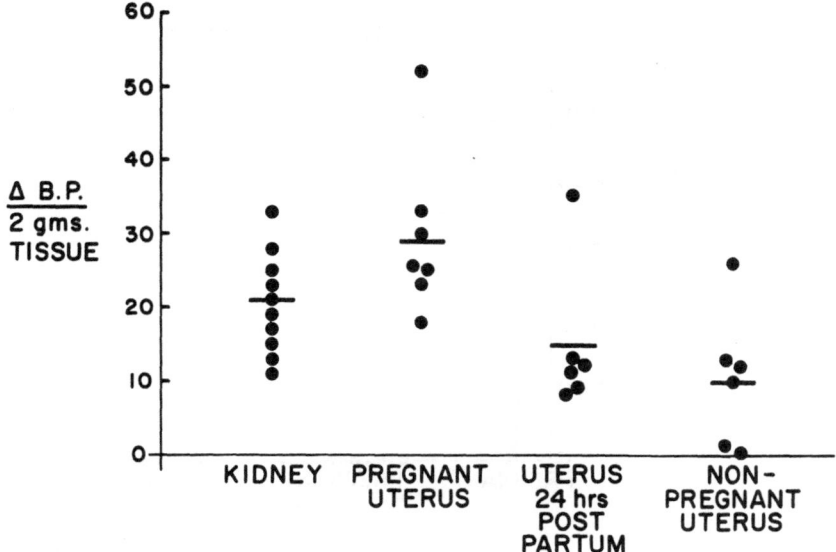

Figure 3. "Pressor activity in kidney and uterine extracts". (Ferris, T.F., Gorden, P. and Mulrow, P.J. Am. J. Physiol. 212: 701, 1967.)

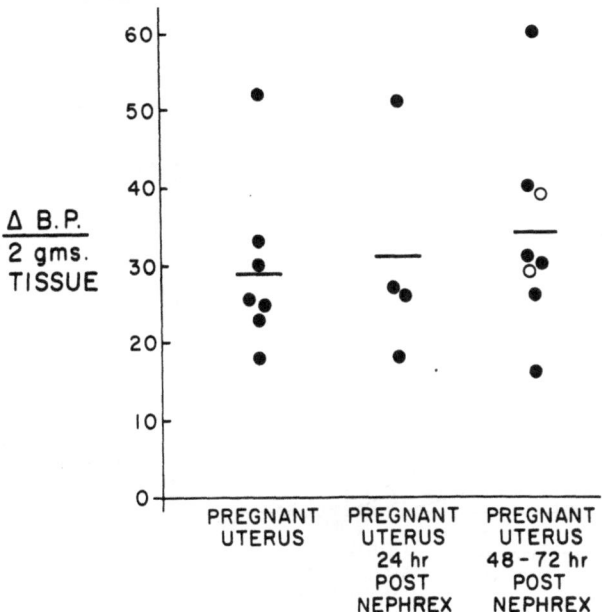

Figure 4. "Effect of nephrectomy on uterine renin concentration. Open circles represent extracts obtained from animals 72 hours postnephrectomy". (Gorden, P., Ferris, T.F. and Mulrow, P.J. Am. J. Physiol. 212:704, 1967.)

PLASMA RENIN ACTIVITY IN RABBITS

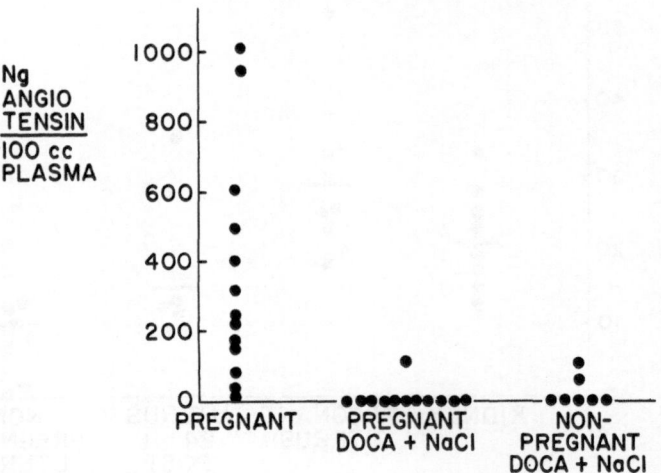

Figure 5. "Comparison of plasma renin activity in DOCA-treated pregnant and non-pregnant animals". (Gorden, P., Ferris, T.F. and Mulrow, P.J. Am. J. Physiol. 212:704, 1967.)

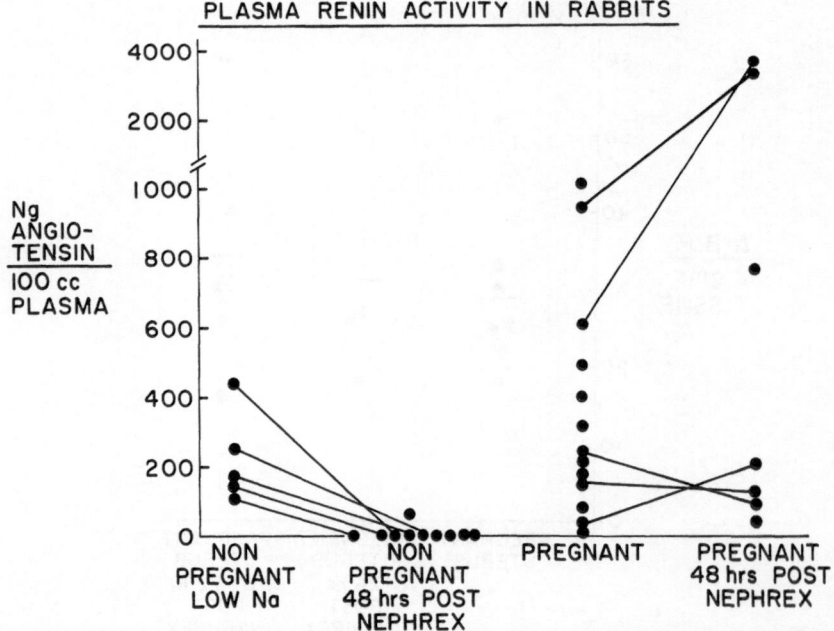

Figure 6. "Effect of nephrectomy on plasma renin activity in the non-pregnant and pregnant animal. Lines connect values obtained from the same animal. Low Na indicates the rabbits were on a sodium deficient diet". (Gorden, P., Ferris, T.F. and Mulrow, P.J. Am. J. Physiol. 212:704, 1967.)

both kidneys (Fig. 3). The presence of large quantities of renin
in the rabbit uterus raises the question of the source of this
material. It was found that administration of desoxycorticosterone
acetate (DOCA) and salt to pregnant rabbits has no effect on the
concentration of uterine renin whereas plasma and renal renin are
markedly reduced; nephrectomy for as long as 72 hours does not
diminish uterine renin (Fig. 4). Although renin derived from the
kidney appears to be the source of plasma renin activity in the
pregnant rabbit (Fig. 5), uterine renin can also contribute to
plasma renin activity (Fig. 6) when the kidneys are removed, suggesting that under certain circumstances renin may leak out of the
uterus into the plasma. Whether this leakage occurs in conditions
other than uremia remains to be elucidated.

The findings suggest that the uterus is a site of renin synthesis. Studies by Bing and Eskildsen (9) showed that oophorectomy
diminished uterine renin while estradiol treatment increased the
renin content without altering the kidney content thus supporting
the concept that the uterus is a site of renin synthesis. Finally,
more direct proof of uterine synthesis of renin was presented by
Symonds and colleagues. They demonstrated the production of renin
by in vitro cultures of human chorion and uterine muscle and this
production continued after several sub-cultures (10).

The physiological role of uterine renin remains an enigma.

REFERENCES

1. Bing, J. and Faarup, P.: Location of renin (or a renin-
like substance) in the submaxillary glands of albino mice. Acta
Path. Microbiol. Scand. 65:203-212 (1965).

2. Bing, J. and Faarup, P.: Location and site of formation
of extrarenal renin. in International Club on Arterial
Hypertension, L'Expansion Scientifique Francaise, Paris, 1966,
p. 75-80.

3. Gross, F., Schaechtelin, G., Ziegler, M. and Berger, M.:
A renin-like substance in the placenta and uterus of the rabbit.
Lancet 1:914-916 (1964).

4. Brown, J.J., Davies, D.L., Doak, P.B., Lever, A.F. and
Robertson, J.I.S.: Plasma renin in normal pregnancy. Lancet ii:
900-901 (1963).

5. Brown, J.J., Davies, D.L., Doak, P.B., Lever, A.F. and
Robertson, J.I.S.: The presence of renin in human amniotic fluid.
Lancet ii:64-66 (1964).

6. Ferris, T.F., Gorden, P., and Mulrow, P.J.: Rabbit uterus as a source of renin. Am. J. Physiol. 212:698-703 (1967).

7. Gorden, P., Ferris, T.F. and Mulrow, P.J.: Rabbit uterus as a possible site of renin synthesis. Am. J. Physiol. 212:703-706 (1967).

8. Anderson, R.C., Herbert, P.N. and Mulrow, P.J.: A comparison of properties of renin obtained from the kidney and uterus of the rabbit. Am. J. Physiol. 215:774-778 (1968).

9. Bing, J. and Eskildsen, P.C.: Influence of estradiol on uterine renin in rabbits. Acta Path. Microbiol. Scand. 72:237-243 (1968).

10. Symonds, E.M., Stanley, M.A. and Skinner, S.L.: Production of renin by in vitro cultures of human chorion and uterine muscle. Nature 217:1152-1153 (1968).

INTERRELATIONSHIPS OF ORAL CONTRACEPTIVES AND HYPERTENSION

James W. Woods

Department of Medicine, University of North Carolina
School of Medicine, Chapel Hill, North Carolina

The large, carefully controlled, prospective studies needed to
define the association between oral contraceptives and hypertension
have not been published and the information to date is largely
anecdotal. That there is an association, however, appears to be
widely accepted among practicing physicians. To our knowledge,
only the 29 cases listed in Table 1 have been reported.

Brownrigg's patient (1) had repeatedly observed blood pressures
of 120/80 over several years, including two pregnancies, until 1961
when Enovid in maximum dosage was begun for the treatment of
endometriosis. Six months later she was seen because of severe
headaches and a 10 pound weight gain. Blood pressure was 200/110
mmHg and there was 1+ proteinuria but no edema. An intravenous
pyelogram was normal. One month after discontinuance of Enovid,
blood pressure, urinalysis and weight had returned to normal and
continued so over the next three months of follow-up. Brownrigg
felt that the acute hypertension occurring in this patient was
"strikingly similar to that which occurs in the more severe toxemia of
pregnancy."

Owen's case (2) was reported in a letter to an editor and had
had an elevation of pressure to a maximum of 160/80 mmHg during
the seventh month of her third pregnancy but her condition had been
normal in all other respects. Enovid was started after delivery.
She returned two months later with headaches and visual disturbances.
Blood pressure was 210/115 mmHg and the urine was negative. A few
weeks after the drug was stopped, headaches had ceased and blood
pressure had fallen to 140/80 mmHg. At this time, she complained
of dysuria and further examination revealed a urinary tract infection. This was treated with antibiotics. On subsequent visits,

Table 1
Association of Oral Contraceptives and Elevated Blood Pressure

Authors	No. of cases	Pre-existing hypertension	Residual hypertension
Brownrigg, 1962[1]	1	0	0
Owen, 1966[2]	1	1	0
Laragh et al, 1967[3]	8	2	4
Woods, 1967[4]	6	3	3
Weinberger et al, 1968[5]	6	2	4
Tyson, 1968[6]	7	0	0
Total	29	8	11

blood pressure ranged between 130/70 and 140/80 and the urine remained clear. In a letter of reply, the Medical Director of G. D. Searle and Company stated that the reported incidence of hypertension in women taking oral contraceptives parallels that in the untreated female population at risk but postulated that some patients particularly likely to develop pre-eclampsia might have an elevation of blood pressure while taking preparations containing estrogen.

Tyson's investigation (6) is of particular interest in that it was a prospective analysis of the blood pressure response in 45 normotensive women receiving Ovulen for varying periods up to eight months. Seven patients or 15.5 percent developed blood pressure elevations above the age-adjusted normal values given in life insurance tables. However, only three or 6.6 percent developed frank hypertension with pressures of 166/104, 146/100 and 130/110 mmHg. Most elevations occurred after the second treatment cycle. The blood pressures of the seven patients returned to normal levels within 30 days of discontinuing the medication. No abnormal blood pressure elevations were observed in 120 women of comparable age who were followed simultaneously in the same clinic in whom the Margulies' intrauterine device was used.

Of the 29 cases listed in Table 1, about a fourth had known pre-existing hypertension which appeared to be aggravated by oral contraceptives and a third had continuing hypertension after discontinuance of the medication. It is impossible to exclude the possibility that others might have had mild labile unrecognized hypertension. It seems clear, however, that some of these patients advanced from a state of normotension to relatively severe hypertention in association with exhibition of oral contraceptives and then reverted to normotensive levels with its discontinuance. In two of Laragh's patients and in one of ours, hypertension was first noted after institution of the drug, improved after cessation, reappeared with resumption of therapy, and again disappeared after

terminating the treatment. An attempt was made to determine
whether there was a correlation between weight and blood pressure
fluctations in these reported patients, but the data were insufficient for this.

If oral contraceptives intensify or precipitate hypertension
in certain susceptible women, by what mechanism might this occur?
The following possibilities are suggested:

1. A direct pressor effect of angiotensin. An increase in
endogenous plasma-renin activity, in renin-substrate concentration,
and in its reactivity to exogenous renin by oral contraceptives
have been found. These increases could exert an important
accelerating influence on the rate of production of angiotensin,
the most powerful pressor substance known.

2. A failure to "escape" from the sodium-retaining effect of
estrogen and/or aldosterone.

Should this hypothesis be confirmed, an explanation for
failure of "escape" and the accumulation of excessive amounts of
salt and water in a minority of women taking oral contraceptives
would be necessary. One explanation might be the presence of pre-
existing renal disease in the form of pyelonephritis, diabetic
nephropathy or nephrosclerosis.

By analogy, pre-eclampsia appears more frequently in the
presence of renal disease, especially chronic nephritis. In
desoxycorticosterone and adrenal regeneration hypertension in rats,
the removal of one kidney or the induction of Masugi nephritis
aggravates the hypertension. Women with diabetes have a higher than
normal incidence of pre-eclampsia and the hypertension which follows
the unilateral wrapping of a rat's kidney is markedly enhanced in
diabetic rats. Perera and Blood (7) found that desoxycorticosterone
produces a rise in blood pressure in subjects with essential hypertension but rarely does so in normotensive individuals.

We studied the effect of oral contraceptives on experimental
hypertension in our laboratory by administering parenteral Enovid
chronically to rats in which one kidney had been removed and the
remaining kidney constricted by a figure-of-eight ligature. Neither
intensification of hypertension nor abnormal weight gain occurred.
They were not given hypertonic saline to drink as is done in the
production of desoxycorticosterone-hypertension in rats and this
might have been important.

In regard to pyelonephritis, the sequence of events in one of
our patients is worthy of mention. This was a 45 year old housewife
with no prior history of hypertension or renal disease. There had
been 4 uneventful pregnancies. In 1963 she was started on an oral

contraceptive. In 1965, she was referred for evaluation of recently
discovered hypertension and severe headaches with diastolic
pressures consistently over 110 mmHg. Asymptomatic bacteruria and
radiological changes suggestive of pyelonephritis in the left kidney
were found. BUN was 29 mg%. There was no edema. Significant
bacteruria disappeared with antibiotic therapy but symptomatic
urinary tract infection recurred in 1967. Birth control pills were
discontinued in April 1966, and over the next few months a 23
pound weight loss occurred and blood pressure fell to 110/70. It
has continued to remain at normal levels to the present time.

Since pyelonephritis has a striking predilection for young
females, since the disease is often asymptomatic, and since it is
notoriously difficult to diagnose, could pyelonephritis be an underlying common denominator? Observations of Mills (8) might lend
tangential support to this speculation. He described three women
who had no signs of heart disease, had never before had edema, were
not hypertensive and had normal values for endogenous creatinine
clearance. They all had in common a history of recurrent urinary
infection, and based on urinary white cell excretion in response to
the administration of pyrogen, were thought to have chronic pyelonephritis. They were unable to escape from the effects of
9α-fluorohydrocortisone, became edematous and developed signs of
congestive heart failure. Mills felt that his patients resembled
those with acute nephritis in showing a raised venous pressure, an
altered Valsalva response and generalized edema involving the face.
They did not become hypertensive which may have been a function
of the rapidity of fluid retention. He was unable to explain these
findings but postulated that the response of the juxtaglomerular
apparatus might have been disturbed by the recurrent urinary infection. It is very difficult to understand the fluid retention in
these patients in the presence of normal creatinine clearance.

Only further investigation can prove whether these speculative
concepts have merit. I suspect that the hypotheses advanced are
far too simple and that the pathogenetic mechanisms involved will
prove to be much more complex. Nevertheless, it would seem that
the apparent interrelationship of oral contraceptives and hypertension offers a very valuable clue and experimental model by which
understanding of etiopathic mechanisms in hypertension, and perhaps
toxemia of pregnancy can be advanced. Carefully controlled studies
of sodium metabolism, blood pressure response and the renin-
aldosterone mechanism during exhibition of the "pill" in women
shown to have appearance or aggravation of hypertension with its
use, in men and women with various degrees of renal impairment and
in women prior to and after removal of the kidneys in anticipation
of renal transplantation are suggested as possible approaches.

REFERENCES

1. Brownrigg, G. M.: Toxemia in hormone-induced pseudopregnancy.
   Canad. Med. Ass. J. 87:408-409 (1962).

2. Owen, G.: Hypertension associated with oral contraceptives.
   Canad. Med. Ass. J. 95:167 (1966).

3. Laragh, J. H., Sealey, J. E., Ledingham, J. G. G. and Newton,
   M. A.: Oral contraceptives. Renin, aldosterone, and high
   blood pressure. J.A.M.A. 201:918-922 (1967).

4. Woods, J. W.: Oral contraceptives and hypertension. The Lancet
   II:653-654 (1967).

5. Weinberger, M. H., Dowdy, A. J., Nokes, G. W. and Luetscher,
   J. A.: Reversible increases in plasma renin activity,
   aldosterone secretion, and blood pressure in women taking oral
   contraceptive preparations. Clin. Res. 16:150 (1968).

6. Tyson, J. E. A.: Oral contraception and elevated blood pressure.
   Amer. J. Obs. Gynec. 100:875-876 (1968).

7. Perera, G. A. and Blood, D. W.: Pressor activity of desoxycorticosterone acetate in normotensive and hypertensive subjects.
   Ann. Intern. Med. 27:401-404 (1947).

8. Mills, I. H.: Sodium retaining steroids in non-oedematous
   patients. Production of oedema and heart failure. The Lancet
   I:1264-1267 (1962).

CLINICAL COURSE AND LABORATORY DATA IN HYPERTENSION

ASSOCIATED WITH ORAL CONTRACEPTIVES

J.A. Luetscher, M.H. Weinberger, A.J. Dowdy and
G.W. Nokes
Department of Medicine, Stanford Medical Center,
Palo Alto, California

During the past two years, four reports have appeared,
indicating that hypertension occurs in some women taking estrogen-
gestagen combinations for control of conception or menstrual irreg-
ularities. Swaab (1) suggested that blood pressure could increase
markedly during the use of oral contraceptives. Laragh (2)
presented data on eleven patients with hypertension during contraceptive administration. In six of these patients, hypertension was
first noted after starting medication. Six of the eight patients
who stopped medication showed improvement or disappearance of the
hypertension. In two cases, hypertension reappeared when medication
was re-instituted. Woods (3) reported six patients with hypertension which was precipitated or aggravated by oral contraceptives.

Tyson (4) reported a prospective study of 51 women observed
before and during administration of ethynodiol diacetate 1 mg. and
mestranol 0.1 mg.. Among the 35 patients followed for five to
eight months, hypertension was present in two patients prior to
medication and remained unchanged. Seven others (15.5%) developed
an elevated blood pressure on medication. Blood pressure rose, in
most instances, after the second treatment cycle, and remained elevated from one to two months until medication was discontinued,

The work was supported by Research Grant AM-03062 from the
National Institute of Arthritis and Metabolic Diseases, NIH, USPHS,
by Training Grant AM-5021 (Dr. Collins), and by a Research Career
Award AM-14176 (Dr. Luetscher) and by a Special Fellowship AM-40790
(Dr. Weinberger). Important assistance was provided by Grant FR-70
from the General Clinical Research Center Branch, and Grant FR-311
(Stanford University Advanced Computer for Medical Research),
Division of Research Facilities and Resources, NIH.

when blood pressure returned to normal after 30 days. None of these patients had a previous history of toxemia or hypertension.

Our interest in this subject was stimulated by the observation that 13 of 80 unselected patients with hypertension were receiving oral contraceptives. Increased plasma renin activity and aldosterone excretion were found in these patients (5).

Hypertension has been observed in at least one patient after ingestion of each of the available combined and sequential estrogen-gestagen combinations. We suspect, but have no proof, that the estrogenic component is responsible for the rise in blood pressure. The increase in blood pressure has varied from moderate to marked. Symptoms have been absent in some cases, while other patients complain of headache, dizziness, and other symptoms.

Both the hypertension and the abnormal laboratory findings returned toward normal when medication was withdrawn (6). Of thirteen hypertensive patients who have discontinued taking oral contraceptives for three months, six patients are normotensive, and five have shown distinct improvement in blood pressure and require either no drugs to control blood pressure or have a lower requirement for such agents. In one case, blood pressure is unchanged following withdrawal of medication; and in another patient, follow-up is inadequate. In several patients, medical records indicate that hypertension occurred during more than one course of administration of estrogen and gestagen. Figure 1 shows the course of the blood pressure in one case. Blood pressure was initially reported to be within normal limits. Hypertension was first observed during a course of combined estrogen-gestagen treatment. Medication was withheld for one year in the course of a planned pregnancy. During this year the patient became normotensive. Hypertension was again noted after the patient re-instituted oral contraceptives and has again subsided when medication was withheld. Although our series is small, we feel that these results indicate that oral contraceptives can induce or aggravate hypertension in a significant number of women. Previous studies have shown increases in circulating renin substrate, renin concentration, and angiotensin generation during pregnancy, when natural estrogen and gestagen levels are increased (7-9). Exogenous estrogen and oral contraceptives have a similar effect (9-11). While the relation of these changes to hypertension remains obscure, active investigation has been stimulated both by a hope of better understanding of the pathogenesis of hypertension, and because measurements of plasma renin and aldosterone are important in the differential diagnosis of hypertension, especially in the identification of cases of primary aldosteronism.

Our results are in good agreement with those of Newton and Laragh (11). Renin substrate, angiotensinogen, is present in normal plasma in a concentration sufficient to produce approximately 1000 ng of angiotensin per milliliter, when the plasma is incubated with an excess of renin. The administration of an oral contraceptive induces a three-to five-fold increase in the concentration of circulating angiotensinogen. Methods for the evaluation of plasma renin activity measure angiotensin released furing incubation of plasma. In the presence of a normal concentration of substrate, the quantity of angiotensin formed is a measure of plasma renin concentration. When substrate is greatly increased, however, the generation of angiotensin is enhanced at physiological levels of renin, both in vivo and in vitro. Since angiotensin is both a potent pressor agent and a stimulus to aldosterone production, the release of increased amounts of angiotensin would be expected to raise arterial pressure and to increase the production of aldosterone.

Newton and Laragh (11) suggested that these effects might also have a negative feedback on renin production. Brown et al (8) measured plasma renin by a method which is not affected by plasma angiotensinogen concentration and found the concentration to be increased during pregnancy. It seemed important to determine whether known stimuli to renin release were affected by estrogens and gestagens. We studied the effects of sodium loading which normally suppressed the release of renin by the kidneys and the secretion of aldosterone by the adrenal cortex. The patients were also studied during sodium deprivation or diuretic administration, which stimulate the secretion of renin and aldosterone. The effect of posture was also studied. Plasma renin activity (i.e., angiotensin generation) was measured by the method of Boucher (12).

When the effects of sodium depletion and assumption of the upright posture are evaluated in a group of patients three months after withdrawal of medication, it is evident that the post-medication pattern of response is very similar to that observed in normotensive controls and in patients with benign hypertension. In these control subjects, plasma renin activity (i.e., angiotensin generation) is lowest in the sodium-loaded, recumbent patient and is increased step-wise by the assumption of the upright posture and by sodium depletion induced by diet or by diuretics.

Angiotensin generation in plasma of patients receiving oral contraceptives is increased as much as five-fold above that observed under similar conditions in the same patients three months after the discontinuance of medication. The average "plasma renin activity" for the group on medication is approximately twice the post-medication average for each set of conditions. The difference between the two groups may be related to increased substrate in the treated group; but the increased plasma renin activity induced by upright posture and by sodium depletion almost certainly reflects increased renin release in response to these normal physiological stimuli.

It seems, therefore, that the increased angiotensin generated during oral contraceptive medication does not suppress the release of renin in the expected fashion.

Aldosterone secretion and metabolism are also affected by oral contraceptives. The secretion rate of aldosterone is stimulated by several factors, including angiotensin, ACTH and potassium. Estrogen can stimulate angiotensin generation, as we have seen. Progesterone in large doses acts as an aldosterone antagonist, and is capable of increasing aldosterone production (13). Combinations of estrogen and gestagen appear to have an additive effect on aldosterone secretion (14). Our observations indicate that most of the combinations, currently used as contraceptives, tend to increase the fraction of aldosterone excreted as the acid-hydrolysable conjugate; but the average effect is small (11.2% on treatment vs. 9.3% post-treatment). Therefore, similar conclusions are reached, regardless of whether secretion or excretion rates are considered.

The average aldosterone excretion is higher during oral contraceptive administration than after three months without medication. In the patients receiving medication, two distinct sub-groups are evident, one excreting unusually large amounts, and the other excreting essentially normal quantities of aldosterone during sodium loading. The patient with normal aldosterone excretion generally had a plasma renin activity below average of the group on medication. Three of the five patients with normal aldosterone excretion were receiving estrogen alone, except for a short period of combined gestagen at the end of the cycle (so-called "sequential" medication). These differences in medication and renin activity may account for lower aldosterone production.

In the patients receiving a low sodium intake and chlorothiazide, oral contraceptive administration was associated with a higher serum potassium level and a higher aldosterone production, compared with levels observed after withdrawal of oral contraceptives. These observations suggest that the oral contraceptives interfere with the action of aldosterone, reduce the secretion of potassium by the distal renal tubule, and thus reduce the potassium-wasting effect of thiazide diuretic. The higher serum potassium concentration, as well as increased angiotensin release, may account for enhanced production of aldosterone.

I do not intend to speculate at this time on a possible causal relation between these interesting laboratory findings and the development of hypertension in patients receiving oral contraceptives. There is no proven connection between increased angiotensin generation or aldosterone production and high blood pressure in the patients. Similar rises in angiotensin generation and aldosterone production are observed in patients whose blood pressure does not rise to abnormal levels on the same medication. The usual decrease in plasma renin and aldosterone levels followed withdrawal of oral contraceptives in one patient who had persistent hypertension. We can not attribute the hypertension to the presence of abnormal renin and aldosterone levels. On the other hand, it would be premature to conclude that these striking alterations in circulating pressor substances have nothing to do with the hypertension. Unusual individual sensitivity, or secondary changes triggered by the increases levels of circulating hormones, could play an important role in the development of hypertension. In any case, it is important to recognize the nature of the changes, and their time relations to the beginning and termination of contraceptive medication, so that confusion does not arise when hypertensive patients are being screened for primary aldosteronism and related conditions.

Finally, it should be noted that hypertension due to oral contraceptives is, at the present time, the most frequently encountered, curable form of high blood pressure in our suburban California community.

REFERENCES

1. Swaab, L.I.: Blood pressure and oral contraception, in Proceedings of Second International Congress on Hormonal Steroids, Milan, Romanoff, E.B. and Martini, L. (eds.) Excerpta Medica Foundation, p. 198.

2. Laragh, J.H., Sealey, J.E., Ledingham, J.G.G. and Newton, M.A.: Oral contraceptives. Renin, aldosterone and high blood pressure. J. Amer. Med. Assoc. 201:918-922 (1967).

3. Woods, J.W.: Oral contraceptives and hypertension. Lancet 2:653-654 (1967).

4. Tyson, J.E.A.: Oral contraception and elevated blood pressure. Amer. J. Obstet. Gynec. 100:875-876 (1968).

5. Weinberger, M.H., Dowdy, A.J., Nokes, G.W. and Luetscher, J.A.: Plasma renin activity and aldosterone secretion in hypertensive patients during high and low sodium intake and administration of diuretic. J. Clin. Endocr. 28:359 (1968).

6. Weinberger, M.H., Dowdy, A.J., Nokes, G.W. and Luetscher, J.A.: Reversible increases in plasma renin activity, aldosterone secretion, and blood pressure in women taking oral contraceptive preparations. Clin. Res. 16:150 (1968).

7. Helmer, O.M. and Griffith, R.S.: The effect of the administration of estrogens on the renin-substrate (hypertensinogen) content of rat plasma. Endocrinology 51:421 (1952).

8. Brown, J.J., Davies, D.L., Doak, P.B., Lever, A.F. and Robertson, J.I.S.: Plasma renin in normal pregnancy. Lancet ii:900 (1963).

9. Helmer, O.M. and Judson, W.E.: Influence of high renin substrate levels on renin-angiotensin system in pregnancy. Amer. J. Obstet. Gynec. 99:9-17 (1967).

10. Crane, M.G., Heitsch, J., Harris, J. and Johns, V.J., Jr.: Effect of ethinyl estradiol (estinyl) on plasma renin activity. J. Clin Endocr. 26:1403 (1966).

11: Newton, M.A., Sealey, J.E., Ledingham, J.G.G. and Laragh, J.H.: High blood pressure and oral contraceptives. Amer. J. Obstet. Gynec. 101:1037-1045 (1968).

12. Boucher, R., Veyrat, R., deChamplain, J. and Genest, J.: New procedures for measurement of human plasma angiotensin and renin activity levels. Canad. Med. Assoc. J. 90:194 (1964).

13. Laidlaw, J.C., Ruse, J.L. and Gornall, A.G.: The influence of estrogen and progesterone on aldosterone excretion. J. Clin.Endocr. 22:161 (1962).

14. Layne, D.S., Meyer, C.J. Vaishwanar, P.S. and Pincus, G.: The secretion and metabolism of cortisol and aldosterone in normal and in steroid treated women. J. Clin. Endocr. 22:107 (1962).

CALCIUM AND SKELETON

THE EFFECT OF ORAL CONTRACEPTIVES ON CALCIUM ABSORPTION

Stanley J. Birge and Louis V. Avioli

Department of Medicine, The Jewish Hospital of St. Louis and Washington University School of Medicine, St. Louis, Missouri

An impressive body of experimental and clinical evidence has accumulated which describes the effects of pharmacological and physiological doses of estrogens and progestogens on calcium and bone metabolism in man. One of the most obvious and glaring observations in this regard is that cyclic therapy of prepubertal subjects with estrogens and progestogens leads to a marked acceleration of epiphysial closure and linear growth with a resultant telescoping of the skeletal growth pattern. Accordingly, the present extensive use of various estrogenic-progestational combinations for the purpose of contraception warrants an objective review of the effects of prolonged therapy with these agents on calcium and mineral metabolism in man. This analysis should include not only any evaluation of hormonal effects in the younger menstruating (and presumably contraceptive prone) population, but also in the older post-menopausal patient since the so-called "oral contraceptive agents" have recently been advocated (and used) for the "therapy" of symptomatic osteoporosis. Subsequent reviews in this symposium will be concerned with the nature and extent of bone mineral and osteoid changes as well as the alterations in calcium and phosphorus homeostasis observed during intervals characterized by increasing circulating levels of estrogens and progestogens. Intrinsic to any scheme proposed to account for these effects is a knowledge of the effects of estrogens and/or progestogens on the intestinal absorption of calcium.

Supported in part by grants AM 11247 and AM 11674 from the National Institute of Arthritis and Metabolic Diseases. Career Research Development Awardee (6-K$_3$-GM-22-676-03).

485

Despite an impressive 20 year history of estrogen "therapy" for osteoporosis only scanty reports exist in humans which describe the effect of this or structurally related hormones on the intestinal absorption of calcium. Unfortunately, the limited available data compiled from human and animal investigations is both contradictory and inconclusive. The majority of studies undertaken in humans during the last two decades devoted to an analysis of estrogens or estrogen-progesterone combinations on calcium metabolism have been limited primarily to utilizing the classical metabolic balance technique. Patients treated with various gonadal steroid combinations and norethandrolone have achieved a "positive" calcium balance with an occasional concomitant fall in serum calcium levels (Table 1) and the data often are interpreted as reflecting an effective increase in calcium absorption. With this investigative approach the intake and fecal output of calcium are measured chemically usually during a short term "balance period" with a stable dietary intake. The dietary calcium which does not appear in the feces is characteristically assumed to have been absorbed by the intestine. These studies invariably disregard the endogenous fecal calcium excretion which normally approximates 130 ± 47 mg per day (1). A knowledge of the endogenous contribution to the total fecal calcium is therefore mandatory for any accurate estimation of calcium absorption. Moreover, since endogenous fecal calcium secretion varies considerably from patient to patient, estimates of the ability of the intestine to absorb calcium during hormonal "therapy" based on chemical balance measurements and on assumed figures for endogenous secretion must be presently regarded as extremely unreliable. It is quite possible that some circumstances prevail wherein the endogenous intestinal calcium may equal or even exceed the dietary calcium. Thus, a reduction or increment in endogenous calcium during periods of estrogen of progestogen administration could significantly affect calculations of calcium absorption based on classical metabolic balance procedures. Accordingly, Nordin (2) (Table 1), while evaluating the effect of short term (two or three weeks) estrogen therapy in osteoporotic patients, noted an increase in calcium balance in eight of eleven subjects with an associated decrease in fecal calcium content. It should be emphasized that the observed small decrease in fecal calcium (approximately 50 mg/day in a 70 kilogram subject) could have been entirely accounted for by a decrease in endogenous calcium rather than by any specific estrogenic stimulation of calcium absorption.

The studies of Lafferty et al (3) in four patients with osteoporosis, although notable in that they represent one of the few attempts to quantitate the true absorption of calcium during estradiol therapy with appropriate corrections for endogenous fecal calcium, are also of equivocal value. No consistent effect of estrogen on calcium absorption was noted after two months of therapy. However, and perhaps of some significance, a decrease in calcium

TABLE 1

EFFECT OF ETHINYL ESTRADIOL ON CALCIUM & PHOSPHORUS BALANCE*

	Calcium		Phosphorus	
	Control	Oestrogen	Control	Oestrogen
	mg/kg/day ± S.E.		mg/kg/day ± S.E.	
Intake	11.59 ±3.3	11.59 ±3.3	17.05 ±2.8	17.05 ±2.8
Faeces	10.94 ±2.8	10.20 ±2.6	7.73 ±1.4	7.70 ±1.3
Urine	2.86 ±0.59	2.04 ±0.50	10.35 ±1.0	8.73 ±0.84
Balance	-2.21 ±0.53	-0.65 ±0.85	-1.03 ±0.82	+0.62 ±0.81

EFFECT OF ETHINYL ESTRADIOL ON PLASMA AND URINARY CALCIUM AND PHOSPHORUS

Parameter	Control Observations		Oestrogen-treated (day 5)		"t"	P
	No.	(Mean ± SE)	No.	(Mean ± SE)		
Plasma Ca(mg/100 ml)	44	9.50 ± 0.06	17	9.21 ± 0.08	2.9	0.01
Plasma P(mg/100 ml)	38	3.43 ± 0.07	15	2.98 ± 0.04	3.5	0.001
Urine Ca/Cr	27	0.17 ± 0.02	15	0.11 ± 0.02	2.0	0.05

*From Young, et al (2).

absorption was apparent after 15 months of estrogen therapy. Later,
Samachson (4), using measurements of gastrointestinal clearance of
^{45}Ca and ^{85}Sr, evaluated calcium absorption in humans during therapy
with either the synthetic estrogen, Mytatrienediol (3-methoxy-
16-methyl-1,3,5 (10)-estratriene-16β, 17β-diol), or the progestogen,
Norlutin (17α-ethinyl - 10-nortestosterone). The results were
again varied, with decreased calcium intestinal clearance (or
absorption) noted in some cases and no changes in others. Despite
the equivocal nature of most of the aforementioned studies in
humans, the bulk of evidence seems to favor an estrogenic inhibition
of calcium absorption. Along these lines, the data obtained by
Schachter and co-workers in the experimental animal may be relevant
(5). These investigators, studying the effect of estradiol and
progesterone administration in the rat, demonstrated a 44% inhibition of calcium transport in the estrogen treated animals with
limited if any effect of progesterone on calcium transport.

Should subsequent studies, designed specifically to evaluate
the effect of estrogens and progestogens on calcium absorption,
verify these interesting but obviously limited observations, the
mechanism whereby estrogens interfere with the intestinal absorption
of calcium may also be uncovered. It is presumptuous at this stage
to incriminate any specific mechanism as accounting for an estrogen-
induced malabsorption of calcium in man, since not only are the
available data unconvincing in this regard, but they have been compiled from experiments which were not specifically designed to
evaluate this parameter of so-called "estrogen effects". One could,
however, postulate that the estrogen-induced malabsorption of
calcium (if indeed verified) results from an inhibition of one, or
all, of many factors known to control or enhance intestinal calcium
absorption. In this regard, the observation of Landau (6) in
patients with hyperparathyroidism and hypercalcemia during estrogen
therapy are of interest (Fig. 1). The observed fall in plasma calcium during the period of estradiol therapy could very well reflect
an inhibition of parathyroid hormone enhancement of the intestinal
absorption of calcium, as well as the postulated estrogenic-inhibi-
tion of bone resorption. Growth hormone, like parathyroid hormone,
has also been shown to effectively increase the intestinal transport
of calcium (5). Hypercalcuria is not uncommonly seen in acromegalic
subjects or during periods of growth hormone administration to
normal subjects (7). Estrogen therapy has been reported to result
in partial or complete reversal of the growth hormone-induced
hypercalcuria (8) in the absence of a reduction in the immunoreactive levels of growth hormone, thus affording the possible
interpretation that the observed fall in urinary calcium reflects
an inhibition of the growth hormone effects at the intestinal
level.

Finally, it becomes increasingly obvious in this symposium
that the varied effects of oral contraceptive medications and

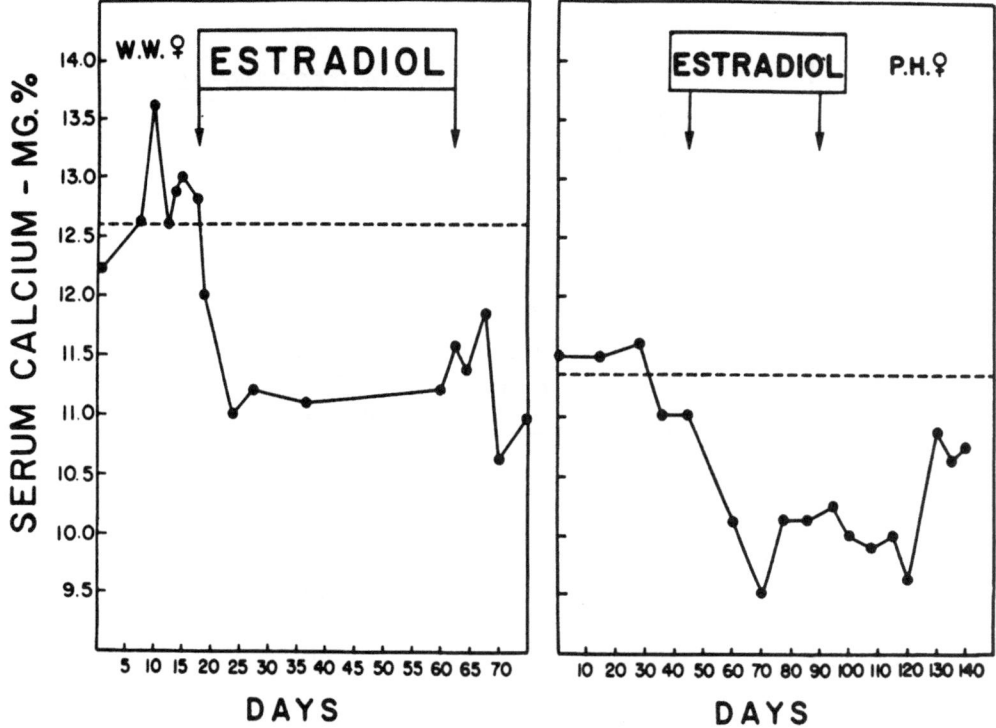

Fig. 1. The effect of estradiol valerate on serum calcium
concentration in two patients with hyperparathyrodism.* The dotted
line in each graph represents the average level of serum calcium in
the pretreatment period. Patient P.H. was given 40 mg/week;
patient W.W., 20 mg/week. *(Reproduced by permission of R.L. Landau,
as published in Annals of Int. Med. 62:1223 (1965).)

estrogens on lipid, protein and carbohydrate metabolism mimic in
many respects the biochemical "side effects" observed with excessive circulating levels of cortisol or any of its synthetic derivatives. Should verification of this similarity obtain, an estrogen-
induced alteration in vitamin D metabolism could also be incrimin-
ated. Recent studies in our laboratory, designed to delineate the
nature of the corticoid-induced decrease in intestinal calcium
transport and the so-called corticoid-vitamin D "antagonism", uncovered a specific defect in vitamin D metabolism in subjects
during prednisone administration (9).

The changes induced in vitamin D metabolism by the prednisone
administration resulted ultimately in a decreased concentration of

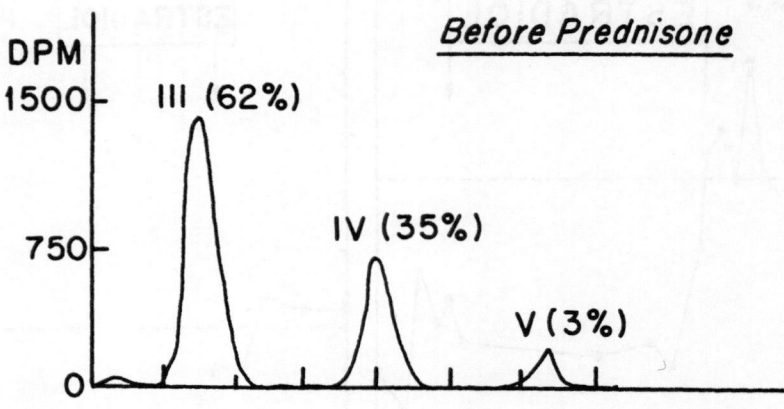

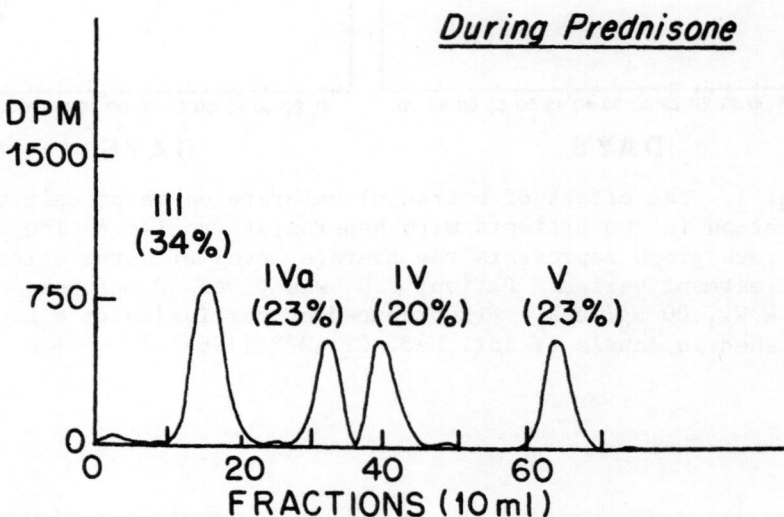

Fig. 2. A. Silicic acid chromatography of the 24-hour plasma chloroform extract from subject JH. The chromatogram was developed with a hyperbolic gradient elution of diethyl ether in n-hexane on multibore columns according to previously published techniques (11). Tritium was measured in aliquots of all column fractions.

B. Effect of prednisone on the distribution of 24-hour plasma chloroform extract from subject JH. The chromatogram was developed as noted above in (A). Tritium was measured in aliquots of all column fractions.

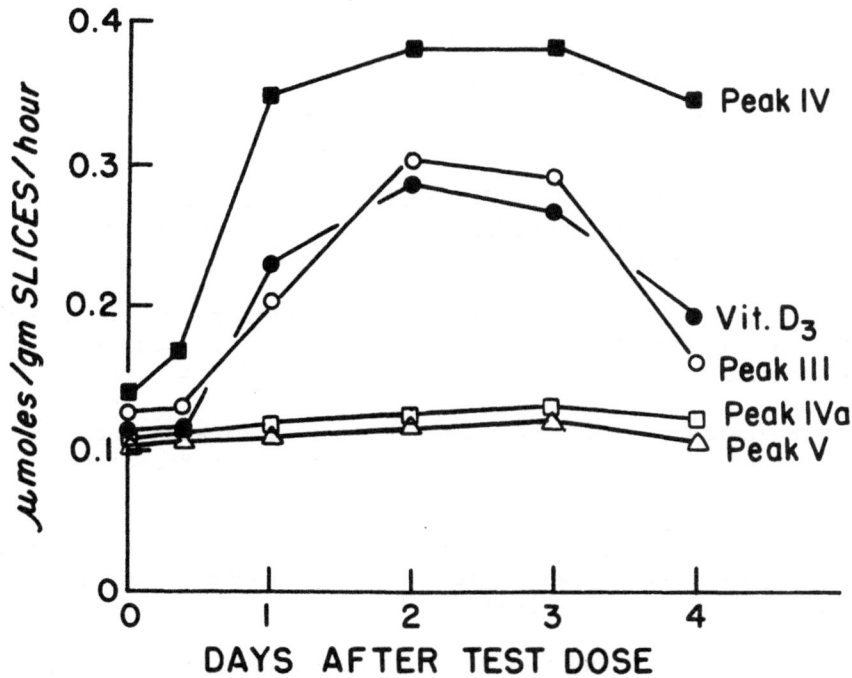

Fig. 3. O$_2$-dependent accumulation of Ca by duodenal slices at various intervals following 0.25 IU of crystalline vitamin D$_3$ and amounts of peak 3 (vitamin D$_3$-^{3}H) and vitamin D$_3$-^{3}H metabolites (peaks 4, 4a, 5) corresponding to 0.25 IU of the parent vitamin according to radioactivity. The amount of each compound tested was estimated on the basis of the specific activity of the parent D$_3$-^{3}H: 176,000 dpm = 1 μg.

25-hydroxy-cholecalciferol, a biologically potent vitamin D metabolite (Fig. 2). As noted in Figure 3, the ability of this metabolite to further the intestinal transport of calcium exceeds that of the parent vitamin D$_3$ compound (9). For reasons which are important but outside the scope of this review, it should be emphasized that 25-hydroxy-cholecalciferol probably also represents the biologically active form of vitamin D$_3$ in man (10).

    In summary, the data presently available do not permit any definite conclusions as to the nature of the effect of estrogens and progestogens on the intestinal absorption of calcium in man. With the ever increasing consumption of these agents for the purpose of contraception as well as their potential incorporation into therapeutic regimens of symptomatic osteoporotic patients, the need for further elucidation of the effects of gonadal hormones on calcium absorption is obvious.

REFERENCES

1. Heaney, R.P.: Endogenous fecal calcium in medical uses of ^{47}Ca. International Atomic Energy Agency Technical Reports Series No. 32, 129 (1964).

2. Young, M.M., Jasani, C., Smith, D.A. and Nordin, B.E.C.: Some effects of ethinyl ostradiol on calcium and phosphorus metabolism in osteoporosis. Clin. Sci. 34:411-417 (1968).

3. Lafferty, F.W., Spencer, G.E. and Pearson, O.H.: Effects of androgens, estrogens and high calcium intakes on bone formation and resorption in osteoporosis. Am. J. Med. 36:514 (1964).

4. Samaechson, J.: The gastrointestinal clearance of strontium - 85 and calcium - 45 in man. Radiation Research 27:64-74 (1966).

5. Finkelstein, J.D. and Schachter, D.: Active transport of calcium by intestine: the effects of hypophysectomy and growth hormone. Am. J. Physiol. 203:873-880 (1962).

6. Landau, R.L. and Kappas, A.: Anabolic hormones in hyperparathyroidism. Annals of Internal Med. 62:1223-1233 (1965).

7. Henneman, P.H., Forbes, A.P., Modawer, M., Dempsey, E.F. and Carroll, E.L.: Effects of human growth hormone in man. J. Clin. Invest. 39:1223 (1960).

8. Schwartz, E., Echemendia, E. and Schiffer, M.: Peripheral metabolic antagonism of estrogen and human growth hormone. J. Clin. Invest. 46:1115 (1967).

9. Avioli, L.V., Birge, S.J. and Lee, S.W.: Effects of prednisone on vitamin D metabolism in man. J. Clin. Endocrin. 28:1341 (1968).

10. Blunt, J.W., DeLuca, H.F. and Schnoes, H.K.: "25-hydroxy-cholecalciferol. A biologically active metabolite of vitamin D_3". Biochemistry 10:3317-3322 (1968).

ESTROGEN EFFECTS ON THE SKELETON

Robert P. Heaney, M.D.

Creighton University School of Medicine
Omaha, Nebraska

INTRODUCTION

Although estrogens have been widely used in the treatment of postmenopausal osteoporosis for the last quarter century, surprisingly little is known of the effects of these hormones on adult skeletal metabolism. Furthermore, as has been usual in endocrine research, more is known of lower animals than of man. I will review the better known (and probably less relevant) skeletal effects of estrogens in birds, mice, and rats, will summarize what is known of estrogen effects in higher mammals and in menopausal women, will review with you our own results using calcium balance and calcium kinetic studies in women, and will conclude with a tentative effort at an explanation of estrogen effects on the adult skeleton.

SKELETAL EFFECTS IN BIRDS AND IMMATURE MAMMALS

During the preparation for egg-laying, birds fill the medullary cavities of their long bones with spongy bone. This is produced by a massive burst of osteoblastic activity at the endosteal surfaces of the bones and can be reproduced by exogenous administration of estrogen in physiological doses (1). This bone stores large quantities of calcium and phosphorus which are to be used in egg production and thus has an obvious physiological importance. During synthesis of the yolk the bone is rapidly resorbed and the plasma calcium rises dramatically. This elevation is entirely in the protein-bound fraction, however, and not in the ionized moiety. Much of the bone phosphorus goes into the yolk, and the calcium into the shell, and the whole system fits together very neatly

493

indeed. In fact, the high plasma calcium probably serves to solu-
bilize the phosphoprotein being transported to the oviduct for
yolk synthesis, rather than the other way around (that is, the
protein carrying the calcium). This is inferred from the fact
that similarly high plasma calcium values are seen in those
amphibia and reptiles which lay soft-shelled eggs (1).

The mouse also demonstrates a spongy accumulation of bone in
the medullary cavities in response to high doses of estrogen, and
as in birds, this too appears to be due to new endosteal bone
formation. Unlike birds, however, this effect is not seen naturally during pregnancy when endogenous estrogen levels are highest,
and has no apparent physiological significance. Curiously, direct
implantation of estrogen within the medullary cavity fails to
reproduce the effect of systemic administration, and hence there
is good reason to wonder if the bone effect is due to estrogens
at all or is instead a response to some extraosseous toxic effect
of estrogen. I stress this point because, except for the mouse,
there is no other known instance of significant stimulation of
new bone formation by estrogens in mammals.

Immature rats given large doses of estrogens show inhibition
of resorption of the primary spongiosa (2). This inhibition applies
only to internal osteoclasts, since remodeling of the external
portion of the metaphyseal funnel continues normally. This is a
pure anti-resorptive effect and is dose dependent. I stress again
that it requires massive doses of hormone and is associated with
significant growth retardation. This effect has not been observed
in guinea pigs, hamsters, rabbits, puppies, or kittens, and, of
course, is seen in rats only during their growth phase.

In all mammals studied the exhibition of estrogens prior to
skeletal maturity produces an accelerated appearance of ossification centers, a slowing of cartilage growth, a reduction in growth
rate of both long and flat bones, and epiphyseal fusion. The
final result of these effects is a smaller than normal adult
skeletal size (1,3). Thus, for example, administration of estrogens alone to a prepuberal castrate girl will produce epiphyseal
fusion without the growth spurt which characterizes normal puberty
and which would have occurred had androgens been given with the
estrogens (4). Nevertheless, despite this veritable mountain of
negative evidence, there still persists a notion that estrogens
somehow stimulate osteoblastic activity in postmenopausal women,
and are responsible for its maintenance in the premenopausal
female.

EFFECTS IN MATURE ANIMALS

All of the results I have cited, with the exception of the
mouse effects, have been observed in immature animals. Virtually
nothing is known of estrogen effects on the adult skeleton. However, the human female, by going through the menopause, becomes
in effect immature again, at least with respect to estrogen levels,
and it is possible in this situation to see effects of estrogens
on calcium and phosphorus metabolism apart from the confusing
features associated with growth. Most notable are four phenomena:

1) There is a distinctly elevated rate of loss of
both cortical and cancellous bone which is associated with the menopause. Although both men
and women begin to lose bone at about age 35,
the rate of loss is much exaggerated in women
as they lose their ovarian function (5, 6).
Although adequately controlled studies have not
yet been performed, there is preliminary evidence that this loss can be retarded to the
level of the male by prophylactic estrogen
treatment (7, 8).

2) There is an elevation of both calcium and
phosphorus in plasma (9). The changes are
small (on the order of a fraction of a mg %),
but are quite real, and are larger in surgically
oophorectomized women than following a spontaneous menopause. Furthermore, these changes can be
reversed by subsequent administration of estrogen
(10).

3) There is decrease in TRP when estrogens are given
to postmenopausal women (11).

4) A positive calcium balance can usually be produced
when estrogens are given to postmenopausal women
(12).

I will attempt to relate these effects in a single mechan-
istic framework in a moment. Before I do so, let me describe
the results of calcium kinetic studies in women given estrogens.
Figure 1 shows both the calcium balance and plasma calcium specific activity curves in a castrated female given estradiol
benzoate. The markedly positive calcium balance is typical and
is essentially the same as that described by Albright and his
co-workers many years ago (11). Note especially in this case

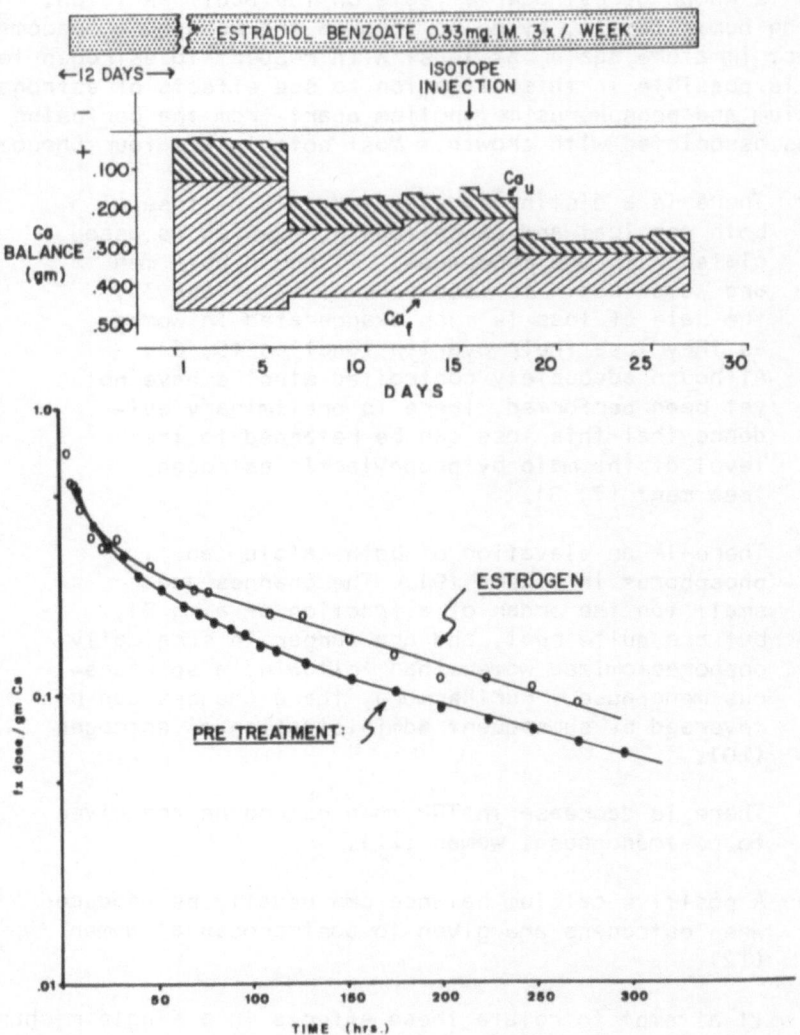

Figure 1. Calcium balance and kinetic data from a 38-year-old female castrate before and after administration of estradiol benzoate.

that both urinary and fecal calcium are reduced and contribute to
the positive balance. The Ca-45 specific activity declined less
rapidly during estrogen treatment than it had during a control
study, indicating decreased turnover of the miscible calcium pool.
Now turnover of the pool, and consequent dilution of tracer contained therein, are produced by inpouring of unlabeled calcium from
the diet and from resorption of bone. As is apparent from the
figure, dietary absorption was increased; hence, bone resorption
must have been decreased even more strikingly than was total turnover. Kinetic calculations based on these curves confirm these
interpretations and reveal that mineral accretion (bone formation)
was not significantly altered in this patient, but that resorption
was reduced almost to zero. It would appear that the anti-
resorptive effect of the estrogen was primary in this case. Had
the renal effect been primary, the consequent retention of calcium
would not have resulted in improved absorption; similarly had the
effect on the intestine been primary, the increased absorption of
calcium should have resulted in hypercalciuria. On the other hand,
direct immediate suppression of bone resorption would be expected
to evoke homeostatic responses which would lead to improved con-
servation of calcium by the kidney and intestine.

One does not see this type of response, however, in women with
normal ovarian function. Table 1 presents data obtained from a 24-
day balance-kinetic study in a normal 25-year-old woman who volun-
teered for a pseudopregnancy study, and who had received 0.4 mg
ethinyl estradiol daily for six weeks and 750 mg of 17-hydroxy-
progesterone caproate weekly for four weeks prior to the isotope
study. Although she experienced mild nausea and breast tenderness,
her calcium metabolism demonstrated essentially no effect despite
a distinctly higher than normal estrogen level: with the exception
of the EFC, which appears to have decreased significantly, all of
the changes noted are within the range of spontaneous variation
from time to time in normal adults.

TABLE 1

Study	Pool (gm)	Turn-over*	A*	R*	Ca_u*	EFC*	α	Bal.*
Control	3.416	0.526	0.288	0.366	0.130	0.108	0.189	-.078
Pseudo-pregnancy	3.480	0.497	0.336	0.383	0.074	0.087	0.132	-.047

* gm/day

TABLE 2

COMPARATIVE RADIOCALCIUM KINETIC DATA IN PATIENTS
WITH ACUTE DISUSE OSTEOPOROSIS
TREATED WITH ANABOLIC STEROID AGENTS

Patient	Miscible Calcium Pool gm/M^2	Bone Formation gm/M^2/day	Bone Resorption gm/M^2/day
P.C.(1)	3.45	0.485	0.772
P.C.(2)	3.64	0.453	0.648
A.A.(1)	4.25	0.491	0.759
A.A.(2)	4.06	0.488	0.627
L.H.(1)	3.72	0.442	0.663
L.H.(2)	3.40	0.382	0.521

When there is a significant non-homeostatic component to bone
resorption as in disuse osteoporosis, it is possible to see effects
of estrogen, androgen, and the anabolic steroids. Several reports
have shown that these agents reduce urine calcium and lessen the
negative calcium balance of this condition (13, 14). Table 2 presents data from our study of patients with acute poliomyelitis
treated with norethandrolone and demonstrates that this so-called
anabolic steroid did not affect bone formation but did produce a
modest reduction in the grossly elevated levels of resorption
which characterize this condition (14).

Thus, we find that estrogens decrease bone resorption in
hypogonadal adults and in some patients with elevated resorption,
and that this reduction is responsible for the calcium balance
effects of the hormone. Although estrogen turns out not to be a
stimulus to osteoblasts as Albright had proposed, its inhibition
of osteoclasts ought to make it equally effective and would in
itself be sufficient theoretical grounds for its use in postmenopausal osteoporosis. Unfortunately, as everyone here knows,
estrogens have not been shown to increase bone mass in osteoporotic patients. At best they stabilize the disease. This failure

does not represent an escape from the anti-resorptive effect:
serial kinetic studies during long-term treatment have shown
that resorption remains depressed. Rather, after 4-6 months of
treatment, formation falls as well, and the bone balance comes
back into equilibrium at a reduced level of turnover (Figure 2).

These findings suggest that bone resorption would be lower
before the menopause than after. Unfortunately, almost no studies
have been directed at this question. Few calcium kinetic studies
have ever been done in normal premenopausal women, and to my
knowledge there are no serial studies using each woman as her own
control. There is some little evidence from morphologic studies
such as those of Jowsey and Frost (17, 18) that bone turnover
reaches its lowest levels at ages 25-35, and that it rises thereafter, but these results have to be considered preliminary.

SUMMARY

Before proposing an integrating hypothesis, let me summarize
the known effects of estrogens on the skeleton.

1) Estrogens stimulate osteoblastic formation of
    medullary bone in egg-laying vertebrates and
    at high doses are associated with a similar
    phenomenon in mice. Also at high doses, they
    suppress remodeling of the primary spongiosa
    in immature rats, but probably in no other
    mammals. I submit that none of these observa-
    tions is particularly relevant to man.

2) Estrogens suppress bone growth in all mammals
    studied, but there are essentially no morpho-
    logic data available on their effects on mature
    bone.

3) Estrogens decrease resorption in hypogonadal
    females, produce a positive calcium balance,
    lower plasma calcium and phosphorus slightly,
    and reduce the TRP.

HYPOTHESIS

These results suggest a direct interference of estrogens
with bone resorption and a secondary, compensatory increase in
PTH secretion with consequent PTH effects on renal calcium clearance and on gastrointestinal calcium absorption. The interference
with resorption appears to occur not at the level of the functioning osteoclast, but at the mesenchymal cell population from which

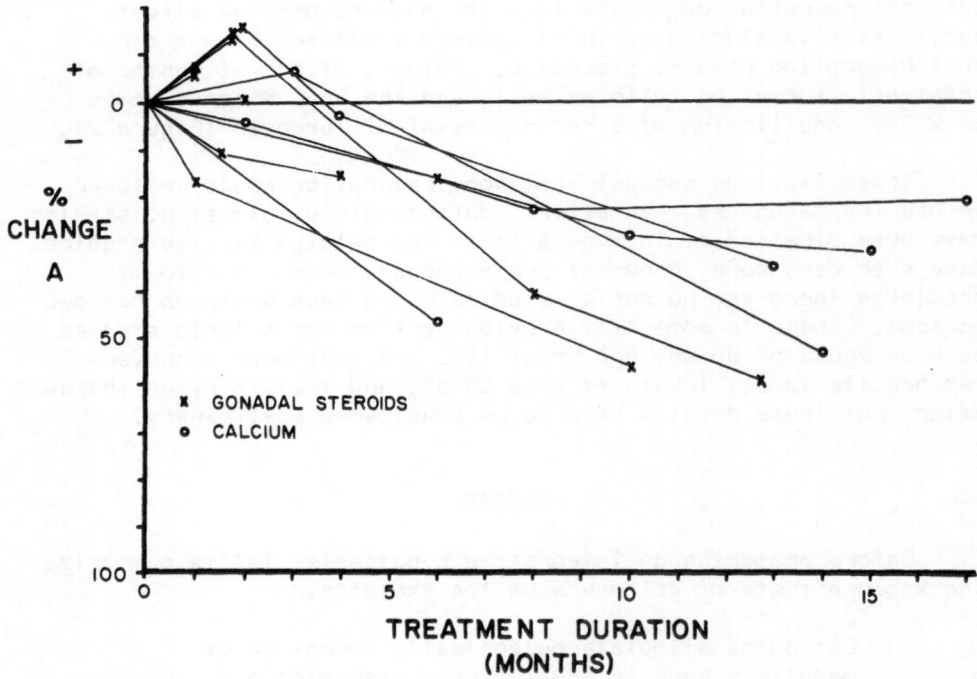

Figure 2. Per cent change in accretion from pretreatment
levels, plotted as a function of treatment duration. Data include
both our own experience and values recalculated from published
material (15, 16).

osteoclasts are recruited. It should be recalled that the classical bone cell functions, i.e., formation and resorption, are
carried out by cells that live only a short while: osteoclasts
for hours to at most one or two days, and osteoblasts for only a
few days to at most one or two weeks. Continued resorption or
formation on any bone surface requires continuous differentiation
of the cell type involved from undifferentiated mesenchymal precursors. Both estrogens and PTH appear to act at the level of the
mesenchymal cell, whereas agents such as calcitonin, fluoride,
and phosphate act more distally, that is, on the functioning
osteoclast itself. The significance of this distinction is that
any agent which interferes with mesenchymal activation may be
expected ultimately to reduce bone turnover and this is exactly
what we have seen happens with long-term estrogen treatment in
osteoporosis. Thus what estrogens appear to do is to stabilize
the bone mass at the level which obtains at the time that they
are administered. Whereas they have not proved to be good treatment for osteoporosis, they may well prove to be very good
prophylaxis.

BIBLIOGRAPHY

1. McLean, F. C. and Urist, M. R.: <u>Bone. Fundamentals of the</u>
    <u>physiology of skeletal tissue</u>. 3rd Ed., pp. 119-124,
    U. Clin. Press, Chicago, Ill. (1968).

2. Budy, A. M., Urist, M. R. and McLean, F. C.: The effect of
    estrogens on the growth apparatus of the bones of
    immature rats. Am. J. Path. <u>28</u>:1143-1167, (1952).

3. Gardner, W. U. and Pfeiffer, C. A.: Influence of estrogens
    and androgens on the skeletal system. Physiol. Rev.,
    <u>23</u>:139-165 (1943).

4. Wilkins, L.: <u>The Diagnosis and Treatment of Endocrine Dis-</u>
    <u>orders in Childhood and Adolescence</u>. 3rd Ed., Ed. R. M.
    Blizzard and C. J. Migeon, Charles C. Thomas, Springfield,
    Ill. (1965).

5. Garn, S. M., Rohmann, C. G. and Wagner, B.: Bone loss as a
    general phenomenon in man. Fed. Proc. <u>26</u>:1729-1736
    (1967).

6. Meema, H. E., Bunker, M. L. and Meema, S.: Loss of compact
    bone due to menopause. Obstet. Gynec. <u>26</u>:333-343
    (1965).

7. Wallach, S. and Henneman, P. H.: Prolonged estrogen therapy
    in postmenopausal women. JAMA <u>171</u>:1637-1642 (1959).

8. Davis, M. E., Strandjord, N. M. and Lanzl, L. H.: Estrogens
    and the aging process: The detection, prevention, and
    retardation of osteoporosis. JAMA <u>196</u>:129-224 (1966).

9. Young, M. M. and Nordin, B. E. C.: Effects of natural and
    artificial menopause on plasma and urinary calcium and
    phosphorus. Lancet <u>2</u>:118-120 (1967).

10. Nordin, B. E. C.: Hormones and Calcium Metabolism. In
    <u>Calcified Tissues 1965</u>, Proc. 3rd European Symp. on
    Calcified Tissues, Ed. H. Fleisch, H. J. J. Blackwood
    and M. Owen, Springer-Verlay, New York, Inc. 1966,
    pp. 226-241.

11. Nassim, J. R., Saville, P. D. and Mulligan, L.: The effect of
    stilbestrol on urinary phosphate excretion. Clin. Sci.
    <u>15</u>:367 (1956).

12. Albright, F. and Reifenstein, E. C., Jr.: The parathyroid
       glands and metabolic bone disease. Baltimore, 1948,
       Williams & Williams Co.

13. Plum, F. and Dunning, M. F.: Amelioration of hypercalciuria
       following poliomyelitis by 17-ethyl, 19-nortestosterone
       (Nilevar). J. Clin. Endocrinol. 18:860 (1958).

14. Heaney, R. P.: Radiocalcium metabolism in disuse osteoporosis
       in man. Am. J. Med. 33:188-200 (1962).

15. Lafferty, F. W., Spencer, G. E. and Pearson, O. H.: Effects
       of androgens, estrogens, and high calcium intakes on
       bone formation and resorption in orteoporosis. Am. J.
       Med. 36:514-528 (1964).

16. Schwartz, E., Panariello, V. A. and Saeli, J.: Radioactive
       calcium kinetics during high calcium intake in osteoporo-
       sis. J. Clin. Invest. 44:1547-1560 (1965).

17. Jowsey, J.: Age changes in human bone. Clin. Orthopaed.
       17:210 (1960).

18. Frost, H. M.: Bone remodelling dynamics. Charles C. Thomas,
       Springfield, Ill. (1963).

EFFECTS OF ESTROGEN ON CALCIUM METABOLISM IN MAN

Eugene Eisenberg

Medical Services, San Francisco General Hospital,
University of California School of Medicine,
San Francisco

Scientific interest in a relationship between gonadal steroids and bone mineral metabolism began when the rapid changes of bone structure that occur during egg-laying in the pigeon were recorded in 1934 (1). As the egg approaches maturity bone formation in the tibias and femurs becomes so intense that these bones become almost solid. This mass of bone is suddenly and rapidly resorbed as calcification of the shell begins. These changes were shown, by classic endocrine studies, to be secondary to cyclic changes in estrogen secretion (2). Similar observations in diverse species, such as chickens, mice, rats, and pocket gophers, showed that gonadal hormones have a variety of effects on bone, including stimulation and inhibition of both bone growth and resorption, as well as no effect.

While some of the variability in response to estrogen is due to variation in age, nutritional status, and prior gonadal status of the animals it is clear that these gross changes in bone are related to species-specific reproductive needs. Their relevance to adult man is unclear and one must be wary of attempts to extend observations of species that show dramatic responses to human bone.

While studying bone disorders in man Albright and his colleagues defined a common clinical condition characterized by decreased mass of bone and fractures occurring after minimal trauma but with no gross abnormality of calcium metabolism and no sign of the increased osteoclastic activity seen in hyperparathyroidism (3). This condition, which he called osteoporosis, was most commonly found in postmenopausal women and in other patients who were deficient in gonadal hormones. In Albright's view loss of bone mass resulted from either "Bone-Formation-Too-Little" or "Bone-Resorption-Too-Great." Since he could find no evidence of the latter,

osteoporosis was attributed to the former. He held that the bones
of man are like those of the pigeon in which estrogen stimulated
osteoblastic proliferation and activity. Support for this theory
was obtained by demonstrating retention of calcium and phosphorus
during administration of estrogens. This concept and its therapeutic corollary were generally but not universally accepted.
Reservations concerning its validity became more widespread when
clinical observation of patients treated with estrogens for 15 years
failed to show an increase in skeletal density. The need for re-
vision of the Albrightian concepts became mandatory when new techniques of studying bone and calcium metabolism suggested other
possible routes in the pathophysiology of osteoporosis. Indeed,
even without this new information some reflection will show that
the decreased mass of bone characteristic of this condition could
result not only from decreased bone formation or increased bone resorption, the two possibilities considered by Albright, but also
from any combination in which resorption is greater than formation
(Fig. 1). While little has been added to the clinical description

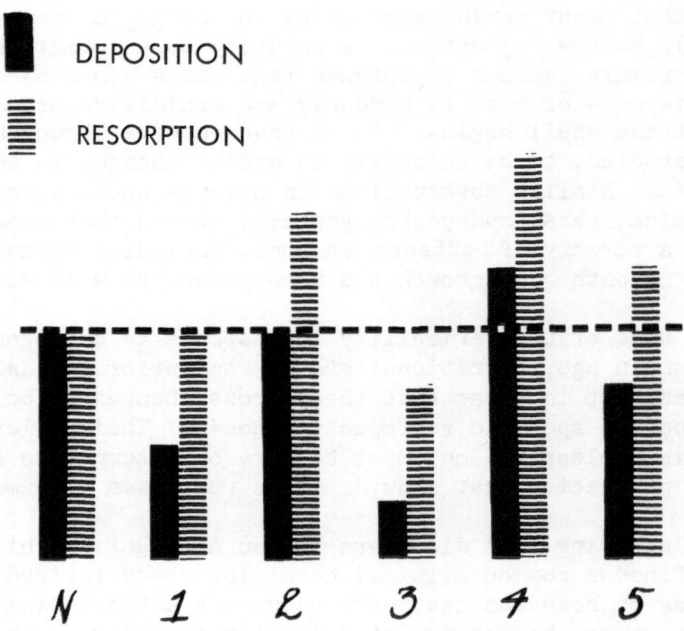

FIVE WAYS TO PRODUCE OSTEOPENIA

Figure 1. Five different combinations of bone formation and resorption rates that would result in osteopenia. Note that the degree
of negative balance is the same in each combination.

of osteoporosis the newer information alluded to indicates that the bone in osteoporosis is qualitatively as well as quantitatively different from normal bone and that control of bone remodeling may vary from normal in any of the ways shown in Figure 1. The causes of these disturbances remain obscure. Because of these questions concerning the nature of osteoporosis we must also reexamine our concepts of the effects of gonadal hormones on bone and calcium. In this presentation I will discuss the status of some of our knowledge in this area but will avoid, as much as possible, the material to be presented by the others on this panel.

The methods available for studying this field now include, in addition to measurement of total and ionized concentrations of calcium and phosphorus in serum and of intake and output of these and other bone minerals, measurement of "bone turnover" and bone density, metabolism of other bone constituents, such as the components of bone matrix, and measurement of hormones that affect bone metabolism. It is not within the scope of this presentation to extensively discuss the technical aspects of the methods and their limitations, but where these factors are very important they will be mentioned briefly.

The first concept we may question is that bone mineral metabolism is normal in postmenopausal osteoporosis. While serum calcium and phosphorus levels are usually in the normal range in patients with osteoporosis it is not unusual to see a slight rise of serum phosphorus especially in a patient who has not yet developed far-advanced bone atrophy (3-5). Even when the serum phosphorus is initially within normal limits estrogen therapy often lowers it slightly (3,6,7). In two recent studies it was shown that postmenopausal women tend to have slight but statistically significant elevation of serum calcium (4,8)(Fig. 2) with no change in the distribution between protein-bound and nonprotein-bound fractions (8).

Measurement of total body balance of calcium and phosphorus has been an attractive tool to many bone clinicians since normally 99% of the body calcium is in bone and therefore gain or loss of body calcium should mean gain or loss of bone. Most balance studies suggest that osteoporotic patients are in equilibrium or in slightly negative calcium balance. I believe it is accurate to state that in most reasonably well performed balance studies (3,9) estrogen therapy often but not always decreases calcium loss from the body, largely because of decreased urinary loss; the effect on fecal calcium is usually minimal. It is just as accurate to state that in many of the balance studies one cannot be certain whether the decreased loss has resulted in positive balance, less negative balance, or mineral equilibrium. Calcium balance must be studied over a long period and even a small but consistent error may accumulate to a significant degree. I will not review the possible sources of such errors but there are several (10). Further uncertainty in interpreting the

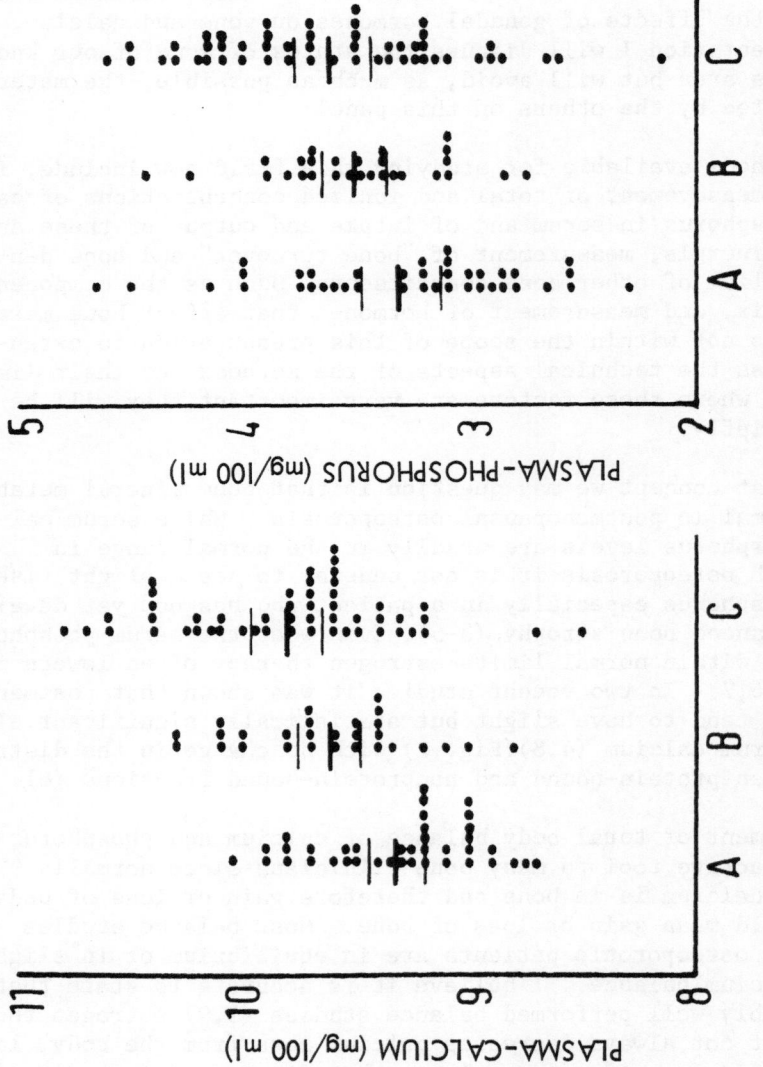

Figure 2. Levels of plasma calcium and phosphorus in A) premenopause,
B) postnatural menopause, and C) postartificial menopause. (Reprinted
from Young, M.M., and B.E.C. Nordin, Lancet 2:118-120, 1967.)

meaning of the calcium retention rises from the fact that most of
the patients studied are subject to cartilaginous and cardiovascular
calcification; for example, the roentgenographic density of the
thoracic aorta often exceeds that of the spine. Along with the
effects on calcium and phosphorus, serum magnesium is reduced by 10%
and urinary magnesium by 40% in women taking mestranol with norethynodrel (11). It is not known whether these are related to effects
on bone or to other effects of the hormone. It should be pointed
out that the few available studies of the effects of progestins on
calcium metabolism yield negative results and that the effects on
bone mineral metabolism observed during administration of estrogen-
progestin combinations can be attributed to the estrogen component.

The next concept we will examine is that of low bone formation
and normal resorption rates in patients with osteoporosis and the
effect of estrogen upon them. Three methods of measuring these
processes in man are 1) analysis of kinetics of bone-seeking iso-
topes, 2) quantitative microradiography, and 3) measurement of appositional movement of tetracycline labels. Careful consideration of
the three techniques reveals that each gives us limited but useful
information.

Most analyses of bone tracer kinetics are calculated by the
"turnover-difference" concept (12,13) which essentially measures
the rate of movement into body depots for the tracer, presumably
the skeleton. The limitations that the possible presence of dystro-
phic or metastatic calcification impose on interpretation of calcium
balance apply here; in addition, we are unable to separate the several processes by which calcium enters bone. These limitations become less significant but are not eliminated when repeated studies
are carried out in the same subjects under varying conditions. In
the technique of quantitative microradiography the relative amount
of bone surface involved in bone formation and in bone resorption
is measured (14). The bone surface is measured in only one dimension
and the results are expressed in linear percentage. There is no direct indication of the rates of bone formation and resorption. Furthermore, there is no way of correcting the figures for the amount
of surface per volume of bone. If, in a given volume of bone, surface area is reduced and the surfaces involved in bone formation
are correspondingly reduced, the percent of surface involved in bone
formation would be reported as a normal figure, thereby disguising
the fact that bone formation is actually reduced in that volume of
bone. This method also suffers from the limitations imposed on any
biopsy technique in that it may not be representative of changes
elsewhere in the body or even in the same bone. The third method
of measuring bone formation is to biopsy bone which has been labeled
with tetracycline. The rate of new bone apposition is measured by
movement of the tetracycline and is expressed as millimeters of new
bone formed per year (15).

In spite of the limitations of each of these methods they have provided us with new ways to qualitatively, if not quantitatively, compare disturbances in calcium metabolism. It is curious that the qualitative concepts derived from them should be so similar even though the theory and methods are so different from each other (Tables 1 and 2 and Fig. 3).

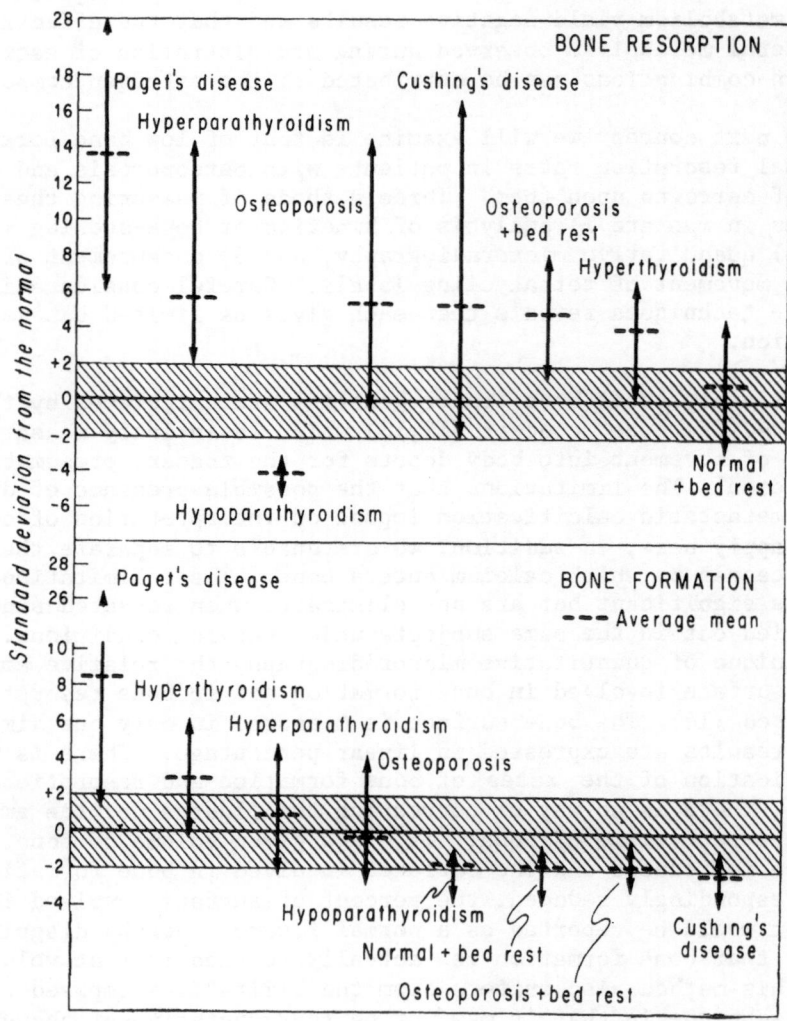

Figure 3. Bone formation and resorption in some disorders of the skeleton as determined by microradiography. (Reprinted from Jowsey, J. In: Calcified Tissues 1965. Springer-Verlag, New York, Fleisch et al, eds., p. 71.)

Table 1. Strontium dynamics in endocrine diseases*

Condition	No. of subjects	Exchange pool (liters)	Excretion rate (liters/day)	"Rate of deposition into bone" (liters/day)
Normal	31	42.7 ± 1.1	3.9 ± 0.2	9.6 ± 0.4
Athletes	11	56.9 ± 2.3	5.8 ± 0.2	15.0 ± 1.0
Nephrolithiasis	11	39.3 ± 2.3	5.7 ± 0.8	7.6 ± 0.6
Osteoporosis				
Postmenopausal	40	33.0 ± 0.9	2.3 ± 0.2	6.4 ± 0.3
Thyrotoxicosis	7	48.9 ± 3.6	27.0 ± 2.2	16.7 ± 2.0
Acromegaly	9	73.8 ± 6.2	5.7 ± 0.5	18.2 ± 2.3
Cushing's syndrome				
< 1 year	2	38.9, 46.1	5.8, 8.6	8.0, 8.8
> 2 years	3	19.8, 24.6, 28.2	3.4, 4.9, 5.1	2.4, 3.1, 3.9

*Values are mean ± S.E. except for Cushing's syndrome where individual values are given.

Table 2. Examples of tetracycline-based, Haversian remodeling parameters in cortical bone.

Disease	No. of cases studied	Bone formation rate %/year	Mu (birth rate) new osteons per year/mm^3	Sigma (osteon formation period) (years)	A_f* number of bone forming sites/mm^2	Mean seam thickness (microns)
Normal at age 50 years	60+	4.0(±2.0)	1.8(±.9)	.19(±.02)	.35(±.15)	7.5(±7.0)
Postmenopausal osteoporosis	7	2.7 D**	1.5 D	2.1 I	1.3 I	6.2 N
Senile osteoporosis	15	2.4 D	1.6 D	2.1 I	1.5 I	6.5 N
Cushing's syndrome (iatrogenic)	18	.6 D	.10 D	.67 I	.05 D	7.5 N
Acromegaly (active)	1	13.0 I	5.5 I	.40 I	5.0 I	7.9 N

*A_f = number of bone forming sites/mm^2 cortical cross section area.
**Abbreviations: I = increased; N = normal; D = decreased.

From Frost, H.M.: Bone dynamics in metabolic bone disease. J. Bone Joint Surg. 48-A:1192, 1966.

Table 1 gives the miscible strontium pool size, the excretion rate from the pool and the rate of strontium deposition into non-exchangeable or very slowly exchangeable depots. Vigorous exercise increases all of these measurements. The athletes were members of a football team. All of these measurements are decreased in patients with clinically and radiologically severe osteoporosis and increased in patients with thyrotoxicosis and acromegaly. Since all of these patients had radiologic osteoporosis we can assume that their bone resorption rate was increased even further above the normal range than was the deposition rate.

The patients with symptoms of Cushing's syndrome for less than one year had increased excretion rates and a slight decrease in bone deposition rate. Since corticoids are not known to increase the absorption of calcium in the intestine, the increased excretion of bone-seeking mineral must come from bone. Those whose clinical course was longer and who had radiologic osteoporosis had less marked elevation of excretion rates and very low deposition rates.

Microradiographic analysis shows similar changes of increased bone surface formation in patients with hyperthyroidism and confirms the conjecture regarding increased bone resorptive activity. The findings in Cushing's disease are likewise confirmatory. The normal figure for bone formation by this technique is not necessarily contradictory, since the reduction in bone deposition by kinetic analysis is about 30% below normal and these patients have lost at least 30% of their bone mass. Hence the bone deposition rate per unit mass of bone would be normal or slightly above normal. The changes shown by analysis of tetracycline labeling are confirmatory also in a qualitative sense (Table 2).

The microradiographic technique has also shown us that osteoporotic bone differs significantly from normal bone in two ways that were not suspected previously. First, there is a good deal of bone with less than usual calcium content (Fig. 4) and secondly, many of the osteons have a central sclerotic ring (Fig. 5), the significance of which is as yet unknown.

The normal to slightly elevated serum level of phosphate and the normal to high urinary excretion of calcium seen in mild to moderate osteoporosis is not consistent with the proposal that this disease develops because of inadequate amounts of dietary calcium and phosphorus or inability to absorb calcium efficiently. It is unlikely that these changes are due to hyperabsorption. They most likely reflect the imbalance of bone formation and resorption shown by any of the combinations in Figure 1. The decrease in urinary calcium seen in patients with advanced osteoporosis is probably a reflection of the small amount of bone mass remaining. Hypercalciuria is less in patients with Cushing's syndrome when the disease has been present for a long time and osteoporosis is severe (Table 1).

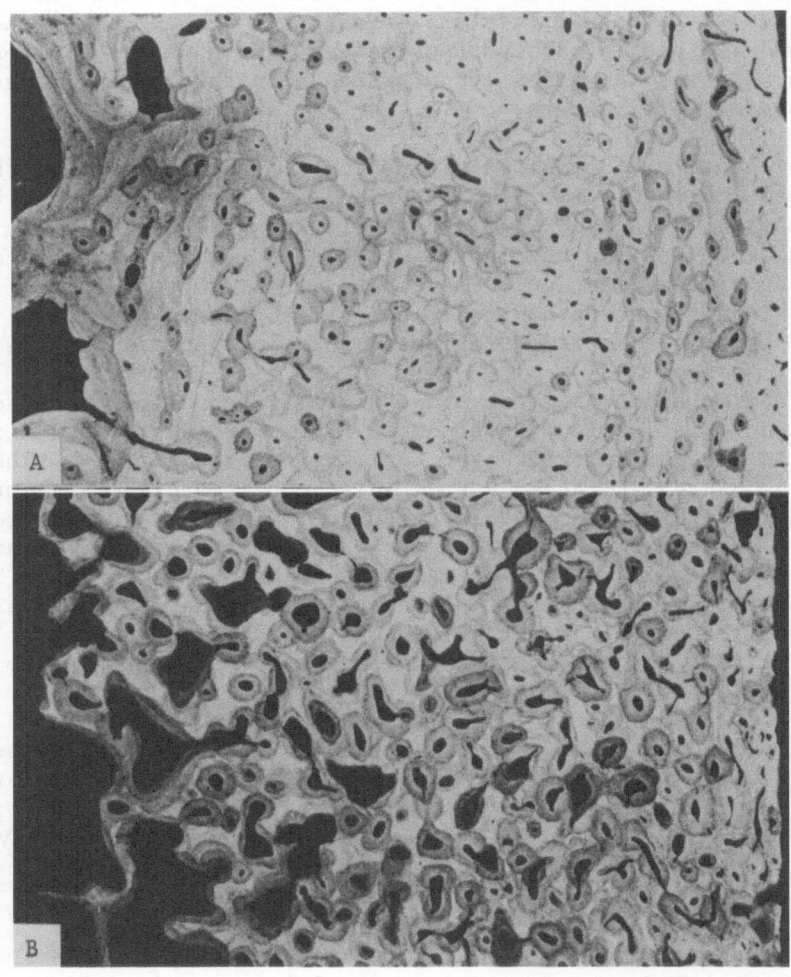

Figure 4. Microradiographs of bone from a 17-year-old male (A) and
a 77-year-old female (B). (Reprinted from Jowsey, J., Clin. Orthoped.
17:214, 1960.)

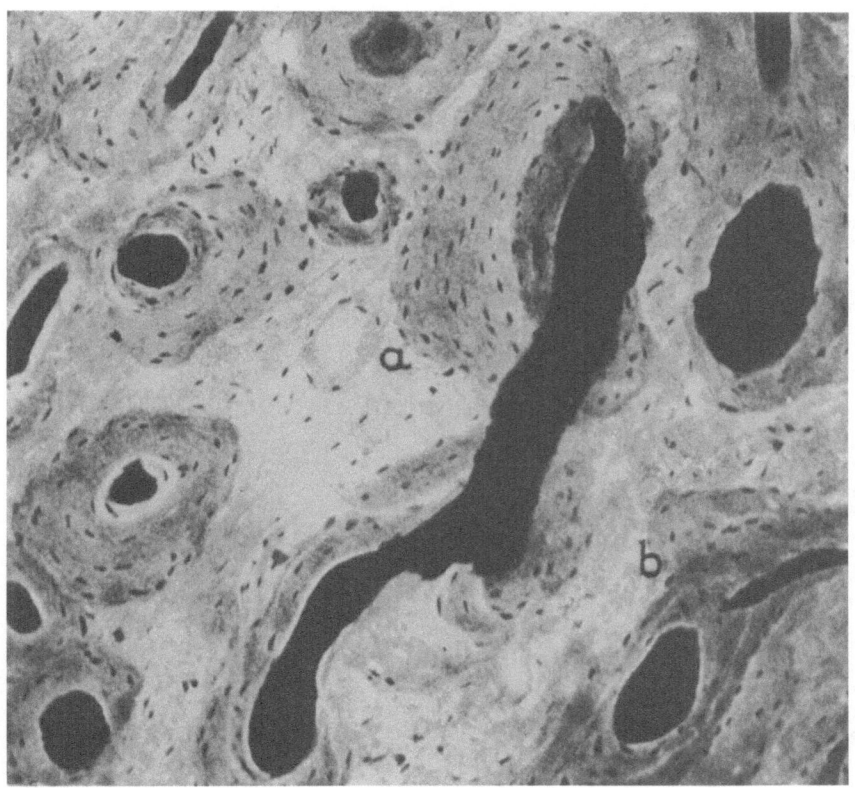

Figure 5. Microradiograph of femoral cortex of an 84-year-old man.
Note the plugged Haversian canal (a) and the filled lacunae (b).
(Reprinted from Jowsey, J., Clin. Orthoped. 17:213, 1960.)

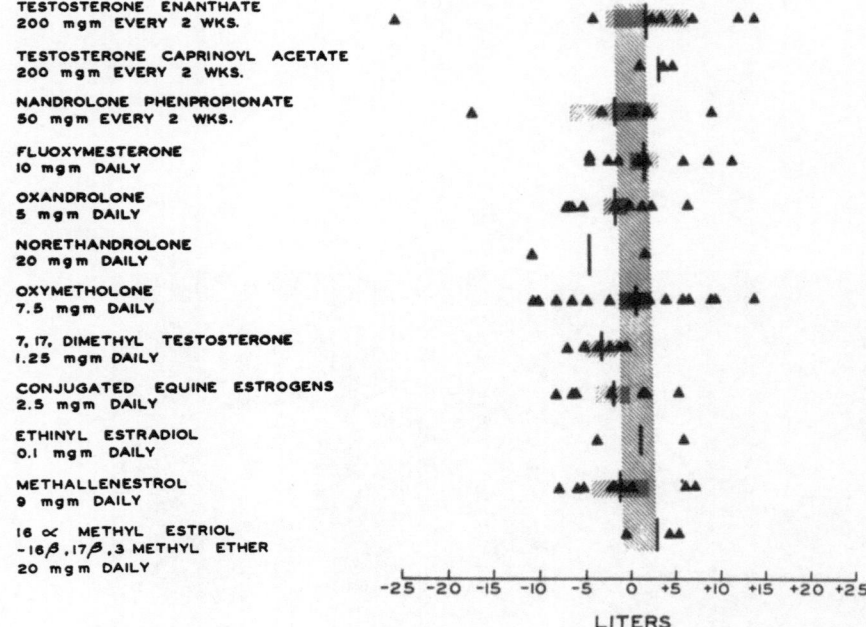

Figure 6. CHANGE IN MISCIBLE POOL OF STRONTIUM

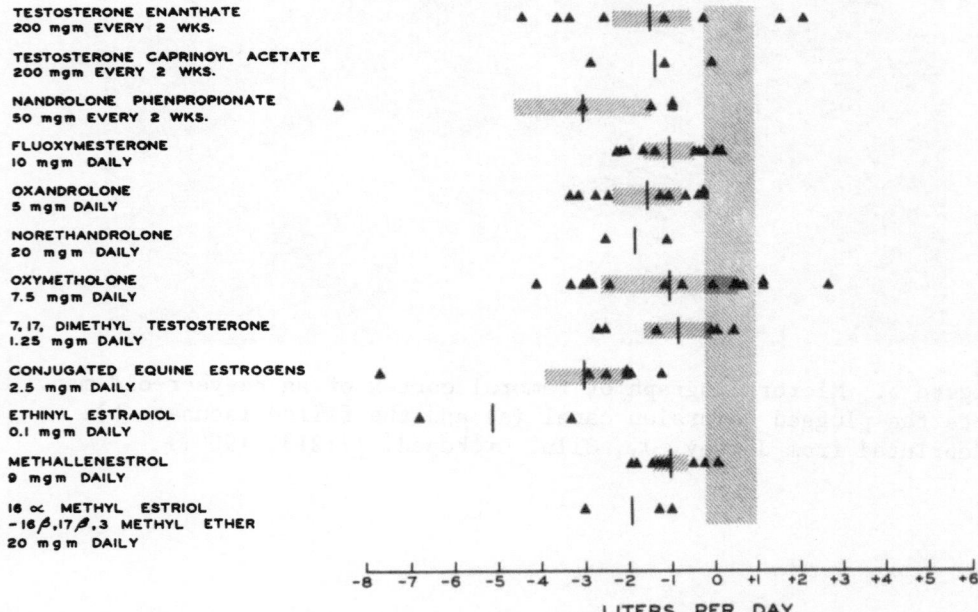

Figure 7. CHANGE IN POOL TURNOVER RATE

Figures 6 & 7. Each ▲ is the change from control value for 1 patient. Vertical bar and horizontal crosshatch is mean ± S.E. Long vertical hatch is mean ± 2 S.D. of change in 34 repeat tests without treatment.

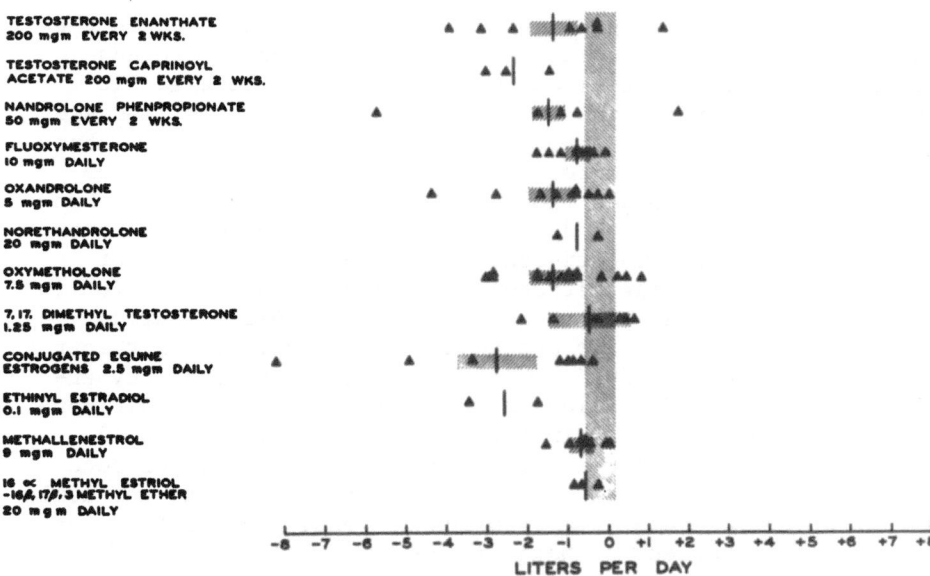

Figure 8.   CHANGE IN URINARY CLEARANCE RATE

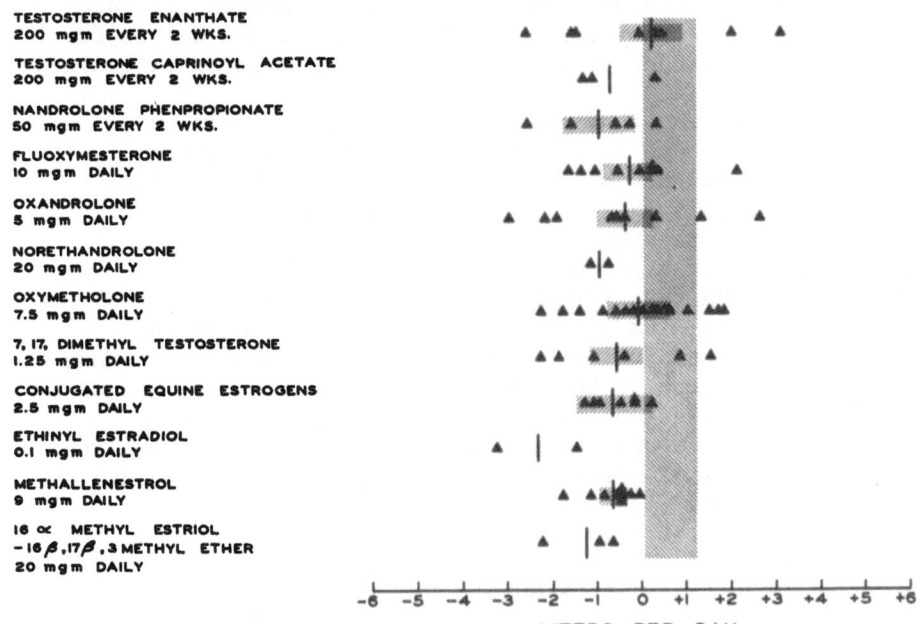

Figure 9.   CHANGE IN "BONE" CLEARANCE RATE

Figures 8 & 9.   Each ▲ is the change from control value for 1 patient.
Vertical bar and horizontal crosshatch is mean ± S.E.   Long vertical
hatch is mean ± S.D. of change in 34 repeat tests without treatment.

What effect does estrogen have on these phenomena seen in the postmenopausal or castrate woman? As already stated, estrogens often decrease urinary calcium and serum phosphorus levels. It seems reasonable to attribute the mild abnormalities sometimes seen in postmenopausal women to a relative deficiency of estrogen. Furthermore, if the slightly increased amounts of bone mineral seen in blood and urine in the postmenopausal woman come from bone then the effect of estrogens is to decrease this egress of mineral from bone. However, the only unequivocal change seen in movement of bone-seeking tracers during estrogen and androgen administration is a decrease in their renal clearance (Figs. 6-9).(16-18) During estrogen therapy there is also a tendency for deposition of tracer into depots to be decreased (Fig. 9). This may represent a cybernetic coupling of bone formation and resorption since in adult bone new bone is made only to fill in a resorption cavity. It could also merely reflect a change in physiochemical reactivity of bone mineral. The change in renal clearance of bone-seeking tracer could be a direct effect on renal hemodynamics or renal tubular function or it could merely reflect a change in bone metabolism that results in a small but significant change in the renal handling of the element. There is no definitive information to separate these possibilities but in twelve experiments during which estrogen was infused directly into a renal artery for up to four hours I was unable to demonstrate a direct effect of estrogens on renal calcium excretion.

In summary I believe that at the present time we can only describe the state of bone and calcium metabolism in postmenopausal osteoporosis and cannot give a clear statement regarding etiology and pathophysiology of the condition. The evidence points to uncompensated bone resorption as an important factor. The clinical correlation of hypogonadism with changes in serum and urine constituents and the fact that some of the biochemical changes are reversible with estrogen treatment lead us to the tentative conclusion, supported by kinetic studies, that estrogens have an inhibiting effect on bone resorption and that they do not stimulate new bone formation in human adults. This conclusion reached by the kinetic studies was recently confirmed by quantitative microradiographic measurement of bone resorption before and during estrogen therapy.(19)

REFERENCES

1. Kyes, P., and T.S. Potter: Physiological marrow ossification in female pigeons. Anat Rec 60:377-379 (1934).
2. Gardner, W.U., and C.A. Pfeiffer: Influence of estrogens and androgens on skeletal system. Physiol Rev 23:139-165 (1943).
3. Albright, F., and E.C. Reifenstein, Jr.: The Parathyroid Glands and Metabolic Bone Disease. Williams and Wilkins, Baltimore, Maryland (1948).

4. Young, M.M., and B.E.C. Nordin: Effects of natural and artificial menopause on plasma and urinary calcium and phosphorus.
   Lancet 2:118-120 (1967).
5. Kelly, P.J., J. Jowsey, B.L. Riggs, and L.R. Elvebach: Relationship between serum phosphate concentration and bone resorption in osteoporosis. J Lab Clin Med 69:110-115 (1967).
6. Pulkkinen, M.O., and K. Willman: Oral contraceptives and
   phosphorus metabolism. Brit Med J 2:574 (1967).
7. Parfitt, A.M.: Changes in serum calcium and phosphorus during
   stilbestrol treatment of osteoporosis. J Bone Joint Surg
   47b:137-139 (1965).
8. Szymendera, J., and S. Madejewicz: Calcium metabolism after
   castration. Lancet 2:1091-1092 (1967).
9. Henneman, P.H., and S. Wallach: A review of the prolonged use
   of estrogens and androgens in postmenopausal and senile osteoporosis. Arch Intern Med 100:715-727 (1957).
10. Goldsmith, N.F., and J.R. Goldsmith: Epidemiological aspects of
    magnesium and calcium metabolism. Arch Environ Health
    12:607-619 (1966).
11. Isakkson, B., and B. Sjögren: Errors inherent in metabolic
    balance studies. Excerpta Med Intern Congr Series No. 83,
    Vol. II. 1965, p. 1041-1049.
12. Heaney, R.P., and G.D. Whedon: Radiocalcium studies of bone
    formation rate in human metabolic bone disease. J Clin Endocr
    18:1246-1267 (1958).
13. Eisenberg, E., and G.S. Gordon: Skeletal dynamics in man
    measured by nonradioactive strontium. J Clin Invest 40:1809-1825
    (1961).
14. Jowsey, J., P.J. Kelly, B.L. Riggs, A.J. Bianco, D.A. Scholz,
    and J. Gershon-Cohen: Quantitative microradiographic studies
    of normal and osteoporotic bone. J Bone Joint Surg
    47a:785-806 (1965).
15. Taylor, T.C., B.N. Epker, and H.M. Frost: The appositional
    rate of Haversian and endosteal bone formation measured in
    tetracycline labeled human ribs. J Lab Clin Med 67:633-639 (1966).
16. Solomon, G.S., W.J. Dickerson, and E. Eisenberg: Psychologic
    and osteometabolic responses to sex hormones in elderly
    osteoporotic women. Geriatrics 15:46-60 (1960).
17. Eisenberg, E.: Effect of steroids on calcium dynamics. In Bio-
    logical Activities of Steroids in Relation to Cancer, G. Pincus
    and E.P. Vollmer, eds. New York, Academic Press. 1960, p.189-197.
18. Eisenberg, E.: Effects of androgens, estrogens and corticoids
    on strontium kinetics in man. J Clin Endocr 26:566-572 (1966).
19. Riggs, B.L., J. Jowsey, and P.J. Kelly: Effect of sex hormones
    on bone metabolism in primary osteoporosis. Clin Res 16:468 (1968).

EFFECT OF ESTROGENS ON THE STRUCTURE OF BONE

Clayton Rich, M. D.

Professor of Medicine, University of Washington
School of Medicine and Chief of Staff, VA Hospital
Seattle, Washington.

The effects of estrogens on the bone of fowl, immature
mice and immature rats are dramatic. In chicks, estrogen
causes formation of new bone originating from the endosteal
surfaces and eventually almost filling the marrow cavity
with trabeculae (1). In normal fowl this is a cyclical phenomenon related to the estrous cycle but can be produced in
cockerels by administering estrogen. A superficially similar growth of new bone, primarily in the metaphysis, but
extending into the diaphysis, can be caused in mice by pharmacological doses of estrogens (2). This effect is not observed normally and the doses of estrogens used are sufficient to inhibit body growth. Simmons (3) and Uelinger (4)
both have measured the uptake of triated thymadine in pre-
osteoblasts after a flash label and found it to be significantly
accelerated, indicating an increase proliferation of these
cells as a result of treatment with estrogens.   Testosterone
appears to inhibit or reverse this action of estrogens, possibly by accelerating bone resorptive activity (5).

Pharmacological doses of estrogens also cause sclerosis
in the metaphysis of the rapidly growing rat. However, in this
case, the cause of the increased amount of bone is a sharp

inhibition of osteoclastic bone resorption rather than increased bone formation, so that the trabeculae of the primary spongiosae are not resorbed and thus contribute to an
unusually dense metaphysis (6, 7). Although the effect of inhibited osteoclastic resorption is most evident at the metaphysis, it appears that osteoclasts are affected generally, since
the diaphysis of rats treated with pharmacological doses for
37 weeks was found to be sclerotic, compared to control animals (8). The effect of estrogens on resorption of the primary spongiosa was neither augmented nor reversed when a
pharmacological dose of testosterone was given in addition to
the estrogens for eight weeks (7).

These observations in chicks, mice and rats emphasized
the magnitude of the effect of estrogens on the skeleton. Although it is probable that estrogen effects are limited to these
species and that other mammals do not show such changes
(7), one should realize that the methods used in the investigations described above are semiquantitative and would show
only relatively marked changes. A small effect on either osteoclastic resorption or osteoblastic formation, which could exert
a significant influence on the skeletal mass in the course of
chronic metabolic disease, would not have been observed.

The findings described above were among the considerations that led Albright to his classic hypothesis that the majority of patients with osteoporosis had this disease directly
because of estrogen deficiency occurring at the time of menopause (9). Several lines of clinical investigation appear to lend
support to this hypothesis, including evidence for a temporal
relationship between menopause and the onset of osteoporosis
and the results of densitometric studies indicating probable
loss of bone at the time of menopause. Additional support
comes from a number of studies which suggest that treatment
with estrogens may reduce the severity of bone loss in osteoporosis. These two points are closely related, but will be examined separately.

RELATIONSHIP BETWEEN MENOPAUSE AND OSTEOPOROSIS

a) Temporal relationship between menopause and osteoporosis. If estrogen deficiency at the time of menopause caused
osteoporosis, one would expect a constant interval between

menopause and osteoporosis, irrespective of the time of menopause. Although there is uncertainty in dating these events,
there have been several studies from which one can evaluate
this relationship. Figure 1 shows the average age at menopause and average age at time of diagnosis of osteoporosis for
the patients in Albright's original series, divided according to
age at time of menopause (9). Although there was a good deal
of variability and overlap in each group, it is apparent that
when these data are so plotted, those patients with onset of
menopause at a very early age had a very long interval between onset of menopause and diagnosis of osteoporosis and
those with menopause occurring late has a short interval; the
average age at the time of the diagnosis of osteoporosis being
nearly the same in all groups. Similar data from a confirmatory series are plotted in figure 2 (10). Thus, when one considers this group of subjects as a whole, there seems to be
little evidence to support what would be expected if estrogen
deficiency at the time of menopause directly caused osteoporosis in the majority of patients.

b) Changes in bone mass at the time of menopause.
Quantitative bone density measurements have been used by
various investigators to examine the possible relationship between bone mass and menopause in large groups of subjects.
All studies of bone mass have shown that there is a gradual
loss of bone at approximately the same rate in man and women,
starting at around the age of 35 years (11, 12). Clearly, this
process cannot be caused by the menopause. Among those
who have examined the possibility that there may be increased
loss of bone at the time of or shortly after menopause, there
is difference of opinion; some discerning an accelerated loss
after menopause (13, 14) and others not (15, 16). The most
suggestive demonstration to date is from work of Meema, who
evaluated muscle and bone mass, both by means of quantitative radiographic densitometry (14). When he compared
these in two groups of women of comparable age but one pre-
and the other post-menopausal, he found muscle mass the
same in both, but bone mass reduced in the latter group. This
is an interesting study because it presents a method for iso-
lating three of the many factors presumed to contribute to
age related bone loss. Assuming that the two groups are
comparable, it demonstrates that there is a definite element
of bone loss at the time of menopause, not accounted for by

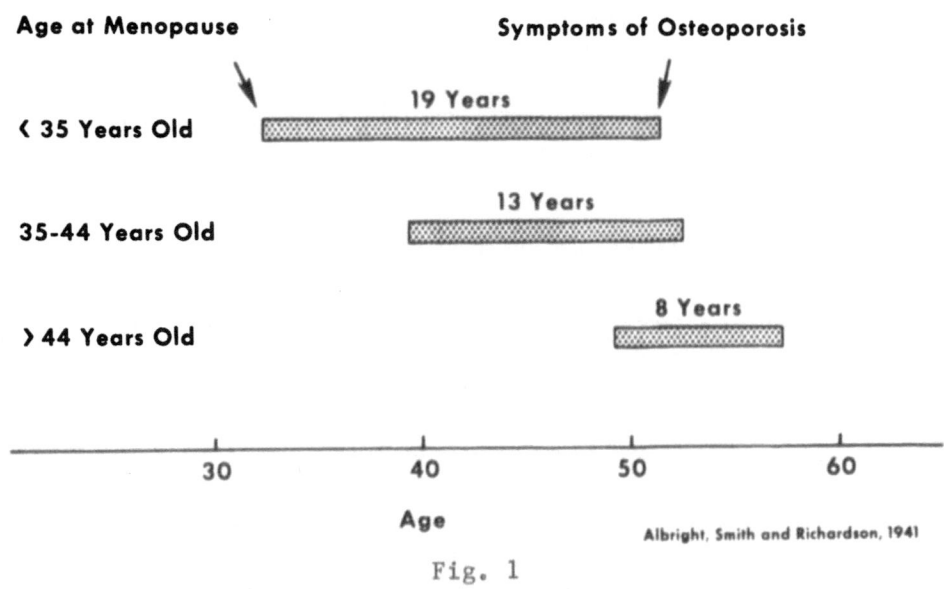

Fig. 1

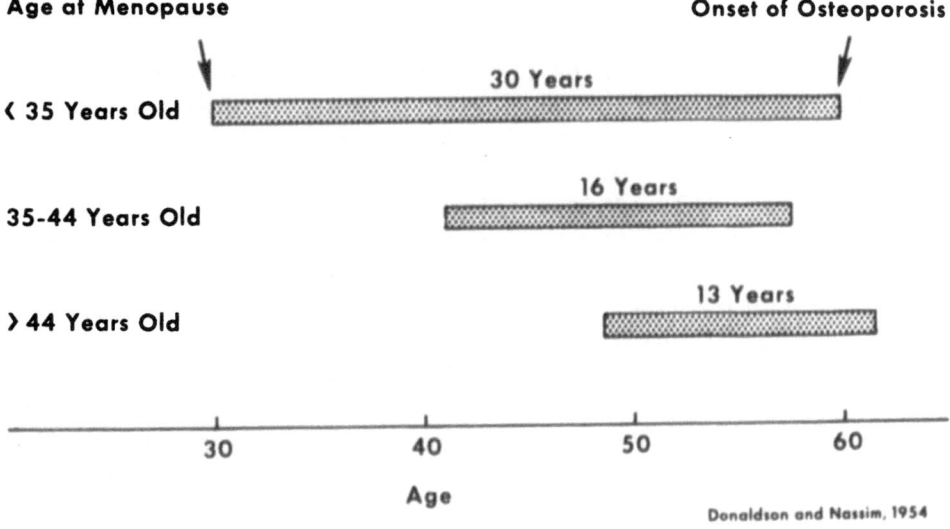

Fig. 2

age or reduction in muscle mass.

Thus, it appears that osteoporosis is not caused directly and simply by estrogen deficiency at the time of menopause but, rather, that estrogen deficiency is the cause of loss of some element of bone mass and that this, along with a number of other contributing factors, all share in the etiology of osteoporosis.

EVIDENCE FOR AN EFFECT OF ESTROGENS ON BONE MASS

There is considerable evidence supporting the concept that estrogen deficiency promotes loss of bone and that treatment with estrogens may confer some benefit on osteoporotic patients. These conclusions are based on several lines of evidence, which are evaluated below.

a) Evidence for decreased morbidity when estrogen treatment is given to osteoporotic patients. This concept is based on clinical observations and one study in which loss of body height was taken as a rough indication of the occurrence of vertebral fractures (17), almost all of which report a favorable effect of treatment. Nevertheless, for the reasons given below, one cannot place much confidence in any of these observations, except for the one study which included a control group of comparable, untreated patients. No difference was observed in symptomatic response between the patients treated with estrogens and those treated with placebos in this controlled study (18). It is predictable that any form of treatment given to osteoporotic subjects under the ordinary clinical situation in an uncontrolled study will likely appear to be beneficial. This is the case because in most subjects, the course of osteoporosis is intermittent; a few weeks or months of symptoms being followed by several or many years of minimal or no symptoms and no fractures. Because the diagnosis usually is made at a time when the patient is symptomatic following a fractured vertebrae, the probable finding if the patient were not treated would be gradual relief of symptoms as the fracture healed, followed by several years of good health. Since treatment usually is started when the diagnosis is made shortly after a fracture has occurred, exactly the same course would be predicted, irrespective of the form of treatment. Thus, one should expect to observe fewer fractures and reduced symptoms in a period of a few years after starting treatment than in the immediate period before treatment. These considerations cause one to have to reject clinical testamonials of therapeutic efficacy which are based upon uncontrolled observations. They also lead to doubt as to how to interpret the study of the effect of estrogens on height. Henneman and Wallach followed their treated group for a total of 100 patient years, during which there were eight instances of loss of height (17). Assuming that this may reflect an incidence of vertebral compression fractures of 8 per hundred patients per year, or 8% per year; would a comparable group selected in the same way, but not treated, have experienced a higher incidence of morbidity than 8% per year or would it have been the same?

b) Evidence for calcium and phosphate retention during treatment of patients with estrogens. There is no question that administration of superphysiological doses of estrogens cause calcium and phosphate retention (17, 19). Therefore, it has been puzzling and disappointing that no discernible increase in bone mass has been observed, even in patients treated with estrogens for many years. An explanation of this apparent delimma may lie in the concept that bone remodelling is an orderly and interrelated process in which osteoclastic differentiation and bone resorption is followed by osteoblastic differentiation and deposition of new bone in the regions of previous resorption (20) and that influences which stimulate or inhibit differentiation of osteoclasts somehow also stimulate or inhibit osteoblastic differentiation. This concept is consistent with an apparent tendency for both of these rates to respond to various stimuli in the same direction, although perhaps not to the same degree, thus tending to maintain a steady state between bone resorption and bone formation.

Figure 3 shows the calcium balance, plotted against weeks of treatment, for all patients treated with either calcium (21) or sex steroids (22) for more than 12 weeks. Isotopic calcium kinetic analysis at the early period after initiation of treatment showed the bone accretion rate to be normal, as it is found to be generally in osteoporosis. In contrast, when these measurements were repeated more than 12 weeks after initiating treatment, the bone accretion rate was found to be low. The

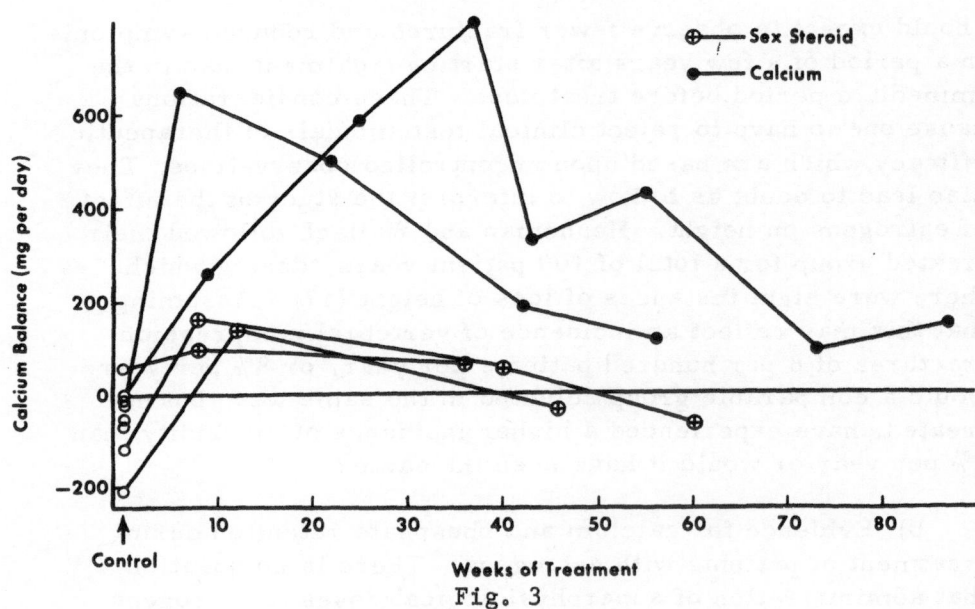

Fig. 3

sequence of events appears to have been an initial reduction
of bone resorption induced by treatment with estrogens or
calcium, followed by a corresponding reduction of bone formation. These results are most consistent with the conclusion that the basic effect of estrogens (or calcium; presumably through a reduction in the circulating level of parathyroid hormone) is to decrease the rate of remodelling in bone.
Assuming that as osteones remodel a resorption cavity first
is formed and new bone is formed in it some time later, the
effect of estrogen would be observed early as reduced resorption and later on as a reduction of both rates.

c) Histological studies. There have been relatively few
quantitative studies of bone formation and resorption in
osteoporosis and only one of the effect of estrogen. However,
they lead to the same conclusions as are described above.
Jowsey has shown that the level of resorptive activity in tra-
becular bone of nonosteoporotic patients increases with increasing age, while the level for bone formation activity remains unchanged. The level of resorptive activity was found
to be 2 to 4 times higher in patients with clinically significant
osteoporosis than in nonosteoporotic patients of the same age
(23). These measurements were of the surface area on which
formation or resorption occurred rather than of the rates of
these two processes. Frost, using the tetracycline labeling

method which allow a direct measurement of the bone formation rate finds that the bone formation rate is approximately the same in osteoporotic patients as in normal subjects and that the absolute rate of bone resorption in osteoporosis is elevated (24, 25).

The only quantitative evaluation of humans treated with estrogen is described in a recently published abstract by Riggs, Jowsey and Kelly (26). They studied 12 osteoporotic patients, of which 11 were postmenopausal, before and after treatment with a physiological dose of estrogens. In 10 of these patients who had been treated for 2 1/2 to 4 months, the level of bone formation was normal. The level of bone resorption was found to be markedly elevated before but had returned almost to normal after 2 1/2 to 4 months of estrogen treatment, thus confirming an immediate effect of estrogens on bone resorption. In two of the patients, the second biopsy was taken after more than one year of treatment. In these patients the level of resorptive activity also had decreased to within or near the normal range, but in these two patients the level of bone formation also was markedly reduced. Thus, these anatomical studies support the concepts described above based on balance and isotopic kinetic measurements; that estrogen treatment will inhibit bone resorptive activity, but that when prolonged treatment with estrogens is given there is a gradual decrease in formation as well, tending to establish a new steady state. These findings also support the concept that estrogens might inhibit the progression of osteoporosis but would not tend to restore bone mass once it has been lost.

d) Effect of estrogens on bone mass. Finally, there are two published studies suggesting that the treatment with physiological doses of estrogens during and after either artificial or natural menopause sustains bone mass at more nearly premenopausal levels. In one of these Davis, Strandjord and Lanzl compared two groups of approximately aged-matched postmenopausal females according to number of years since the menopause (27). One group was treated with replacement dose of estrogens and the other was not. They found a very significantly increased rate of bone loss between the 5th and 10th year after menopause in the untreated group. Subsequently the rate of loss of bone in the two groups was comparable and, therefore, the bones in the untreated group remained lighter. This suggests that estrogen deficiency may have contributed to the loss of some quantum of the mass of the skeleton and that loss of this portion of the skeletal mass was prevented by treatment with estrogens. In a somewhat similar study, Meema found that patients treated with replacement doses of estrogen for more than two years following surgical menopause lost a smaller amount of bone mass than did untreated patients, the former maintaining about the same skeletal mass as did normal subjects of the same sex and age (28). These studies would appear conclusive if the two groups of patients studied were comparable. On the other hand, if the treated groups represented a specially selected group of patients; for instance, a group of ambulatory healthy patients in a practice in which all patients were treated with estrogens, whereas the control group represented patients referred from the inpatient ward services of a hospital, then there would be no basis for deciding whether the differences in bone density were due to estrogen deficiency or to extraneous factors, such as differences in nutritional state or the presence of various diseases for which hospital admission had been necessary. Although the criteria for selection of patients are not given in one of these studies (27), the two studies lead to the same conclusions as can be derived from the morphological work; that maintenance therapy with estrogens can reduce the rate of bone loss in post-menopausal women.

CONCLUSIONS

1. Estrogen deficiency appears to result in accelerated bone resorption. This leads to loss of an appreciable amount of bone soon after the menopause.

2. Post-menopausal bone resorption is one of the factors that contributes to age related bone loss and osteoporosis but does not appear to be the major cause of these processes.

3. Physiological or low pharmacological doses of estrogens tend to counteract the accelerated rate of bone resorption observed in post-menopausal osteoporosis.

4. Prolonged treatment with estrogens probably slows the rate of bone remodelling, so that both the rate of formation and resorption is slower.

REFERENCES

1. Pfeiffer, C. A., and Gardner, W. U. Skeletal changes and blood serum calcium level in pigeons receiving estrogens. Endocrinology 23, 485 (1938).

2. Silberberg, M., and Silberberg, R. The difference in the response of skeletal tissues to estrogen in mice of various ages. Anat. Record 80, 347 (1941).

3. Simmons, D. J. Cellular changes in the bones of mice as studied with triated thymidine and the effects of estrogen. Clin. Orthopaed. 26, 176, (1963).

4. Uehlinger, E. On the influence of thyroxine, thiouracil, cortisone, estrogen and testosterone on endochondral ossification utilizing autoradiography, in Calcified Tissues 1965, H. Fleisch, H. J. J. Blackwood and M. Owen, eds. Springer-Verlog, New York, (1966) p. 243.

5. Barker, D. J. and Crossley, J. N. Effect of testosterone on oestrogen-induced bone formation in mice. Nature 194, 1088 (1962).

6. Day, H. G. and Follis, R. H., Jr. Skeletal changes in rats receiving estradiol benzoate as indicated by histological studies and determinations of bone ash, serum calcium and phosphate, Endocrinology, 28, 83, (1941)

7. Budy, A. M., Urist, M. R. and McLean, F. C. The effect of estrogens on the growth apparatus of the bones of immature rats. Am. J. Path. 28, 1143, (1952).

8. Bernick, S. and Ershoff, B. H. Histochemical study of bone in estrogen - treated rats. J. Dent. Res. 42, 981, (1963).

9. Albright, F., Smith, P. H. and Richardson, A. M. Postmenopausal osteoporosis: Its clinical features. J. Am. Med. Assoc. 116, 2465 (1941).

10. Donaldson, I. A. and Nassim, J. R. The artificial menopause with particular reference to the occurrence of spinal porosis. Br. Med. J. 1, 1228 (1954).

11. Garn, S. M. , Rohmann, C. G. and Nolan, P. , Jr. The developmental nature of bone changes during aging in Relations of Development and Aging. J. E. Burren, ed. C. C. Thomas, Springfield, Ill. (1964).

12. Arnold, J. S. , Bartley, M. H. , Tont, S. A. and Jenkins, D. P. Skeletal changes in aging and disease. Clin. Orthopaed. 49, 17 (1966).

13. Jasani, C. , Nordin, B. E. C. , Smith, D. A. and Swanson, I. Spinal osteoporosis and the menopause. Proc. Royal Soc. Med. 58, 441 (1965).

14. Meema, H. E. Menopausal and aging changes in muscle mass and bone mineral content. J. Bone and Joint Surg. 48A, 1138 (1966).

15. Smith, R. W. , Jr. Dietary and hormonal factors in bone loss. Federation Proc. 26, 1737 (1967).

16. Baylink, D. J. , Vose, G. P. , Dotter, W. E. and Hurxthal, L. M. Two new methods for the study of osteoporosis and other metabolic bone disease. II. Vertebral bone densitometry. Lahey Clin. Bull. 13, 217 (1964).

17. Henneman, P. H. , and Wallach, S. A review of the prolonged use of estrogens and androgens in postmenopausal and senile osteoporosis. Arch. Internal Med. 100, 715 (1957).

18. Solomon, G. F. , Dickerson, W. J. and Eisenberg, E. Psychologic and osteometabolic responses to sex hormones in elderly osteoporotic women. Geriatrics 15, 46 (1960).

19. Albright, F. , and Reifenstein, E. C. , Jr. The Parathyroid Glands and Metabolic Bone Disease: Selected Studies. (1948) Williams & Wilkins Company, Baltimore.

20. Hattner, R. , Epker, B. N. and Frost, H. M. Suggested sequential mode of control of changes in cell behavior in adult bone remodelling. Nature, 206, 489 (1965).

21.   Schwartz, E., Panariello, V. A. and Saeli, J.   Radio-
       active calcium kinetics during high calcium intake in
       osteoporosis.   J. Clin. Invest. 44, 1547 (1965).

22.   Lafferty, F. W., Spencer, G. E., Jr. and Pearson, O. H.
       Effects of androgens, estrogens and high calcium intakes
       on bone formation and resorption in osteoporosis. Am. J.
       Med. 36, 514 (1964).

23.   Jowsey, J., Kelly, P. J., Riggs, B. L., Bianco, A. J., Jr.,
       Scholz, D. A., and Gershon-Cohen, J.   Quantitative micro-
       radiographic studies of normal and osteoporotic bone.   J.
       Bone Joint Surg. 47A, 785 (1965).

24.   Villanueva, A., Frost, H., Ilnicki, L., Frame, B., Smith,
       R. and Arnstein, R.   Cortical bone dynamics measured by
       means of tetracycline labeling in 21 cases of osteoporosis.
       J. Lab. Clin. Med. 68, 599 (1966).

25.   Wu, K., Jett, S. and Frost, H. M.   Bone resorption rates
       in rib in physiological, senile, and postmenopausal osteo-
       poroses.   J. Lab. Clin. Med. 69, 810 (1967).

26.   Riggs, B. L., Jowsey, J. and Kelly, P. J.   Effect of sex
       hormones on bone metabolism in primary osteoporosis.
       Clin. Res. 16, 468 (1968).

27.   Davis, M. E., Strandjord, N. M. and Lanzl, L. H.   Estrogens
       and the aging process: The detection, prevention, and retarda-
       tion of osteoporosis.   J. Am. Med. Assn. 196, 219 (1966).

28.   Meema, H. E., and Meema, S.   Prevention of postmenopausal
       osteoporosis by hormone treatment of the menopause.   Can.
       Med. Assoc. J. 99, 248 (1968).

EFFECTS OF ESTROGENS AND PROGESTERONES ON COLLAGEN METABOLISM

Stephen M. Krane, M.D.

Departments of Medicine, Harvard Medical School and
Massachusetts General Hospital, Boston, Mass.

In attempting to evaluate effects of estrogens and progestational compounds on bone, it is important to consider how the components of the organic matrix may be affected. Bone consists of
an inorganic mineral phase, which comprises approximately two
thirds of the weight of the tissue, and an organic phase which is
largely the protein collagen. Today I shall discuss selected
studies on the effects of estrogens and progesterones on metabolism of collagen not only in bone but in other connective tissues
as well. It is necessary, however, to review briefly some aspects
of the chemistry and biology of collagen (1,2) in order to evaluate the results of such studies.

Collagen is among the most abundant proteins in animal tissues. In the form in which it exists at physiological temperature,
ionic strength and pH, collagen is remarkably resistant to attack
by proteolytic enzymes. Its amino acid composition is unique with
a high content of glycine and proline, the presence of hydroxyproline and hydroxylysine, the low content of tyrosine and the absence
of tryptophan and cystine. The collagen molecules are composed of
three polypeptide chains, each of which has a molecular weight of
approximately 100,000. Each of these polypeptide chains in the
native state is in the form of a left-handed helix and the three
chains together are then coiled about a central axis in a right-
handed super helix. Collagen molecules in solution are thus in
the form of rigid rods of dimensions of approximately 2800 x 15 Å,
and of approximate molecular weight 300,000. The polypeptide
chains (called α chains) are held together in the native molecule
by hydrogen bonds and other short-range forces. The α chains are
of approximately the same size and have similar but not identical

amino acid compositions, usually with two chains the same (α_1) and one different (α_2). In some molecules two α chains are linked covalently near the amino-terminal end to produce β components, probably through an α, β-unsaturated aldehyde formed by the condensation of two lysyl-derived aldehydes (3).

In the tissues most of the collagen is in the form of insoluble fibrils, which are composed of the collagen molecules aligned head to tail and laterally in such a fashion as to be staggered at approximately one quarter of the length of the molecule. The molecules interact with their neighbors through a variety of forces including covalent bonds. When a tissue containing collagen is minced and suspended in cold, neutral salt solutions a small fraction of the collagen will be solubilized. Increasing the ionic strength may result in an additional increment of collagen solubilized; a further fraction may be obtained by decreasing the pH using organic acids such as citric or acetic. Finally, a fraction of collagen remains which is insoluble in all of these solvents and can be rendered soluble only by heating beyond the denaturation temperature or by using denaturing agents such as urea, lithium chloride or guanidine hydrochloride.

An index of the rate of collagen synthesis can be obtained by measuring the incorporation of a radioactively labeled amino acid present in high concentration, such as glycine. Incorporation of a labeled amino acid such as proline or lysine is also useful since these substances are hydroxylated to hydroxyproline and hydroxylysine, respectively, after incorporation into the polypeptide chain. Neither hydroxyproline nor hydroxylysine are reutilized for collagen synthesis and therefore their excretion provides some measure of collagen metabolism. Of course, changes in the rate of incorporation of a labeled amino acid into a protein in vivo must be interpreted in relation to the size of the free amino acid precursor pool. Using radioisotopes of these amino acid precursors it has been shown that the collagen that is soluble in cold neutral salt solutions is the most recently synthesized and has the higher proportion of α chains to β components. Insoluble collagens are formed by some maturation process, in which the more soluble collagens are the precursors. This maturation involves formation of intramolecular and intermolecular bonds although these processes may not be interdependent. As mentioned previously, the intramolecular covalent bond is an α, β-unsaturated aldehyde probably formed by the condensation of the aldehydes corresponding to the δ-semialdehyde of α-aminoadipic acid. This aldehyde is formed through the oxidation of the side chain of specific lysyl residues. These observations pertain to the soft tissue collagens; there are probably several differences in maturation of collagens from bone which will not be discussed here.

The synthesis and maturation of collagen may be altered by a variety of factors including rate of growth. For example, if

young guinea pigs are fasted and fail to gain weight for even two
days, the amount of collagen extracted from their skin is strikingly decreased (4). Several drugs affect collagen synthesis and
maturation the most interesting of which is β-aminopropionitrile
and related compounds. β-aminopropionitrile is the active substance present in the sweet pea, lathyrus odoratus, that produces
the disorder known as osteolathyrism when administered to animals
(5). Depending upon such factors as age of the animal, species,
and duration of treatment a variety of changes results such as de-
formities of skeleton, hernias and dissecting aneurysms of the
aorta. The collagen in lathyritic animals is defective as shown
by a striking increase in the neutral salt-soluble fraction and
relative decrease in the insoluble fraction, decrease in the formation of β-components and disordered maturation of the collagen.
With this agent, synthesis of the lysyl-derived aldehyde precursor
of the intramolecular crosslink is inhibited (3). Other substances
such as penicillamine produce lathyrism by a mechanism which differs from that resulting from the use of β-aminopropionitrile,
i.e. the aldehydes are formed but stable crosslinks are disrupted
(3,6,7). Penicillamine, used in the treatment of Wilson's disease
in man, has in some instances resulted in skin lesions characterized by friability and ulceration over pressure points. Biopsies
of skin from such patients have shown the expected chemical lesion
with increased percentage of soluble collagen and an increased
ratio of α chains to β components as compared to normal (8).

In considering the effects of estrogens and progesterones on
collagen metabolism in order to relate such effects to the use of
oral contraceptive agents, it must be emphasized that different
species react differently as well as different tissues in the same
animal. In addition, some investigators have examined effects of
replacement doses and others pharmacological doses. Extrapolation
to the use of these agents in humans may not be possible.

One study in which 17 β-estradiol benzoate over a wide range
of dosage was given to rats for 2 weeks was reported by Smith and
Allison (9). The content of collagen in the skin, uterus and femurs was measured. The amount of collagen per total skin was decreased at all dose levels as a result of estrogen treatment. Although the dry, fat-free weights of the femurs remained unchanged
the collagen per femur was found to increase at the higher dose
levels of estrogens. Unfortunately all doses resulted in failure
of the animals to gain weight normally. Thus the specificity of
the changes observed in the skin was not established.

A slightly different approach is that of Kao et al (10).
They measured the collagen formed in implanted sponges over a period of 4 weeks, then assayed collagen synthesis in a sample of
the sponge incubated in vitro with ^{14}C-lysine by measuring labeling of protein-bound lysine and hydroxylysine. Normal and oophor-

ectemized rats were treated with vehicle only or with estradiol
benzoate twice weekly in doses ranging from 1 to 300 μg. The
total collagen per sponge was decreased 20 to 25% as a result of
estrogen treatment, consistent with the findings of Smith and Allison (9) mentioned previously. However the specific activities of
hydroxylysine and lysine in collagen in the in vitro incubation
system, were significantly greater in the samples from the animals treated with the 300 μg doses of estradiol. Although the
collagen was not purified for these analyses it was concluded that
estrogens stimulated synthesis as well as catabolism of collagen.

More recently Henneman (10) has examined the effects of estradiol on collagen metabolism in guinea pigs of various ages. Granulomas were induced by the subcutaneous injection of carrageenan and
the effect of estrogen on total and soluble collagen measured in
skin, granuloma, aorta and bone. In both young and old animals estrogens decreased the amount of collagen in skin and granuloma
while increasing bone mass and bone collagen. On the basis of
analysis of fractions containing hydroxyproline soluble in 0.15$\underline{M}$
and 0.5$\underline{M}$ NaCl and 0.5$\underline{M}$ sodium citrate and the specific activity in
fractions after administration of ^{14}C-proline, it was suggested
that estrogens stimulated collagen synthesis, turnover and maturation. A further suggestion was offered that a proline-rich precursor was formed as a result of estrogen therapy. Unfortunately,
the collagens soluble in the various fractions were not isolated
and purified and therefore it is not possible to conclude that the
proline-rich material was actually related to collagen and not to
other proteins. Also it is not certain in these experiments
whether estrogens affected the weight gain of the guinea pigs;
rate of growth markedly influences collagen metabolism in these
animals (4).

However, it appears from these studies that estrogens do decrease the collagen in skin and granulation tissue in rats and
guinea pigs whereas bone collagen may increase under the same circumstances. The decrease in skin collagen may be associated with
increased turnover. Few studies are available in humans in regard to collagen metabolism as effected by estrogens. Only indirect information can be obtained from measurement of total urinary
hydroxyproline excretion. In short-term studies a slight decrease
in hydroxyproline excretion resulted from the administration of
0.2 mg of ethinyl estradiol daily to osteoporotic women (12).
Larger decrements were noted in women given doses of estradiol and
estriol calculated to be similar to amounts secreted in late pregnancy (13). Whether these decreases are due to decrease in collagen degradation or decrease in synthesis and in which collagenous
structure remain to be determined.

The effects of progestational agents on collagen metabolism
have not been extensively investigated. However, the results of

a recent study by Kühn et al (14) are of considerable interest.
Rats were given 0.5 mg of progesterone subcutaneously each day for
14 days without altering the general appearance of the animals or
their rate of weight gain. At the end of this period the rats were
given ^{14}C-glycine and groups of animals killed at intervals from
0.5 to 9 days. Samples of skin were removed and analyzed for
total collagen content (hydroxyproline) as well as the collagen
which could be extracted into cold solutions of neutral salt or
weak acid. The specific and total activities of ^{14}C-glycine were
measured in each fraction. Progesterone increased the amount of
collagen in the neutral salt extracts from 6.10 to 6.93% and decreased that in the acid-soluble fraction from 2.14 to 1.72%. The
specific activity of the neutral salt soluble collagen was increased by progesterone treatment up to the fifth day and then
fell off to values below that of the control animals. However,
the specific activities of the acid-soluble and insoluble collagen were lower in the treated than in the control animals throughout the whole experiment. These observations suggest that the
formation of insoluble and acid-soluble collagen was inhibited by
progesterone whereas total synthesis was stimulated by the hormone.
The inhibition of formation of insoluble collagen (formation of
intermolecular crosslinks) was therefore similar to that produced
by β-aminopropionitrile, although the lathyrogenic effects of the
latter are much more striking.

These studies, although preliminary, suggest that in rats
progesterone is a mild lathyrogen. The type of chemical lesion
is not yet known. Whether or not effects of continued administration of progestational agents would produce a similar response
in humans cannot be predicted from these studies. It has been
possible to show using punch biopsy specimens (8) that a drug such
as penicillamine which is lathyrogenic in animals does alter the
cross-linking (ratio of α chains to β components) and solubility
of human skin collagen. Such techniques might also be used to
assay the possible lathyrogenic effects of progesterone in man.

Summary

Studies in animals have shown that estrogens decrease the
collagen content of skin and granulomas whereas bone collagen is
not decreased. These alterations may be accompanied by increase
in "turnover" of collagen. Progesterone in rats is a mild lathyrogen, and interferes with generation of crosslinks and maturation
of collagen. It is not known whether long-term use of combinations of estrogens and progesterones will produce similar defects
in collagens in humans.

REFERENCES

1. Ramachandran, G.N. and Gould, B.S. (Eds.) A Treatise on Col-
    lagen. Academic Press, London and New York, 1968. Vol. 1, 2A
    and 2B.
2. Seifter, S. and Gallop, P.M.: The structure proteins, in
    The Proteins, H. Neurath (Ed.). Academic Press, New York,
    1966, pp. 153-458.
3. Piez, K.A.: Cross-linking of collagen and elastin. Ann. Rev.
    Biochem. 37:547-570, 1968.
4. Gross, J.: Studies on the formation of collagen.II. The in-
    fluence of growth rate on neutral salt extracts of guinea pig
    dermis. J. Exp. Med. 107:265-277, 1958.
5. Tanzer, M.L.: Experimental lathyrism. Int. Rev. Connective
    Tissue Res. 3:91-112, 1965.
6. Nimni, M.E. and Bavetta, L.A.: Collagen defect induced by
    penicillamine. Science 150:905-907, 1965.
7. Nimni, M.E.: A defect in the intramolecular and intermolecu-
    lar cross-linking of collagen caused by penicillamine. I.
    Metabolic and functional abnormalities in soft tissues. J.
    Biol. Chem. 243:1457-1466, 1968.
8. Harris, E.D., Jr. and Sjoerdsma, A.: Effect of penicillamine
    on human collagen and its possible application to treatment
    of scleroderma. Lancet 2:996-999, 1966.
9. Smith, Q.T. and Allison, D.J.: Changes of collagen content
    in skin, femur and uterus of 17 β-estradiol benzoate-treated
    rats. Endocrinol. 79:486-492, 1966.
10. Kao, K.-Y.T., Hitt, W.E. and McGavack, T.H.: Connective
    tissue XIII. Effect of estradiol benzoate upon collagen
    synthesis by sponge biopsy connective tissue. Proc. Soc.
    Exp. Biol. Med. 119:364-367, 1965.
11. Henneman, D.H.: Effect of estrogen on in vivo and in vitro
    collagen biosynthesis and maturation in young and old female
    guinea pigs. Endocrinol. 83:678-690, 1968.
12. Young, M.M., Jasani, C., Smith, D.A. and Nordin, B.E.C.:
    Some effects of ethinyl oestradiol on calcium and phosphorus
    metabolism in osteoporosis. Clin. Sci. 34:411-417, 1968.
13. Katz, F.H. and Kappas, A.: The effect of natural estrogens
    on hydroxyproline excretion in man. J. Clin. Invest. 44:
    1063, 1965.
14. Kühn, K., Stecher, K., Iwangoff, P., Hammerstein, F., Dur-
    ruti, M., Holzmann, H. and Korting, G.W.: Studies on the
    metabolism of collagen III. The incorporation of (^{14}C) gly-
    cine into the collagen of rats treated with progesterone.
    Biochem. Z. 343:528-536, 1965.

VASCULAR SYSTEM

THROMBOEMBOLISM AND CONTRACEPTIVE MEDICATION: INCIDENCE

AND MECHANISM

Anthony P. Fletcher and Norma Alkjaersig

Washington University School of Medicine
St. Louis, Missouri

The nature of this morning's meeting on blood and vascular
changes resulting from contraceptive medication differs sharply
from those previously held. Earlier we have considered significant
biochemical changes resulting from contraceptive medication, changes
which, in the main, appeared reversible or potentially reversible
on discontinuation of medication and which were, generally speaking,
clinically asymptomatic.

This morning we discuss the possibility that contraceptive
medication may, directly or indirectly, induce or precipitate a
number of serious non-reversible, or only partially-reversible,
clinical syndromes, which include thrombophlebitis, pulmonary embolism, cerebral thrombosis and possible other thromboembolic complications. The occurrence of such disease states, in gross form, is
readily obvious, but neither the exact relationship of contraceptive medication to these disease states, nor the biochemical mechanism involved, is presently clear.

Since certain special facets in the field will be considered
in detail by the other contributers--Doll, the epidemiological
studies, Wessler, the induction and effects of blood hypercoagulability in the experimental animal, Astrup and Brakman, certain
of the effects of steroid administration on blood and tissue fibrinolytic activity, and Haslam, the effect of steroid administration
on platelets, it will be my function to attempt to set these
special subjects in general perspective and also to cover additional
areas of relevance.

Though the epidemiological data will later be discussed in

detail, I shall cite certain epidemiological incidental data to
define the potential magnitude of the problem. The latest English
epidemiological findings (1) suggest first that on a mortality
basis, the excess mortality in otherwise healthy women from pulmonary embolism or other thromboembolic complications, attributable to
the use of contraceptive drugs, will be approximately 1.3 per
100,000 users per year in those women aged 20-34 and 3.4 per 100,000
users per year when aged 35-45. Furthermore, there are strong
grounds for suspicion that contraceptive medication may increase
the risk of incurring cerebral thrombosis and possibly also myocardial infarction.

On a morbidity basis, Vessey and Doll (2) concluded that for
otherwise healthy women on contraceptive medication, the risk of
hospital admission for venous thromboembolic complications was
approximately nine fold greater than for women not receiving the
medication. Overall, the latest English figures suggest that approximately one in 2,000 women who are using oral contraceptives
will be admitted to the hospital each year with "idiopathic" venous
thromboembolism compared to an incidence of about one in 20,000
cases among untreated women.

While I am sure that Dr. Doll will be the first to agree that
the most urgent need in this field is for the obtaining of further
data, these cited figures may suffice to define roughly the quantitative aspects of these problems. If these figures are accepted,
they represent, despite the human suffering implied in their statement, a relatively low incidence of complicating thromboembolism.
Such an incidence forces consideration of two distinct investigative possibilities: First, that contraceptive agents induce, in
all or the majority of patients, some hypothetical biochemical alterations predisposing subjects to thromboembolism. Second, that
the medication may unmask a small subject population, genetically
or otherwise susceptible to thromboembolism, which alone will show
biochemical changes suggestive of impending thrombosis.

If this latter possibility obtains, and it cannot be excluded,
two implications follow. First, investigation of a large unselected population may not, since the number of non-susceptible persons
will be large and the number of presumed susceptible subjects small,
yield homogeneous or reliable information on the cause of thrombosis and, second, in these circumstances, we should be prepared
to accept the reliability of an association between thromboembolism
and contraceptive medication on solid epidemiological evidence
alone, even in the absence of significant laboratory data on the
mechanisms involved.

However, not all are in agreement with the epidemiological
data and their interpretation. For instance, Drill and Calhoun (3)

have recently advanced the extreme view that epidemiological data
purporting to establish an association between chronic contraceptive medication and thromboembolism are either faulty or misinter-
preted and that no significant problem exists. I find this latter
conclusion hard to accept and think that Doctors Doll and Seigel
will later convince us that a very real problem is involved.

In many ways, the problem of vascular and blood coagulation
changes attributable to contraceptive medication is analogous to
that posed by the relationship of carcinoma of the lung to smoking.
In each instance, the primary evidence for both the existence of
the problem and for its quantification rests on epidemiological
study; in neither instance, is there certainty as to the precise
mechanism of these effects. Moreover, in both cases, the epidemiological data and findings either were, or are, in dispute.

The present _positive_ epidemiological data can be summarized
as follows:

1. Women in the younger age groups in whom the spontaneous
occurrence of thromboembolism is relatively rare, receiving contraceptive medication, incur an increased rate of morbidity and mortality from the development of thromboembolic disease.

2. Medication risks increase as the subject becomes older,
in line with the known higher risk of developing spontaneous throm-
bcembolism.

3. While the thromboembolic lesions occur predominantly in
the venous system, there are reasonable grounds for suspecting
that arterial lesions may also occur and lead to either cerebrovascular insufficiency or myocardial infarction.

On the negative side, no satisfactory data are available to
answer the extremely important question as to whether the risk of
developing thromboembolism increases with treatment duration, and
since medication may presumably be needed for one or more decades,
extreme urgency attends the answering of this question. Also, the
epidemiological data have been obtained from examination of hospital statistics and we are all too aware that in situations of this
sort, thromboembolic complications may occur in patients who are
neither hospitalized, nor in many cases, diagnosed. While at
present the importance of these uncertainties cannot be weighed, it
is possible that additional epidemiological data could demonstrate
that the magnitude of the thromboembolic disease problem produced
by contraceptive drugs is greater than presently realized.

The present data do not permit decision as to whether any
particular oral contraceptive preparation carries higher risks than

others, but it is suspected that the oestrogen content of the
preparation may be largely responsible for the increased risk of
thromboembolism. The evidence for this supposition is indirect
for though there are studies indicating that high dosage oestrogen
therapy may, under certain circumstances, predispose to thromboembolism in men---the Veterans Administration study on the treatment
of carcinoma of the prostate with oestrogen (4) and trials of oestrogen therapy post-myocardial infarction (5,6)---the evidence for
such effects of oestrogen administration in women is less. However,
recently this phenomenon has been observed in women receiving high
dosage oestrogen therapy for suppression of lactation following
delivery. In both studies (7,8), it was claimed that high dosage
oestrogen therapy clearly increased the risk of thromboembolism,
though the estimates of increased risk varied from ten-fold to
three-fold. I have not shown the detailed data, since again, the
dosage range was far higher than that used for contraceptive purposes and the data obtained retrospectively from hospital records
were rather complex. Nevertheless, these recent findings are of
a rather striking and suggestive nature.

PATHOLOGICAL EVENTS IN THROMBOSIS

While several important approaches to the thrombosis problems
will be outlined this morning, our interpretation of the scientific
findings is hindered by ignorance concerning the precise events
precipitating thrombosis in man (9-11). We know a good deal concerning the functions of blood platelets, blood coagulation both
normal and abnormal, the fibrinolytic enzyme system, mechanisms of
hemostasis, clearance of activated blood coagulation factors, the
role of the reticuloendothelial system, blood rheology, fluid
mechanics, the effects of alterations in lipid metabolism on coagulation function, and other factors of relevance to the thrombosis
problem. However, though knowledge of the precipitating factors
in thrombosis is increasing, especially with respect to those
causative in microthrombosis, understanding of these factors in
producing clinically evident or macrothrombosis, is still
incomplete.

Essentially, we now appreciate from in vitro experiments,
from animal experimental model studies, and also from extensive
clinical and pathological human studies, that not only is thromboembolism often a clinically-silent process, (a fact that, of
course, has been known for many years) but that microthrombosis,
or non-clinically-evident thrombosis, must be inferred to occur
and resolve spontaneously with considerable frequency in the human.
As with all such terms, microthrombosis requires definition. This
term, a useful though imprecise one, is customarily used by path-
ologists and others studying the microcirculation to describe a
lesion due to mechanical, electrical, or other trauma; a lesion,

which has as a minimal descriptive basis, selective platelet
deposition at the trauma site. Through common usage and experience,
the term microthrombosis carries a connotation of reversibility,
for such platelet deposits are notoriously unstable. The second
stage of microthrombosis, the stabilization of the platelet mass
by fibrin, is also reversible; and indeed, the fibrinolytic enzyme
system may aid in the resolution of such lesions. How frequently
microthrombosis leads to macrothrombosis or indeed, to clinically-
evident thrombosis is uncertain. Unfortunately, the circumstances
favoring resolution or progression of the lesion are unclear. It
is also acknowledged that even when vessels are wholly occluded by
thrombotic deposits, total or partial resolution may still occur
through the actions of the fibrinolytic enzyme system or through
cellular enzyme systems. Thus, thrombosis must be regarded as a
dynamic rather than static state and especially when discussing
thrombosis in the clinical context, equal weight should be given
both to those factors that precipitate the condition and to those
factors acting to resolve lesions and preventing their occurrence
as clinically-evident thromboembolism.

No discussion of thrombosis is complete without reference to
the intuitive understanding of the problem displayed by Virchow
approximately a century ago. His famous triad is shown below
(Fig. 1) and states that thrombosis must arise from either: a)
changes in the blood; b) changes in the vessel wall; or c) changes
in blood flow. We now realize that thrombosis is a multifactorial
disease process and we may, also with confidence, add one further
factor to the triad, a factor undescribed in Virchow's time: the
influence of the plasma fibrinolytic system in resolving the initial thrombotic process.

VIRCHOW TRIAD

Thrombosis arises from:

    (a). Changes in blood.
    (b). Changes in vessel wall.
    (c). Changes in blood flow.

    (d). Changes in plasminogen-plasmin
         (fibrinolytic) enzyme function.

Figure 1

Things have, of course, become considerably more complicated since Virchow's original statement on this problem and in Figure 2, the famous triad has been updated. For instance, changes in the blood may include platelet abnormalities, the influence of plasma lipids, stress resulting in the release of catecholamines, which may alter platelet adhesiveness, antigen-antibody reactions, the effect of endotoxin, and numerous other factors. Conditions in the vessel wall might include: damage, the exposure of collagen which will result in platelet adhesiveness to it, exposure of plaque lipid with similar effects, and also the effects of change of the vessel wall on thrombosis. The effects of flow will include the well-known influence of turbulence, stasis, the effect of branching sites in the vascular tree, and atheroma due to hemodynamic stresses. Factors tending to resolve thrombi will include: instability of the initial platelet plug due to diminished platelet adhesiveness, and also the powerful effects of the fibrinolytic enzyme system in resolving fibrinous masses. Obviously, this is not an all-inclusive list and merely indicates some of the many factors which may be involved in the development of clinical thromboembolism.

CAUSES OF THROMBOSIS

Changes In

BLOOD	Platelet Abnormality
	Plasma Lipids
	Catecholamines (Stress)
	Antigen-Antibody Reaction, Etc.
	Blood Hypercoagulability
VESSEL WALL	Injury
	Exposure of Collagens
	Effects of Electrical Charge
	Exposure of Plaque Lipid
FLOW	Turbulence
	Stasis
	Branching Sites
	Atheroma Localized Through Hemodynamic Effects

Figure 2

Figure 3 shows the general stages of thrombus formation in vivo and emphasizes the potential reversibility of the process at its several stages. Platelets adhere to collagen or other non-endothelial surface exposed by vessel injury or disease, release of platelet ADP and other factors causes localized platelet aggregation and the presence of a reactive platelet surface with the release of platelet coagulation factors induces consolidation into a white platelet thrombus. Fibrin is layed down with the formation of a red thrombus, cross-linking of the fibrin fibrils is produced by coagulation Factor XIII, fibrin stabilizing factor, a transamidase. Such a thrombus may either extend or resolve and even if persistent, may eventually be recanalized through cellular mechanisms.

THROMBUS FORMATION

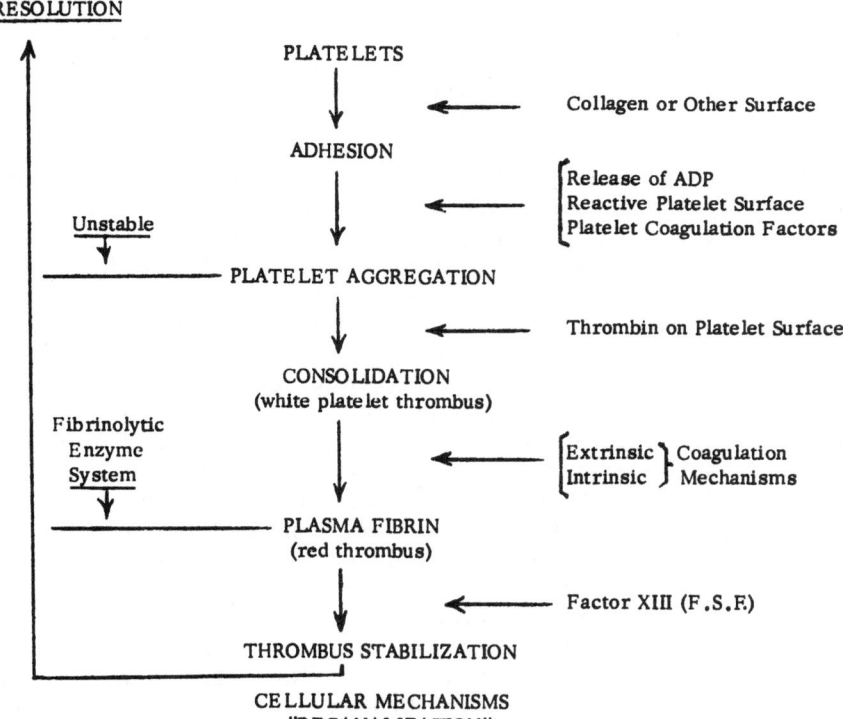

Figure 3. Mechanism of in vivo thrombus formation. Thrombosis is a dynamic state and mechanisms contributing to thrombus resolution are equally as significant as those contributing to thrombus propagation. The chief mechanisms responsible for resolution are those of platelet mass instability, the fibrinolytic enzyme system and cellular mechanisms.

The relative role and importance of abnormality in the various factors shown and others not shown in the genesis of a clinically-evident thrombotic lesion is unclear; it is also known that the relative importance of the different factors may vary in the genesis of arterial and venous lesions. For instance, on both histological and experimental grounds, it would be inferred that blood hypercoagulability would be of considerably greater significance in the genesis of venous, rather than arterial, lesions. Similarly, platelet factors are presently considered to be of greater relevance in the genesis of arterial lesions than in venous thrombosis.

BLOOD HYPERCOAGULABILITY

Increase of various blood coagulation system components has sometimes been referred to as blood hypercoagulability with the implication that such hypercoagulability may predispose to thromboembolism. Thus, the finding that significant increases in certain blood constituents occur during pregnancy has been used in explanation of thromboembolism occurring late in pregnancy or post-partum. For similar reasons, many investigators have studied blood coagulation during contraceptive medication. Thus, the concept of blood hypercoagulability merits consideration; shown in Figure 4 is a modern coagulation scheme known as the McFarlane "cascade" or the Ratnoff "waterfall" theory. Schemes of this nature tend to produce glazing of the eyes in non-coagulationists, but this scheme is reasonably simple and illustrates two points. First, this scheme implies that following the activation of factor XII or Hageman factor by surface contact, each successive blood coagulation factor in the reaction sequence is activated by a preceding enzymatic reaction and that the whole cascade of reactions acts as a powerful biochemical amplifier - the great multiplicity of stages providing a corresponding increase in response to an initial stimulus. Second, there are two distinct pathways by which prothrombin may be activated to thrombin and clot fibrinogen: (A), the so-called intrinsic blood coagulation system in which all the coagulation components required for the reaction are confined to the blood and which is triggered by activation of Hageman factor (Factor XII) following surface contact and (B), the extrinsic coagulation system which is triggered by tissue thromboplastin. Despite extensive speculation on this point, it is not entirely clear that these' two systems have discrete _in vivo_ functions. But, since both mechanisms share a final common pathway through factor X, or Stuart Prower factor, the existence of two distinct mechanisms increases the number of stimuli that may trigger the coagulation response.

Not all the experimental predictions inherent in the cascade hypothesis have been confirmed, and it is presently considered that the blood coagulation mechanism is best represented by a reduced cascade hypothesis (Fig. 5).

CASCADE HYPOTHESIS

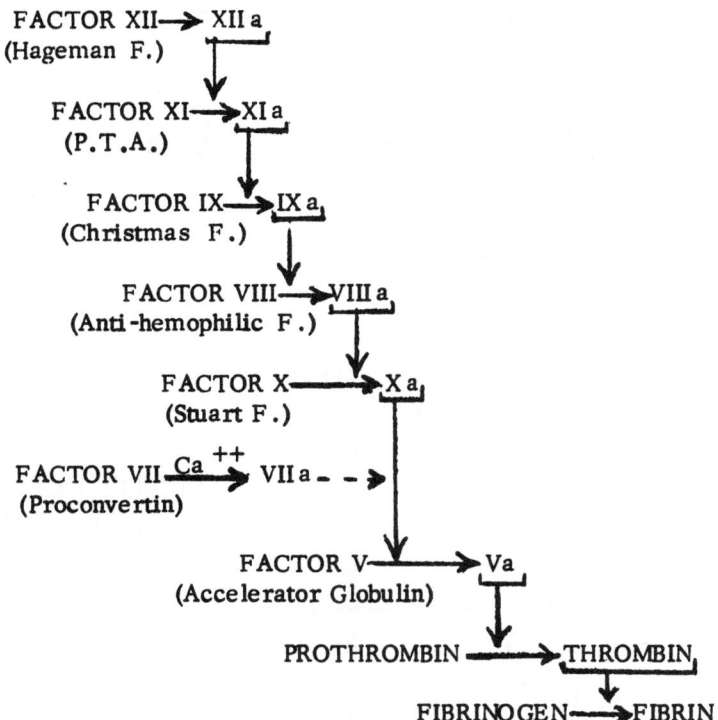

Figure 4. The "cascade" hypothesis of blood coagulation implies the existence of a powerful biochemical amplifier mechanism – each separate blood coagulation function (except factor XII) being activated by the preceding enzymatic step. The Roman numerals designate the known blood coagulation factors; "a" denotes activation. Common synonyms are included beneath the Roman numeral.

This scheme, following that of Esnouf (12), fits well with the present evidence and suggests that, while blood coagulation does involve a substantial degree of biochemical amplification, only three enzymatic steps and possibly a fourth, are involved in the amplifier system. Enzymatic steps involved, prior to the conversion of fibrinogen to fibrin, in the intrinsic system, constitute factor XII (Hageman factor), factor X, (Stuart Prower factor) and prothrombin; possibly also, factor IX, or Christmas factor, may also be involved in an enzymatic activation step. The other known components of the blood coagulation system, namely, factors XI (plasma thromboplastin antecedent), VIII (the antihemophilic factor), and V (labile factor), may act as high molecular weight co-factors to their respective enzymes and may also increase the specificity

of each stage. The dotted line in the scheme represents the effect
of thrombin in increasing the biological activity of both factors
V and VIII, a synergism which can be demonstrated both in plasma
and in partially purified systems.

REDUCED CASCADE HYPOTHESIS

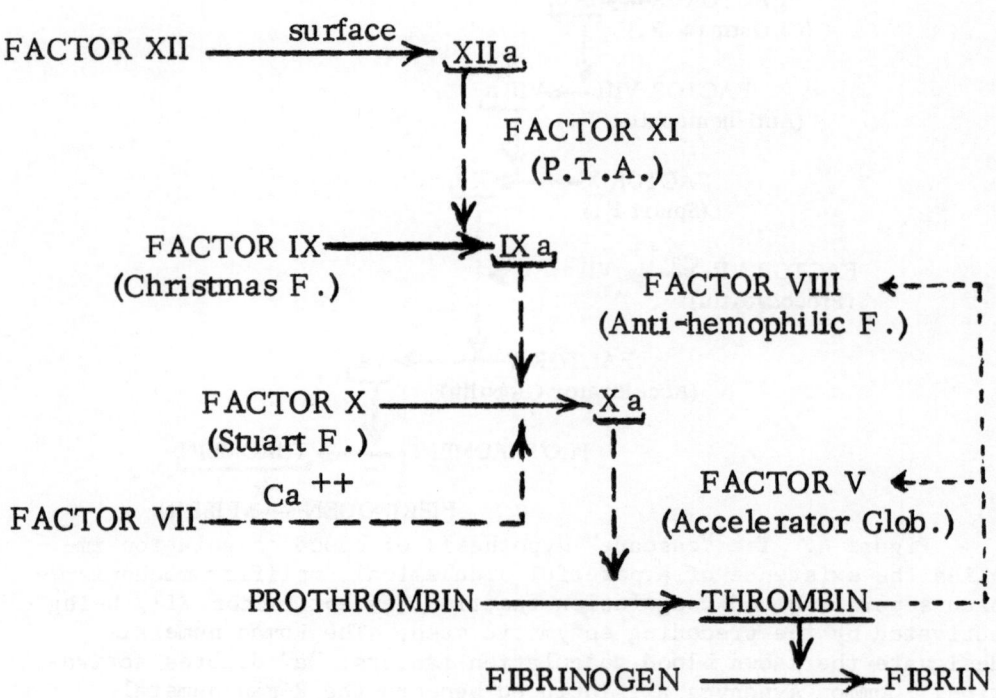

Figure 5. Reduced "cascade" hypothesis of blood coagulation
retains the concept that coagulation involves a biochemical amplifier mechanism but suggests that only three, or possibly four,
enzymatic steps are involved. Other coagulation factors act as
high molecular weight co-factors. Dotted lines indicate that
thrombin potentiates the actions of factors V and VIII.

Relatively sensitive, though rather poorly reproducible, assay
methods are available for the quantification of all these blood
factors and certain tests of overall coagulation function are also
available. Moreover, the complexity of the system and the uncertainties as to its detailed operation make interpretation of
clinical data difficult. Similarly, individual levels of blood

coagulation factors may vary quite widely without demonstrable
alteration in blood coagulation system function. For example,
physiological levels of factor VIII or IX may vary from 50-150% of
the average value and other factors in the range of 70-130% of
normal.

Thus, study of relatively large groups of individuals, both
treated and untreated with the pill, are required to demonstrate
significant alteration in individual coagulation factor concentration. Moreover, as will be emphasized in Wessler's presentation
on the experimental production of hypercoagulability, activated
blood factors are rapidly cleared from the circulation and experimental production of blood hypercoagulability does not necessarily
lead to thrombosis unless additional factors, such as blood stasis,
are present. Also, the studies of Crumb and Ratnoff (13), in which
Hagemann factor activation was induced in rabbits by ellagic acid
infusion, indicate that notable blood hypercoagulability, easily
demonstrable by in vitro testing, is well tolerated unless additional thrombosis-inciting factors, such as total blood stasis, are
also employed.

These latter studies emphasize, in elegant fashion, the importance of powerful in vivo inhibitory mechanisms, antithrombins,
etc., preventing generalized intravascular coagulation. That
Hagemann factor constitutes the trigger to the intrinsic blood
coagulation system is known, but its systemic in vivo activation,
as apart from its activation in local sites, where conditions are
condusive to clotting, does not produce intravascular coagulation.

Thus, while blood hypercoagulability exists in both systemic
and local forms, it cannot be justifiably diagnosed, together with
the implication of thrombosis predisposition, merely because unac-
tivated blood coagulation factor concentrations are increased. A
large number of blood coagulation studies performed on subjects on
contraceptive medication have been reported, but since the results
are in general accord, I shall quote data from only three representative studies to display the range of variation.

The study by Sise (14) involved subjects receiving either
Enovid or C-Quens therapy, significant differences not being observed. Moreover, during long-term (6-12 months) therapy with
C-Quens, except for shortening of the partial thromboplastin time,
a result which is somewhat suspect in view of the fact that the
reagents had to be changed during the study, the findings in the
subjects receiving C-Quens did not differ significantly from control studies. Though certain of the individual factor assays
showed minor variation while the subjects received medication, the
author concludes "none of these changes were of a magnitude which
would not be encountered in normal persons and the degree of change
was not considered significant in relation to thromboembolism".

A smaller number of patients was studied in the Mayo Clinic
report (15) but the study possesses the useful advantage that the
assay data are quoted in comparison with the same investigator's
findings in pregnant subjects. Essentially, the data obtained with
12 subjects receiving contraceptive medication from nine months to
five years indicate that the various contraceptive medications employed cause only an increase in the one-stage prothrombin time
largely accounted for by relatively modest increase in plasma factor VII concentration. In contrast, the pregnant subjects at term
showed a greater than two-fold increase in factor X concentration,
a three-fold increase in factor VII concentration, and significant
increases in plasma fibrinogen.

Thus, in this study, as in the last, the oral contraceptives
induced only modest changes in coagulation function, changes that
appear unlikely to be responsible for increased evidence of thromboembolism in patients receiving the medication. Moreover, the
Mayo Clinic workers, in a comparison between 12 patients receiving
contraceptive medication and admitted to the hospital for thromboembolism and 12 similarly-medicated patients without thrombosis,
noted no difference in coagulation function, as measured by the
conventional coagulation screening tests.

The data by Poller, Tabiowa and Thompson (16) represent an
investigative study in which substantially positive changes in
blood coagulation factors were found. Using the preparations,
Norinyl-1 and Ortho-Novum, one containing half the hormone concentration of the other, it was observed that both coagulation factors
VII and X rose substantially with long-term medication. However,
neither instance did the concentration increases recorded reach
the levels customarily obtained in the third trimester of pregnancy.
Nor on the basis of these data, is the increase in coagulation
factors VII and X dose dependent.

Taken overall, studies on blood coagulation changes with women
on contraceptive medication indicate that, with the exception of
plasma fibrinogen, such medication induces coagulation changes
similar to those seen in the pregnant woman at term but of a considerably more modest nature. On the basis of present data, they
would not appear to be of significance in predisposing to thromboembolism.

Though comparatively little accurate data are available on
levels of plasma factor XIII in those receiving contraceptive
medication, the subject merits brief consideration.

Plasma factor XIII, the enzyme precursor activated by thrombin into a plasma transamidase, stabilizes clots both mechanically

FIBRIN STABILIZATION REACTION

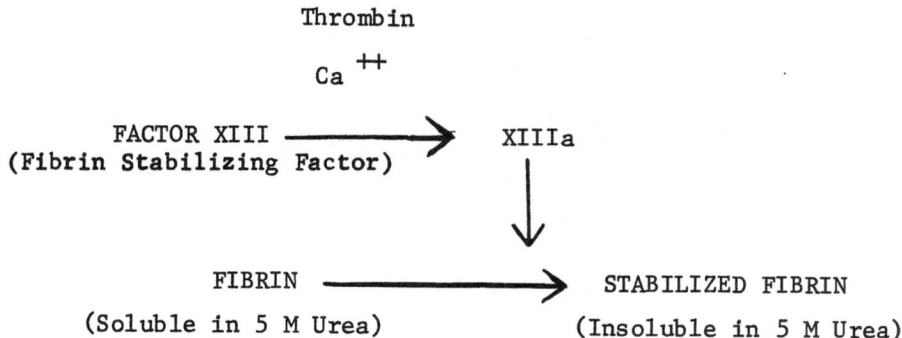

Figure 6

and biochemically and substantially increases their resistence to
lysis (17). Consequently, alterations in plasma factor XIII could
be of significance in altering lysis rates of microthrombi. However, we have recently shown: a) that plasma factor XIII concentration falls steadily with duration of pregnancy, reaching about
50% of normal at term (18); and b) that in a small number of patients receiving long-term contraceptive medication, plasma factor
XIII was not significantly altered. Thus, contraceptive medication, which has been shown to mimic the blood coagulation changes
induced by pregnancy, is unlikely to influence the incidence of
thromboembolism through such a mechanism.

Nevertheless, clinical experience suggests that neither assays
for individual coagulation factors nor conventional assays for
overall coagulation function will necessarily reveal evidence relevant to the diagnosis of blood hypercoagulability. One reason for
this unfortunate state of affairs is that activated blood factors
are rapidly cleared from the blood stream with half lives measured
in minutes. For this reason, a new method for the diagnosis of
blood hypercoagulability has been developed in our laboratory over
the last three years and Figure 7 shows its basis (19,20).

In its simplest form, the technique is an adaption of the
Allison-Humphrey immunodiffusion procedure (21) for the determination of protein antigen diffusion constants applied to the examination of the physical state of fibrinogen in plasma.

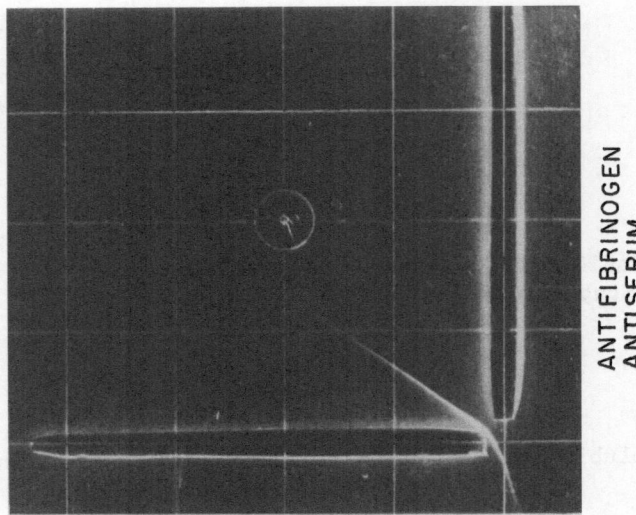

HUMAN PLASMA
$\tan\theta = (Dg/Db)^{1/2}$;
$Db = 3.8 \times 10^{-7} cm^2/sec.$

Figure 7. Allison-Humphrey immunodiffusion procedure for determination of antigen (proteins) $D_{20,w}$.

The Allison-Humphrey procedure involves the immunodiffusion of antigen, which may be contained in biological fluid, against specific antiserum. Antigen and antibody are placed in troughs at right angles to each other and a linear precipitin line forms, the angle of which, in relation to the antigen trough, is measured. Using suitable gel concentrations, protein gel diffusion is equivalent to free diffusion and by determination of the angle of the precipitin line, the antigen diffusion constant may be determined by means of the formula shown at the bottom of Figure 7.

Shown in Figure 8 are $D_{20,w}$ values, with standard deviations, for a number of fibrinogen derivatives, ranging from that of a small polymer, the upper limit of methodological accuracy, to that of the smallest fibrinogen derivative containing an antigenic determinant. The method, in skilled hands, is highly reproducible and enables the physical state of fibrinogen or its derivatives to be determined in plasma or in gel-sieved fractions of plasma (22).

The rationale for the use of this method to detect blood
hypercoagulability or a thrombosing tendency of any significant
degree, is simple. If the blood coagulation system is activated
in such systemic fashion as to produce even the mildest clotting,
fibrin monomer will be formed. Such monomer in low concentration
may undergo three fates: A. Possibly it could polymerize mas-
sively and be deposited as intravascular fibrin. B. More likely,
it could polymerize to a limited degree with other monomer units
to form polymers of small size, or C. most certainly and most
likely, because of its low concentration, it could polymerize with
normal fibrinogen molecules, forming a fibrinogen dimer by the
method proposed by Scheraga and Laskowski some years ago (23).
Consequently, if either of the two latter circumstances occurs,
small fibrinogen polymers or more probably, fibrinogen dimers, will
circulate in vivo. Since these moieties have substantially larger
molecular weights than fibrinogen itself and consequently, considerably smaller $D_{20,w}$'s, they may be detected in unfractionated
plasma by this method (19). All that can be said presently is that
the method has been extensively evaluated in our laboratory in a

DIFFUSION COEFFICIENTS OF FIBRINOGEN AND ITS BREAKDOWN PRODUCTS

	Free Diffusion $D_{20,w}$	Immuno Diffusion $D_{20,w}$
Polymer		0.94
Dimer		$1.46 \pm .12$
Fibrinogen	1.98	$1.99 \pm .17$
Fibrinogen First Derivative	2.52	$2.55 \pm .11$
Intermediates		$3.02 \pm .13$
		$3.74 \pm .05$
		$4.24 \pm .17$
Final Product 5.27S	5.3	$5.28 \pm .20$
3S	7.3	

Figure 8. $D_{20,w}$ values for fibrinogen and its derivative determined by Allison-Humphrey method and free diffusion.

wide variety of clinical states, including a most instructive
experience with a heat-stroke epidemic in St. Louis, where a substantial number of patients died late from either pulmonary embolism or myocardial infarction. In a number of instances, this
method alone, both in this epidemic and in other clinical conditions, has enabled us to make a diagnosis of blood hypercoagulability and predict either thromboembolic complication or thromboembolic death (22). As yet, we have not applied this method to
the study of blood hypercoagulability in those receiving contraceptive medications, but we shall do shortly. I have mentioned
this procedure for it provides a new approach to an extremely
significant disease problem, the solution to which has long been
handicapped by inadequate methodology.

FIBRINOLYTIC ENZYME SYSTEM

Figure 9 illustrates the _in vivo_ mode of action of the plasminogen-plasmin or fibrinolytic enzyme system. Since Astrup and
Brakman will consider the effects of contraceptive medication on
this system, I shall make only general comments concerning its
physiological significance (24-25).

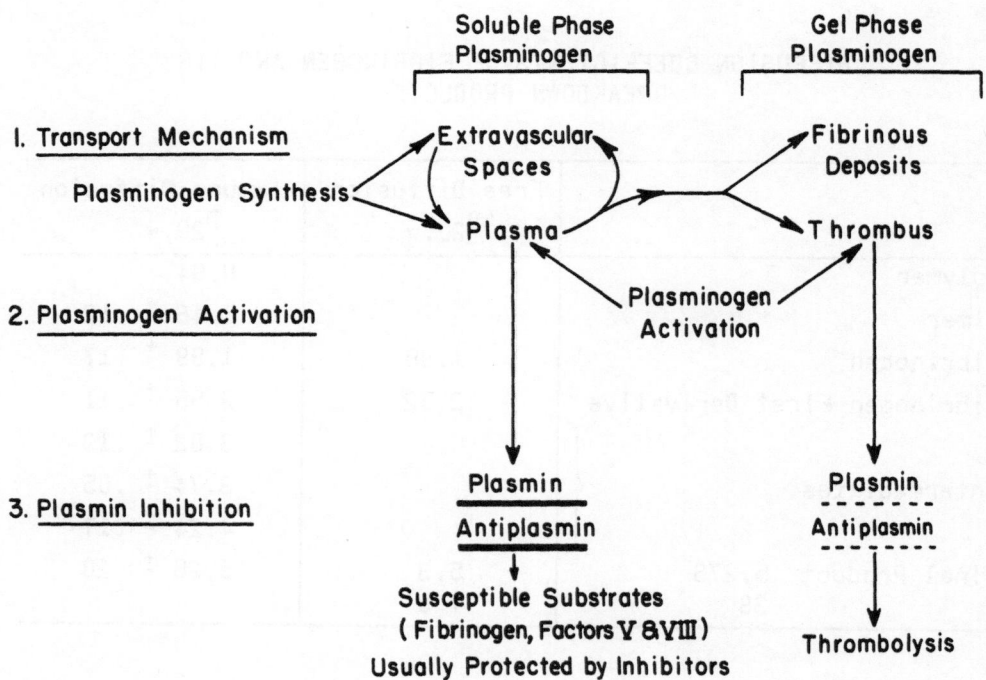

Figure 9. Illustrates the dual "phase" concept of plasminogen-
plasmin system (fibrinolytic enzyme system) function.

Plasminogen is a serum globulin which, on activation by specific kinases or activators, is converted into the enzyme plasmin--a
proteolytic enzyme of wide specificity having comparable properties to trypsin. Indeed, informative analogy may be drawn between
the trypsinogen-trypsin system, activated specifically by entero-
kinase and the plasminogen-plasmin system, activated by its own
specific kinases.

Enzymatic reactions of the proteolytic type are essential to
biological function. Nevertheless, when such reactions occur in
the intravascular compartment and involve enzymes such as plasmin,
which possess relatively non-specific substrate requirement, they
may present peculiar hazards to the organism. However, in vivo,
because of certain biological properties of the plasminogen-plasmin
system, this relatively non-specific enzyme normally produces a
single highly-specific action - fibrinolysis.

Following its synthesis, plasminogen is distributed in the ex-
travascular spaces and in the plasma. When clotting occurs, either
extra- or intravascularly, the fibrin deposit or thrombus contains
plasminogen which is in intimate spatial relationship with the
fibrin fibril.

Consequently, plasminogen in a plasma clot system exists, in
a physical sense, as a dual-phase system: plasminogen in plasma
constituting the soluble phase and plasminogen in the clot, the gel
phase. As a result of this physical distribution, the biochemical
consequences of plasminogen activation in the two phases are entirely different. Plasminogen activation in the soluble plasma
phase (provided it is slow) produces no detectible effects on susceptible substrates contained in plasma, for plasmin is rapidly
inhibited by plasma-antiplasmin on its formation. Thus, the inhibitory actions of antiplasmins protect plasmin-susceptible substrates in plasma from proteolysis.

Plasminogen activation in the clot or gel phase produces an
entirely different result. Fibrin is now the major substrate and
thrombolysis, or clot dissolution, proceeds, because of the intimate spatial relationship of clot plasminogen and fibrin fibrils,
relatively independent of plasma inhibitors. In this manner, the
actions of the enzyme plasmin, though themselves relatively non-
specific with respect to substrate requirements, may in vivo be restricted to a circumscribed locus and a particular substrate, fibrin.

Specific kinases, or activators, of the plasminogen-plasmin
system are listed below (Fig. 10). All these specific kinases
possess exceptionally high gel/soluble phase activation ratios and
consequently produce a marked preferential action on gel phase, as
opposed to soluble phase, plasminogen. Consequently, these kinases

act primarily to lyse thrombi and fibrinous deposits and in
physiological concentrations exert only a minimal effect on plasma
plasminogen.

All organs, tissues and blood vessels, with the exception of
the liver and full-term placenta, contain varying concentrations
of extractable plasminogen activator. Release of such stored activator, either locally or into the circulation, is crucial to effective plasminogen-plasmin function and the production of thrombolysis
or clot lysis. If the activator is released into the plasma, it is
termed plasma activator and the plasma concentration of this moiety
is critically related to overall plasma thrombolytic activity.

BIOLOGICAL ACTIVATORS FOR FIBRINOLYTIC SYSTEM

1. Tissue Activators

2. Plasma Activator

3. Activators in other biological fluids

   a. Urokinase in urine

   b. Activators in tears, sweat and
       fluids from other secretory
       epithelium.

Figure 10

Plasminogen activator is normally present in plasma in very
low concentration and in this complex biochemical milieu, even
such simple assay manipulations as sample dilution are best avoided
if physiologically relevant data are to be obtained.

Figure 11 illustrates radiochemical assay procedure for plasminogen activator present in plasma or other biological fluids.
Clots containing I^{125} or I^{131} labeled fibrinogen are formed as
shown in the lower left-hand corner of the figure. After washing
to remove unincorporated isotope, the clot is incubated with
freshly-drawn plasma for 30 or more minutes. It is then separated
and the degree of clot dissolution quantified by assay of isotope
released into the plasma supernatant. By alteration of the clot
composition, particularly with respect to clot plasminogen concentration, the method may be made extremely sensitive and capable of
detecting very low levels of plasminogen activator, present in the
plasma of normal resting man (26,27). Furthermore, the method
yields meaningful assay results, even in the presence of activator
inhibitors or other inhibitors.

Assay of Plasma Thrombolytic Activity with I¹³¹ Tagged
Plasma Clots.

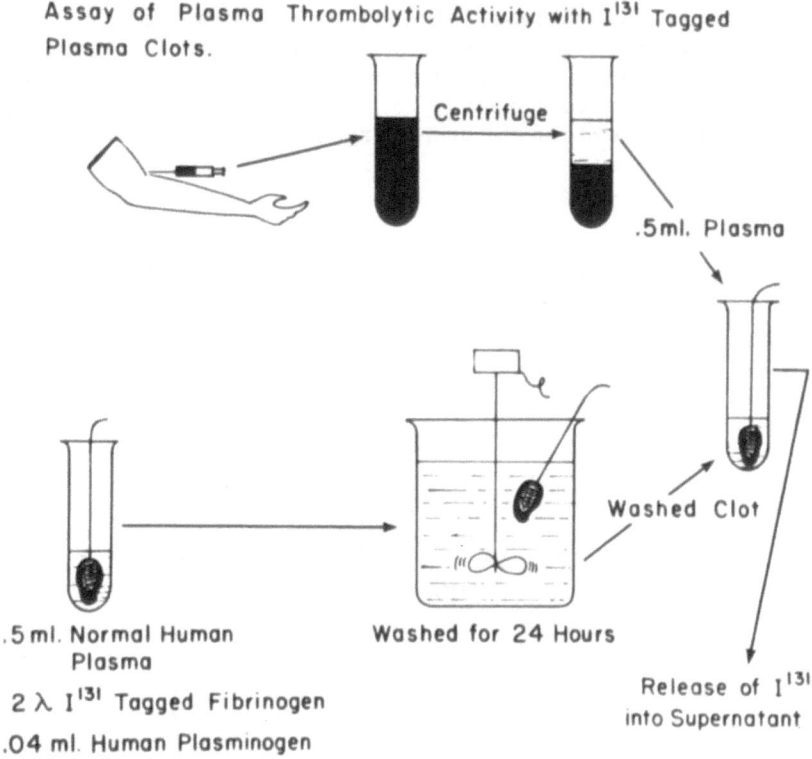

Figure 11. Radiochemical assay of plasma thrombolytic
activity.

The next two figures (12 and 13) show the levels of plasma-
plasminogen activator in normal resting man and in patients suffering from a variety of disease states (27). Activator activity
(the ordinate) is expressed in micrograms fibrin lysed under the
assay conditions employed.

Figure 12 demonstrates that the plasma of normal resting man
contains low but significant quantities of plasminogen activator.
Under these assay conditions, which mimic physiological conditions,
this finding significantly documents the constant potential of the
plasminogen-plasmin system to induce the lysis of microthrombi and
prevent their increase to a size sufficient to produce clinical
disease. It is to be emphasized that levels of plasminogen activator may vary considerably in man; for instance, stimuli such as
exercise or ischemia may cause transient 10- to 20-fold increases
in activator level (Fig. 12, at right). Thus, the full potential

of this enzyme system to lyse intravascular thrombi may not be
revealed by activator assays in the resting state. Nevertheless,
sufficient concentrations of plasminogen activator are present in
normal resting plasma to effect lysis of microthrombi without additional activator release from other organs.

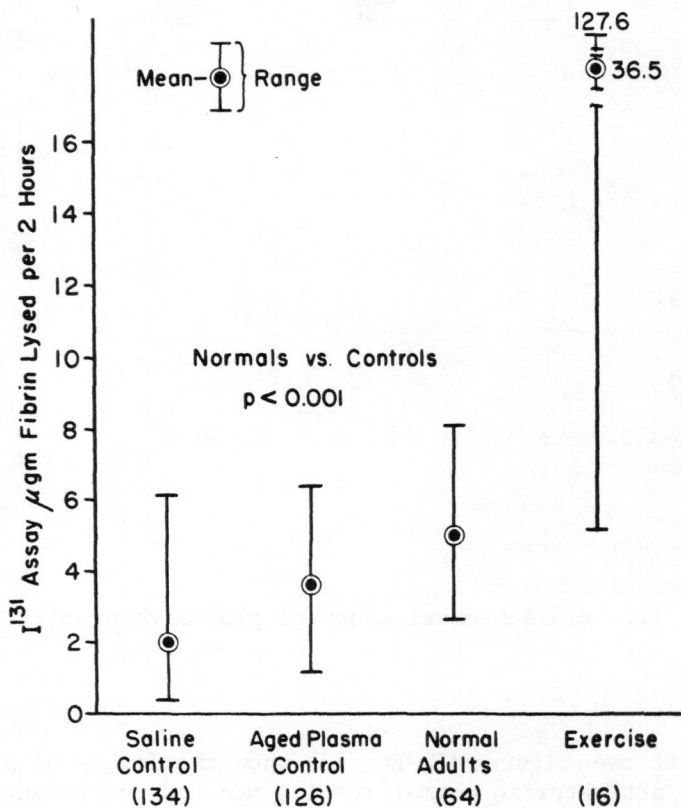

Figure 12. Radiochemical assay of plasma thrombolytic activity in resting man and after exercise.

Figure 13, similar to the last, shows activator assays in
normal adults and in patients suffering from congestive cardiac
failure, cancer and atherosclerosis - all conditions where the risk
of developing thromboembolic complications is higher than normal.
Activator levels determined under these conditions did not differ
significantly from normal.

However, these data should not be interpreted as indicating
that failure of the plasminogen-plasmin system function is unlikely
to predispose to the development of thromboembolic complications.

These patients may not have been at particular risk of developing thromboembolic complications.

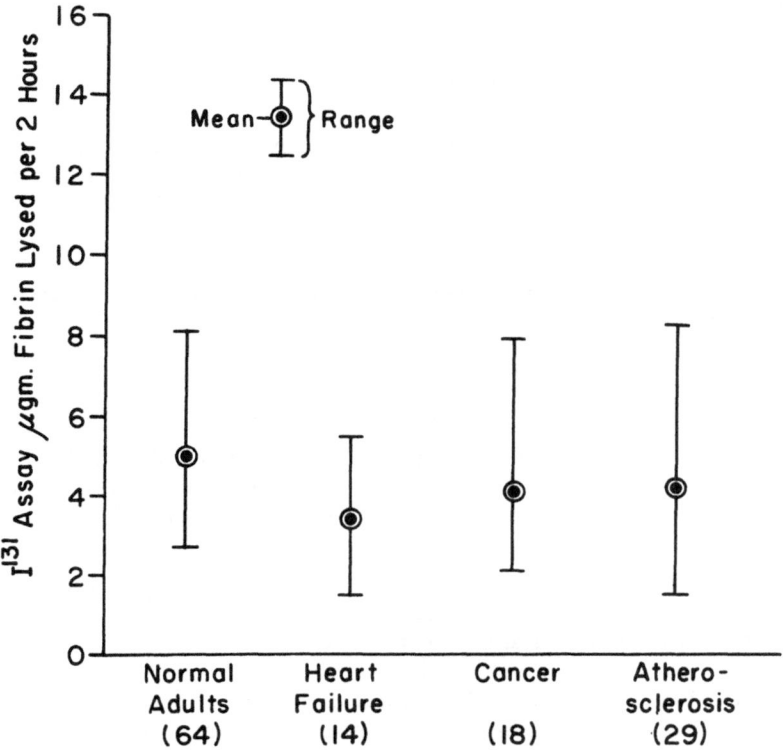

Figure 13. Radiochemical assay of plasma thrombolytic activity in a number of disease entities, heart failure, cancer, atherosclerosis, in which thromboembolism occurs with high relative frequency.

Moreover, there is additional powerful indirect evidence to indicate that the plasminogen-plasmin enzyme system is of unusual physiological significance in preventing microthrombi from growing and becoming clinically evident. The importance of adequate investigative effort in this area, in patients taking the contraceptive pill, is underscored by the fact that plasma activator concentration falls in the pregnant state.

In this brief introductory survey of a very complex problem, I have tried to set in perspective those factors which are both of relevance and which are also susceptive to investigation. However, there are significant omissions, particularly with respect to consideration of blood rheology, hemodynamic functions and vessel wall alteration. While restriction on time partially accounts for neglect of these potentially relevant factors, lack of adequate methodology is also culpable.

REFERENCES

1. Inman, W.H. and Vessey, M.P.: Investigation of deaths from pulmonary, coronary and cerebral thrombosis and embolism in women of childbearing age. Brit. Med. J. 2:193 (1968).

2. Vessey, M.P. and Doll, R.: Investigation of relation between use of oral contraceptives and thromboembolic disease. Brit. Med. J. 2:199 (1968).

3. Drill, V.A. and Calhoun, D.W.: Oral contraceptives and thromboembolic disease. J.A.M.A. 206:77 (1968).

4. The Veterans Administration Co-operative Urological Research Group. Treatment and survival of patients with cancer of the prostrate. Surg. Obstet. Gyn. 124: 1011 (1967).

5. Oliver, M.F. and Boyd, G.S.: Influence of reduction of serum lipids on prognosis of coronary heart-disease. A five year study using oestrogen. Lancet ii:499 (1961).

6. Stamler, J., Pick, B., Katz, L.N., Pick, A., Berkson, D.M. and Century, D.: Effectiveness of oestrogens for therapy of myocardial infarction in middle-aged men. J. Am. Med. Assoc. 183: 632 (1963).

7. Daniel, D.G., Campbell, H. and Turnball, A.C.: Puerperal thromboembolism and suppression of lactation. Lancet ii:287 (1967).

8. Jeffcoate, T.N.A., Miller, J., Roos, R.F. and Tindall, V.B.: Puerpal thromboembolism in relation to the inhibition of lactation by oestrogen therapy. Brit. Med. J. 4:19 (1968).

9. Mustard, J.F., Roswell, H.C. and Murphy, E.A.: Thrombosis. Amer. J. Med. Sci. 248:469 (1964).

10. Mustard, J.F. and Packman, M.A.: The biochemistry of primary hemostasis. Page 306 in Plenary Session Papers XII. Congress International Society of Hematology, New York, (1968).

11. Mitchell, J.R.A.: The pathogenesis of thrombosis. Page 321 in Plenary Session Papers XII. Congress International Society of Hematology, New York (1968).

12. Esnouf, M.P.: Biochemical aspects of blood coagulation. Page 315 in Plenary Session Papers XII. Congress International Society of Hematology, New York (1968).

13. Crumb, J.D. and Ratnoff, O.D.: Activation of Hageman factor by solutions of ellagic acid. J. Lab. Clin. Med. 62:1006 (1963).

14. Sise, H.: Anovulatory hormones and blood coagulation. In Blood Coagulation, Thrombosis and Female Hormones. Editors: T. Astrup and I.S. Wright. James F. Mitchell Foundation, Washington, D.C., 1968, p. 19.

15. Owen, C.A., Thompson, J.H., Jr., Bowie, W., Didisheim, P. and Spittell, J.A.: Coagulation studies during pregnancy and hormone treatment. In Blood Coagulation, Thrombosis and Female Hormones. Editors: T. Astrup and I.S. Wright. James F. Mitchell Foundation, Washington, D.C., 1968, p. 24.

16. Poller, L., Tabiowa, A. and Thompson, J.M.: Effects of low-dose oral contraceptives on blood coagulation. Brit. Med. J. 2:218 (1968).

17. Gormsen, J., Fletcher, A.P., Alkjaersig, N. and Sherry, S.: Enzymatic lysis of plasma clots: the influence of fibrin stabilization on lysis rates. Archives of Biochem. and Biophys. 120:654 (1967).

18. Coopland, A., Fletcher, A.P. and Alkjaersig, N.: Reduction of plasma factor XIII (fibrin stabilizing factor) concentration during pregnancy. J. Lab. Clin. Med. (In Press).

19. Fletcher, A.P.: The problem of intravascular fibrinolytic reaction. In Platelets: Their Role in Hemostasis and Thrombosis. Editors: K.M. Brinkhous, I.S. Wright, J.P. Samlier, H.R. Roberts and S. Hinnon. Thromb. et diath. Haemorrh. Suppl. 26:343 (1967).

20. Fletcher, A.P. and Alkjaersig, N.: Plasma fibrinogen and hemostatic function (pathological and genetic disorders) Progress in Hematology (Editors: E.B. Brown and C.V. Moore), 5:246 (1966).

21. Allison, A.C. and Humphrey, J.H.: A theoretical and experimental analysis of double diffusion precipitin reaction in gels and its application characterization of antigens. Immunology 3:95 (1960).

22. Alkjaersig, N., Fletcher, A.P. and Bachmann, F.: In Preparation.

23.   Scheraga, H.A. and Laskowski, M., Jr.:   The fibrinogen-fibrin conversion.   Advances in Protein Chemistry 12:1 (1957).

24.   Alkjaersig, N., Fletcher, A.P. and Sherry, S.:   The mechanism of clot dissolution by plasmin.   J. Clin. Invest. 38: 1086 (1959).

25.   Fletcher, A.P., Alkjaersig, N. and Sherry, S.:   Fibrino-lytic mechanisms and the development of thrombolytic therapy. Am. J. Med. 33:738 (1962).

26.   Fletcher, A.P.:   Measurement of plasma thrombolytic activity:isotopic method.   In Blood Coagulation, Hemorrhage and Thrombosis:Methods of Study. Editors: L.A. Kazal and L.M. Tocantins.   Grune and Stratton, 1964, p. 254.

27.   Sawyer, W.D., Fletcher, A.P., Alkjaersig, N. and Sherry, S.:   Studies on the thrombolytic activity of human plasma. J. Clin. Invest. 39:426 (1960).

EFFECTS ON THE VASCULAR SYSTEM AND BLOOD: EPIDEMIOLOGICAL STUDIES

Richard Doll and Martin Vessey

Medical Research Council's Statistical Research Unit,
115 Gower Street, London, W.C. 1.

In 1961, Dr. W.M. Jordan, a general practitioner in Suffolk, published the first report in the medical press of a woman developing a thrombo-embolic disorder while taking an oral contraceptive (1). The patient was a 40 year old nurse who was given Enovid for the control of recurrent endometriosis. The treatment had to be abandoned after several weeks because of severe vomiting and ten days later (one week after the vomiting had stopped) the patient developed a left-sided pleurisy. Bilateral pulmonary embolism was diagnosed by chest x-ray and electrocardiogram and the patient recovered. No clinical evidence was found of thrombosis in the legs and it was concluded that she had had "a silent thrombosis secondary to the dehydration and vomiting, caused by Enovid". Since that time many hundreds of cases of deep vein thrombosis and pulmonary embolism have been reported in medical journals throughout the world and thousands have been reported to the manufacturers, the Food and Drug Administration in the United States, and the Committee on Safety of Drugs in Great Britain. Most of these reports relate to deep vein thrombosis in the lower limbs or to pulmonary embolism, but others relate to cerebrovascular accidents, coronary thrombosis, mesenteric and other arterial thromboses, and the Budd-Chiari syndrome.

All these conditions also occur in young women who do not use oral contraceptives and, by themselves, the reports provide no significant evidence that oral contraceptives are a cause of thrombo-embolic disease. Even the fact that thrombo-embolic conditions have been reported in association with the use of oral contraceptives far more frequently than any other complication (Table 1), carries little weight, as it must be anticipated that doctors will

TABLE 1

REACTIONS TO ORAL CONTRACEPTIVES REPORTED TO THE
COMMITTEE ON SAFETY OF DRUGS, 1964 TO MID-1968

A

Reaction	Number Reported	
	cases	deaths
Amenorrhea	36	
Other menstrual disorders	79	
Breast disorders	37	
Weight gain	118	
Oedema	46	
Depression	144	1
Headache	266	
Migraine	15	1
Nausea, vomiting	67	
Pigmentation	49	
Change in libido	127	
Total	984	2
Abortion	3	
Pregnancy	21	
Total	1008	2

TABLE 1 (Continued)

REACTIONS TO ORAL CONTRACEPTIVES REPORTED TO THE
COMMITTEE ON SAFETY OF DRUGS, 1964 TO MID-1968

B

Reaction	Number Reported	
	cases	deaths
Thyroid disorders	11	
Diabetes, hyperglycaemia	9	1
Porphyria	2	1
Neutropenia, aplastic anaemia, etc.	16	1
Cerebrovascular thrombosis, haemorrhage, etc.	174	33
Hypertension	66	2
Thrombophlebitis	595	30
Pulmonary embolism	355	96
Coronary thrombosis	76	46
Other thrombosis	39	5
Other heart disorders	78	7
Other vascular disorders	43	1
Periarteritis nodosa	1	1
Jaundice	75	4
Skin disorders	145	1
Hair disorders	44	
Tumors	16	
Other	550	6
Foetal malformation	23	
Total	2318	235

Total persons affected (A + B) 2864, deaths 194

Note: (i)   Including a small proportion of reactions to oestrogens
(other than stilboestrol) given alone for other purposes.

(ii) Including some reports of two or more reactions in the
same subject; for example, the death reported in association
with migraine was also associated with cerebral thrombosis.
The total number of affected persons (A + B) was 2,864 and
the total number of deaths (A + B) 194.

report most readily those conditions that have already been
publicized as possible effects of the treatment.

For further progress, we need to make an estimate of the incidence of disease in women who are using oral contraceptives and to
compare it with the incidence in women who are not using them, but
who are otherwise equally at risk from other causes. This was, of
course, immediately appreciated and several such comparisons have
been made. Drill (2) compared the incidence of thrombo-embolism
reported in clinical trials undertaken to assess the efficacy of
oral contraceptives with that reported in routine statistics and
found no evidence of excess morbidity in the oral contraceptive
users. Further comparisons were made by one of the principal
manufacturers (3), a Committee of the American Food and Drug
Administration (4,5) and the British Committee on the Safety of
Drugs (6). These investigators relied on the voluntary submission
of reports of the occurrence of thrombo-embolism by doctors who
were responsible for treating the patients and all found either
that the reported incidence was less than the estimated normal incidence in women of similar age in the country as a whole or that
the excess, if there was one, was not statistically significant.
It is, however, now evident that the reporting of thrombo-embolism
by doctors, on a voluntary basis, has been far from complete.

CLINICAL SERIES

Somewhat different results have been obtained by physicians
who have reviewed their total clinical experience over a period of
time. This method, which assumes a knowledge of the normal use of
oral contraceptives in the population, has been particularly applicable to cerebrovascular disease which is normally rare in women
of child-bearing age who are not pregnant and which, when it occurs
in such women, tends to be referred for specialist investigation.
Bergeron and Wood (7), for example, reviewed the records of all
women aged 20-45 years who had cerebral angiograms performed at
the Neurological Institute of New York in the years 1960 and 1966.
In the first period, 58 women had non-occlusive disease and two
had occlusive disease (one in association with pregnancy). In the
second period, 55 women had non-occlusive disease and nine had
occlusive disease (none in association with pregnancy). In the
first period, neither of the women with occlusive disease had been
using oral contraceptives; in the second period, eight of the nine
had been doing so. Similar, but less striking, results have been
reported in the United States (8,9), and in Great Britain (10,11).
Only Jennett and Cross (12) in Great Britain have reported negative
results. Striking though some of the figures are it is not easy
to interpret them. The reported cases can be only a small proportion of the total that have occurred in each area and it is
difficult to avoid the suspicion that negative series would have

been less likely to attract attention and so be less likely to be
reported.

CONTROLLED STUDIES

More conclusive evidence has been obtained by investigators
who have studied groups of patients with thrombo-embolic disease
and have compared the results with those obtained from a control
group of women who have been specifically selected as suitable for
comparison with the affected patients.

METHODS

In one such study the Royal College of General Practitioners
(13) sought the cooperation of sixty doctors who were known to have
maintained a diagnostic index of the conditions for which patients
had consulted them. For each year for which records were kept the
doctors were asked to prepare a list of names of all women aged
15 to 49 years who had attended with a new episode of vascular disease affecting the central nervous system, arteriosclerotic heart
disease, arterial embolism and thrombosis, phlebitis, thromphlebitis
or pulmonary embolism. For each affected patient two control
patients were also to be selected consisting of (i) the woman on
the doctor's National Health Service list who, being of the same
marital and parity status and in the same five-year group, was
nearest to the affected patient in alphabetical order on the list;
and (ii) a woman selected from the doctor's disease index according
to specified rules, who matched the affected patient in the same
way in respect of marital and parity status and age, and who had
attended in the same year as the affected patient, but for a
specified minor condition (i.e. wax in the ears, acute upper respiratory infection, disease of the teeth or gums, gastroenteritis,
or sprain of the upper limb). Each doctor was asked to seek an
interview with all the affected and control patients and to record
information concerning the patients' obstetric and contraceptive
history at or previous to the relevant episode (or, in the case of
women selected from the doctor's list, at or previous to the date
of the episode in the life of the patient for whom she was the
matched control). In the event, twenty-nine doctors agreed to participate and collected the data for 147 patients and 294 controls
who had attended at some time before the end of June, 1966.

In another study, Vessey and Doll (14) investigated patients
who had been admitted to hospital with a similar thrombo-embolic
disease. Cooperation was sought and obtained from 19 general hospitals of more than 300 beds situated in one of the 15 regions into
which England and Wales are divided for hospital administration,
and which maintained a sufficiently detailed diagnostic index. At
each hospital, the index was searched and the case notes reviewed

relating to all women with appropriate diagnoses who (i) had been
admitted to hospital in 1964-1966; and (ii) were aged 16 to 40
years inclusive. All women who satisfied these criteria were included unless they (i) were single or widowed; (ii) had an evident
predisposing reason for developing the disease – that is, were
suffering from some other relevant acute or chronic disease or had,
within the previous three months, been pregnant, undergone a surgical operation, or suffered trauma requiring hospital treatment;
(iii) were post-menopausal or sterilized; or (iv) could not be
interviewed because they had died during their stay in hospital.
For each patient with deep vein thrombosis or pulmonary embolism,
two control patients were selected who had been diagnosed as
suffering from an acute medical or surgical condition or had been
admitted to hospital for an elective operation, and who matched the
affected patient in regard to hospital, date of admission, age,
parity, and absence of any of the attributes used to exclude patients from the affected series. The selected patients were then
interviewed in their homes, or in a few instances when the patients
had moved too far away, were asked to complete a postal questionnaire. If there was any doubt about the eligibility of a patient
for inclusion, an abstract was prepared omitting any reference to
contraceptive habits, and the decision was made by an independent
colleague. Altogether, data were obtained for 80 patients with
thrombo-embolic disease and 116 controls.

In a third study, Inman and Vessey (15) investigated all the
deaths that occurred in England, Wales and Northern Ireland during
1966 in women aged 20 to 44 years in which thrombosis or embolism
of the pulmonary, cerebral, or coronary vessels was referred to on
the death certificate. Deaths were excluded when the thrombosis or
embolism was a terminal event of some other fatal disease, or when
investigation failed to support the diagnosis, and also when the
woman was unmarried, widowed, separated, or divorced, and living
alone. Detailed case histories for the remaining patients, including the history of the use of oral contraceptives and other drugs,
were sought from the patient's general practitioner, and amplified
by reference to hospital casenotes, family planning records, and
court depositions. For comparison, each general practitioner was
also asked to give information about the age, marital status, parity
and current use of oral contraceptives of two to six other women
in his practice, who were in the same broad age group as the women
who had died and whose records were filed in proximity to the position where the records of the dead women were normally kept.
Altogether, information was obtained relating to 309 women who had
died and 1116 other married women who were aged 20 to 44 years and
were not known to have been pregnant at the time of death or, in
the case of living women, at the time the information was obtained.
Fourteen of the fatal cases (4.5 percent) and 118 of the control
women (10.6 percent) had to be omitted because of inadequate

TABLE 2

SUPERFICIAL THROMBOPHLEBITIS

(Expected Numbers in Parentheses)

Source of data	No. of affected women with a history of oral contraceptives:		Total Number of:		Relative risk: users to non-users
	used	not used	affected women	control women	
G.P. consultation	11 (4.0)	61 (68.0)	72	144	3.1 to 1

TABLE 3

DEEP VEIN THROMBOSIS AND PULMONARY EMBOLISM

(Expected Numbers in Parentheses)

Source of data	No. of affected women with a history of oral contraceptives:-		Total Number of:		Relative risk: users to non-users
	used	not used	affected women	control women	
G.P. consultation	5 (2.0)	15 (18.0)	20	40	3.0 to 1
Inpatients	26 (5.0)	32 (53.0)	58	116	8.6 to 1
Deaths, women without predisposing cause	16 (4.2)	10 (21.8)	26)		8.3 to 1
			)		
			)	998	
Deaths, women with predisposing cause	9 (6.8)	40 (42.2)	49)		1.4 to 1

TABLE 4

"CEREBRAL THROMBOSIS"

(Expected Numbers in Parentheses)

Source of data	No. of affected women with a history of oral contraceptives:-		Total Number of:		Relative risk: users to non-users
	used	not used	affected women	control women	
G.P. consultation	1 (0.5)	2 (2.5)	3	6	-
Inpatients	5 (1.0)	4 (8.0)	9	116*	10.0 to 1
Deaths, women without predisposing cause	5 (1.5)	5 (8.5)	10)	998*	5.7 to 1
Deaths, women with predisposing cause	0 (1.5)	16 (4.5)	16)		-

*The same control groups as in Table 2.

information about parity or the use of oral contraceptives. The
results, therefore, relate to 295 women who had died of thromboembolic disease and 998 control women who were attended by the same
general practitioners.

RESULTS

The results of these three studies are summarized in Tables
2-5. Each Table relates to a single group of diseases and all have
been set out in the same way. Table 2 shows the data for superficial phlebitis. For this condition evidence was obtained only in
the general practitioners' study. The numbers of women with superficial phlebitis who were using oral contraceptives and those who
were not are given in comparison with the numbers expected from
the experience of the control series. In this study, the expected
numbers have been obtained directly from the whole group of control
women, as these were selected to match the affected patients in regard to age, parity, and year of illness - three factors which, in
Britain, are closely associated with the use of oral contraceptives
(13,15). The Table also shows an estimate of the risk of developing
superficial phlebitis in women who are using oral contraceptives
relative to that in women who are not (11/61 divided by 4.0/68.0,
or 3.1 to 1).

Table 3 shows similar data for deep vein thrombosis and pulmonary embolism. All three series are represented and the data
relating to fatal attacks are shown separately for women with and
without known predisposing conditions. The control women in the
hospital in-patient study were selected, as in the general practitioner study, to match the affected patients for age, parity, and
year of illness and the expected numbers have been calculated directly from the control series as a whole. In the study of deaths,
the control women were not matched in this way and the expected
numbers have been calculated separately for each age and parity
group and then summed. The relative risks estimated from the in-
patient data and the data for women who died without known predisposing cause are closely similar; they are somewhat larger than
that estimated from the general practitioners' study, and much
larger than that for death from pulmonary embolism in women with a
known predisposing cause (recent surgery, prolonged immobilization,
previous thrombo-embolism, etc.). It should be noted, however,
that in the case of women with predisposing causes, the estimated
risk is not a valid one because of the nature of the control series,
which consisted of normal women and not women with similar predisposing conditions. The true risk in this group would be much
larger if the presence of a predisposing condition reduced sexual
activity and hence the frequency of use of contraceptives.

Table 4 shows the data for "cerebral thrombosis". The numbers

TABLE 5

CORONARY THROMBOSIS

(Expected Numbers in Parentheses)

Source of data	No. of affected women with a history of oral contraceptives:-		Total Number of:		Relative risk: users to non-users
	used	not used	affected women	control women	
G.P. consultation	0 (0.5)	7 (6.5)	7	14	-
Inpatients	0 (0.7)	13 (12.3)	13	116*	-
Deaths, women without predisposing cause	18 (11.4)	66 (72.6)	84)		1.7 to 1
			)	998*	
Deaths, women with predisposing cause	5 (12.6)	105 (97.4)	110)		0.4 to 1

*The same control groups as in Table 2.

are small in all series, but there is a clear association with the use of oral contraceptives in the in-patient series and in the series of deaths without predisposing cause (hypertension, previous cerebrovascular accident, etc.). The control women in the in-patient study had not been selected to match the patients with cerebral disease and the expected numbers were, therefore, estimated separately for each age, parity, and year of illness group and summed. The relative risks estimated from these results are similar to those for deep vein thrombosis and pulmonary embolism.

Table 5 shows the data for coronary thrombosis. In all the series the expected numbers have been estimated as previously for "cerebral thrombosis". No series shows any marked association with the use of oral contraceptives and the women who died from coronary thrombosis in the presence of a predisposing cause (hypertension, previous stroke or coronary thrombosis, diabetes mellitus, etc.) tended to have used them less often than expected.

INTERPRETATION

The associations demonstrated in the Tables between the use of oral contraceptives and the development of superficial phlebitis, deep vein thrombosis and pulmonary embolism, and "cerebral thrombosis" are statistically highly significant (in two cases, $P < 0.001$) and evidence has been presented in the original papers to show that they are likely to be real and not due to bias in the design or conduct of the studies. It is not possible to review all the evidence here, but it may be noted (i) that the frequency of use of oral contraceptives recorded in the control series corresponds reasonably well with the frequency that would be estimated from knowledge of available supplies at the relevant periods in Britain, and (ii) that women were included in all the affected series only for objective reasons, and any subsequent decision to exclude them was taken independently and in ignorance of their contraceptive practice.

It is, of course, possible that the general practitioners may have tended to diagnose phlebitis more readily in women who were using oral contraceptives than in other women and they may have been more inclined to send women to hospital with deep vein thrombosis, pulmonary embolism, or "cerebral thrombosis" (or the hospital physician may have diagnosed these conditions more readily) when the women were using oral contraceptives. It is remotely possible that a similar bias may also have affected the series of deaths. Two pieces of evidence, however, suggest that this type of bias is unlikely to be the explanation of the results, at least so far as the study of hospital in-patients is concerned. First, if diagnostic bias had accounted for the results, the association would presumably have been more marked when the diagnosis was least

TABLE 6

RELIABILITY OF DIAGNOSIS OF DEEP VEIN THROMBOSIS
AND PULMONARY EMBOLISM IN HOSPITAL INPATIENTS BY
CONTRACEPTIVE USE

Diagnosis	No. of affected women with a history of oral contraceptives:-		Per cent with history of use
	used	not used	
possible	3	8	27%
probable	15	23	39%
certain	9	3	75%
all categories*	27	34	44%

*Totals differ from those in Table 3 because of the inclusion of three additional cases (see Vessey and Doll (14)).

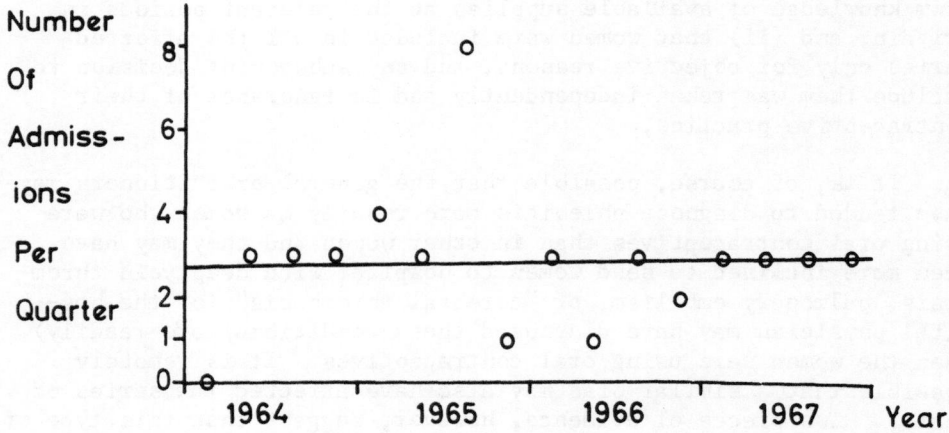

Fig. 1. Number of married women, aged 16 to 40 years, who were not using oral contraceptives, admitted to hospital with "idiopathic" deep vein thrombosis or pulmonary embolism, per quarter (19 hospitals, 1964 to 1967).

well confirmed. In fact, the reverse was true and, as is shown in
Table 6, the more definite the diagnosis the more marked was the
association. Secondly, admission rates showed no evidence of any
association with publicity about adverse effects. The study of
hospital in-patients has been continued to cover hospital admissions during 1967 and provisional figures for the year are now
available. Figures 1 and 2 show the numbers of cases of deep vein
thrombosis and pulmonary embolism admitted each quarter throughout
the four years of the study. Figure 1 shows that the number of
admissions of women who were not using oral contraceptives remained
fairly constant. Figure 2 shows a progressive increase in the
number of admissions of women who were using oral contraceptives
which corresponds fairly closely to an increase in the proportion
of women using them in the general population over the same period
from about 3 percent to about 12 percent. The arrows indicate the
periods of maximum publicity (the publication of a letter from the
Committee on Safety of Drugs in the medical press in November 1965,
and a statement by the Minister of Health in April and the publication of a report by the Medical Research Council in May, 1967)
and the graph shows no evidence of any gross distortion in the
following periods, such as would be expected if the risk of admission was seriously biased by knowledge of the woman's contraceptive habits.

If we conclude, as we believe we must, that the association is
real, we have to consider whether it reflects cause and effect or
is due to the existence of a common factor which is associated both
with the use of oral contraceptives and with the development of
disease. In principle, it is impossible to decide this question on
the sort of data we have been considering. For a firm decision, it
would be necessary to have data that had been obtained experimentally, by allocating to women the use or non-use of the contraceptives at random, subsequently ensuring (perhaps even more difficult)
that their behavior was unaffected by the allocation, and then observing the incidence of disease in the two treatment groups. In
practice, this is impossible and we have to reach a decision as
best we can on the basis of circumstantial evidence. Fortunately,
experience has shown that if we take sufficient care we are not
likely to be misled.

First, we may note that the association is very much closer
for venous thrombosis, pulmonary embolism, and "cerebral thrombosis"
than for coronary thrombosis. It is, therefore, more likely that
the relationship with coronary thrombosis, if indeed there is one at
all, is a secondary epiphenomenon. In our data (14), there was a
suggestion that women who used oral contraceptives smoked more
heavily than women who did not, and this might account for these
results. If this is so, we may anticipate that the relationship
will disappear as the proportion of users increases. No such

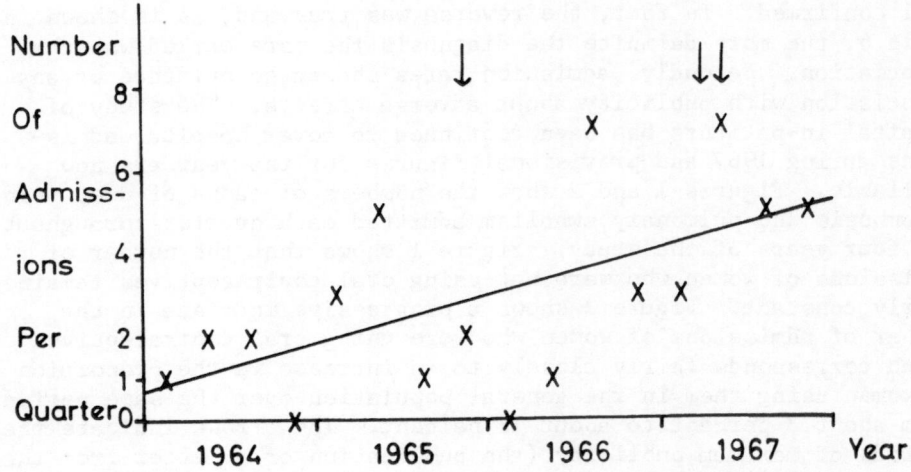

Fig. 2. Number of married women, aged 16 to 40 years, who had been using oral contraceptives within the previous four weeks, admitted to hospital with "idiopathic" deep vein thrombosis or pulmonary embolism, per quarter (19 hospitals, 1964 to 1967). Arrows indicate periods of greatest press publicity.

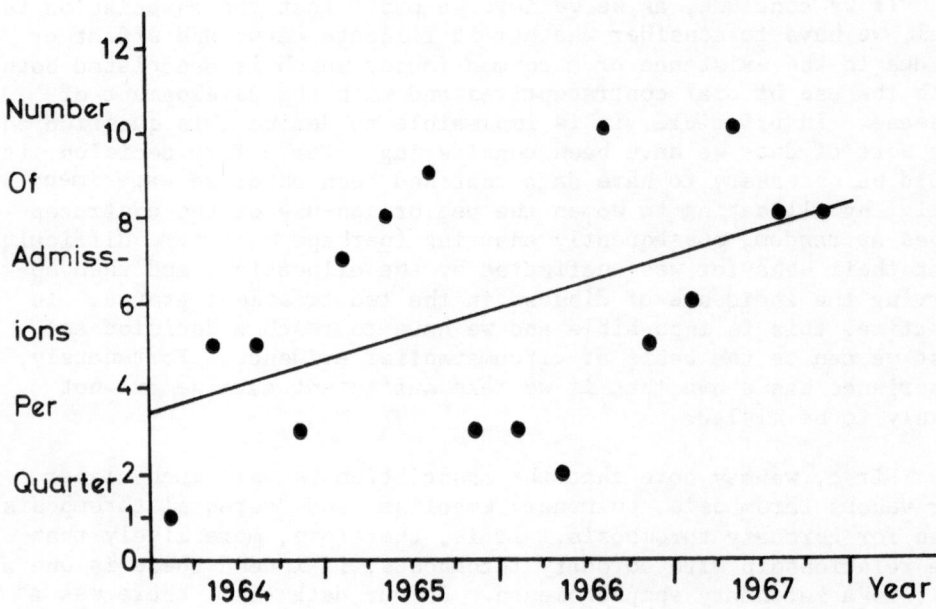

Fig. 3. Number of married women, aged 16 to 40 years, admitted to hospital with "idiopathic" deep vein thrombosis or pulmonary embolism per quarter, including cases associated with the use of oral contraceptives (19 hospitals, 1964 to 1967).

factor could account for the association with venous thrombosis or "cerebral thrombosis" and neither could any other that we were able to examine.

Secondly, we must ask whether a cause and effect relationship is compatible with other epidemiological evidence; whether, for example, the incidence of these conditions has increased pari passu with the increase in the use of oral contraceptives. Review of the trends in national mortality statistics did not, at first, suggest that they had (16,17). It was not realized, however, at the time these reviews were carried out, what little effect current practices would have been expected to have on national mortality rates and Vessey and Weatherall (18) have now shown that the British vital statistics for venous thromboembolic diseases are fully compatible with the estimates of the small increase in mortality that would be expected in the light of the data obtained by the Committee on Safety of Drugs (15). So, we may note, are hospital admission rates in England (Fig. 3).

Thirdly, we must consider whether the evidence is compatible with other data obtained when the individual hormones are administered independently, and whether they make biological sense in the light of their known physiological effects. This last will be discussed by others, but we note that there is accumulating evidence that, in other circumstances, oestrogens alone may be capable of precipitating thrombosis (19-21). The dose of oestrogens has, however, been much larger than that used in oral contraceptives and the site in which thrombosis has occurred has not been the same in all the reports.

CONCLUSION

We conclude that, on existing evidence, the most likely interpretation is that the use of oral contraceptives contributes to the development of venous thrombosis, pulmonary embolism and cerebral thrombosis, including in the latter thrombosis of arterial origin, but that it does not contribute significantly to the development of coronary thrombosis. In our study we were unable to obtain any indication that the thrombosis affected individuals who were particularly susceptible for genetic reasons (14) and, although this remains an important possibility, it seems more likely that the effect of the preparation is to increase the level of risk in all who use them.

This conclusion has been challenged by Drill and Calhoun (22) who collected statistics from the literature and found that the incidence of "thrombophlebitis" was much the same irrespective of whether oral contraceptives had been used or not. These authors, however, postulate figures for the use of oral contraceptives in

England that do not correspond to English experience, dismiss figures as unacceptable that do not accord with their hypothesis, and compare figures for "thrombophlebitis" that relate to different entities. Their argument is, therefore, not convincing.

Some difficulties do, of course, remain. The most outstanding are, perhaps, the apparent discrepancy between the dose of oestrogen given by itself or as a contraceptive and the size of the apparent effect, the fact that coronary thrombosis has been reported as an effect of oestrogens alone but not of oral contraceptives, and that oral contraceptives are associated with the development of thrombosis in the veins and the cerebral arteries but not with thrombosis in the coronary arteries. In our opinion, these discrepancies indicate the need for further research, but they do not justify overthrowing conclusions that have been reached from detailed investigation of controlled series.

REFERENCES

1. Jordan, W.M.: Pulmonary embolism. Lancet ii:1146 (1961).

2. Drill, V.A.: Oral Contraceptives. McGraw Hill. New York, U.S.A. (1966).

3. Searle and Co.: Proceedings of the Conference on Thrombolic Phenomena in Women. G.D. Searle and Co. Chicago. U.S.A. (1962).

4. Food and Drug Administration: Final report on Enovid by the Ad Hoc Committee for the evaluation of a possible etiologic relation with thromboembolic conditions: Food and Drug Administration Washington, D.C., U.S.A. (1963).

5. Food and Drug Administration: Report on the oral contraceptives. Advisory Committee on Obstetrics and Gynecology. Food and Drug Administration. Washington, D.C., U.S.A. (1966).

6. Cahal, D.A.: Safety of oral contraceptives. Brit. Med. J. 2:1180 (1965).

7. Bergeron, R.T. and Wood, E.H.: Oral contraceptives and cerebrovascular complications. Radiology. In press. (1969).

8. Shafey, S. and Scheinberg, P.: Neurological syndromes occuring in patients receiving synthetic steroids (oral contraceptives). Neurology 16:205-211 (1966).

9. Cole, M.: Strokes in young women using oral contraceptives. Arch. Intern. Med. 120:551-555 (1967).

10. Illis, L., Kocen, R.S., McDonald, W.I. and Mondkar, V.P.:
Oral contraceptives and cerebral arterial occlusion. Brit. Med. J.
2:1164-1166 (1965).

11. Bickerstaff, E.R. and Holmes, J.M.: Cerebral arterial
insufficiency and oral contraceptives. Brit. Med. J. 1:726-729
(1967).

12. Jennett, W.B. and Cross, J.N.: Influence of pregnancy and
oral contraceptives on the incidence of strokes in women of childbearing age. Lancet i:1019-1023 (1967).

13. Royal College of General Practitioners: Oral contraception
and thromboembolic disease. J. Roy. Coll. Gen. Practit. 13:267-279
(1967).

14. Vessey, M.P. and Doll, R.: Investigation of relation
between use of oral contraceptives and thromboembolic disease.
Brit. Med. J. 2:199-205 (1968).

15. Inman, W.H.W. and Vessey, M.P.: Investigation of deaths
from pulmonary, coronary and cerebral thrombosis and embolism in
women of childbearing age. Brit. Med. J. 2:193-199 (1968).

16. Swyer, G.I.M.: Oral contraceptives, thrombosis and cyclical factors affecting veins. Brit. Med. J. 1:355 (1966).

17. World Health Organization: Clinical aspects of oral
gestogens. Techn. Rep. Ser. Wld. Hlth. Org. No. 326 (1966).

18. Vessey, M.P. and Weatherall, J.A.C.: Venous thromboembolic disease and the use of oral contraceptives. A review of
mortality statistics in England and Wales. Lancet ii:94-96 (1968).

19. Oliver, M.F.: Thrombosis and oestrogens. Lancet ii:510
(1967).

20. Bailar, J.C.: Thromboembolism and oestrogen therapy.
Lancet ii:560 (1967).

21. Daniel, D.G., Campbell, H. and Turnbull, A.C.: Puerperal
thromboembolism and suppression of lactation. Lancet ii:287-289
(1967).

22. Drill, V.A. and Calhoun, D.W.: Oral contraceptives and
thromboembolic disease. J. Amer. Med. Assn. 206:77-84 (1968).

ORAL CONTRACEPTIVES AND EXCESS MORTALITY FROM VENOUS AND

PULMONARY THROMBOEMBOLISM IN THE UNITED STATES

Daniel G. Seigel, S. D., and Robert E. Markush. M. D.

National Institutes of Health, Bethesda, Maryland

Analysis of trends in mortality from thromboembolic disorders in women in the reproductive ages was motivated by two types of information. The first is that the proportion of women who are using oral contraceptives is large, estimated in a national survey in 1965 to be 15% of married women under age 45 (1). The second is that the risk of death from pulmonary embolism or cerebral thrombosis has been reported to be increased by a factor of 8 in these women (2). The combination of a large proportion of oral contraceptive users with such an increased risk should produce a doubling in the overall national mortality from these causes for women in the childbearing ages.

That a large increase should be expected is an important pre-condition to the analysis of mortality data. There are too many severe limitations in the use of such data to permit study of small effects. These limitations include a) the inherent difficulty in selecting an underlying cause, especially when more than one disease process is present, b) the complex of factors that lead to unreliable death certificate diagnosis such as certifiers who are unfamiliar with the medical history of the decedent, c) the bias that physicians may bring to the diagnosis of a condition in a young woman who has been using oral contraceptives, and d) changes in other factors occurring simultaneously that may also affect mortality levels.

We have reviewed mortality trends (3,4) from several rubrics of the International Classification of Disease (ICD), notably ICD Categories 420, Arteriosclerotic heart disease, including coronary disease, 332, Cerebral embolism and thrombosis, and 460-468, Diseases of veins and other diseases of circulatory system. We tried to determine whether death rates from these causes in recent years

TABLE 1 - Difference Between Observed and Expected Mean Annual
Percent Change in Mortality for U. S. Women Ages 15-64, by
Color and Five-Year Age Group, During 1962-66 in Three
Categories of Underlying Cause

Age	ICD #332 Cerebral Embolism and Thrombosis	ICD #420 Arteriosclerotic Heart Disease	ICD #460-468 Diseases of Veins, etc.
White			
15-19	(- 9.8)	(+39.4)	(-16.8)
20-24	(-15.4)	+ 8.1	(+ 4.4)
25-29	(+ 6.0)	+ 0.5	+ 3.5
30-34	(- 2.2)	+ 1.1	+ 9.3
35-39	-15.4	+ 3.5	+13.7
40-44	- 0.2	- 0.4	+12.5
45-49	+ 1.9	- 0.5	+ 1.2
50-54	- 6.4	+ 0.1	+ 5.4
55-59	- 3.5	+ 0.3	- 0.2
60-64	- 3.1	- 1.1	- 2.1
Non-white			
15-19	(-40.3)	(-19.9)	(- 1.6)
20-24	(- 6.9)	(+ 5.8)	(+ 4.5)
25-29	(+15.6)	+ 0.3	(+ 0.7)
30-34	(+25.3)	+10.1	+14.7
35-39	(-23.8)	+ 4.5	+13.2
40-44	- 0.5	+ 0.5	+ 2.1
45-49	- 7.9	+ 7.2	+16.4
50-54	- 1.5	- 0.5	- 0.8
55-59	- 8.3	+ 1.5	+ 0.8
60-64	+ 0.4	- 6.0	- 9.6

NOTE: Entries based on small numbers are enclosed in parentheses.

in women in the reproductive ages are greater than one would expect. Estimates of expected rates were derived from the experience of women in the years prior to the marketing of the oral contraceptives, and from trends in men. Table 1 shows the differences between the observed annual percent change in mortality, by age, for whites and non-whites and those which we estimated as expected changes (3). Entries that are positive signify that the observed rates are increasing relative to the expected rate of change; those that are negative indicate a rate of change in rates in recent years that is less than would be expected. Neither ICD 332 nor ICD 420 shows a consistent pattern of relative increases in women in the reproductive ages. For ICD 460-468, on the other hand, each five-year age group 20-45 shows some relative increase, both in white and non-white. Outside these ages, moreover, negative changes occur. Furthermore, the increases are not trivial. White females in the ages 20-45 are showing increases of from 3 to 14 percent greater each year than one might have predicted.

The mortality data were also used to estimate the relative risk of death from ICD 460-468 (4) for women in each age group (Table 2). By relative risk we mean the ratio of mortality rates in women using the oral contraceptives and those who are not. It should be clear that mortality rates were not available separately for these two groups. The estimates were made using the information on the proportion of the population using these drugs and the excess in mortality that appears to be present. The relative risks range from 3 to 9, with the exception of whites age 40-44 and non-whites 35-39. These values are not directly comparable to the estimates yielded by the British studies, which included women without a prior history of thromboembolism, and were concerned with thromboembolic disease appearing anywhere on the death certificate. It

TABLE 2 - Estimated Relative Risks

in 1966 for Diseases of Veins, Etc., (ICD 460-468),

by Age and Color

Age	20-24	25-29	30-34	35-39	40-44
White	4	5	6	8	22
Non-white	4	3	9	17	6

TABLE 3 - Estimated Excess Deaths, by Year, for Combined Ages

20-44 From Diseases of Veins, Etc., (ICD 460-468),

with Four Assumptions* for Expected Deaths

	1962	1963	1964	1965	1966
Observed Deaths	389	422	492	565	669
Expected Deaths					
Assumption 1	314	325	341	345	349
Assumption 2	315	324	346	351	360
Assumption 3	328	355	393	414	438
Assumption 4	333	363	406	431	458
Excess Deaths					
Assumption 1	75	97	151	220	320
Assumption 2	72	98	146	214	309
Assumption 3	61	67	99	151	231
Assumption 4	56	59	86	134	211
Average of Estimates of Excess	66	80	121	180	268

* Expected slope of mortality rates in women 1962-66 given by:

Assumption 1: Slope of mortality rates in women, 1957-61.

Assumption 2: Slope of mortality rates in women, 1957-1961,
multiplied by ratio of mean of rates in women,
1962-66 and mean of rates in women, 1957-1961.

Assumption 3: Slope of mortality rates in men 1962-66.

Assumption 4: Slope of mortality rates in men, 1962-66
multiplied by ratio of mean of rates in women,
1962-66, and mean of rates in men, 1962-66.

is impressive then that the values obtained are of the same order
of magnitude as those yielded in the case-control analyses, in which
a relative risk of eight times was demonstrated. The very high
value of relative risk for whites age 40-44 arises from allocating
the increased mortality at that age to low estimates of oral
contraceptive use. It has been suggested to us that administration
of estrogens to premenopausal women became more common at about
the same time as the oral contraceptive began to be used, and has
increased in medical practice. One can speculate that there is a
much broader base of hormonal use in women over age 40 than is
indicated by surveys of family-planning practice.

A third way to use the mortality data to indicate the relationship between oral contraceptive usage and mortality from ICD
Category 460-468, which we have not reported elsewhere, is in
the form of estimates of excess numbers of deaths (Table 3). The
expected number of deaths for each five-year age group was computed
separately for non-whites and whites using four different assumptions as to what these rates should have been. Two assumptions
were that the slope of rates of women in 1962-66 should be that of
men in the same time period or that of women 1956-61. The other
two assumed that the relative slope, that is the slope divided by
the mean rate, should be the same as the relative slope in these
same two groups. Finally the expected deaths were summed over the
ages 20-44 and compared with the observed deaths. In all cases
there was an excess in the observed number of deaths, the excess
increasing with each year. By 1966 from a third to a half of all
deaths were in excess of what one would expect. The means of these
estimates of excess deaths is also provided. They increase to a
level in 1966 of 268 deaths.

In summary, review of mortality data reveals an increase in
rates for ICD 460-468 that is greater than one would expect from
the experience of other comparison groups. The excess mortality
produces estimates of relative risk that are of the same order of
magnitude as that found in case-control studies of deaths in Great
Britain and might account for an excess of 268 U. S. deaths in
1966. These data are regarded as supplementary to the British
studies, and tend to strengthen their conclusions concerning the
effect of oral contraceptive use on thromboembolic diseases of
veins.

REFERENCES

1. Ryder, N. B., and Westoff, C. F.: Use of oral contraception in
   the United States, 1965. Science 153:1199-1205 (Sept 9) 1966.

2. Inman, W. H. W., and Vessey, M. P.: Investigation of deaths from pulmonary, coronary, and cerebral thrombosis and embolism in women of child-bearing age, Brit. Med. J. 2:193-199 (April 27) 1968.

3. Markush, Robert E., and Seigel, Daniel G.: Oral contraceptives and mortality trends from thromboembolism in the United States. Amer. J. Public Health (In Press).

4. Seigel, Daniel G., and Markush, Robert E.: Oral contraceptives and relative risk of death from venous and pulmonary thrombo-embolism in the United States. Submitted for publication.

HYPERCOAGULABILITY

Stanford Wessler and E. Thye Yin

Department of Medicine, The Jewish Hospital of St. Louis
and the Washington University School of Medicine,
St. Louis, Missouri

The concept that altered coagulation of the blood plays a role in thrombosis has a respectable lineage. Richard Wiseman was perhaps the first to apply the newly acquired knowledge of the circulation to the etiology of intravascular coagulation. In 1676, Wiseman described the properties of a thrombus and stated that intravascular coagulation was related, in part, to systemic alterations in the circulating blood (1). This concept, however, was destined to dominate neither the investigation of Wiseman's day, nor of subsequent generations. Although Virchow almost 200 years after Wiseman mentioned hypercoagulability almost, as it were, in passing (2), data in support of the concept were not forthcoming.

Since 1944 new clotting factors have been discovered in rapid succession, largely by the recognition of congenital deficiency states in specific patients. The identification of each new clotting factor has raised the possibility that abnormalities in this factor might be found among patients with thromboembolism. It has been suggested, for example, that venous thrombosis may result post-partum or while on antiovulatory drugs from increases in Factors VII or X (3,4), that thrombosis after trauma may be caused by elevation of Factor VIII (5), and postoperatively by an increased adhesiveness of platelets (6).

In fact, alterations in in vitro coagulation assays found among patients with thrombosis have led some investigators to conclude that the observed changes represent evidence of "systemic hypercoagulability" that is causally related to thrombus formation.

Supported in part by NIH Grant HE 09326 and, in part, by the Stella H. Shoenberg Research Fund.

Support for this concept has been collected from at least three
types of observations: the absence or relative rarity of phlebitis
among patients with congenital deficiencies in specific clotting
factors, the prophylactic efficacy of anticoagulant drugs, and
plasma elevations of clotting factors in the immediate post-partum
period.

   Objections to the validity of these arguments can be readily
marshalled. Thus, the data on patients with congenital deficiencies are scanty and include few individuals in the older age groups.
Moreover, thrombosis has been observed in patients with low levels
of Factors I, V, VII, VIII, and XII (7,8). In regard to anticoag-
ulent therapy, the fact that interference with clotting reactions
can prevent thrombosis, does not establish a priori that the basis
for this effect is related to the prevention of any systemic hypercoagulability. Pregnant women in the third trimester have coagulation factor elevations of the same order as that found in the
immediate post-partum period yet a smaller incidence of phlebitis
is observed during pregnancy than following delivery. In addition,
many patients develop phlebitis without any detectable change in
their coagulation profile; whereas others show changes in clotting
factors that appear to be consequent rather than causal to the
thrombosis (9,10).

   Rokitansky (11) and subsequently Astrup (12) intimated that
the intravascular deposition of fibrin can initiate the atherosclerotic lesion. Duguid has suggested that thrombosis precedes
atherosclerosis (13). The rapid turnover of clotting factors and
the demonstration by electron microscopy of fibrin on normal vessels
are often cited as evidence in support of the concept that thrombosis may precede intimal damage (14-16). Evidence has also been
brought forward that platelets participate in the process of continuous coagulation (17). However, Hjort and Hasselbach have noted
that the rapid turnover of clotting factors does not necessarily
indicate their consumption in continuous coagulation; for the life
span of factors unconsumed in clotting is as short as those which
are; and spontaneous or induced hypercoagulable states do not
affect the turnover of clotting factors (18). More recent investigations of platelet consumption suggest that platelets complete
their life span chiefly by senescence rather than by utilization in
the clotting process (19).

   There is one type of relatively uncommon situation in man in
which demonstrable intravascular coagulation occurs. This is the
defibrination syndrome or consumptive coagulopathy in which diffuse
fibrin deposition in the microvasculature and occasionally frank
thrombosis in large vessels occur. The inciting causes are unknown,
but the phenomenon is observed among patients with metastic carcinoma, leukemia, giant hemangioma, purpura fulminans, drug reactions,

FIGURE 1

MODIFIED DIAGRAM OF CLOTTING MECHANISM

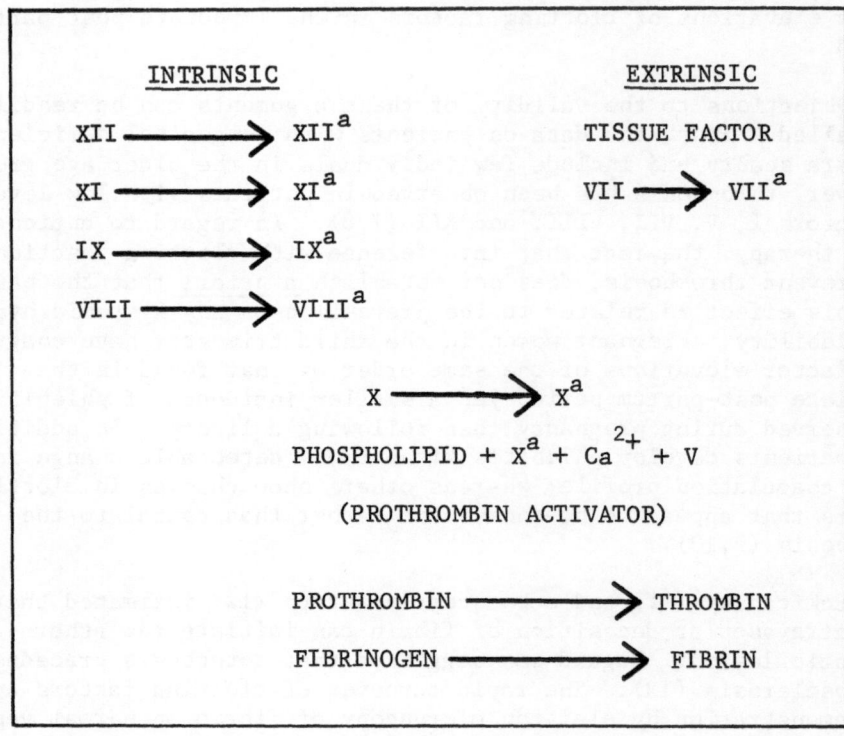

TABLE 1

FACTOR X

NON-ACTIVATED		ACTIVATED	
units infused	stasis thrombus	units infused	stasis thrombus
2.5	0	2.5	0
5.0	0	5.0	+
50.0	0	10.0	+
158.0	0	20.0	+
315.0	0	30.0	+
630.0	0	50.0	+

hemorrhagic shock, following snake bites, after transfusions of
mismatched blood, and during extracorporeal shunts (20). The clinical picture and laboratory findings are different, however, from
the usual patient with venous or arterial thrombosis. Experimentally, consumptive coagulopathies may be produced by infusion of
tissue thromboplastin or thrombin and by the generalized Shwartzman
reaction (21,22).

Although it is clear that most thrombi begin as a platelet
nidus; to make platelet aggregation irreversible, thrombin is
necessary and to cause the massive propagation of the thrombus, the
elaboration of fibrin is required. In both of these latter roles,
activation of the clotting mechanism appears essential. Thus, even
if clotting factors do not serve as trigger mechanisms in the initiation of intravascular coagulation, they may be important in the
fixation and growth of the thrombus.

The effective evaluation of thrombogenicity requires an understanding of clotting reactions; the purification of individual
coagulation factors at least to the point where they are rid of
contaminating clot-promoting acitivty; and, finally, a reproducible
animal model for measuring thrombus formation.

Although it might reasonably be argued that a several-fold
increase in a circulating clotting factor would set the stage for a
greater and more rapid explosion of enzyme coagulation kinetics,
no experiments in man or animals have provided evidence to support
this hypothesis.

We have recently completed some experiments that demonstrate
that it is not the quantity per se, but the species of a clotting
factor that is responsible for the initiation of thrombosis (23).

From among the thirteen clotting factors given Roman numerals
by the International Nomenclature Committee, Factor X, also known
as intermediate product I and autoprothrombin C in both its non-
activated and activated forms, was chosen for this study because
of its unique position in the clotting scheme and because kinetic
studies have suggested that it is the pivotal enzyme in the elaboration of prothrombin activator.

Figure 1 is a diagramatic representation of the clotting
mechanism modified for the purposes of this presentation. Factor X
occupies a unique place at the headwaters of the final common pathway, whereby activation either of the intrinsic system or the
extrinsic system leads via the so-called enzymic cascade to the
activation of Factor X. Activated Factor X in combination with
phospholipid, Factor V and calcium then results in the formation of
prothrombin activator and the subsequent generation of fibrin.

    It was first necessary to obtain highly purified fractions of plasma rich in either non-activated or activated Factor X and devoid of other clotting factors. For this purpose, Factor X, in its non-activated form, was prepared from bovine plasma by a modification of the technique of Duckert, Yin and Straub (24), utilizing DEAE-cellulose and Sephadex gel filtration. The resulting fraction of non-activated Factor X has a specific activity of 25,000 units per mg tyrosine and is devoid of all known clotting factors, including activated Factor X.

    Activated bovine Factor X was then prepared in our laboratory from commercial thrombin by a step-wise chromatographic technique on DEAE-cellulose resulting in the complete separation and partial purification of both thrombin and activated Factor X (25). This activated Factor X fraction did not clot a standard fibrinogen solution during twenty-four hours either at 22° or 37° C, with or without added calcium, or after the removal of the citrate by dialysis against 0.14 M sodium chloride. This resulting fraction of activated Factor X has a specific activity of 22,000 units per mg tyrosine, is devoid of other clotting factors, and is biologically indistinguishable from that derived from activation of highly purified non-activated Factor X by either venom or trypsin (25).

    These two activities (non-activated and activated Factor X), which have different physical constants, were then compared for their thrombogenic effects in a reproducible animal model developed for this purpose in our laboratory. In brief, a segment of a fasted rabbit's jugular vein is freed from its surrounding structures. One ml of saline, containing in this instance ten units of activated Factor X is injected into the marginal ear vein in two seconds. Five seconds after the infusion, the previously freed jugular vein segment is isolated with ligatures. When the contents of the segment are examined ten minutes later, a cast delineating the isolated segment is observed. Thrombi also invariably form behind the distal ligature, where stasis is incomplete. Such thrombi are not produced, however, by the infusion of this amount of activated Factor X alone or isolation of the vein segment alone.

    In an examination of infusions of human serum into rabbits with which the technique of stasis-induced thrombosis was originally standardized, it was demonstrable that the formation of thrombotic casts in isolated vein segments was dose dependent (26). This technique has permitted the determination of the relative quantities of thrombogenic activity in different plasma and serum fractions.

    A comparison of the thrombogenicity of non-activated and activated bovine Factor X is shown in Table 1. Whereas amounts of non-activated Factor X as great as 630 units failed to induce stasis thrombi; activated Factor X in quantities as small as five

units was fully thrombogenic. Stated differently, the infusion
into a rabbit of an amount of activated Factor X equivalent to the
amount of activated Factor X that can be derived from ten ml of
bovine plasma was thrombogenic; whereas an infusion of non-activated
Factor X equivalent to the injection of more than one liter of
bovine plasma was inert.

That lipids exert important effects on in vitro clotting and
in vivo coagulation is well established (27-30). Although a role
for lipid in several reactions in the clotting scheme have been
suggested, it is only in the formation of prothrombin activator
that there is general agreement on a lipid requirement. If,
instead of activated Factor X alone, a mixture of activated Factor
X and cephalin is infused, two additional effects on thrombus
formation are observable. First, as shown in Table 2, thrombi
that require for their formation five units of activated Factor X
alone, can now be induced with only 0.3 units of activated Factor X,
if phospholipid is added to the activated X before infusion -- a
more than ten-fold increase in sensitivity. Secondly, as seen in
Table 3, the duration of the hypercoagulability induced by activated Factor X alone is prolonged from five seconds to 200 seconds
if phospholipid is added -- a forty-fold increase. Control experiments have demonstrated that cephalin is not itself thrombogenic
and when mixed with non-activated Factor X before infusion does not
confer thrombogenicity on the inactive form of this clotting factor.
These findings suggest that there is an instantaneous formation of
prothrombin activator in vivo when the activated Factor X-cephalin
fraction is infused: the other factors, Factor V and calcium,
being already present in circulating blood and not representing
rate-limiting reactions in the formation of prothrombin activator.
These observations are consistent with the view that activated
Factor X is the prime activator of prothrombin (31,32) and with
data indicating that activated Factor X, (because of the added
variable of adsorption onto a lipid surface) does not function in
the coagulation sequence as part of a simple enzyme-substrate relationship exemplified by the so-called cascade scheme of coagulation
(33). The specificity of the role of lipid is further emphasized
by other data from our laboratory indicating that cephalin does not
enhance the thrombogenicity of infusions of purified thrombin (34).

These experiments also demonstrate that hypercoagulability is
not related to the total quantity of a specific clotting factor in
the circulation, but rather to whether it is circulating as an
activated species. These data confirm the view that hypercoagulability should be defined as a state in which activated products or
intermediates, normally absent from circulating blood, are found
intravascularly or are released from tissues (7).

TABLE 2

INFUSATE		STASIS THROMBUS
X^a units	CEPHALIN (μgP)	
5.0	none	+
2.5	none	0
2.5	2	+
1.3	2	+
0.6	2	+
0.3	2	+
0.2	2	0

TABLE 3

INFUSATE X^a + CEPHALIN	LIGATION DELAY AFTER INFUSION (SECONDS)	STASIS THROMBUS
130 units	5	+
X^a alone	10	+
5 units X^a	5	+
PLUS	10	+
2 μg P	40	+
CEPHALIN	80	+
	120	+
	160	+
	200	+
	240	0

It is, perhaps, a truism to state that venous thrombosis is dependent on coagulation of the blood. From this concept, however, has been derived the thesis that patients with thrombosis have an augmented tendency to clot which has been termed "hypercoagulability". As we have seen, increased levels of clotting factors in the non-activated form cannot initiate intravascular coagulation. This can only be achieved by the appearance of the activated species in the circulation. When, however, even in experimental situations, an activated species appears in the circulation, it is opposed promptly and successfully by compensatory mechanisms that are very potent. For we now recognize that the fluidity of the circulating blood is controlled, in part, by the release of plasminogen activator from endothelial cells (35), by circulating inhibitors to thrombin and Factor X (36), by the liver clearance of certain activated clotting factors (37), and by the rate of blood flow (38).

As one reviews the area of thrombosis, it is difficult to escape the fact that some kind of "hypercoagulability" must be present to account for the propagation of red thrombi particularly in the venous circulation, but also in the peripheral arteries.

While it is very tempting to believe in systemic hypercoagulability, proof of its existence is man remains elusive. Even in the consumptive coagulopathies, the initiating mechanism is not understood. Proof will require the recognition of the transient presence of an activated clotting factor in the circulating blood.

While attempts to demonstrate the existence of systemic hypercoagulability remain unavailing, the possible role of local hypercoagulability in the augmentation of the platelet thrombus is essentially unexplored. In the experimental thrombus produced by vessel damage, the platelet plug is usually completed before fibrin deposition is noted. Apparently, the initial small amounts of thrombin believed to form locally are enough to make platelet aggregation irreversible, but insufficient to result in the conversion of fibrinogen to fibrin. The quantity of fibrin formed presumably depends upon the amount and rate of thrombin elaboration, which in turn is related to the extent to which the extrinsic and intrinsic coagulation systems are activated. Local hypercoagulability, by which is meant the focal but intravascular accumulation of activated clotting factors, may play a critical role in thrombus growth. If this is the manner in which hypercoagulability expresses itself in venous thrombosis, it would account for the failure to find the activated factors in the systemic circulation. Even if hypercoagulability exists systemically, there remain many checks and balances which would tend to return the clotting mechanism to normal very promptly. In this regard, evidence that a thrombus has formed may possibly be determined retrospectively from recognition of "markers" such as circulating breakdown products of fibrin that might persist after the activated species has been neutralized.

Finally, two observations appear warranted: first, we must
determine what are the biologic stimuli to the activation of the
clotting proteins, particularly Factor X; and, second, further
progress in understanding the thrombotic process will require
animal models that integrate data being accumulated by biologists,
chemists, and flow engineers.

REFERENCES

1. Wiseman, R.: Several Chirugical Treatises, 2nd ed.,
Norton and Macock, London, 1676, p. 64.

2. Virchow, R.: Gesammelte Abhandlugen zur Wissenschaftlichen
Medicin. Frankfurt, Meidinger Sohn, 1856, p. 219.

3. Pechet, L. and Alexander, B.: Increased clotting factors
in the gravid: a hypercoagulable state. New Eng. J. Med. 265:
1093 (1961).

4. Hougie, C., Rutherford, R.W., Banks, A.L. and Coburn, W.A.:
Effect of a progestin-estrogen oral contraceptive on blood clotting
factors. Metabolism 14:411 (1965).

5. Egeberg, O.: Changes in the coagulation system following
major surgical operations. Acta Med. Scand. 171:679 (1962).

6. Wright, H.P.: Changes in adhesiveness of blood platelets
following parturition and surgical operations. J. Path. Bact.
54:461 (1942).

7. Duckert, F. and Streuli, F.: Role of coagulation in
thrombosis. In Pathogenesis and Treatment of Thromboembolic
Diseases. International Symposium, Basle, Switzerland, 1966, Ed.
F. Duckert, p. 185.

8. Ratnoff, O.D., Busse, R.J., Jr. and Sheon, R.P.: The
demise of John Hageman. New Eng. J. Med. 279:760 (1968).

9. McDonald, L. and Edgill, M.: Coagulability of the blood
in ischaemic heart disease. Lancet ii:457 (1957).

10. MacFarlane, R.G.: In General Pathology, 2nd ed. Edited by
H. Florey, W.B. Saunders, London, 1959, p. 156.

11. Rokitansky, K.: A Manual of Pathological Anatomy (Trans-
lated by G.E. Day) London, Sydenham Society, Vol. 4, 1852, p. 261.

12. Astrup, T.: Neure Aspekte in der Blutgerinnung und der
Fibrinolyse und ihren Beziehungen zur Koronarthrombose und
Koronarsklerose. Wien. Ztschr. f. inn. Med. 39:373 (1958).

13. Duguid, J.B.: Thrombosis as a factor in the pathogenesis of coronary atherosclerosis. J. Path. Bact. 58:207 (1946).

14. Copley, A.L.: Thrombosis and Embolism. Schwabe, Basle, 1955, p. 458.

15. Roos, J.: Blood coagulation as a continuous process. Thromb. Diath. Haemorrh. 1:471 (1957).

16. Astrup, T.: Connective Tissue, Thrombosis and Atherosclerosis. Academic Press, New York, 1959, p. 223.

17. Adelson, E., Rheingold, J.J., Parker, O., Buenaventura, A. and Crosby, W.H.: Platelet and fibrinogen survival in normal and abnormal states of coagulation. Blood 17:267 (1961).

18. Hjort, P.P. and Hasselback, R.: A critical review of the evidence for a continuous hemostasis in vivo. Thromb. Diath. Haemorrh. 6:558 (1961).

19. Aster, R.H. and Jandl, J.H.: Platelet sequestration in man. I. Methods. J. Clin. Invest. 43:843 (1964).

20. Mersky, C., Johnson, A.J., Kleiner, G.J. and Wohl, H.: The defibrination syndrome: clinical features and laboratory diagnosis. Brit. J. Haemat. 13:528 (1967).

21. McKay, D.G.: Disseminated Intravascular Coagulation. An Intermediary Mechanism of Disease. Harper and Row, New York, 1965.

22. Hardaway, R.M., Watson, H.E. and Weiss, F.H.: Alterations in blood coagulation mechanisms after intra-aortic injection of thrombin. Arch. Surg. 81:983 (1960).

23. Wessler, S. and Yin, E.T.: Experimental hypercoagulable state induced by Factor X: Comparison of non-activated and activated forms. J. Lab. Clin. Med. 72:256-260 (1968).

24. Duckert, F., Yin, E.T. and Straub, W.: Separation and purification of the blood clotting factors by means of chromatography and electrophoresis. Preparative methods. In Proc. VIII Colloquium. Protides of Biological Fluids. H. Peeters, ed. Elsevier Publishing Co., Amsterdam, 1961, p. 41.

25. Yin, E.T. and Wessler, S.: Bovine thrombin and activated Factor X: Separation and purification. J. Biol. Chem. 243:112-117 (1968).

26. Wessler, S., Reimer, S.M. and Sheps, M.C.: Biologic assay of a thrombosis-inducing activity in human serum. J. Appl. Physiol. 14:943 (1959).

27. Howell, W.H.: The nature and action of the thromboplastic (zymoplastic) substances of the tissues. Am. J. Physiol. 31:1 (1912).

28. MacFarlane, R.G., Trevan, J.W. and Atwood, A.M.P.: Participation of a fat soluble substance in coagulation of the blood. J. Physiol. 99:78 (1946).

29. Poole, J.C.F.: Fats and blood coagulation. Brit. Med. Bull. 14:253 (1958).

30. Connor, W.E., Hoak, J.C. and Warner, E.D.: Massive thrombosis produced by fatty acid infusion. J. Clin. Invest. 42:860 (1963).

31. Milstone, J.H.: Thrombokinase as prime activator of oprthrombin: historical perspectives and present status. Fed. Proc. 23:742 (1964).

32. Barton, P.G., Jackson, C.M. and Hanahan, D.J.: Relationships between Factor V and activated Factor X in the generation of prothrombinase. Nature 214:923 (1967).

33. Hemker, H.C. and Muller, A.D.: Kinetic aspects of the interaction of blood clotting enzymes. V. The reaction mechanism of the extrinsic clotting system as revealed by the kinetics of one-stage estimations of coagulation enzymes. Thromb. Diath. Haemorrh. 19:368-382 (1968).

34. Yin, E.T. and Wessler, S.: Investigation of the apparent thrombogenicity of thrombin. Thromb. Diath. Haemorrh. (In press)

35. Ashford, T.P., Freiman, D.G. and Weinstein, M.C.: The role of the intrinsic fibrinolytic system in the prevention of stasis thrombosis in small veins: an electron microscope study. Am. J. Path. 52:1117 (1968).

36. Yin, E.T. and Wessler, S.: Evidence for a naturally occurring plasma inhibitor of activated Factor X: its isolation and partial purification. Thromb. Diath. Haemorrh. (In press)

37. Spaet, T.H.: Studies on the in vivo behavior of blood coagulation product I in rats. Thromb. Diath. Haemorrh. 8:276 (1962).

38. Merrill, E.W.: Rheology of human blood: in vitro observations and theoretical considerations. National Research Conference on Thrombosis. (In press).

INFLUENCE OF HORMONES ON TISSUE AND BLOOD FIBRINOLYTIC ACTIVITY

Tage Astrup

Director of Research, Institute for Medical Research
The James F. Mitchell Foundation, Washington, D.C.

Resolution of fibrin deposits in the living organism is caused by a specific process of fibrinolysis. An enzyme precursor, plasminogen, present in the circulating blood, is converted by activators into the blood protease, plasmin, the enzyme in the body primarily attacking fibrin. Activators of plasminogen are present in the blood or in tissues. Their effects in blood are balanced by large amounts of inhibitory compounds. Some organs and tissues are particularly rich in plasminogen activator, while only few contain inhibitory agents except for such inhibitors as are derived from the blood present in the organ or in the interstitial fluid. The biochemistry and physiology of the tissue plasminogen activator has recently been reviewed (1), as has the role of the fibrinolytic system in tissue repair (2).

Fibrin formation is an early stage in tissue repair. The fibrin deposit forms a hemostatic barrier preventing extravasation of blood. It also prevents the spreading of an invasive process, thus limiting the area affected by the tissue injury. It forms the fabric on which fibroblasts migrate and lay down collagen in the process of organization of the coagulum. In this repair process fibrinolysis assists by limiting the amount of fibrin remaining at a site of injury, thus impeding excessive formation of reparative connective tissue. This particular role in tissue repair makes fibrinolysis a fundamental physiological process. We see the resolution of clots in the blood vessels by fibrinolytic agents as an extension of the role of fibrinolysis in tissue repair, -modified according to the specific conditions prevailing in the walls of blood vessels caused by their anatomical structure, their histochemical properties and the presence of blood.

Supported by NIH Grant HE-05020.

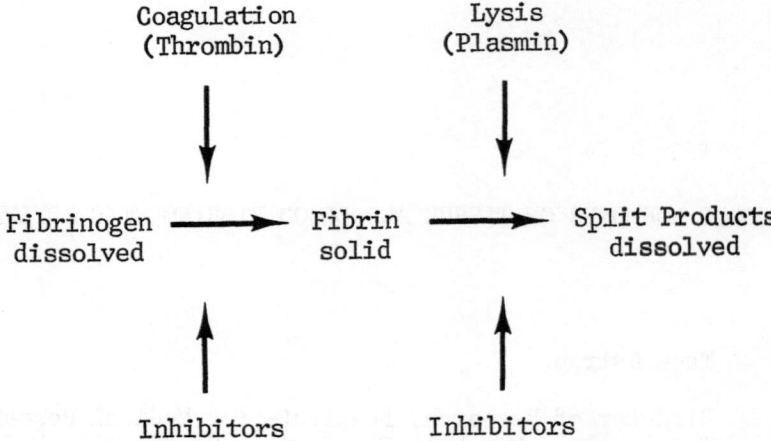

Figure 1. The dynamic hemostatic balance in the body. Fibrin
formation and deposition regulated by clot promoting and fibrinolytic agents and by inhibitors.

The equilibrium between fibrin formation and fibrin resolution
in the body is in a dynamic hemostatic balance as schematically
described in Figure 1.

The regulation of the formation and resolution of fibrin by
compounds released from injured tissue and interacting with humoral
components is depicted in Figure 2.

Tissue thromboplastin locally released from injured cells
interacts with blood coagulation components to form thrombin. In
a similar manner a fibrinolytic agent released from tissues acts
as an activator of plasminogen converting it to the fibrin splitting protease, plasmin. It is believed that in the mammalian
organism the cellular release of thromboplastin and plasminogen
activator plays a decisive role in local tissue repair because
both components are bound to particulate cellular material. However, we should not forget the existence of an intrinsic system
of blood coagulation acting by the formation of a plasma thromboplastin from humoral components initiated by platelet agglutination
and disruption, as well as a similar system of fibrinolysis involving the formation of a plasminogen activator in the circulating
blood. In certain localizations and in some animal species where
active agents are low in concentration or missing, fibrin formation
and resolution depend upon these intrinsic systems (3). Hence, it
is possible to explain many deviations in normal tissue repair in
various organs or animal species by considering the content of
thromboplastin and plasminogen activator in their tissues as well

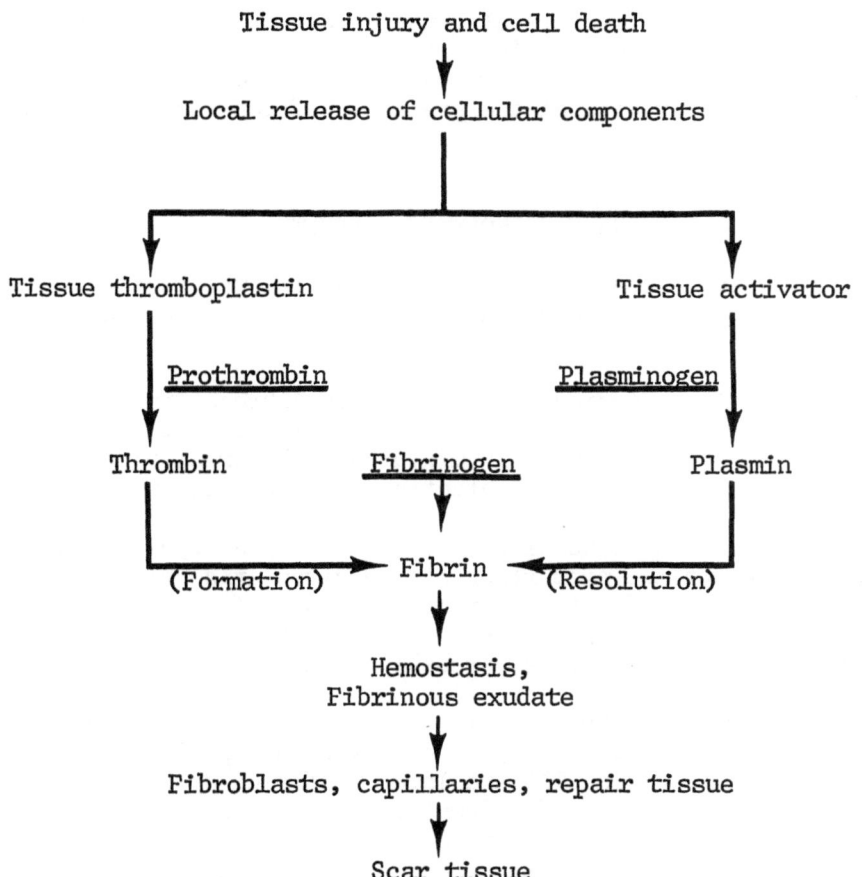

Figure 2. Role of blood coagulation and fibrinolysis in regulating connective tissue formation in tissue repair. Humoral components are underlined.

as the composition of their intrinsic systems of blood coagulation and fibrinolysis. In view of these interrelations it becomes important to elucidate the influence of extraneous influences on the compositions of the cellular and humoral systems of blood coagulation and fibrinolysis. This is a field of research which is just beginning to be systematically studied, -first because of a lack of suitable assay methods, and secondly because animal species differ in their response among themselves and from man. Among information urgently needed is data describing the influence of hormone administration upon fibrin formation and fibrin resolution. The present article will give a brief survey of studies aimed at the elucidation of the influence of hormones on

tissue fibrinolysis. In particular the effect of steroid sex
hormones will be dealt with. The effects of these on blood
coagulation and fibrinolysis in blood have been recently reviewed
(4) and will be dealt with at the present conference by Dr. Pieter
Brakman.

UTERINE FIBRINOLYTIC ACTIVITY

The fluidity of menstrual blood contrasting the rapid
coagulation of blood from a normal wound has aroused curiosity
from earliest times.

The subject was studied and reviewed by Albrechtsen (5).
Whitehouse (6) was first to report on the lytic activity of
menstrual blood observing that in mixtures with normal blood,
coagulation was followed by liquefaction. Since then, the fibrinolytic property of menstrual blood has been repeatedly confirmed
and its relation to uterine tissues and the ovarian cycle studied.
Its independence on the properties of the circulating blood was
demonstrated when blood obtained from incisions of the uterus
clotted normally (7, 8, 9). This suggested that the cause of the
fluidity was of a local nature, probably related to the endometrium.

The presence of a fibrin-splitting, trypsin-like enzyme in
human endometrial tissues was first observed in experiments by
Halban and Frankl (10) in 1910 and later confirmed by Caffier (11).
Saline or aqueous extracts of endometrial tissues also contained
fibrin-splitting agents (12, 13). Later, the fibrinolytic activity
of the endometrium was found to be caused by a plasminogen activator
(14, 15). The concentration of this activator increases in the
secretory phase thus implying the existence of a mechanism of
hormonal regulation. Interestingly, in 1910 Halban and Frankl (10)
had already observed an increase in fibrin-splitting properties of
the endometrium in the secretory stage, an observation confirmed by
Caffier (11) and Page, Glendening and Parkinson (13). The activity
in the myometrium is also caused by an activator of plasminogen
(14, 16) which is present in higher concentrations than in the
endometrium, though not fluctuating with the menstrual cycle.

Albrechtsen (17) observed an activator of plasminogen in
menstrual blood and found it to be stable at acid reaction, and,
therefore, similar to the activator present in tissues, and
probably originating in the endometrial tissue and liberated
during the late secretory stage by tissue necrosis. These results
were recently confirmed by Rybo (18, 19) who drew attention to the
fact that lysosomes of the glandular epithelium of the endometrium
became progressively more fragile in the secretory phase. He
suggested a release of fibrinolytic activity from these lysosomes
caused by steroid hormones. However, new investigations (see

below) have shown that the endometrial glandular epithelium is not fibrinolytically active.

Using a histochemical fibrin slide technique, Todd (20) observed that the tissue plasminogen activator is related to small vessels, in particular veins and venules, and that the high activity in the human myometrium is caused by its rich vascularization. He found fibrinolytic activity in the endometrium in the proliferative phase related to blood vessels in the basal layer (21) though he also observed plasminogen activator in the superficial endometrium at the time of menstrual shedding. This superficial activity was more diffuse than the focal myometrial and basal endometrial activity. He assumed the superficial activity to be related to an exudative process possibly originating in the injured tissue and becoming "trapped in the spongework of the epithelium" (21, 22).

A relation between increased fibrinolysis and decrease in estrogen level has been suggested by several authors beginning with Caffier in 1930 (11). Luginbuhl and Picoff (23) confirmed Todd's histological observations of a focal lysis related to vessels in the deeper layers of the endometrium as well as of a superficial lysis of more diffuse character related to the onset of menstruation. They suggested that a drop in progesterone and/or estrogen levels could lead to the release or production of an activator of plasminogen. It is of interest in this respect to recall the many reports on a hemostatic effect of estrogen preparations, chiefly in the form of the preparation "Premarin". The beneficial effects of estrogen on certain forms of uterine bleeding reported by Greenblatt and Barfield (24) could possibly be caused by the prevention of endometrial necrosis with impairment of release of plasminogen activator. Though some forms of habitual abortion and uterine bleeding during pregnancy are believed to be caused by a deficiency in progesterone production, it should also be recalled that beneficial results have also been reported after estrogen (25). Such results would fit into the pattern of a hormonal effect on the release of endometrial fibrinolytic activity reported here. The concept is supported by the observation (13, 14, 15) that the normal human placenta or decidua are fibrinolytically inactive. In contrast, a number of samples of decidua from spontaneous abortions contained varying concentrations of plasminogen activator. The absence of fibrinolytic activity in the normal human placenta was confirmed by Beller et al (26) using the histochemical fibrin slide technique.

In animal species endometrial tissue has been found fibrinolytically active (27, 28). Page, Glendening and Parkinson (13) reported that the fibrinolytic activity in the rabbit uterus decreased after castration, remained unchanged when estrogen and

progesterone was administered, and increased after discontinuation
of estrogen treatment. They concluded that the concentration of
"fibrinolytic enzymes" in the rabbit uterus increased when the
level of estrogen in blood decreased. It is now known that the
active compound is an activator of plasminogen. Because of the
variation in activity related to the hormonal state of the animal,
the data reported by Page et al. (13) probably reflects changes in
the endometrial lining of the rabbit uterus, since the myometrium
would probably change little in activity if results from studies
on man are applicable to animal experiments.

Albrechtsen (29) has studied the effect of castration and
estradiol administration on the plasminogen activator concentration
in the rat uterus. There was no change in uterine concentration of
plasminogen activator after castration, though the total amount was
decreased because of the smaller size of the uterus. Administration
of estradiol raised the weight of the uterus but did not change the
activator concentration (expressed in units per gram fresh tissue).
However, in animals killed 17 to 56 days after the last injection
of estradiol-dipropionate, when the uterine weight was still nearly
normal and vaginal smears showed the animals to be in late estrus,
the concentration of activator as well as its total amount (average)
per uterus was increased. It was assumed that this change reflected
the composition of the endometrium and was related to an estrogen
withdrawal phase. The reason why this phenomenon had escaped notice
in the studies of the castrated animals possibly could be that it
is of transient occurrence, and that in the castrated group studied
the uterine weights had reached a stage far below normal indicating
that the hormonal effect had long disappeared.

Using the histochemical fibrin slide technique, Kwaan and
Albrechtsen (30) confirmed the localization of fibrinolytically
active sites to vessels in the myometrium and the endometrium in
the rat uterus. The activity in the endometrium varied with its
vascularization during the estrus cycle. Endometrial glands were
always inactive. Myometrial arteries were fibrinolytically active.
After estradiol-dipropionate intramuscularly the proliferative
endometrium contained numerous active vessels. Later, after estrogen
withdrawal, there was a further increase in fibrinolytic activity
around endometrial vessels. Two months later the uterus was atrophic
with little fibrinolytic activity. Treatment with progesterone
intramuscularly after estrogen gave a histological picture as in
the secretory phase with a highly vascular endometrium, but the
fibrinolytic pattern was different with few active sites, though
the activity of myometrial vessels had not changed significantly.
This contradicts the report by Page, Glendening and Parkinson (13)
of a lack of effect of progesterone on the fibrinolytic activity
of the rabbit uterus. It is apparent that progesterone exerts a
specific influence on the fibrinolytic activity of endometrial

vessels. Perhaps this observation could be related to the formation
of decidual tissue and represents a phase simulating pregnancy,
since Albrechtsen (15) had found human decidua fibrinolytically
inactive. Kwaan and Albrechtsen (30) also noticed sites of fibrinolytic activity where there was loss of continuity of the epithelial
lining at the endometrium and where active vessels came into close
contact with the lumen. They thought, like Todd (21) in his studies
of the human endometrium, that this activity originated in the endothelium of broken vessels close to the surface of a hyperemic
endometrium.

Recent observations have pointed to a different source of the
diffuse endometrial activity in man reported by Todd (21), and of
the activity at discontinuities of the endometrial lining in rat
mentioned by Kwaan and Albrechtsen (30). In studies on the rat
uterus Tympanidis and Astrup (31) observed a transient appearance
of high fibrinolytic activity at the surface epithelium of the
endometrium at estrus. The activity was of a more diffuse
character than that usually seen related to vessels and seemed to
occur in association with cellular degeneration and desquamation
along the epithelial lining. At diestrus, proestrus and metestrus
fibrinolytic activity was usually localized only to the vessels of
the myometrium and endometrium with no activity along the surface
epithelium. These results show a definite correlation between the
induction of endometrial fibrinolysis and a brief phase in the
ovarian cycle of the rat and they suggest a relation to certain
epithelial cells in addition to the known relation to vascular
endothelial cells. The observation by Kwaan and Albrechtsen (30)
that glandular endometrial cells are fibrinolytically inactive was
confirmed. Also, fibrinolytic activity was observed particularly
around small arteries while veins usually were inactive, while
Todd (20) studying human endometrium and myometrium reported
activity around the veins.

Pandolfi and Astrup (32) recently noted that corneal epithelial
cells become fibrinolytically active, presumably during a process
of degeneration. Next, it was found that vaginal epithelial cells
go through a phase in which they are fibrinolytically active (33).
These findings are of interest when evaluating the results of a
study of the fibrinolytic activity of the human uterine tube (34)
in which relatively high concentrations of plasminogen activator
were found in the mucosal layer of the tube. The muscular and
peritoneal layers still had higher activity, presumably caused by
their high vascularity. It was also thought that the activity in
the mucosal layer reflected its content of fibrinolytically active
vessels. However, a study of the rat oviduct using the histochemical technique, Tympanidis and Astrup (35), revealed that in
addition to the fibrinolytically active vessels, mostly arteries,
fibrinolysis also occurred along the surface epithelium of the

mucosa, suggesting an epithelial origin for fibrinolysis. The distribution in the tissues of the oviduct did not vary with the ovarian cycle or during pregnancy, suggesting at this localization an independence from the influence of steriod sex hormones. It is known that the surface epithelium of the oviduct has a low renewal rate. This could possibly explain variations in localization of fibrinolytic activity, since active sites were often seen adjacent to inactive areas. The observations mentioned above may imply that fibrinolytically active sites indicate areas where epithelial necrosis and cellular desquamation are in progress. In a study of the pregnant rat uterus diffuse fibrinolytic activity was observed in the decidua and placenta during early pregnancy (36). At mid-pregnancy numerous fibrinolytically active vessels appeared in the placenta. Later, most of them disappeared again and at term only a few active vessels remained. The myometrium and parametrium continued to contain fibrinolytically active vessels. These observations unequivocally demonstrate that the development of fibrinolytic activity in different tissues may follow different patterns of regulation. As mentioned, Albrechtsen (15), using an extraction method, had found normal human decidua and placenta at term to be inactive, while samples of decidual tissue from spontaneous abortions frequently were fibrinolytically active. At earlier stages of pregnancy plasminogen activator was observed in the human placenta by Phillips, Butler and Taylor (14) and Phillips and McKay (37). It was suggested that presence of tissue plasminogen activator in the placenta could assist in the removal of subsyncytical deposits of fibrin, thereby preventing the development of necrotic areas during middle pregnancy. It is interesting in this connection to mention that Picoff and Luginbuhl (38) reported the presence of fibrin in a number of samples of endometrial tissue, namely in 64 instances among 691 specimens, representing 9% of total. Among these, 60 specimens were from a group of 434 patients with a history of abnormal bleeding, equal to 13.3%. There were only four samples from the remaining 257 patients with normal menses representing 1.5%. It is apparent that in most individuals fibrin was absent even in the pathological samples and, as mentioned above, this points to an effect of the plasminogen activator present in the normal and hyperplastic endometrium. Fibrin deposits are frequently observed in placental tissues and can be experimentally induced in the rat placenta (39). Its occurrence can be explained by the low fibrinolytic activity of the placenta at term. Perhaps the occurrence of fibrin deposits in the endometrium stroma could be related to samples with abnormally low fibrinolytic activity. Thrombotic processes have also been reported in the normally highly fibrinolytic myometrium, namely in relation to the presence of myomata, and occasionally leading to disseminated intravascular fibrin deposition (40). It should be recalled here that in contrast to the high concentrations of plasminogen activator in the normal myometrium, there is

considerably lower fibrinolytic activity in myomatous tissue (41).
The degeneration of myoma during pregnancy is reported to be a
common phenomenon, which might suggest a correlation with the
changes known to occur in blood coagulation and fibrinolysis
during pregnancy as reviewed by Dr. Pieter Brakman (42).

In a study of the effects of estradiol, progesterone and
gonadotrophins on the uterus of the juvenile rat, Tympanidis and
Astrup (43) found large differences in the qualitative effects
of these hormones. In the untreated three week old rats fibrinolytic activity was localized to vessels, mostly arteries, in the
immature myometrium and endometrium, while the endometrial surface
epithelium was inactive. After estrogen administration the pro-
liferating endometrium showed, in addition to the active vessels,
a diffuse zone of lysis along its epithelial lining, and fibrinolytically active desquamated cells appeared in the lumen. After
injection of chorionic or serum gonadotrophin (Physex and Antex,
Leo Pharmaceuticals, Copenhagen, respectively) a tremendous
increase in uterine weight occurred and the endometrium became
hypertrophic but remained fibrinolytically inactive with no
cellular desquamation. It is difficult to explain the findings
after gonadotrophin stimulation in relation to the effects produced
by estradiol and progesterone. There are large qualitative
differences even if stimulation by gonadotrophin is supposed to be
mediated through ovarian hormones. Detailed investigations are
required in order to elucidate these interrelations.

The fibrinolytic properties of endometrial tissue have also
been observed by cultivation in vitro. Ingemanson (44) tried to
overcome this by adding lysine ethyl ester as an inhibitor of
fibrinolysis. This method was also applied by Kullander and
Källén in the cultivation in vitro of normal human endometrial
tissue (45) and uterine carcinoma tissue (46). They confirmed the
lack of fibrinolytic activity in the normal decidua. Maurer,
Rounds and Raiborn (47) studied the effect of estradiol on calf
endometrial tissue in vitro preserving the surface endothelium.
Estradiol had no stimulating effect on the isolated epithelial
cells.

In a discussion of the fibrinolytic activity of the endometrium
and its hormonal regulation, it should be recalled that uterine
secretions have been found fibrinolytically active. Kross (48)
and Huggins, Vail and Davis (12) observed liquefaction of fibrin
clots by secretions from the rat uterus. The production of endometrial secretion in the ligated uterus of the mouse was reported
to be stimulated by estrogens and inhibited by androgens (49).
Progesterone enhanced secretion but decreased its protein concentration. They noticed an anticoagulant effect of the fluid
and used the term "uterone" to describe the secretion collected.

Earlier, Greenberg (50, 51) had reported on an anticoagulant in
the human myometrium and related this to the incoagulability of
menstrual blood. He used the term "hysterin" for the compound
involved. Later, Harpel and Bang (52) reported the presence of a
plasminogen activator in mouse uterine fluid. The activator
decreased in concentration after administration of estradiol and
disappeared completely after progesterone (53). In a further
study, Harpel, Homburger and Treger (54) reported on the effects
of a contraceptive hormone preparation (Enovid®) and its separate
components (mestranol and norethynodrel) on the mouse uterine
fluid. The results did not parallel those previously obtained
with estradiol and progesterone, but the active doses used were
also smaller, in particular doses of the gestagen. Studied
separately, these two hormones only had a slightly decreasing
effect on the fibrinolytic activity of the uterine fluid. In
combination (i.e. Enovid®) the total effect was more pronounced
and led to a nearly complete repression of fibrinolytic activity.
This difference between the combined preparation and the individual
compounds is an interesting observation corresponding to a similar
finding made during our own studies of the effects of Ortho-Novum®
on the blood fibrinolytic system (55). Harpel et al (54) observed
decreased fibrinolytic activity concomitant with an increase in
endometrial glandular activity indicating that production of fibrinolytic agents did not depend upon glandular secretion. This is in
agreement with our finding that fibrinolysis was never related to
glandular structures of the endometrium. In women fibrinolytic
activity was observed in cervical mucus (56) from which it disappeared during ovulation and after Stilbestrol.

VAGINAL FIBRINOLYTIC ACTIVITY

Vaginal epithelial cells may also acquire fibrinolytic
activity (33, 57). This is caused by an activator of plasminogen
and is under hormonal regulation. In frozen sections from the
adult rat vagina a diffuse zone of fibrinolytic activity appears
along the mucosal lining in the animals in anestrus. The activity
disappears during estrus and leaves a cornified, vaginal epithelium
with no fibrinolytic activity. In smears fibrinolytically active
epithelial cells are related to the proliferative stage with
nucleated cells. Cornified, anuclear, epithelial cells are inactive though in early phases of cornification an occasional
fibrinolytically active anuclear cell can be seen. Smears prepared
from seven week old animals show fibrinolytically active nucleated
cells, as do smears from animals 10 days after ovariectomy with or
without hysterectomy. The latter experiment demonstrates that the
vaginal fibrinolytic activity does not originate in the uterine
secretion. The independency of the vaginal and endometrial activities also is indicated by the fact that endometrial fibrinolytic

activity is highest in the secretory phase (man) or in late estrus (rat) when the vaginal epithelium is inactive. This difference is particularly marked because of the brief and transient nature of the endometrial surface activity appearing during estrus (31). In three week old rats the vaginal epithelium is fibrinolytically inactive (43) but becomes active after estrogen as well as after gonadotrophin, in the latter case proceeding in some cases to complete cornification and loss of activity. Widespread cellular desquamation of the vaginal mucosa occurs after gonadotrophin, which is in contrast to the endometrium, -a further indication that the cellular response to hormonal stimulation with release of fibrinolytic activity differs. There are also fibrinolytically active epithelial cells in human vaginal smears (58) but so far a specific pattern has not emerged because of large individual differences. It is quite possible that such individual variations could be caused by differences in susceptibility to the hormones. Genetic differences in the response of different strains of mice to estrogen have been reported by several authors (59). It is, however, interesting and significant that there was a marked increase in number of fibrinolytically active cells in smears obtained from postmenopausal women. The occurrence after estrogen of fibrinolytically active epithelial cells in the vaginal mucosa is possibly related to the increase in proliferation and turn-over rate (60). Likewise, the transient appearance of diffuse activity of the endometrial surface epithelium was also related to cellular necrosis and degeneration. Perhaps the phase of cellular degeneration is more prolonged in the vagina with cells in different phases of migration and proliferation, thereby delivering fibrinolytically active cells over a longer period. This could perhaps explain why the vaginal epithelium responds with fibrinolytically active cells in a phase different from the endometrium, since the phase of cellular necrosis might differ in the two organs. The marked effects related to estrogen with-drawal could also be better understood since many more epithelial cells would suddenly reach the stage of degeneration. As corneal epithelial cells do become fibrinolytically active after mechanical injury (32), it is worth relating this to an old report of mechanically induced hyperplasia and cornification of the vaginal mucosa in the rat and mouse (61).

FIBRINOLYTIC ACTIVITY OF MALE GENITAL SYSTEM

Relatively little is known about the fibrinolytic systems in the male genital organs and the elucidation of a possible hormonal regulation is only in its early beginning.

As early as 1943 Huggins, Vail and Davis (12) reported that saline extracts of the human prostatic gland were able to liquefy

a human fibrin clot. This observation was later confirmed by
other authors. Albrechtsen (16) found the fibrinolytic activity
to be caused by an activator of plasminogen. The prostate is
among the organs with the highest concentrations of plasminogen
activator. Though saline extracts of prostatic tissue has considerable fibrinolytic activity, most of the activity remains in the
sediment which can be extracted by molar potassium thiocyanate
solutions. Thermostability curves showed the activator to be of
stable tissue activator type, though the saline extracts also
contained some labile activator probably originating from blood
components present in the interstitial fluid in the gland (62).
The report by Tagnon, Whitmore and Shulman (63) of increased
fibrinolytic activity in the circulating blood in cases of
prostatic carcinoma created great interest and has been confirmed
by several later investigators. Tagnon suggested that a prostatic
fibrinolysin originating in the diseased tissue could appear in
the circulating blood in a similar manner as the acid phosphatase.
Saline extracts of prostatic cancer tissue (including tissue from
metastases) were found fibrinolytically active (64). Later Tagnon
reported (65) that the increased fibrinolytic activity in blood
disappeared after administration of estrogen, while testosterone
showed an opposite effect. Ladehoff and Rasmussen (66) determined
the concentration of plasminogen activator in hyperplastic prostate
tissue and found high concentrations particularly in the "surgical
capsule" (mean: 824 units per gram), and also high values in the
nodular tissue (444 units per gram) and in solitary adenomas
(395 units per gram). They observed increased blood fibrinolytic
activity during the first two hours after surgical enucleation.
Todd (67) demonstrated fibrinolytically active sites related to
the veins of the human prostate similar to the occurrence in
other organs. The fibrinolytic activities observed in saline
extracts of the prostate (62) are not higher than those observed
for some other organs (68), where fibrinolytic activity, as
indicated by Todd's investigations, is related to vascular
structures. Hence, there is no proof that the fibrinolytic
activity occurring in the prostate is related to the prostatic
secretion, such as has been assumed by several investigators,
including ourselves, or that this is the source of the fibrinolytic
activity in seminal plasma (69). There are now indications to
the contrary.

    Röhl (70) has reviewed the behavior of prostatic tissue
cultivated in vitro using addition of a fibrinolysin inhibitor as
described before (44). He studied the influence of androsterone
in cultures and found no effect in tissues from hyperplastic
prostates but observed a stimulation of prostatic carcinoma growth.
The presence of estrogen in tissue culture caused a decrease in
fibrinolytic activity (71), while the growth rate of prostatic
epithelium (rat) in vitro was not influenced by estradiol, andro-

sterone or testosterone (72). In organ cultures of the rat ventral
prostate testosterone was reported to delay regressive changes and
release of p-nitrophenol phosphate phosphatase activity, while
estradiol enhanced phosphatase activity (73).

Human seminal plasma is highly fibrinolytic (74) due to the
presence of a plasminogen activator (75, 76) which belongs to the
stable tissue activator type (69). This was thought to support
the assumption shared by most investigators that fibrinolytic
agents in seminal plasma originated in the fibrinolytically active
prostate. However, Harvey in 1949 (77) found no correlation between fibrinolytic activity of seminal fluid and the amount of
prostatic secretion. Ying et al (78) found that specimens of
semen might have higher fibrinolytic activity than prostatic
secretions, obtained by prostatic massage from the same person.
When Todd (67) reported that fibrinolytic activity in the prostate
was related to the veins, it became evident that the prostatic
secretion could contribute little to the fibrinolytic activity of
seminal plasma. Von Kaulla and Shettles (79) suggested that the
fibrinolytically active seminal plasma could assist in the process
of fertilization by enhancing the ability of the sperm cell to
penetrate the egg membrane. In many species (rodents) the semen
clots and forms a vaginal plug, for references see (80). It has
been suggested that leukocytes are active in the resolution of
the clotted semen. However, the fibrinolytic activity of leukocytes is weak (81). Huggins and Neal (74) found the fibrinolytic
activity of semen to remain after passing through a sterilization
filter thus excluding the sperm cells as a significant source of
activity. Buruiana (82) is often quoted for the demonstration of
trypsin activity in sperm cells but his experiments deal with semen
expressing trypsin activity in units per ml.

We have recently observed plasminogen activator in the heads
of sperm cells from rat, rabbit and man (83). This observation
revives the old problem of a possible involvement of proteolytic
enzymes in the process of fertilization. This is of particular
interest in the present context because in many mammalian species
sperm cells require a period of residence in the genital tract of
an animal in estrus in order to acquire the capacity to fertilize
the ovum. This process of maturation is called sperm capacitation.
The nature of this process is still unknown. However, Kirton and
Hafs (84) have reported that the secretion accumulating in the
ligated uterus of a rabbit in estrus could induce sperm capacitation
in vitro as well as in utero. They suggested a carbohydrate
splitting enzyme to be active in the capacitation process, since a
beta-amylase preparation produced partial capacitation. However,
the amounts of beta-amylase in the uterine fluid amounted to only
one-sixth of the concentration in blood serum which is unable to
produce capacitation. Hence, this concept would seem highly

conjectural. A concept could more naturally be built around the
presence of fibrinolytic activity in the endometrium, its periodic
release from the surface epithelium during the ovarian cycle, and
the presence of fibrinolytically active agents in uterine secretions.
Interestingly, sperm capacitation is also known to take place after
incubation in the anterior chamber of the eye or the bladder of the
male or female (85), -sites which are known to be fibrinolytically
active (1). It is worth recalling that the epithelial lining of
the uterine tube is fibrinolytically active (35). Furthermore,
Hamner, Jones and Sojka (86) reported that progesterone-treated
animals were unable to induce capacitation of sperm cells. As
mentioned, progesterone suppresses the fibrinolytic activity of
the surface epithelium of the endometrium (43) and the production
of plasminogen activator in the uterine secretion (53). Recently,
chorion gonadotrophin was reported to enhance uterine capacitation
of rabbit sperm cells (87), which might correlate with our observation of the effect of gonadotrophins on the endometrium (43).
Capacitated rabbit sperm cells lose their fertilizing ability after
treatment with rabbit seminal plasma or epididymal fluid. These
"decapacitated" sperm cells recover their fertilizing capacity
after incubation in utero (88). The need of sperm capacitation
has not been proved in all animal species or in man. However, the
presence of a decapacitation factor in small amounts in human
seminal plasma has recently been described (89). Perhaps the
high fibrinolytic activity of the human seminal fluid excludes
a need for sperm capacitation in man. Attention should be drawn
to the finding that a washing of sperm cells was required to
demonstrate plasminogen activator (83), and that a protease
inhibitor could be demonstrated in the wash water. An inhibitor
of trypsin has also been observed in human seminal plasma, though
in small amounts, when compared to its fibrinolytic activity (69).
A relation between fibrinolysis (endometrial or seminal) and
sperm capacitation as suggested here could possibly explain the
decrease in fertility observed in rats treated with epsilon-amino-
caproic acid, an inhibitor of fibrinolysis (90). It is obvious
that much additional experimental data are required to fully
substantiate this concept.

                                COMMENTS

     The effect of contraceptive hormone preparations is commonly
believed to consist in the establishment of a simulated state of
pregnancy, conception being chiefly prevented because of the lack
of ovulation. Recent studies have revealed specific effects of
estrogen and progestins on the fibrinolytic activity of the endometrium. Vascular fibrinolytic activity was little influenced.
Pregnancy converts the endometrium to a fibrinolytically inactive
decidual tissue. Administration of progestin suppresses the

epithelial fibrinolytic activity of the endometrium and of uterine fluid. It seems quite possible that the contraceptive effects of progestins are caused by a combination of effects consisting in the prevention of ovulation and the suppression of the production and release of fibrinolytic activity from the endometrium, thereby impeding sperm capacitation and implantation of the fertilized ovum. Thus, there would be a triple role of progesterone in the process of conception, perhaps explaining the surprisingly high efficacy of hormonal contraception. This three-fold effect may vary in different animal species and could be less in man because of the high fibrinolytic activity of human seminal plasma. It is possible that a fourth effect has to be added to this, namely a decrease of fibrinolytic activity in the circulating blood, such as observed during pregnancy (91) or after progestin (42, 92). One wonders whether this decrease in circulating fibrinolytic activity could be due to a lack of release into the blood stream of agents from a transient fibrinolytically active endometrium. If so, this could be a possible explanation for an increase in vulnerability to thrombosis. It is apparent that the presentation of these new data opens new avenues of research in the field of hormonal regulation of fibrinolysis, its effect on fertilization and conception, and its possible role in thrombosis. It is also evident that at this early stage these data pose more problems than they supply answers, and that a complete elucidation of these problems is a major undertaking requiring the collaborative efforts by many investigators from several different disciplines.

Supported by grant HE-05020 from the United States Public Health Service, National Institutes of Health, National Heart Institute.

REFERENCES

1. Astrup, T.: Tissue activators of plasminogen. Fed. Proc. 25: 42-51 (1966).

2. Astrup, T.: Blood coagulation and fibrinolysis in tissue culture and tissue repair. Biochem. Pharmacol. Supplement: 241-257 (1968).

3. Astrup, T.: Fibrinolytic mechanisms in man and animals. In: Dynamics of Thrombus Formation and Dissolution, International Symposium, Washington, D.C., August 31, 1968, in print.

4. Astrup, T. and Wright, I.S. (editors): Blood Coagulation, Thrombosis, and Female Hormones - Transactions of a Symposium. James F. Mitchell Foundation, Washington, D.C., 1968.

5. Albrechtsen, O.K.: Fibrinolytic activity in the organism.
   Acta Physiol. Scand. 47 (Supplementum 165): 1-112 (1959).

6. Whitehouse, H.B.: The physiology and pathology of uterine
   haemorrhage. Lancet 1: 877-885 (1914).

7. Christea, G.M. and Denk, W.: Ueber Blutgerinnung während der
   Menstruation. Wien. Klin. Wschr. 23: 234-243 (1910).

8. Zondek, B.: Ueber Menstrualblut. Z. Geburtsh. Gynäk. 83:
   870-874 (1921).

9. Kross, I.: Uterine secretion: A brief investigation of its
   nature in the human being. Amer. J. Obstet. Gynec. 7: 310-
   313 (1924).

10. Halban, J. and Frankl, O.: Zur Biochemie det Uterusmukosa.
    Gynäk. Rundschau. 4: 471-484 (1910).

11. Caffier, P.: Die Rolle des menschlichen Uterus als mesoder-
    males Verdauungsorgan. Münch. Med. Wschr. 77: 389 (1930).

12. Huggins, C., Vail, V.C. and Davis, M.E.: Fluidity of menstrual
    blood; proteolytic effect. Amer. J. Obstet. Gynec. 46: 78-
    84 (1943).

13. Page, E.W., Glendening, M.B. and Parkinson, D.: Cyclic
    biochemical changes in the human endometrium with specific
    reference to the fibrinolytic system. Amer. J. Obstet. Gynec.
    62: 1100-1105 (1951).

14. Phillips, L.L., Butler, B.C. and Taylor, H.C.: A study of
    cytofibrinokinase and fibrinolysin in extracts of tissue from
    human myometrium, endometrium, decidua and placenta. Amer. J.
    Obstet. Gynec. 71: 342-349 (1956).

15. Albrechtsen, O.K.: The fibrinolytic activity of the human
    endometrium. Acta Endocr. 23: 207-218 (1956).

16. Albrechtsen, O.K.: The fibrinolytic activity of human tissues.
    Brit. J. Haemat. 3: 284-291 (1957).

17. Albrechtsen, O.K.: The fibrinolytic activity of menstrual
    blood. Acta Endocr. 23: 219-226 (1956).

18. Rybo, G.: Plasminogen activators in the endometrium.
    I. Methodological aspects. Acta Obstet. Gynec. Scand. 45:
    411-428 (1966).

19. Rybo, G.: Plasminogen activators in the endometrium.
    II. Clinical aspects. Variation in the concentration of
    plasminogen activators during the menstrual cycle and its
    relation to menstrual blood loss. Acta Obstet. Gynec. Scand.
    45: 429-450 (1966).

20. Todd, A.S.: The histological localisation of fibrinolysin
    activator. J. Path. Bact. 78: 281-283 (1959).

21. Todd, A.S.: Some topographical observations on fibrinolysis.
    J. Clin. Path. 17: 324-327 (1964).

22. Todd, A.S.: Localization of fibrinolytic activity in tissues.
    Brit. Med. Bull. 20: 210-212 (1964).

23. Luginbuhl, W.H. and Picoff, R.C.: The localization and
    characteristics of endometrial fibrinolysis. Amer. J. Obstet.
    Gynec. 95: 462-467 (1966).

24. Greenblatt, R.B. and Barfield, W.E.: The effect of intravenous
    estrogen in uterine bleeding. J. Clin. Endocr. 11: 821-832
    (1951).

25. Snaith, L.: Oestrogen therapy in habitual abortion. Proc.
    Soc. Study Fertil. 1: 32-34 (1950).

26. Beller, F.K., Goessner, W. and Herrschlein, H.J.: Tissue
    activator of the fibrinolytic system in placental tissue.
    Obstet. Gynec. 20: 117-119 (1962).

27. Champy, C. and Morita, J.: Recherches sur les culture de
    tissus. Observations sur les cultures de testicule et
    d'ovaire chez les mammifères, les Oiseaux et les Batraciens.
    Arch. Exp. Zellforsch. 5: 308-340 (1928).

28. Galstjan, S.: Über die Verwandlungen des epithels der
    Gebärmutter im Explantat. Arch. Exp. Zellforsch. 13: 635-
    660 (1933).

29. Albrechtsen, O.K.: Effect of estradiol on fibrinolytic
    activity of rat uterus. Proc. Soc. Exp. Biol. 94: 700-702 (1957).

30. Kwaan, H.C. and Albrechtsen, O.K.: Histochemical study of
    fibrinolytic activity in the rat uterus in normal and
    hormonally induced estrus. Amer. J. Obstet. Gynec. 95:
    468-473 (1966).

31. Tympanidis, K. and Astrup, T.: Transient appearance of
    fibrinolytic activity at the epithelium of the rat uterus.

J. Clin. Path. 22: in print (1968).

32. Pandolfi, M. and Astrup, T.: A histochemical study of the
     fibrinolytic activity; cornea, conjunctiva, and lacrimal
     gland. Arch. Ophthal. 77: 258-264 (1967).

33. Astrup, T., Henrichsen, J., Tympanidis, K. and King, A.E.:
     Fibrinolytically active vaginal epithelial cells. Nature 214:
     297-298 (1967).

34. Astrup, T., Beller, F.K., Glas, P. and Rasmussen, J.:
     Fibrinolytic activity of the human uterine tube. Obstet.
     Gynec. 25: 853-857 (1965).

35. Tympanidis, K. and Astrup, T.: Localization of fibrinolytic
     activity in the rat oviduct. Obstet. Gynec. 31: 727-731 (1968).

36. Tympanidis, K. and Astrup, T.: Fibrinolytic activity of the
     pregnant uterus, decidua, and placenta in rat. Obstet.
     Gynec. in print (1969).

37. Phillips, L.L. and McKay, D.G.: Profibrinolysin activator
     in the rat placenta. Amer. J. Obstet. Gynec. 87: 56-62 (1963).

38. Picoff, R.C. and Luginbuhl, W.H.: Fibrin in the endometrial
     stroma: Its relation to uterine bleeding. Amer. J. Obstet.
     Gynec. 88: 642-646 (1964).

39. McKay, D.G.: The placenta in experimental toxemia of pregnancy.
     Obstet. Gynec. 20: 1-22 (1962).

40. Hnat, R.F., Anderson, G.G. and Alonzo, D.R.: Diffuse intra-
     vascular coagulation associated with a degenerating myoma
     during pregnancy. Obstet. Gynec. 29: 207-210 (1967).

41. Rasmussen, J., Roberts, H.R. and Astrup, T.: Fibrinolytic
     activity of the normal and fibromyomatous human uterus.
     Surg. Gynec. Obstet. 118: 1277-1280 (1964).

42. Brakman, P.: Effect of contraceptive hormone preparations
     on plasma fibrinolytic activity. This Conference.

43. Tympanidis, K. and Astrup, T.: Hormonal influence on
     fibrinolytic activity of uterus and vagina in the juvenile
     rat. Acta Endocr. in print (1968).

44. Ingemanson, B.: A method of reducing the fibrinolytic activity
     of endometrium cells in plasma clot tissue culture.
     Experientia 15: 159 (1959).

45. Kullander, S. and Källén, B.: The fibrinolytic activity of human endometrium studied in tissue culture. I. Normal endometrial and decidual tissue. Acta Obstet. Gynec. Scand. 40: 1-15 (1961).

46. Kullander, S. and Källén, B.: The fibrinolytic activity of human endometrium studied in tissue culture. II. Carcinoma of the uterine body. Acta Obstet. Gynec. Scand. 40: 234-243 (1961).

47. Maurer, H.R., Rounds, D.E. and Raiborn, Ch.W.: Effects of oestradiol on calf endometrial tissue in vitro. Nature 213: 182-183 (1967).

48. Kross, I.: Uterine secretion - an experimental investigation into its effect upon coagulation of the blood. Surg. Gynec. Obstet. 36: 217-219 (1923).

49. Homburger, F., Bernfeld, P., Treger, A., Grossman, M.S. and Harpel, P.: Endometrial secretions. Ann. N.Y. Acad. Sci. 106: 683-691 (1963).

50. Greenberg, E.M.: Fourth stage of labor; account of physiology and clinical aspects of postpartum uterus during first post-placental hour. Amer. J. Obstet. Gynec. 52: 746-755 (1946).

51. Greenberg, E.M.: "Hysterin" - A hysterogenous clot-dissolving substance. Bull. N.Y. Acad. Med. 6: 397-398 (1948).

52. Harpel, P.C. and Bang, N.U.: Uterone, coagulation and fibrinolysis. Fed. Proc. 23: 240 (Abstract 836) (1964).

53. Harpel, P., Bang, N.U., Homburger, F. and Treger, A.: Plasminogen activator in mouse uterine fluid: Its suppression by estradiol and progesterone. Proc. Soc. Exp. Biol. Med. 122: 1192-1195 (1966).

54. Harpel, B., Homburger, F. and Treger, A.: Mouse uterine fluid plasminogen activator, acid phosphatase, and contraceptive hormones. Amer. J. Physiol. 215: 928-931 (1968).

55. Brakman, P., Albrechtsen, O.K. and Astrup, T.: Blood coagulation, fibrinolysis, and contraceptive hormones. J. Amer. Med. Ass. 199: 69-74 (1967).

56. Beller, F.K. and Weiss, G.: The fibrinolytic enzyme system in cervical mucus. Fertil. and Steril. 17: 654-662 (1966).

57. Henrichsen, J. and Astrup, T.: Fibrinolytically active rat
    vaginal epithelial cells. J. Path. Bact. 93: 706-710 (1967).

58. Tympanidis, K., King, A.E. and Astrup, T.: Fibrinolytically
    active cells in human vaginal smears. Amer. J. Obstet. Gynec.
    100: 185-193 (1968).

59. Gardner, W.U.: Sensitivity of the vagina to estrogen: Genetic
    and transmitted differences. Ann. N.Y. Acad. Sci. 83: 145-
    159 (1959). (Monograph: The Vagina, O.V. St. Whitelock,
    editor).

60. Peckham, B., Ladinsky, J. and Kiekhofer, W.: Autoradiographic
    investigation of estrogen response mechanisms in rat vaginal
    epithelium. Amer. J. Obstet. Gynec. 87: 710-714 (1963).

61. Wade, N.J. and Doisy, E.A.: Cornification of vaginal epith-
    elium of ovariectomized rat produced by smearing. Proc. Soc.
    Exp. Biol. Med. 32: 707-709 (1935).

62. Rasmussen, J. and Albrechtsen, O.K.: Characterization of the
    fibrinolytic components in the human prostate. Scand. J.
    Clin. Lab. Invest. 12: 261-268 (1960).

63. Tagnon, H.J., Whitmore, W.F. and Shulman, N.R.: Fibrinolysis
    in metastatic cancer of the prostate. Cancer 5: 9-12 (1952).

64. Tagnon, H.J., Whitmore, W.F., Schulman, P. and Kravitz, S.C.:
    The significance of fibrinolysis occurring in patients with
    metastatic cancer of the prostate. Cancer 6: 63-67 (1953).

65. Tagnon, H.J., Schulman, P., Whitmore, W.F. and Leone, L.A.:
    Prostatic fibrinolysin, study of a case illustrating the
    role in hemorrhagic diathesis of cancer of the prostate.
    Amer. J. Med. 15: 875-884 (1953).

66. Ladehoff, A. and Rasmussen, J.: Fibrinolysis and thrombo-
    plastic activity in relation to hemorrhage in transvesical
    prostatectomy. Scand. J. Clin. Lab. Invest. 13: 231-244 (1961).

67. Todd, A.S.: Fibrinolysis autographs. Nature 181: 495-496
    (1958).

68. Albrechtsen, O.K.: The fibrinolytic agents in saline extracts
    of human tissues. Scand. J. Clin. Lab. Invest. 10: 91-96
    (1958).

69. Rasmussen, J. and Albrechtsen, O.K.: Fibrinolytic activity
    in human seminal plasma. Fertil. and Steril. 11: 264-277 (1960).

70. Röhl, L.: Prostatic hyperplasia and carcinoma studied with tissue culture technique. Acta Chir. Scand. Supplementum 240: 1-88 (1959).

71. Källén, B. and Röhl, L.: The fibrinolytic activity of human hyperplastic prostate studied in tissue culture. Acta Chir. Scand. 118: 240-245 (1960).

72. Bengmark, S., Ingemanson, B. and Källén, B.: Endocrine dependence of rat prostatic tissue in vitro. Acta Endocr. (Kbh.) 30: 459-471 (1959).

73. Lasnitzki, I., Dingle, J.T. and Adams, S.: The effect of steroid hormones on lysosomal activity of rat ventral prostate gland in culture. Exp. Cell Res. 43: 120-130 (1965).

74. Huggins, C. and Neal, W.: Coagulation and liquefaction of semen. J. Exp. Med. 76: 527-541 (1942).

75. von Kaulla, K.N. and Shettles, L.B.: Relationship between human seminal fluid and the fibrinolytic system. Proc. Soc. Exp. Biol. Med. 83: 692-694 (1953).

76. Lundquist, F., Thorsteinsson, T. and Buus, O.: Purification and properties of some enzymes in human seminal plasma. Biochem. J. 59: 69-79 (1955).

77. Harvey, C.: Fibrinolysin in human semen. Proc. Soc. Study Fertil. 1: 11 (1949).

78. Ying, S.H., Day, E., Whitmore, W.F. and Tagnon, H.J.: Fibrinolytic activity in human prostatic fluid and semen. Fertil. and Steril. 7: 80-87 (1956).

79. von Kaulla, K.N. and Shettles, L.B.: Beitrag zur Kenntnis des proteolytischen Fermentsystems im menschlichen spermaplasma, mucus cervicalis, Tubarschleimhaut und Liquor folliculi. Klin. Wschr. 32: 468-472 (1954).

80. Price, D. and Williams-Ashman, H.G.: The accessory reproductive glands of mammals. In Sex and Internal Secretions, W.C. Young (editor), The Williams and Wilkins Co., Baltimore, 1961, pp. 366-448.

81. Astrup, T., Henrichsen, J. and Kwaan, H.C.: Protease content and fibrinolytic activity of human leukocytes. Blood 29: 134-138 (1967).

82.   Buruiana, L.M.:   Sur l'activite hyaluronidasique et
      trypsinique du sperme.   Naturwissenschaften 43: 523 (1956).

83.   Tympanidis, K. and Astrup, T.:   Fibrinolytic activity of rat,
      rabbit and human sperm cells.   Proc. Soc. Exp. Biol. Med.
      129: 179-182 (1968).

84.   Kirton, K.T. and Hafs, H.D.:   Sperm capacitation by uterine
      fluid or beta-amylase in vitro.   Science 150: 618-619 (1965).

85.   Noyes, R.W., Walton, A. and Adams, C.E.:   Capacitation of
      rabbit spermatozoa.   J. Endocr. 17: 374-380 (1958).

86.   Hamner, Ch.E., Jones, J.P. and Sojka, N.J.:   Influence of
      the hormonal state of the female on the fertilizing capacity
      of the rabbit spermatozoa.   Fertil. and Steril. 19: 137-143
      (1968).

87.   Wettemann, R.P. and Hafs, H.D.:   Sperm capacitation in estrous
      rabbits injected with HCG or LH.   Fed. Proc. 27: 567
      (Abstract 1975) (1968).

88.   Weinman, D.E. and Williams, W.L.:   Mechanism of capacitation
      of rabbit spermatozoa.   Nature 203: 423-424 (1964).

89.   Pinsker, M.C. and Williams, W.L.:   Spermatozoan decapacitation
      factor (DF) in human seminal plasma.   Proc. Soc. Exp. Biol.
      Med. 129: 446-448 (1968).

90.   Melander, B., Gliniecki, G., Granstrand, B. and Hanshoff, G.:
      Biochemistry and toxicology of amikapron, the antifibrino-
      lytically active isomer of AMCHA (A comparative study with
      epsilon-aminocaproic acid).   Acta Pharmacol. (Kbh.) 22:
      340-352 (1965).

91.   Brakman, P.:   The fibrinolytic system in human blood during
      pregnancy.   Amer. J. Obstet. Gynec. 94: 14-20 (1966).

92.   Brakman, P.:   Fibrinolysis in blood during pregnancy and
      hormone treatment.   In Blood Coagulation, Thrombosis, and
      Female Hormones-Transactions of a Symposium, T. Astrup and
      I.S. Wright (editors), James F. Mitchell Foundation,
      Washington, D.C., 1967, pp. 27-32.

EFFECT OF CONTRACEPTIVE HORMONE PREPARATIONS ON PLASMA FIBRINOLYTIC ACTIVITY

Pieter Brakman

Senior Investigator, Institute for Medical Research,
The James F. Mitchell Foundation, Washington, D.C.

The variety of metabolic processes discussed at this conference indicates the growing interest in the effects of gonadal
hormones on the organism. The introduction of progestational
hormones with estrogen as oral contraceptives and the widespread
use of these drugs has provided the biologist with almost unlimited
material for study. Simultaneously, the unwanted side effects make
the secondary effects of these hormones of importance to the
clinician.

Coagulation and fibrinolysis are fundamental processes and,
for a long time, investigators have been interested in knowing
whether these processes are influenced by fluctuations in hormone
levels in normal physiological conditions. Early in this century
increased coagulation at the time of delivery was reported (1)
while a retardation during menstruation was noted (2). However,
at that time little was known about coagulation mechanisms and the
methods used were of questionable value. Gram's observation (3)
on increased fibrinogen concentration during pregnancy was one of
the first contributions in a series of more detailed observations
of changes in coagulation factors during pregnancy. Numerous
reports on changes of coagulation factors during pregnancy now
exist and it has been well established that pregnancy is associated with high levels of fibrinogen, factors VII, VIII and X.
More information, however, is needed on blood coagulation during
delivery and puerperium. Hormonal fluctuations occurring during
the normal ovarian cycle have occasionally been associated with
minor changes in coagulation factors (4, 5). An increase in
fibrinogen concentration before menstruation, supposedly related
to the increased urinary estrogen secretion, was also reported (6).

Supported by NIH Grant HE 05020 and a grant-in-aid from
the National Foundation for Research in Medicine.

Others were unable to demonstrate an influence of the ovarian cycle
on the coagulation system (7, 8). The wide range of individual
observations often makes it difficult to evaluate a trend in the
obtained results. From the fact that anticoagulant therapy is
possible, it can be deduced that many of the coagulation factors
are present in excess and are normally not needed to maintain the
integrity of the organism. This makes it obvious that the biological importance of minor changes is extremely difficult to evaluate.

Particularly elucidating the effect of pregnancy on coagulation
was the observation that a patient, deficient in factor X, improved
during pregnancy (9). This observation culminated in the demonstration that administration of a progestational hormone to the
deficient patient brought the level of factor X to nearly normal (10).
Similarly, it has been demonstrated (11) that two potential carriers
of hemophilia A had normal factor VIII levels when taking Enovid
and low levels when not treated. Although these observations may
aid in the elucidation of the physiological homeostasis of blood
clotting components, they do not provide the key since the doses of
hormones used would be unphysiological in man.

Reports on the effects of oral contraceptives on blood coagulation are controversial. This can be attributed in part to methodology and also to the widely varying design of the different studies.
Furthermore, the doses employed can be an influence as was clearly
demonstrated in increased fibrinogen concentrations in patients
receiving high doses of Enovid for treatment of endometriosis (12,
13), while the use of the same drug as a contraceptive did not give
such an increase. There is good reason to believe that oral contraceptives produce similar changes in blood coagulation, with the
exception of fibrinogen concentration, as seen in pregnancy (14, 15).

Conversion of fibrinogen to the gel-like substance, fibrin,
is regulated by the coagulation mechanism. Fibrin is not a permanent structure and, even after functioning as a hemostatic barrier
and as a network for ingrowing fibroblasts in tissue repair, it has
to be removed. For this purpose there exists in the organism the
so-called fibrinolytic system. In Figure 1 it is seen that several
activating and inhibiting substances regulate this system. The
inactive protease precursor in blood, plasminogen, can be activated
to the proteolytic enzyme plasmin, which digests fibrin. Studies
on fibrinolysis during normal pregnancy have shown a decreased
spontaneous fibrinolytic activity (16, 17). It has been suggested
that this decrease could have been caused in part by an increase
in inhibitory activity. An increase in serum antitrypsin was
already reported in 1909 (18). It is of interest to mention
that in 1914 plasma from pregnant donors was seen to reduce
fibrinolytic activity in tissue culture (19). An increase in
antiplasmin was also reported (20) while our own studies showed an
increase in selective inhibition in urokinase-induced fibrinolysis.

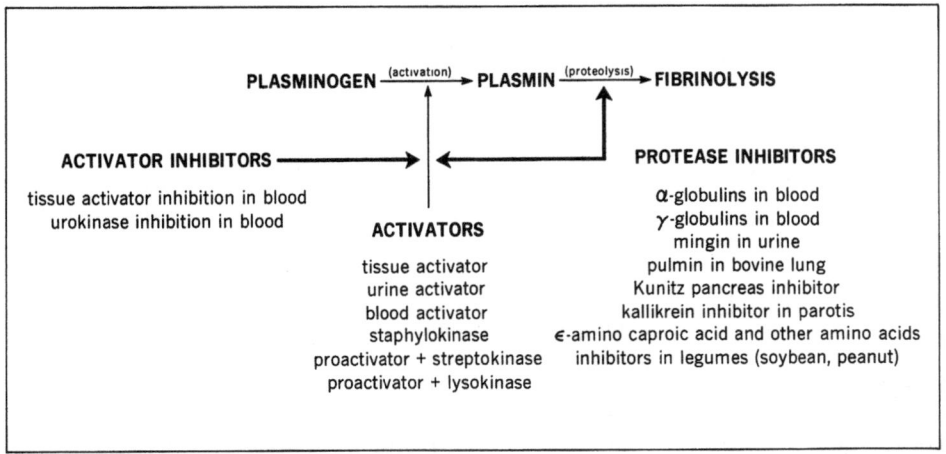

Figure 1. Scheme of the fibrinolytic system.

COMPARISON OF RESULTS OF PLASMA SAMPLES COLLECTED DURING

THE OVARIAN CYCLE AND THE POSTMENOPAUSE VERSUS MEN

	Follicular Phase	Luteal Phase	Menstruation	Postmenopause
Fibrinogen	n	n	n	↑
Euglobulin	n	n	n	n
Plasminogen	n	n	n	n
Urokinase Inhibition	n	n	n	n

n = normal, ↑ = increased

Figure 2. Summary of results of studies in normal women.

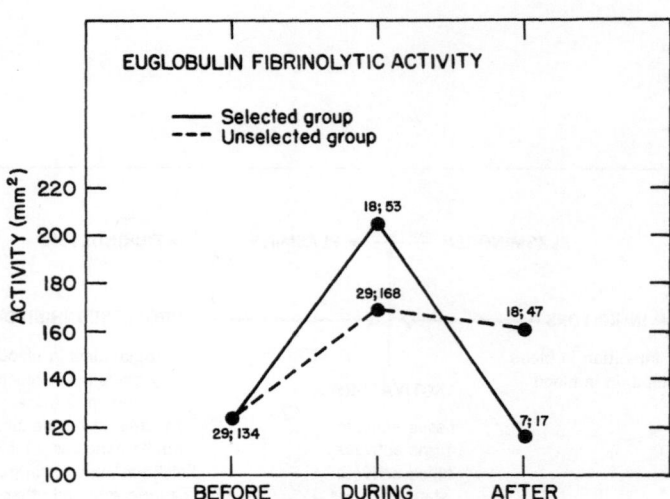

Figure 3. Plasma euglobulin fibrinolytic activity before, during, and after treatment with Ortho Novum. Ordinate: fibrinolytic activity expressed as product in square millimeters of two perpendicular diameters of lysed area (mean of triplicate). The numbers in the figure correspond to: number of individuals; number of determinations (modified from Reference 15).

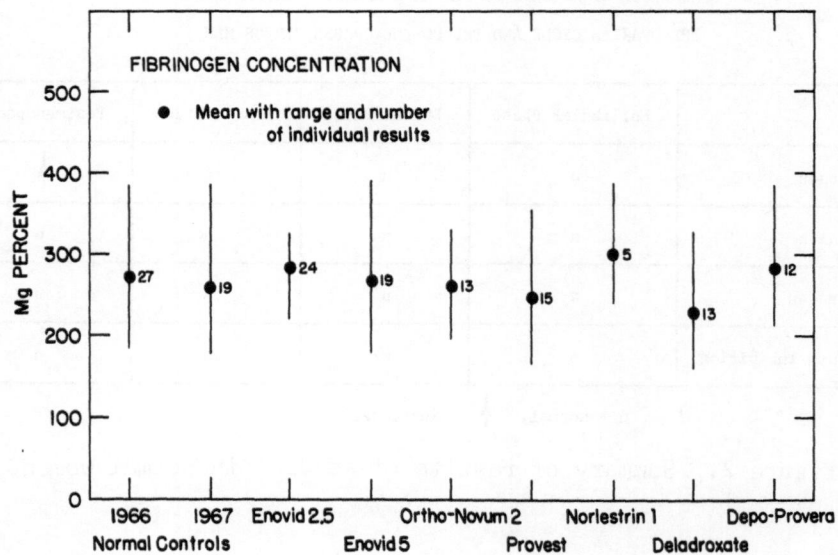

Figure 4. Fibrinogen concentration in women receiving oral or parenteral contraceptives. Ordinate: concentration in milligrams per 100 ml (modified from References 22 and 32).

This increase in inhibition is particularly noticeable in the third trimester (21, 22). Normal plasminogen levels have been described in pregnancy (17, 23) but slightly elevated levels are also reported (24, 25).

Increased fibrinolytic activity of the circulating blood during menstruation has been recorded (26, 27) but other authors (28, 29) were unable to confirm this. Our own studies also failed to demonstrate an increase in fibrinolytic activity of the circulating blood during menstruation (8) and showed no change in fibrinolysis, plasminogen and inhibition of urokinase-induced fibrinolysis during the ovarian cycle. Furthermore, in a comparative study between men and women, no significant differences were found in the fibrinolytic system (8, 15). Figure 2 reviews our results indicating no effect of the ovarian cycle on fibrinolysis. The increased fibrinogen concentration seen in postmenopausal women agrees with a reported increase of fibrinogen with age (30).

This information provides a baseline for the evaluation of the effects of oral contraceptives on blood coagulation and fibrinolysis. The effect of such treatment was investigated in a study of 29 normal women in the childbearing age and receiving Ortho-Novum (15). Blood samples were collected at weekly intervals in periods before, during, and after treatment. Data obtained in the periods before and during treatment were significantly different. However, no marked changes were observed between results obtained during and after treatment, while some significant changes were seen between results before and after treatment. The reason for this unexpected observation became clear when test results from some of the individuals were graphically plotted against time. Noticeable changes did not occur immediately after starting treatment nor immediately after cessation of treatment. This observation indicated the existence of a time relationship between duration of treatment with oral contraceptives and the changes in components studied.

The results presented in Figure 3 are from blood samples obtained from all participants (unselected group) and from women treated for four weeks or more. The after-treatment in the selected group represents blood samples obtained in the period from four to seven weeks after discontinuation of treatment. The fibrinolytic activity, measured in the plasma euglobulin fractions, increased during treatment with a statistical significance at the one per cent level. This observation of increased fibrinolytic activity during treatment with oral contraceptives agreed with results of a preliminary study (31). In this study of women receiving Enovid-5 for more than six months, the results also showed an increased fibrinogen concentration and a normal plasminogen level. The latter two observations were not in agreement with observations after treatment with Ortho-Novum (15) and this discrepancy as well as the lack of agreement with results reported in the literature

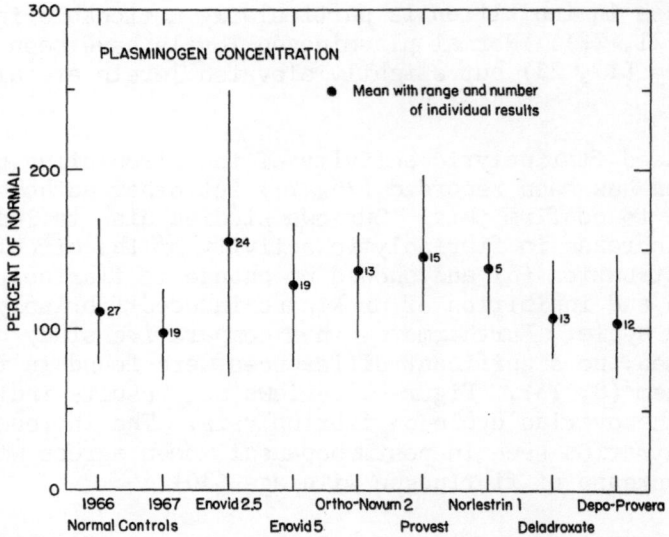

Figure 5. Plasminogen concentration in women receiving oral or
parenteral contraceptives expressed as percentage of normal pooled
plasma (modified from References 22 and 32).

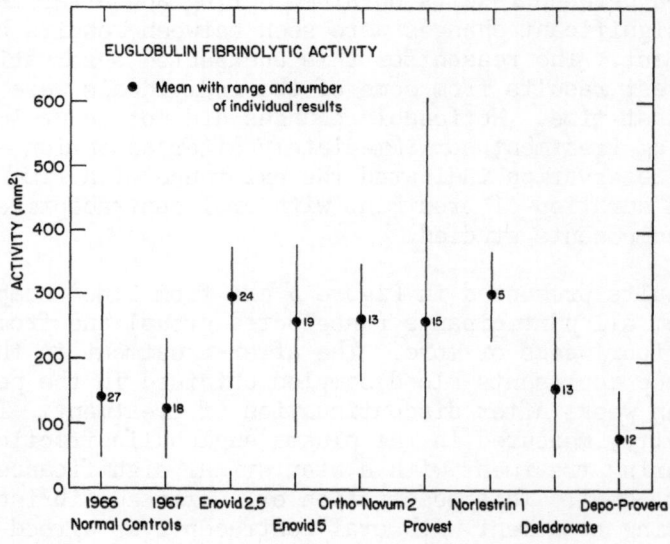

Figure 6. Plasma euglobulin fibrinolytic activity in women
receiving oral or parenteral contraceptives. Ordinate: activity
expressed as product in square millimeters of two perpendicular
diameters of lysed area (mean of triplicate) (modified from
References 22 and 32).

initiated the study of several different contraceptives (22, 32).

Two groups of healthy women, the first mainly comprised of
women four to eight weeks post partum and the second of women using
loop or diaphragm, constituted the normal control group. Groups
receiving oral contraceptives (Enovid 2.5, Enovid 5, Ortho-Novum 2,
Provest, Norlestrin) had received these for a period ranging from
six months to five years. Women receiving long-acting parenteral
preparations (Deladroxate, Depo-Provera) had been treated from
three to 18 months. In none of the women treated in this study
were changes in fibrinogen concentration observed (Figure 4).
Plasminogen concentration was elevated in women receiving oral
contraceptives but not in those receiving the parenteral preparations (Figure 5). Plasma euglobulin fibrinolytic activity increased after the use of oral contraceptives, remained normal after
a parenteral preparation containing estrogen and progestin (Deladroxate),and decreased after a parenteral preparation consisting
solely of a progestin (Depo-Provera) (Figure 6). A similar decrease in fibrinolytic activity was observed during pregnancy (17).
A search for an increase in inhibition against urokinase similar
to that occurring during pregnancy (21) proved negative and also
the increase in fibrinogen, normal for pregnancy, did not occur.

The finding that oral contraceptive hormones are able to
produce changes in fibrinolysis in blood is of great interest.
It emphasizes the observation that these hormones can produce
changes in the body separate from those directly related to their
target organs. The observed changes differ from the impairment
in fibrinolysis seen during pregnancy. Also of interest is the
observation that a parenteral long-acting, estrogen-progestin
preparation does not cause any change in fibrinolysis whereas a
parenteral long-acting progestin causes a decrease in fibrinolytic
activity. Our results are summarized in Figure 7 where the changes
occurring in pregnancy are also presented for the purpose of
comparison. The decreased fibrinolytic activity seen after the
use of progestin might indicate that the increase in activity after
oral treatment with the combined preparations could be caused by
the estrogen component.

In our earlier study (15) of the effect of Ortho-Novum, the
individual components of this drug were also investigated in a small
group of women. Four women received estrogen (0.1 mestranol, 17 α-
ethinylestradiol 3-methyl ester) for one or two cycles. Treatment
with estrogen is difficult in women of the childbearing age and,
therefore, these studies are very limited. Seven other women
received progestin (2 mg norethindrone) for two cycles. Progestin
preparations were especially prepared free from estrogen. Compared
with the large number of changes that occurred in coagulation and
fibrinolytic studies after treatment with a mixture of progestin
and estrogen (Ortho-Novum), surprisingly few changes were found
after treatment with the two hormones separately. A main difference

COMPARISON OF PREGNANCY, ORAL CONTRACEPTIVES (PROGESTIN-ESTROGEN MIXTURE),

AND PARENTERAL CONTRACEPTIVES VERSUS NORMAL

	PREGNANCY	ORAL CONTRACEPTIVES	PARENTERAL CONTRACEPTIVES	
			Progestin-Estrogen	Progestin
Fibrinogen	↑	n	n	n
Plasminogen	n	↑	n	n
Euglobulin	↓	↑	n	↓
Urokinase Inhibition	↑	n	-	n

n = normal,   ↑ = increased,   ↓ = decreased

Figure 7. Summary of results of studies in pregnant women and in women receiving oral or parenteral contraceptives.

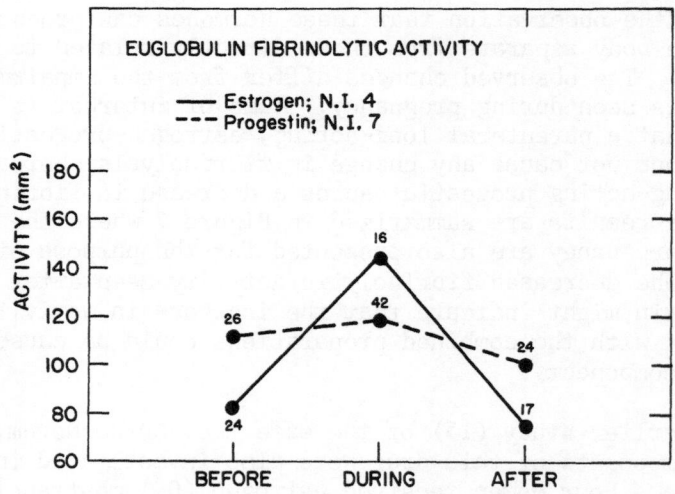

Figure 8. Plasma euglobulin fibrinolytic activity before, during and after treatment with estrogen or progestin. Ordinate: see Figure 6. "N.I." indicates number of individuals. The numbers in the figure correspond to number of determinations (modified from Reference 15).

in this comparison was the purity of the progestin preparation,
which was free of estrogen. Owing to the fact that results in the
two small groups receiving the separate hormones were handled
similar to the results in the much larger study of 29 women receiving the hormone mixture, the findings in the two small groups are
difficult to evaluate. A clear tendency for increased fibrinolytic
activity after estrogen treatment can be seen in Figure 8. Though
in a few women a tendency of decreased activity was noted after
progestin treatment, this was not nearly comparable to the decreased
fibrinolytic activity seen after treatment with parenteral progestin
(Depo-Provera). The above observations would indicate that the
estrogen component in oral contraceptives is responsible for the
increase in fibrinolytic activity. This would fit with the early
observations by Phillips et al (33, 34). Increased fibrinolytic
activity in an euglobulin fraction prepared after treatment with
estrogen was also reported by Japanese investigators (35). This
is inconsistent with Tagnon's observation (36) of decreased fibrinolytic activity after estrogen treatment in a patient with prostatic
carcinoma and metastatic disease. However, results obtained in
patients with cancer might not provide a safe basis for evaluating
a hormonal effect in normal individuals. This is illustrated in
one of our own studies of a patient being treated with stilbestrol
for carcinoma of the prostate*. In Figure 9 is shown that during
a three month period this patient had a normal plasminogen concentration and extremely elevated fibrinogen concentration. This
high fibrinogen concentration is reminiscent of the increase in
fibrinogen seen by Gillman et al (37) in gonadectomized male rats
after treatment with estrogen. Gonadectomy had also been performed
in the patient described here. The euglobulin fibrinolytic activity
was increased on two occasions while a normal activity was seen in
the last test (Figure 9). The latter sample was taken one month
prior to death but, in comparison with the two earlier observations,
there were no special clinical observations which might explain
why the fibrinolytic activity had returned to a normal level.
This example adds further caution to drawing conclusions from
material obtained in the study of pathological conditions.

Fearnley (38) has established that male hormones can induce
increased fibrinolytic activity in men and women and recently he
has shown a similar effect of estrogen (39). The enhancing effect
of testosterone on fibrinolysis was confirmed in a study of male
patients with ischemic heart disease and reduced fibrinolytic
activity at pretreatment (40). Experiments with male and female
hormone treatment in gonadectomized rats (37) have also been reported.
In these experiments it was shown that fibrinolytic activity of
plasma of males was only affected by gonadectomy and that only in
gonadectomized females was significant change in fibrinolytic
activity seen after hormone treatment. It seems, therefore, that
it cannot be taken for granted that the gonadal hormones will act

*Courtesy of Dr. John J. Lynch, Washington, D.C.

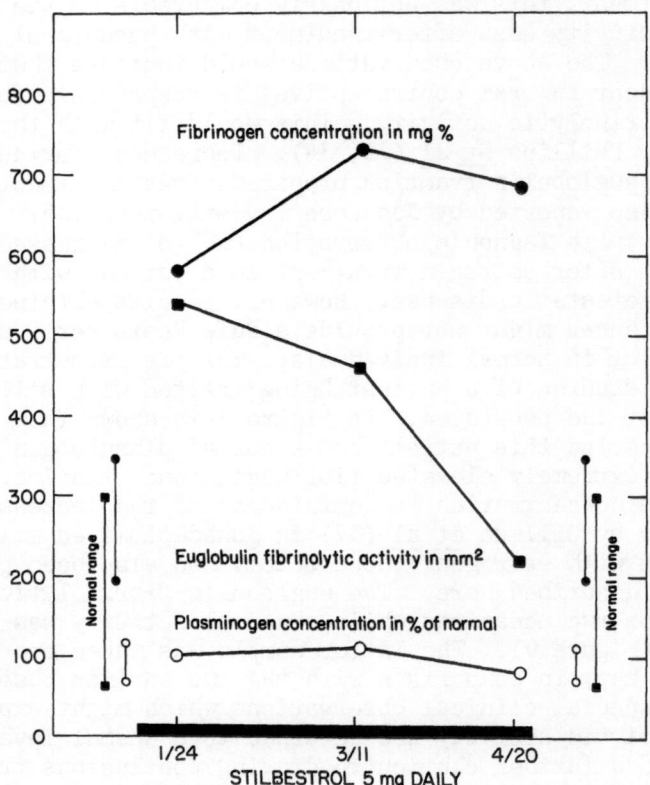

Figure 9. Fibrinogen and plasminogen concentration and fibrinolytic activity in a patient receiving stilbestrol for carcinoma of the prostate with metastasis. Blood samples were collected at approximately six week intervals.

similarly on the different metabolic processes in men and women. Perhaps a large part of the early research in this area has been too disease oriented without properly knowing the normal pattern of response of the body.

Young women have a marked lower incidence of coronary heart disease than do young men and, from the observation that women who have undergone oophorectomy in the childbearing age experience an increased incidence of arteriosclerotic heart disease, it could be inferred that the female gonads may provide protection against factors involved in heart disease.

In view of the lower incidence of fatal coronary occlusion in women, and despite the difficulties in designing a study evaluating prophylactic treatment with estrogens in men, such therapy has been tried in patients who already had evidence of serious cardiovascular disease. The study of Oliver and Boyd (43) did not show a beneficial effect of treatment with ethinylestradiol in survivors of a first myocardial infarction while in another project, after use of conjugated estrogens, an improvement of survival rate was observed (44). In the latter study rather low doses of estrogen were employed and feminizing effects were minimal. In a third study using high doses of estrogen (Premarin) a significant increase in survival rate was found (45). However, in this study it is reported that in a group of 60 men treated with 10 mg Premarin daily, 13 recurrent infarctions were seen within two months, while only four occurred in the control group of 64 patients.

Little is known about the role of progestin in these processes but a reduction in the atherogenesis of the cholesterol diet in rabbits treated with norethynodrel has been reported (46). To exclude the possibility that the estrogen present in norethynodrel is responsible, this observation needs confirmation with a study using a preparation free of estrogen.

Reports on the sporadic occurrence of cases of thromboembolism in apparently normal women using female hormones as oral contraceptives have raised a question of the safety of their use and have further emphasized the need to have detailed knowledge about the occurrence of thromboembolism in an apparently normal population. Evidence has been presented (47) that the use of Stilbestrol to suppress lactation causes an increased risk of thromboembolism. Whether such an increase exists in a larger population than reported on needs still to be confirmed. It seems, however, that treatment with estrogen cannot be considered without some risk. This is also apparent from a report on thromboembolism and estrogen treatment in the palliative treatment of carcinoma of the prostate (48, 49). In this study was shown an increased risk of death from cardiovascular disease or cerebrovascular accident after estrogen treatment.

The possibility of a relationship between oral contraceptives and increase of thromboembolism remains unclear. Reports from England would indicate that a slight increase in thrombosis after the use of oral contraceptives indeed exists (50). However, the same conclusion was not reached in a recent study reported in the JAMA (51). The authors of this report found no increase in thrombophlebitis or death from thromboembolism after the introduction of oral contraceptives. Moreover, these authors do not agree with the conclusions reached by the English investigators. The reassuring thing about this controversy is the fact that if an increased risk of thromboembolism exists after treatment with oral contraceptives, this increase is so small that it is difficult to prove. Apparently thrombosis is very rarely seen during treatment with oral contraceptives, whereas changes in coagulation and fibrinolysis are the rule. The changes occurring in blood coagulation during treatment with oral contraceptives resemble the potential enhancement of blood coagulation during normal pregnancy. On the other hand, the changes observed in the fibrinolytic system differ from the impairment found in pregnancy. The relative infrequency of thrombosis despite all the changes in coagulation and fibrinolysis seems to indicate that no direct relationship exists between the observed changes in blood and the incidence of thrombosis. The possibility exists that the changes make the organism more vulnerable to injury. Such a situation has been shown to exist in rabbits (52). After pretreatment with oral contraceptives the rabbits, like pregnant rabbits, were more vulnerable to the induction of the generalized Shwartzman reaction. Such a consequence of treatment with oral contraceptives, though of an indirect nature, would show a positive correlation with the observed changes in blood and with the hormone treatment.

It is obvious that considerably more information must be collected on the effects of the different hormones in both normal men and women before their secondary actions on the body are understood. Such information is urgently needed.

Acknowledgment: The kind cooperation of Dr. Aquiles J. Sobrero and his staff of the Margaret Sanger Research Bureau, New York, N.Y., is gratefully acknowledged.

REFERENCES

1. Dienst, A.: Kritische Studien über die Pathogenese der Eklampsie auf Grund pathologisch-anatomischer Befunde, Blut- und Harnuntersuchungen eklamptischer Mütter und deren Früchte. Arch. Gynäk. 65: 369-464 (1902).

2. Birnbaum, R. and Osten, A.: Untersuchungen über die Gerinnung des Blutes während der Menstruation. Arch. Gynäk. 80: 373-383 (1906).

3. Gram, H.C.: The results of a new method for determining the fibrin percentage in blood and plasma. Acta Med. Scand. 56: 107-161 (1922).

4. Robinson, A.J.: Clotting Factors and Fibrinolysis in Relation to Menstruation, Pregnancy, and the Use of Contraceptive Drugs. Thesis, University of North Carolina, Chapel Hill, 1965.

5. Sise, H.: Anovulatory hormones and blood coagulation. In Blood Coagulation, Thrombosis, and Female Hormones, Washington, D.C., (editors: T. Astrup and I.S. Wright), 1967, pp. 19-23.

6. Turksoy, R.N., Phillips, L.L. and Southam, A.L.: Influence of ovarian function on the fibrinolytic enzyme system. I. Ovulatory and anovulatory cycles. Amer. J. Obstet. Gynec. 82: 1211-1215 (1961).

7. Egeberg, O. and Owren, P.A.: Oral contraception and blood coagulability. Brit. Med. J. 1: 220-221 (1963).

8. Brakman, P., Albrechtsen, O.K. and Astrup, T.: A comparative study of coagulation and fibrinolysis in blood from normal men and women. Brit. J. Haemat. 12: 74-85 (1966).

9. Brody, J.I. and Finch, S.C.: Improvement of factor X deficiency during pregnancy. New Engl. J. Med. 263: 996-999 (1960).

10. Haber, S.: Norethynodrel in the treatment of factor X deficiency. Arch. Intern. Med. 114: 89-94 (1964).

11. Schiffman, S. and Rapaport, S.I.: Increased factor VIII levels in suspected carriers of hemophilia A taking contraceptives by mouth. New Engl. J. Med. 275: 599 (1966).

12. Beller, F.K. and Porges, R.F.: Blood coagulation and fibrinolytic enzyme studies during cyclic and continuous application of progestational agents. Amer. J. Obstet. Gynec. 97: 448-459 (1967).

13. Nilsson, I.M. and Kullander, S.: Coagulation and fibrinolytic studies during use of gestagens. Acta Obstet. Gynec. Scand. 46: 286-303 (1967).

14. Owren, P.A.: Blood coagulation, thrombosis, and contraceptive hormones. In Blood Coagulation, Thrombosis, and Female Hormones, Washington, D.C., (editors: T. Astrup and I.S. Wright), 1967, pp. 11-15.

15. Brakman, P., Albrechtsen, O.K. and Astrup, T.: Blood
coagulation, fibrinolysis and contraceptive hormones. J. Amer.
Med. Ass. 199: 69-74 (1967).

16. Biezenski, J.J. and Moore, H.C.: Fibrinolysis in normal
pregnancy. J. Clin. Path. 11: 306-310 (1958).

17. Brakman, P.: The fibrinolytic system in human blood during
pregnancy. Amer. J. Obstet. Gynec. 94: 14-20 (1966).

18. Gräfenberg, E.: Der Antitrypsingehalt des mütterlichen
Blutserums während der Schwangerschaft. Münch. Med. Wschr. 56:
702-704 (1909).

19. Maccabruni, F.: Esperienze di coltivazione "in vitro" del
cancro uterino umano. Ann. Ostet. Ginec. 36: 57-65 (1914).

20. Guest, M.M.: Profibrinolysin, antifibrinolysin, fibrinogen
and urine fibrinolytic factors in the human subject. J. Clin.
Invest. 33: 1553-1559 (1954).

21. Brakman, P. and Astrup, T.: Selective inhibition in human
pregnancy blood of urokinase induced fibrinolysis. Scand. J. Clin.
Lab. Invest. 15: 603-609 (1963).

22. Brakman, P.: Fibrinolysis in blood during pregnancy and
hormone treatment. In Blood Coagulation, Thrombosis, and Female
Hormones, Washington, D.C., (editors: T. Astrup and I.S. Wright),
1967, pp. 27-32.

23. Shaper, A.G., Macintosh, D.M., Evans, C.M. and Kyobe, J.:
Fibrinolysis and plasminogen levels in pregnancy and the puerperium.
Lancet 2: 706-708 (1965).

24. Phillips, L.L. and Skrodelis, V.: The fibrinolytic enzyme
system in normal hemorrhagic and disease states. J. Clin. Invest.
37: 965-973 (1958).

25. Hedner, U. and Nilsson, I.M.: Determination of plasminogen in
human plasma by a casein method. Thrombos. Diathes. Haemorrh. 14:
545-561 (1965).

26. Smith, O.W. and Smith, G.V.S.: A fibrinolytic enzyme in
menstruation and late pregnancy toxemia. Science 102: 253-254 (1945).

27. Dausset, J., Bergerot-Blondel, Y. and Colin, M.: Fibrinolyse
du sang péripherique au cours du flux menstruel physiologique.
Transactions of the 6th Congress of the European Society of
Haematology, Copenhagen, 1957, pp. 490-493.

28. Macfarlane, R.G. and Biggs, R.: Observations on fibrinolysis. Spontaneous activity associated with surgical operations, trauma, etc. Lancet 2: 862-864 (1946).

29. Beller, F.K., Goebelsmann, U., Douglas, G.W. and Johnson, A.: The fibrinolytic system during the menstrual cycle. Obstet. Gynec. 23: 12-16 (1964).

30. Hume, R.: The relationship to age and cerebral vascular accident of fibrin and fibrinolytic activity. J. Clin. Path. 14: 167-171 (1961).

31. Brakman, P. and Astrup, T.: Effects of female hormones, used as oral contraceptives, on the fibrinolytic system in blood. Lancet 2: 10-12 (1964).

32. Brakman, P., Sobrero, A.J. and Astrup, T.: Effects of different systemic contraceptives on blood fibrinolysis. Amer. J. Obstet. Gynec. in print (1968).

33. Phillips, L.L., Skrodelis, V. and Furey, C.A.: The fibrinolytic enzyme system in prostatic cancer. Cancer 12: 721-730 (1959).

34. Phillips, L.L., Turksoy, R.N. and Southam, A.L.: Influence of ovarian function on the fibrinolytic enzyme system. II. Influence of exogenous steroids. Amer. J. Obstet. Gynec. 82: 1216-1220 (1961).

35. Nagayama, M., Maki, M., Kikuchi, I., Kanbe, K., Sasaki, K. and Sasaki, Ky.: Effect of estrogens on blood clotting and plasmin systems. Tohoku J. Exp. Med. 86: 219-230 (1965).

36. Tagnon, H.J., Schulman, P., Whitmore, W.F. and Leone, L.A.: Prostatic fibrinolysin. Study of a case illustrating role of hemorrhagic diathesis of cancer of the prostate. Amer. J. Med. 15: 875-884 (1953).

37. Gillman, T., Naidoo, S.S. and Hathorn, M.: Sex differences in plasma fibrin, fibrinolytic capacity and lipids as influenced by ingested fat, gonadectomy and hormone implants; possible implications for pathogenesis of coronary occlusion. Clin. Sci. 17: 393-408 (1958).

38. Fearnley, G.R.: Fibrinolysis. Edward Arnold (Publishers) Ltd., London, 1965.

39. Fearnley, G.R., Chakrabarti, R., Hocking, E.D. and Evans, J.F.: Fibrinolytic effects of diguanides plus ethyloestrenol in occlusive vascular disease. Lancet 2: 1008-1011 (1967).

40. Winther, O.: Testosterone and fibrinolytic activity. Scand. J. Clin. Lab. Invest. Suppl. 93: 207-210 (1966).

41. Oliver, M.D. and Boyd, G.S.: Effect of bilateral ovariectomy on coronary-artery disease and serum lipid levels. Lancet 2: 690-694 (1959).

42. Higano, N., Robinson, R.W. and Cohen, W.D.: Increased incidence of cardiovascular disease in castrated women. New Engl. J. Med. 268: 1123-1125 (1963).

43. Oliver, M.F. and Boyd, G.S.: Influence of reduction of serum lipids on prognosis of coronary heart-disease. Lancet 2: 499-505 (1961).

44. Stamler, J., Pick, R., Katz, L.N., Pick, A., Kaplan, B.M., Berkson, D.M. and Century, D.: Effectiveness of estrogens for therapy of myocardial infarction in middle-age men. J. Amer. Med. Ass. 183: 632-638 (1963).

45. Marmorston, J., Moore, F.J., Kuzma, O.T., Magidson, O. and Weiner, J.: Effect of Premarin on survival in men with myocardial infarction. Proc. Soc. Exp. Biol. 105: 618-620 (1960).

46. Gore, I., Iwanaga, Y. and Gore, H.: Inhibition of dietary atherosclerosis in rabbits by Norethynodrel. J. Atheroscler. Res. 7: 361-366 (1967).

47. Daniel, D.G., Campbell, H. and Turnbull, A.C.: Puerperal thromboembolism and suppression of lactation. Lancet 2: 287-289 (1967).

48. Veterans Administration Co-operative Urological Research Group: Treatment and survival of patients with cancer of the prostate. Surg. Gynec. Obstet. 124: 1011-1017 (1967).

49. Bailar, J.C.: Thromboembolism and oestrogen therapy. Lancet 2: 560 (1967).

50. Subcommittee of the Medical Research Council: Risk of thromboembolic disease in women taking oral contraceptives. Brit. Med. J. 2: 355-359 (1967).

51. Drill, V.A. and Calhoun, D.W.: Oral contraceptives and thromboembolic disease. J. Amer. Med. Ass. 206: 77-84 (1968).

52. Buitrago, B. and Jensen, O.M.: The effect of an oral contraceptive as a preparatory mechanism in the generalized Shwartzman reaction in rabbits. Acta Path. Microbiol. Scand. 73: 323-337 (1968).

THE ROLE OF BLOOD PLATELETS IN THROMBOSIS IN RELATION TO THE EFFECTS OF CONTRACEPTIVE STEROIDS ON PLATELET FUNCTION

R.J. Haslam

Department of Pathology, McMaster University,
Hamilton, Ontario, Canada

Recent epidemiological studies (1,2) have shown that use of oral contraceptives of the combined progestin and estrogen type is associated with a considerably increased risk of venous thromboembolism and cerebral thrombosis, though an association between coronary thrombosis and contraceptive use has not yet been statistically proven. As the preparations used contain one of a wide variety of progestins combined with one of only two similar estrogens (ethynyl estradiol or mestranol), it is probable, if a causal relationship exists, that the harmful component is the estrogen. This conclusion is supported by reports that use of synthetic estrogens alone to suppress lactation (3) or in the treatment of carcinoma of the prostate (4) is associated with increased risk of venous thrombosis and pulmonary embolism. A wide range of both experimental and clinical studies have established the importance of blood platelets in both hemostasis and arterial thrombosis but, although there is considerable evidence for altered platelet function in venous thrombosis and in conditions predisposing thereto, platelets have often been ignored in this latter context. In an attempt to redress the balance this paper will be devoted mainly to an assessment of the possible roles for platelets in venous thrombosis and pulmonary embolism with particular emphasis on the effects of contraceptive steroids on platelet function.

BLOOD PLATELETS AND VASCULAR INJURY

The effects of injury to a blood vessel are most readily studied in the microcirculation (e.g., of the rat mesentery), where events within the vessel can be followed directly with the light microscope, but basically similar processes occur in large arteries

and veins. Injury to the vessel endothelium results in the immediate deposition of platelets at the injury site. If for instance
an arteriole is transected, platelets build up around the margins
of the cut vessel until after a variable period, usually a few
minutes, blood flow is blocked. A hemostatic plug is then said to
be formed. Observations with the electron microscope have shown
that such a plug is comprised mainly of platelets, which adhere
closely to each other and to the damaged vessel wall. Fibrin
interspersed with red cells is found around the periphery of the
plug and has an important stabilizing function (5,6). The pathogenesis of an arterial thrombus has many features in common with
the formation of a hemostatic plug. Thus, such a thrombus usually
develops in response to a lesion of the arterial wall - often a
break in the endothelium covering an atherosclerotic plaque (7) -
and consists of layers and masses of closely adherent platelets
surrounded by polymorphs and a dense fibrin meshwork (white
thrombus), which alternates with a finer fibrin network containing
trapped red cells (red thrombus) (8). The structure of venous
thrombi is more variable but in general the proportion of red
thrombus is much larger and platelet masses may be largely confined
to the site of origin of the thrombus in a valve pocket (9).
Although in morphological terms the difference between arterial and
venous thrombi is one of degree rather than kind, an important
difference may exist in that propagation of a venous thrombus by
blood coagulation may have to occur before it becomes clinically
significant.

     During the last ten years, there has been considerable progress
in our understanding of hemostasis and thrombus formation at the
molecular level. When the vascular endothelium is damaged, platelets adhere to exposed collagen fibres (10) and to the basement
membrane (11) rather than to damaged endothelial cells per se.
This process leads to a selective release of platelet granule constituents, especially adenosine diphosphate (ADP), which is itself
capable of inducing platelet aggregation, so that a large mass of
platelets accumulates. Exposure of collagen may also activate the
intrinsic pathway of blood coagulation (12), so that fibrin formation occurs as soon as the platelet mass is large enough to prevent
the rapid removal of activated clotting factors in the flowing
blood. In the transected arteriole this may not occur until the
platelet plug has stopped the blood flow, but in a large vein it
may occur more rapidly if there is stasis. Fibrin formation is
centered around the platelet masses, probably because the interaction of the platelets with collagen and ADP results in an increased
availability of the clot promoting phospholipid (platelet factor 3)
that they contain. In some vessels thrombin formation may be initiated by release of tissue thromboplastin from the damaged vessel
wall but there is evidence from experiments with dogs deficient in
various clotting factors that the intrinsic pathway of thrombin

generation is more important than the extrinsic pathway, at least
in hemostasis (13). This simplified account of the role of
platelets in hemostasis and thrombosis forms an adequate basis for
a more detailed consideration of platelet function in venous
thrombosis.

FACTORS CONTRIBUTING TO VENOUS THROMBOSIS

It is still customary to consider this problem in terms of
Virchow's triad of a local vascular injury, an abnormality of the
blood and venous stasis. It is clear that stasis alone is insufficient to cause thrombosis or intravascular clotting but exerts an
important permissive role in the presence of other precipitating
factors. In this connection it is important to note that there is
evidence that oral contraceptive or estrogen treatment reduces the
rate of venous flow by increasing venous distensibility (14,15).
The relative importance of vascular injury and 'hypercoagulability'
remains uncertain though work in Wessler's laboratory has clearly
shown that 'stasis thrombi' can be produced by injection of activated clotting factors in the absence of endothelial damage (16).
The problem is whether or not this model is relevant to clinical
venous thrombosis in which there is no convincing evidence of
systemic as opposed to local hypercoagulability. Equally, it is
certain that a large vascular injury can initiate the formation of
a propagating thrombus in a vein, particularly if the blood flow
is sluggish. The problem here is whether a sufficient vascular
injury is associated with clinical venous thrombosis. In cases of
severe trauma or thrombophlebitis this may be so, but histological
examination of the vessel wall in bland venous thrombosis (the
majority of cases) has not revealed any obvious injury or disease
(17). However, the presence of platelet masses in the valve
pockets (9) may be construed as evidence of local injury. The work
of Robertson et al (18) suggests that external pressure no greater
than is likely to occur during everyday activities may damage veins
sufficiently to initiate thrombus formation. Baumgartner et al
(11) have shown that in the marginal ear vein of the rabbit a
minimal injury to the endothelium sufficient only to expose the
basement membrane causes platelet deposition and subsequent fibrin
formation. Paterson (19) has recently suggested that venous hypertension caused by stasis may distend the endothelium of the valve
pockets to the point at which injury occurs. There is evidence
that release of permeability factors from the platelets themselves
could aggravate a primary endothelial injury (5). These considerations suggest that is possible that endothelial damage is the
initiating factor in bland venous thrombosis, even if propagation
of the thrombus depends on abnormalities of the circulating blood.
Relevant changes in the blood may include not only activation of
clotting factors but also inhibition of fibrinolysis and enhanced
platelet reactivity. This last possibility will now be discussed
in detail.

PLATELET FUNCTION AND VENOUS THROMBOSIS

A variety of techniques have been developed for assessment of platelet function in man. Only one, measurement of platelet survival and turnover with isotopically labelled platelets, relates to platelet function as a whole in the normal environment. Measurements of bleeding time and in vivo platelet adhesiveness have been useful mainly in assessing defects in hemostasis. In many studies platelet adhesion to glass surfaces or platelet responsiveness to ADP and other aggregating agents have been examined in anticoagulated blood or platelet-rich plasma. One general conclusion emerges from the work discussed below, in spite of many minor inconsistencies, namely that patients with acute venous thrombosis or with a predisposition to venous thrombosis show abnormal platelet function in one or more tests. The problem remains of whether this is a result of the pathogenic process or contributes directly to it.

Platelet Survival Studies

A marked reduction in the mean platelet half-life and an increased platelet turnover or consumption have been demonstrated in patients with thrombophlebitis (20,21) and following major surgery (21,22). Studies in which platelets were labelled with DFP[32] in vivo have indicated that platelet survival is also reduced in patients showing the complications associated with atherosclerosis (23,24), though this effect has not always been observed when platelets labelled in vitro with Cr[51] were used (21,25). Recently Gorelick et al (24) have reported that the mean platelet half-life in both normal males and survivors of myocardial infarction is directly related to the rate of endogenous estrogen production and have suggested that endogenous estrogens may possibly help to protect men against arterial disease through effects on the platelet economy. A reduced platelet survival and increased platelet turnover presumably reflect an increased utilization of platelets in hemostasis, in thrombus formation or in blood coagulation but do not indicate whether or not platelet reactivity is itself increased.

Platelet Adhesiveness

A variety of in vitro methods of quantitating platelet adhesion have been developed. All depend on the decrease in platelet count on exposure of blood to a large glass surface - for instance in a rotating glass bulb (26) or in a column of glass beads (27). In actual fact, these methods probably measure mainly platelet aggregation induced by ADP released from those platelets which do adhere to the glass and from damaged red cells (28). It is, therefore, not surprising that similar results are obtained when the adhesiveness to glass of platelets in platelet-rich plasma is measured after the addition of low concentration of ADP (29). It is obvious that

these methods will detect not only changes in the intrinsic platelet
behavior, but also the effects on platelet function of alterations
in the plasma and red cells.

Increases in platelet adhesiveness have been demonstrated both
during acute venous thrombosis (30,31) and during quiescent periods
in patients suffering from recurrent venous thrombosis or recurrent
pulmonary embolism (32). Hume and Chan (31) found that a mathematical function derived from measurements of platelet adhesiveness,
together with the hematocrit and partial thromboplastin time of
dilute plasma permitted a good discrimination between individuals
with and without active venous thrombosis.

Surgical trauma is among the most important of the conditions
which predispose to venous thromboembolism and has been shown to
lead to a marked increase in platelet adhesiveness (26,33,34). The
time after operation at which the peak adhesiveness appears to occur
seems to depend on the method of measurement (34) but a correlation
has been observed (33) between the magnitude of the increase in adhesiveness and the appearance of clinical signs of thrombosis a few
days later. These observations suggest that the enhanced platelet
adhesiveness may play a role in the development of venous thrombosis.
It is probable that the release into the circulation of large numbers of young platelets is responsible for the post-operative increase in platelet adhesiveness (26). Thus, a marked increase in
platelet count occurs and reaches a maximum around the tenth day
after operation. Furthermore, experimental studies in rabbits have
shown that young platelets selectively adhere to collagen fibers
(35) or to glass (36).

There appears, as yet, to be no convincing evidence of increased platelet adhesiveness in women taking oral contraceptives.
In one report, oral contraceptive therapy was found to increase
platelet adhesiveness in the presence of an encephalitogenic factor
(37), but the significance of this observation is doubtful. Hilden
et al (38) observed no significant difference from the controls in
women taking Delpregnin (megestrol acetate and mestranol) and
Elkeles et al (39) were unable to detect any effect on platelet
adhesiveness of treating men with synthetic estrogens or Premarin,
though they found marked changes in other tests of platelet function
(see below). It is, of course, possible that changes in platelet
adhesiveness are only seen in the very few women taking oral contraceptives who subsequently develop venous thrombosis.

Platelet Aggregation

This phenomenon is usually studied in stirred platelet-rich
plasma and is measured in terms of the decrease in optical density
caused by addition of ADP (40) or other aggregating agents, such as
thrombin, adrenaline, 5-hydroxy tryptamine (HT) or collagen fibers.

While this technique has proved a valuable research tool, it has
usually only been possible to demonstrate significant differences
in thromboembolic disease by careful comparison of large groups of
patients and controls (41). However, Emmons and Mitchell (42)
found an increase in the rate and extent of clumping by ADP and
other agents after surgical operations and Elkeles et al (39) have
recently shown that treatment of males with estrogens enhances the
platelet aggregation response to low concentrations of ADP or
noradrenaline.

Platelet Electrophoretic Mobility

Hampton and Mitchell (43) have reported that low concentrations
(0.05 µg/ml) of ADP or noradrenaline cause an increase in the
electrophoretic mobility of platelets, while higher concentrations
cause a decrease in mobility. They claim (44) that in acute conditions the sensitivity of platelets to both ADP and noradrenaline
is enhanced so that 0.005 µg/ml or less causes the maximum increase
in mobility, while in chronic arterial disease the sensitivity to
ADP alone is increased. However, as a recent report (45) has denied
that this increase in electrophoretic mobility occurs, confirmation
of this interesting work by other laboratories using more sophisticated equipment is clearly required.

Bolton, Hampton and Mitchell (46) have recently used the
electrophoretic technique to study the effects of oral contraceptives on platelets. They found changes closely resembling those
occurring in arterial disease, in that there was an increased
sensitivity to ADP, apparently due to the effect of a labile plasma
component on abnormal low density lipoprotein lecithin, and they
suggested that this interaction generates lysolecithin which affects
the platelet membrane. The abnormal sensitivity to ADP developed
gradually over the first week of a treatment cycle and disappeared
between cycles. A contraceptive preparation containing a progestin
only (chlormadinone) did not affect the electrophoretic response
to ADP. Elkeles, Hampton and Mitchell (39) have now reported that
synthetic estrogens enhance ADP sensitivity in men in a similar
manner to oral contraceptives containing estrogens in women. The
estrogen component of the oral contraceptive is thus implicated in
both a change in platelet reactivity and in the pathogenesis of
venous thrombi. It is therefore of great interest that these
authors found that a natural conjugated estrogen (Premarin) did not
induce a change in platelet sensitivity to ADP and suggest that a
combination of a progestin and a natural estrogen might prove to
be a safer, and yet effective, oral contraceptive.

POSSIBLE SECONDARY ROLE FOR PLATELETS IN PULMONARY EMBOLISM

Experiments in rabbits have shown that the lethality of pulmonary emboli is greatly increased if the animals' platelets are

sensitized to thrombin by a prior injection of adrenaline (47).
The mechanism apparently involves release of 5-HT from platelets
adhering to the embolus. While the relevance of these findings to
man is uncertain they emphasize that platelets may have a continuing
role throughout the course of venous thromboembolism.

ORAL CONTRACEPTIVES, PLASMA LIPIDS AND PLATELET FUNCTION

Changes in the plasma lipids other than abnormality of low
density lipoprotein lecithin reported by Bolton et al (46) may also
directly or indirectly affect platelet function in women taking
oral contraceptives. Thus, the shift in the plasma lipids toward
the post-menopausal or male pattern, which certainly occurs with
some preparations (48,49), may accelerate the development of atherosclerosis with the result that coronary thrombosis becomes an
increasing hazard. If these lipid changes mainly reflect residual
androgenic activity of the progestin component of the pill, as has
been suggested (49), they may not contribute to the development
of venous thrombosis, which seems to depend on the estrogen component. However, estrogens have been shown to mobilize fatty acids
in experimental animals (50) and Wynn and Doar (51) found some
elevation of plasma non-esterified fatty acids (NEFA) in women
taking oral contraceptives. In this context it is important to
note that rapid hormonal mobilization of NEFA in the rabbit can
promote venous thrombosis, probably by activation of Hageman
factor (52).

EFFECTS OF ESTROGENS ON HEMOSTASIS

There have been a number of reports that treatment with estrogens is beneficial in hemostatic disorders associated with defective
platelet function (53-56). For instance, Akman et al (55) found
that estradiol succinate restored the in vivo platelet adhesiveness
to normal within one hour in von Willebrand's disease and in primary and secondary thrombocytopathy. More recently Gorelick and
Read (56) have reported that Norlestrin therapy markedly improved
platelet adhesiveness in von Willebrand's disease and in a case of
Glanzmann's thrombasthenia. At present it is unclear whether or
not these effects can be related to the changes in electrophoretic
response to ADP described above. It is certainly surprising that
such widely different platelet defects should respond to the same
agents. The current view on the mode of action of estrogens is
that they initiate transcription of DNA and so ultimately act
through control of the synthesis of new proteins. Although there
is residual protein synthesis in platelets there is little or no
DNA, so it is unlikely that estrogens act directly on the platelet.

CONCLUSION

Our present knowledge is fully consistent with the view that platelet reactions play an important role not only in hemostasis and arterial thrombosis, but also in venous thrombosis. In addition, there is suggestive evidence, particularly from post-operative patients, that changes in platelet adhesiveness can contribute directly to the development of thromboembolism. However, while oral contraceptives and estrogens appear to increase platelet sensitivity to aggregating agents, the difficulty of correlating these changes, which occur in all women taking the pill, with the occurrence of thromboembolism in a very small minority remains.

REFERENCES

1. Inman, W.H.W. and Vessey, M.P.: Investigation of deaths from pulmonary, coronary and cerebral thrombosis and embolism in women of childbearing age. Brit. Med. J. 2:193 (1968).

2. Vessey, M.P. and Doll, R.: Investigation of relation between use of oral contraceptives and thromboembolic disease. Brit. Med. J. 2:199 (1968).

3. Daniel, D'.G., Campbell, H. and Turnbull, A.C.: Puerperal thromboembolism and suppression of lactation. Lancet ii:287 (1967).

4. Veterans Administration Co-operative Urological Research Group: Treatment and survival of patients with cancer of the prostate. Sug. Gynecol. Obst. 124:1011 (1967).

5. Mustard, J.F.: Recent advances in molecular pathology: A review - Platelet aggregation, vascular injury and atherosclerosis Exp. Molec. Path. 7:366 (1967).

6. Mustard, J.F.: Hemostasis and thrombosis. Seminars in Hematology 5:91 (1968).

7. Constantinides, P.: Plaque fissures in human coronary thrombosis. J. Atheroscler. Res. 6:1 (1966).

8. Poole, J.C.F. and French, J.E.: Thrombosis. J. Atheroscler. Res. 1:251 (1961).

9. Paterson, J.C.: Deep venous thrombosis. In Blood Vessels and Lymphatics. Abramson, D.I. (ed.) Academic Press, N.Y. p.688 (1962).

10. Spaet, T.H. and Zucker, M.B.: Mechanism of platelet plug formation and role of adenosine diphosphate. Amer. J. Physiol. 206 1297 (1964).

11. Baumgartner, H.R,, Tranzer, J.P. and Studer, A.: An electron microscopic study of platelet thrombus formation in the rabbit with particular regard to 5-hydroxy-tryptamine release. Thromb. Diath. Haemorrh. 18:592 (1967).

12. Niewiarowski, S., Bankowski, E. and Rogowicka, I.: Studies on the absorption and activation of the Hageman factor (factor XII) by collagen and elastin. Thromb. Diath. Haemorrh. 14:387 (1965).

13. Hovig, T., Rowsell, H.C., Dodds, W.J., Jorgenson, L. and Mustard, J.F.: Experimental hemostasis in normal dogs and dogs with congenital disorders of blood coagulation. Blood 30:636 (1967).

14. Neistadt, A., Schwartz, R.W. and Schwartz, S.I.: Norethynodrel with mestranol and venous blood flow. J. Amer. Med. Assoc. 198:784 (1966).

15. Goodrich, S.M. and Wood, J.E.: The effect of estradiol - 17β on peripheral venous distensibility and velocity of blood flow. Amer. J. Obst. Gynecol. 96:407 (1966).

16. Wessler, S.: Experimental coagulation thrombus. In Pathogenesis and Treatment of Thromboembolic Diseases. Thromb. Diath. Haemorrh. Suppl. 21:177 (1966).

17. Paterson, J.C. and McLachlin, J.: Precipitating factors in venous thrombosis. Surg. Gynecol. Obst. 98:96 (1954).

18. Robertson, H.R., Moore, J.R. and Mersereau, W.A.: Observations on thrombosis and endothelial repair following application of external pressure to veins. Canad. J. Surg. 3:5 (1959).

19. Paterson, J.C.: personal communication, 1968.

20. Mustard, J.F., Murphy, E.A., Robinson, G.A., Rowsell, H.C., Ozge, A. and Crookston, J.H.: Blood platelet survival. Thromb. Diath. Haemorrh. Suppl. 13:245 (1964).

21. Abrahamsen, A.F.: Platelet survival studies in man. Scand. J. Haemat. Suppl. 3: (1968).

22. Adelson, E., Rheingold, J.J., Parker, O. Buenaventura, A. and Crosby, W.H.: Platelet and fibrinogen survival in normal and abnormal states of coagulation. Blood 17:267 (1961).

23. Murphy, E.A., and Mustard, J.F.: Coagulation tests and platelet economy in atherosclerotic and control subjects. Circulation 25:114 (1962).

24. Gorelick, M., Harkness, R.A., Ismail, A., Morse, W.I. and Shane, S.J.: Sex hormone metabolism and platelet economy in male survivors and myocardial infarction. Canad. Med. Assoc. J. 98:119 (1968).

25. O'Neill, B. and Firkin, B.: Platelet survival studies in coagulation disorders, thrombocythemia and conditions associated with atherosclerosis. J. Lab. Clin. Med. 64:188 (1964).

26. Wright, H.P.: Changes in adhesiveness of blood platelet following parturition and surgical operations. J. Path. Bact. 54:461 (1942).

27. Hellem, A.J.: The adhesiveness of human blood platelets in vitro. Scand. J. Clin. Lab. Invest. 12: Suppl. 51 (1960).

28. Harrison, M.J.G. and Mitchell, J.R.A.: The influence of red blood cells on platelet adhesiveness. Lancet ii:1163 (1966).

29. Hellem, A.J., Odegaard, A.E. and Skalhegg, B.A.: Investigations on adenosine diphosphate (ADP) induced platelet adhesiveness in vitro. I. The ADP-platelet reaction in various experimental conditions. Thromb. Diath. Haemorrh. 10:61 (1963).

30. Bobek, K. and Cepelak, V.: Laboratory diagnosis of venous thrombosis. Acta Med. Scand. 160:121 (1958).

31. Hume, M. and Chan, Y.K.: Examination of the blood in the presence of venous thrombosis. J. Amer. Med. Assoc. 200747 (1967).

32. Hirsh, J. and McBride, J.A.: Increased platelet adhesiveness in recurrent venous thrombosis and pulmonary embolism. Brit. Med. J. 2:797 (1965).

33. Bygdeman, S., Eliasson, R. and Johnson, S.R.: Relationship between post-operative changes in adenosine diphosphate induced platelet adhesiveness and venous thrombosis. Lancet i:1301 (1966).

34. Bennett, P.N.: Post-operative changes in platelet adhesiveness: J. Clin. Path. 20:708 (1967).

35. Hirsh, J., Glynn, M.F. and Mustard, J.F.: The effect of platelet age on platelet adherence to collagen. J. Clin. Invest. 47:466 (1968).

36. Evans, G. and Mustard, J.F.: Platelet-surface reaction and thrombosis. Surgery 64:273 (1968).

37. Caspary, E.A. and Peberdy, M.: Oral contraception and blood platelet adhesiveness. Lancet i: 1142 (1965).

38. Hilden, M., Amris, C.J. and Starup, J.: The haemostatic mechanism in oral contraception. Acta. Obst. Gynecol. Scand. 46: 562 (1967).

39. Elkeles, R.S., Hampton, J.R. and Mitchell, J.R.A.: Effect of oestrogens and human platelet behavior. Lancet ii:315 (1968).

40. Born, G.V.R.: Aggregation of blood platelets by adenosine diphosphate and its reversal. Nature 194:927 (1962).

41. O'Brien, J.R., Heywood, J.B. and Heady, J.A.: The quantitation of platelet aggregation induced by four compounds: a study in relation to myocardial infarction. Thromb. Diath. Haemorrh. 16:752 (1966).

42. Emmons, P.R. and Mitchell, J.R.A.: Post-operative changes in platelet clumping activity. Lancet i:71 (1965).

43. Hampton, J.R. and Mitchell, J.R.A.: Effect of aggregating agents on platelet electrophoretic behavior. Brit. Med. J. 1:1074 (1966).

44. Hampton, J.R. and Mitchell, J.R.A.: A transferable factor causing abnormal platelet behavior in vascular disease. Lancet ii:764 (1966).

45. Grottum, K.A.: Influence of aggregating agents on electrophoretic mobility of blood platelets from healthy individuals and from patients with cardiovascular diseases. Lancet i:1406 (1968).

46. Bolton, C.H., Hampton, J.R. and Mitchell, J.R.A.: Effect of oral contraceptive agents on platelets and plasma phospholipids. Lancet i:1336 (1968).

47. Thomas, D.P., Gurewich, V. and Stuart, R.K.: Epinephrine potentiation of platelet aggregation: its effect on death from experimental pulmonary embolism. J. Lab. Clin. Med. 71:955 (1968).

48. Aurell, M., Cramer, K. and Rybo, G.: Serum lipids and lipoproteins during long term administration of an oral contraceptive. Lancet i:291 (1966).

49. Wynn, V. Doar, J.W.H. and Mills, G.L.: Some effects of an oral contraceptive on serum lipid and lipoprotein levels. Lancet ii:720 (1966).

50. Laron, Z. and Kowadlo-Silbergeld, A.: Fat mobilizing effect of oestrogens. Acta Endocr. 48:125 (1965).

51. Wynn, V. and Doar, J.W.H.: Some effects of oral contraceptives on carbohydrate metabolism. Lancet ii:715 (1966).

52. Hoak, J.C., Poole, J.C.F. and Robinson, D.S.: Thrombosis associated with the mobilization of fatty acids. Amer. J. Path. 43:987 (1963).

53. Jacobson, P.: Spontaneous hemorrhage; clinical entity, with special reference to epistaxis. Arch. Otolaryng. 59:523 (1954).

54. Carré, I.J., Campbell, S., Nicholl, B. and Carson, N.A.J.: Prolonged bleeding time and A.H.G. deficiency. A case treated with oestrogens. Brit. Med. J. 2:682 (1961).

55. Akman, N., Bayrak, G., Berkarda, B. and Ulutin, O.N.: The effect of oestradiol succinate on in vivo platelet adhesion. New Istanbul Contrib. Clin. Sci. 8:106 (1965).

56. Gorelick, M.M. and Read, H.C.: Effect of estrogen-progestin compounds on platelet-surface reactions and coagulation factors in bleeding disorders. Reported to Canad. Soc. Clin. Invest. 1968.

CENTRAL NERVOUS SYSTEM

THE ROLE OF PROGESTINS AND PROGESTERONE IN BRAIN FUNCTION

AND BEHAVIOR

Bert S. Kopell, M.D.

Department of Psychiatry, Stanford University School
of Medicine

The extensive use of synthetic progestins as components of
contraceptive preparations has focused interest on the effects of
these substances on the central nervous system and on behavior.
Recently the effects of progesterone and its metabolites on behavior has been reviewed by Hamburg (1), who emphasized that major
clinical problems often occur during the postpartum period, the
premenstrual period and menopause. These are periods of not only
profound psychological meaning to the woman but also periods of
dramatic changes in the levels of circulating sexual hormones, in
general, and progesterone, in particular.

Section I of the presentation will be a review of some effects
of progestinal agents on the central nervous system (CNS). The
emphasis will be on mechanisms that mediate behavior rather than
those which are concerned with homeostases and feedback. This review will not include discussion of the role of the central nervous
system in the ovulation-blocking action of progestinal agents
though work in this area may be cited in other contexts. The evidence for the CNS's involvement in this action was reviewed by
Rothchild (2). The more broad issue of the control of gonadotropin
secretion was recently reviewed by Flerko (3). In section II we
will examine the role of progesterone and progestational agents in
sexual and nonsexual behavior in infraprimate mammals. The effects
of these hormones on the sexual and nonsexual behavior of human
and infrahuman primates will be examined in section III.

I wish to express my deep appreciation to David A. Hamburg
for his valuable contributions.

I. THE EFFECTS OF PROGESTERONE AND PROGESTINS ON BRAIN FUNCTION

There are many ways of evaluating the effects of these substances on the brain. We have somewhat arbitrarily divided these
techniques into six major categories which are: (1) electroshock
seizure threshold; (2) incidence of spontaneous seizures; (3) hypnotic action; (4) electroencephalography, sleep and arousal; (5)
EEG After Reaction threshold and EEG Arousal threshold; (6) single
unit and multi-unit recordings in hypothalamus. The effects of
progesterone and progestinal agents on the CNS as measured by each
method will be reviewed separately.

1. Electroshock Seizure Threshold

The electroshock seizure threshold is obtained by measuring
the minimal current necessary to cause convulsions in experimental
animals: Although the information obtained is of a general nature
and tells us little about the specific mechanisms of action, it
can be of great clinical interest. The technique is described in
detail by Woodbury and Swinyard (4). The application of this
method to hormone research has recently been summarized by
Woodbury (5).

Spiegel and Wycis (6) were the first to show anti-convulsant
effect of progesterone in immature female rats. Woolley and Timiras
reported that 500 μg progesterone per hundred grams body weight
quickly raises the seizure threshold in ovariectomized female rats
(7). This effect lasted 21 days. Progesterone had, however, no
immediate effect on seizure threshold in castrated male rats. In
both male and female rats progesterone tended to lower the seizure
threshold after about three weeks. The effect of estrogens was to
lower the seizure threshold. In a recent study Stitt and Kinnard
(8) studied the effects of progesterone, estrogen and certain progestins on seizure threshold of intact female rats. Progesterone
in the same dosage used by Woolley and Timiras had no effect but
medroxy-progesterone plus ethinyl estradiol (a combination used as
an anti-fertility agent "Provest") did lower the threshold. Norethynodrel plus mestranol (Enovid) also lowered the threshold for
seizures. In both combinations different progestin to estrogen
ratios were tested and it was found that the combinations became
less effective in lowering seizure threshold as the progestin to
estrogen ratios increased. Another example of the antagonistic
effect of estrogens and progestins was demonstrated by Woolley and
Timiras who showed that in intact rats convulsive reactivity was
lowest during diestrus, higher during proestrus, and highest during
estrus.

2. The Incidence of Spontaneous Seizures

As early as 1895 Gowers suspected a relationship between the incidence of epileptic seizures and the phase of the menstrual cycle (5). More recently Laidlaw (9) demonstrated in human epileptics a decreased incidence of seizures during the luteal phase and exacerbations during the premenstrual period. He explained that the decreased incidence was due to the anesthetic effect of progesterone while the increase was attributed to progesterone withdrawal.

Logothetis et al (10) also described increased seizure incidence in the premenstrual, menstrual and immediate postmenstrual period. They felt that this increase was due to rising estrogen level rather than falling progesterone level. In support of this interpretation they showed that estrogens tend to activate the EEG of epileptics. Hamburg suggests that the estrogen to progesterone ratio rather than absolute hormone levels affects the probability of seizures (1).

3. Hypnotic Action

In 1927 Cashin and Moravel (11) found that high doses of cholesterol produced anesthesia. Selye (12) in 1941 reported that at pharmacological dosage no steroid was found to be a "better anesthetic" than progesterone, and that progesterone was a more effective anesthetic in females than in males. In human subjects (13) 500 mg injected intravenously was a highly effective anesthetic while 100 mg was ineffective. Recently a metabolite of progesterone 3-β-hydroxy-5β-pregnane-20-one (pregnanolone) was found to surpass thiopental in relative hypnotic potency (14). Pregnanolone was also more effective in the cat than pentobarbitol in producing sleep spindles, suppressing the arousal response from the reticular formation, and suppressing rhinencephalic seizures (15). Comparing the onset of activity and the potency of progesterone and some of its metabolites has led Gyermek to the conclusion that progesterone exerts its hypnotic action through pregnanolone. Three progestins commonly used as constituents of anti-fertility agents (norethynodrel, norethisterone and lynestrenol) have very little anesthetic effect (16).

The quality of sleep induced by exogenous progesterone was studied by Heuser (17). He reported that 30 to 100 µg crystal progesterone applied to the pre-optic area of the forebrain produced a state that resembled normal sleep more closely than a state of anesthesia in that there were periods of both slow wave sleep and paradoxical sleep, the latter being markedly reduced in states induced by Nembutal. Systemic progesterone (150 mg per kg intraperitoneally) produced a normal sleep pattern which however,

became more like barbiturate induced sleep as the dose of progesterone was increased.

4. The EEG, Sleep and Arousal

Lindsley and Rubenstein (18) first found that in some women
the alpha frequency varied during the mid-menstrual period. Dusser
de Barrenne and Gibbs (19) reported slowing of the alpha after the
beginning of flow while Gibbs and Reid (20) showed that when progesterone is high during the last week of pregnancy, there was a
marked slowing compared to the postpartum frequency. However, in
post-menopausal women, Cress and Greenblatt (21) were unable to
alter the EEG frequency with injection of progesterone. How the
interaction of progesterone and estrogen influences the frequency
of the EEG was demonstrated in rats by Arai et al (22), who showed
that 300 µg progesterone reduced the EEG frequency in intact female
rats while lower doses were ineffective. In spayed rats 75 µg was
sufficient to cause slowing. Pre-treatment of spayed rats with
estrogen raised the minimum effective dose to 300 µg. Bayer (23),
reported that one to two hundred µg progesterone produced spindling
and a decrease in diencephalic background activity in rats. The
same dosage had no effect on rabbits. Deactivation in rats was
always accompanied by a rise in blood pressure. They concluded
that EEG effects of hormones were non-specific and reflected
changes in brain excitability which were activated by changes in
blood pressure. The long term effects of progesterone-estrogen
combinations found in oral contraceptives on the EEG was investigated by Matsumoto (24) who demonstrated in their patients both
generalized and localized sleep spindles which though not found in
normal controls were found in women suffering from amenorrhea and
anovulatory periods. They suggest that the contraceptives produce
these spindles by their action on the hypothalamus.

5. The EEG After-Reaction Threshold and EEG Arousal Threshold

The EEG after-reaction is an electroencephalographic pattern
which was first observed in the female following coitus (hence
the term). It was described in the rabbit by Sawyer and Kawakami
(25), in the cat by Porter et al (26) and in the rat by Barraclough
(27). This particular EEG pattern is now recognized as consisting
of a short episode of slow wave sleep followed by a period of
paradoxical sleep. It can be induced by coitus, vaginal probing
and conditional stimulation (28) as well as by low frequency direct
stimulation of various hypothalamic areas (29). The minimum amount
of voltage needed to elicit this pattern has been referred to as
the "EEG after-reaction threshold."

When one electrically stimulates the reticular formation,
there is a tendency for the EEG to change to an alerted or aroused

pattern (30). The threshold of this response is referred to as the
"EEG arousal threshold." In general, the threshold of these two
systems parallel each other. When they diverge, it would appear
that the arousal threshold is more closely related to sexual behavior while the after-reaction threshold is more intimately linked
with pituitary activation (31). In a series of experiments
Kawakami and Sawyer (32) have shown that in estrogen primed animals,
progesterone first lowers then raises both thresholds. If the animal is not primed with estrogen, progesterone loses its biphasic
effect and will then tend to raise both the EEG after-reaction
threshold and the EEG arousal threshold. Kawakami and Sawyer also
investigated the effects of both norsteroids and progesterone derivatives used in oral contraceptives on both EEG thresholds. They
found that at ovulation blocking dosages, the norsteroids had no
effect on EEG arousal while both progesterone derivatives as well
as norsteroids elevate the EEG after-reaction threshold. The progesterone derivatives synergize with estrogens, and like progesterone, exert a biphasic influence on both thresholds. The long
acting progesterone derivatives prolong both phases of the biphasic
response. From the above we may conclude that progesterone and its
derivatives depress the ability of signals originating in the hypothalamus or the reticular formation from evoking alterations in the
electrical activity of the cortex. This effect on the reticular
formation suggests that the influence of progesterone on both levels
of consciousness and seizure threshold may be mediated by the reticular formation since this region plays an important role in maintaining consciousness (30) and mediating stimuli that play a role
in convulsive activity (33).

6. Single Unit and Multi-Unit Activity of the Hypothalamus

     The study of the mode of action of progesterone on the CNS has
been advanced by the utilization of single unit recording techniques. Barraclough and Cross (34) reported a selective depression
of responses of lateral hypothalamic neurons to cervical probing
when the rat receives a slow intravenous infusion of 400 µg progesterone. On the other hand, increased firing of independent units
due to cold, smell, light and noise were not depressed by progesterone infusion. Cross and Silver (35) report that in pseudo-
pregnant rats the percentage of hypothalamic neurons excited by
cervical probing was only one-fourth the number previously observed
in cyclic rats. Removal of the ovaries of these pseudo-pregnant
rats (these ovaries are a source of a large amount of progesterone)
resulted in a four-fold increase in the percentage of neurons responding to cervical probing. In the ovariectomized rat initially
responsive hypothalamic neurons ceased to be excited by cervical
stimulation thirty minutes after the intravenous infusion of 400 µg
progesterone. The authors claim that the pattern of firing was
specific to stimuli from the cervix since little differences were

recorded in the percentage of hypothalamic neurons excited by other
stimuli such as pain or cold in cyclic, pseudo-pregnant and
ovariectomized pseudo-pregnant rats.

Ramirez et al (36) contested the interpretations of the above
findings, arguing that the effect of progesterone is to induce
generalized inhibitory changes in brain activity and that individual neurons as well as groups of neurons reflect this non-specific
depression. A third interpretation is suggested by Komisaruk et
al (37), who state "progesterone in this preparation is thus considered to exert differential effects on neurons through a non-
specific depression of arousal. Since the activity of individual
neurons is bound more or less closely to the arousal level, neurons
are differentially affected by the general depression induced by
progesterone." The aim of much of the work cited above was to investigate the mechanisms by which progesterone influences the
secretion of gonadotropin. Although there are several interpretations of the mechanism, there is general agreement that circulating progesterone levels influence the activity of the hypothalamus and the reticular formation.

The hypothalamus and the reticular formation both have close
anatomical and functional relationships with the rhinecephalon or
limbic lobe. In 1937 Papez (38) suggested that the limbic lobe
may be the anatomical substrate of emotions. More recently many
workers have confirmed that emotional and visceral functions are
mediated in this region (39). Kawakami and Terasawa (40) studied
the effects of progesterone on the excitability, sensitivity and
conduction of pathways from the peripheral nerves, the reticular
formation and limbic system to the hypothalamus. They found that
the conduction from the limbic nuclei to the hypothalamus was influenced by changing estrogen-progesterone ratios. These relationships are, however, complex in that hippocampus to hypothalamus
conduction in inhibited by estrogen and enhanced by progesterone
while the reverse is true of responses in the hypothalamus evoked
by stimulation of the amygdala. His conclusions were that during
estrogen dominance over progesterone (i.e., during estrous), the
reticular formation caused a facilitation of transmission of soma-
tosensory afferent impulses to the higher center while it had an
inhibitory effect on the transmission of viscero-sensory afferent
impulses. Conversely, when progesterone's influence exceeded that
of estrogen, i.e., during pregnancy, the role of the reticular
formation was reversed. The transmission of peripheral somato-
sensory afferent impulses to the highest centers was inhibited
while transmission of viscero-sensory afferent impulses was facilitated. A squiggle on the oscilloscope is not an emotion any more
than a woman is a rabbit; so as we move to behavior and particularly to human behavior, we do so with utmost caution.

II. BEHAVIOR IN INFRA PRIMATE MAMMALS

1. Effects of Progesterone on Sexual Behavior

We will define sexual behavior in the female as that behavior which leads to and includes adopting a position which facilitates mounting and intromission on the part of the male. The role of progesterone in influencing this behavior varies with species, individuals and strains (41). In the mouse (42), rat (43), guinea pig (44) and hamster (45) progesterone will work synergistically with estrogen. In these rodents spaying will lead to the immediate cessation of sexual behavior. After being primed with estrogen a systemic injection of progesterone will induce a return of sexual behavior within a few hours. These new patterns of behavior are indistinguishable from previously observed behavior. The role of the central nervous system in mediating this effect of progesterone was demonstrated by Kent and Liberman (45) who showed that progesterone injected alone directly into the lateral ventricle of spayed hamsters induced an oestrus pattern which had not occurred when the same dose of progesterone was injected subcutaneously. However, in the ewe (46) the order must be reversed, and progesterone must precede estrogen in order for oestrus to occur. In some species such as the rabbit and the cat (47) estrogen alone is sufficient to induce estrous patterns.

On the other hand, there is also evidence that in some species progesterone inhibits female sexual behavior and acts antagonistically with estrogen. For example, in the rabbit, postpartum oestrus is suppressed by progesterone (48), and implants of progesterone inhibit estrogen induced oestrus in the ferret (49). Lunde (50) showed that even in rats estrogen alone can induce sexual behavior if the male is sufficiently insistent and if the experimenter is sufficiently patient. He also reports that excessive stimulation during the experimental procedure could have the same effect in inducing sexual behavior. Lunde's findings were supported by those of Edwards et al (51) who demonstrated that in spayed rats estrogen alone could lead to sexual receptivity and that the role of progesterone could be either inhibitory or facilitory depending on the dosage and the timing.

Two hypotheses which attempt to reconcile the antagonistic and facilitory effects of progesterone on sexual behavior have been evaluated by Phoenix et al (47). The first hypothesis proposes that the inherent action of progesterone is antagonistic to sexual behavior, and the facilitory action depends on prior conditioning with estrogen. An alternate theory suggested by Sawyer and Everett (52) proposes that progesterone alone has both antagonistic and facilitory phases of action, and the decisive variable is related to the timing of administration. Neither theory can

account for all the data. Phoenix et al (67) do however feel that
the temporal relationship of the activity of progesterone and
estrogens as well as species differences deserve more study.

2. Non-sexual Effects of Progesterone on Infra Primate Mammals

The effects of progesterone on maternal behavior was demonstrated by Zarrow et al (53). The ten-day-old natural young of a
lactating rat were removed and replaced by new-born foster young.
A single injection of two mg progesterone given to the foster
mother increased the percentage of survivors in the foster litter.
The authors ascribe the increased survival to both increased lactation and "increased maternal care".

Progesterone also seems to play a role in aggressive behavior
in the female. The aggressive behavior that spayed hamsters showed
when approached by males decreased after injections of estrogens
followed by progesterone. Estrogen alone seemed to increase the
agressive behavior while progesterone alone had no effect (54).

Behavioral alterations which seem closely related to the
hypnotic effects of progesterone and its derivatives have been
described by Gyermek (14) and Campbell (55). Gyermek measured the
minimum amount of progesterone and progesterone derivatives needed
to reduce avoidance performance in rats. As expected, the threshold was much lower for some of the 5β-pregnane derivatives than
for progesterone. Campbell showed in the rabbit that the rate of
self-stimulation of the septal area increased after a two mg subcutaneous injection of progesterone. His results were interpreted
as evidence of inhibition by progesterone since in order to maintain the same "subjective" inhibition, the animal had to increase
the rate of self-stimulation.

When a response learned in a particular chemical state is more
likely to occur when the subject is in that particular state than
when he is not, we have an example of "state-dependent learning"
or "drug dissociation" (56). It has been shown that progesterone
can discriminatively control behavior through state-dependent
learning (57). Spayed rats were trained to run a maze one way
when receiving progesterone and another way when receiving a saline
placebo. They were then given progesterone or saline, and it was
observed that the drug state influenced how they ran the maze.
These findings suggest a possible mechanism by which complicated
behavioral response patterns such as premenstrual tension or post-
partum depressions may be induced by changes in hormonal patterns.

III. BEHAVIOR OF HUMAN AND NON-HUMAN PRIMATES

1. Sexual Behavior

There is evidence that progesterone following estrogen inhibits the sexual response of the spayed rhesus monkey (58). More recent work by Michael and his group have shown that bilateral ovariectomy of female rhesus monkeys abolishes all rhythmic variation in the sexual behavior of male monkeys (59). The mechanism by which progesterone inhibits sexual receptivity was also studied (60). It was found that progesterone activates a refusal mechanism on the part of the females. As Michael points out (59), the rhesus monkey belongs to the group of old world monkeys and apes which are, unlike other animals, but like women, in having a thirty day cycle with a clearly difined menstruation. Rather than having a period of heat or oestrus, they, again like humans, copulate during the entire cycle. It is therefore of particular interest to note that in intact rhesus females, sexual activity as measured by the number of male mountings reached its peak a day or two prior to ovulation. This peak was followed by a marked decrease during the luteal phase. Some monkeys showed a second peak during the premenstrual period. These findings are consistent with several studies of the human menstrual cycle. McCance et al (61), studied the percentage of 167 normal women who reported on various symptoms on each day of their cycle. The greatest percentage of women showed "sexual feelings" between the ninth and the fifteenth day of an average 28 day cycle. Moos et al (62) studied variations in symptoms and mood during two menstrual cycles in fifteen married nulliparous women. He reports that the average self-rated sexual arousal level was highest on the fourteenth day with some rise on the 25th day.

Benedek (63) described qualitative as well as quantitative changes in sexual drive through the menstrual cycle. She describes the first part of the cycle as a build up of active object directed heterosexual tendencies. At the time of ovulation, this heterosexual tension is released. The sense of relaxation and well being is described by her "as if the psychic apparatus has registered the somatic preparations for pregnancy. The emotional concern shifts to the body and its welfare. This is a high hormone phase, since both estrogen and progesterone are produced. Yet the active heterosexual tendencies appear to be masked by a psychological expression of the preparation for motherhood." It is interesting that Benedek also describes increase in heterosexual interest in the premenstrual period. She claims that it is different qualitatively from the heterosexual interest expressed at the time of ovulation. Benedek's conclusions, which contend that during the estrogen phase the woman is oriented toward her environment while during the progestin phase she is oriented inward toward her body,

finds neurophysiological support in the work of Kawakami and
Terasawa (40) cited earlier in this review. They conclude that
during the estrogen phase peripheral afferent impulses were facilitated and viscero-sensory impulses were inhibited while during
periods of progesterone dominance the reverse was true. Rhesus
monkeys and humans are not the only primates who show maximum sexual activity at mid-cycle. Yerkes and Elder (64) describe a lack
of sexual interest in the chimpanzee during the progesterone phase
following increased sexual activity at mid-cycle.

The effects of progesterone and synthetic progestin on the
libido in young healthy males has also been studied (65). Nilevar,
Norlutin, Enovid and progesterone all caused either reduction or
disappearance of libido. This loss was accompanied by testicular
atrophy and azoospermia. After the drugs were discontinued, sexual libido returned with testicular function. The onset and the
recovery time of these agents varied with the individual preparation. The effect of progesterone is probably not primary but
mediated by gonadotropin inhibition.

2. Non-Sexual Behavior

Grooming behavior in primates is related to the individual
status within the primate society (66). It has been shown by
Michael (67) that rhythmic fluctuations of grooming time in both
male and female rhesus monkeys were related to the female's menstrual cycle. Grooming time in mid-cycle was minimal for females
and maximal for males. Bilateral ovariectomy of the female of a
pair abolished all rhythmic variation and reduced the male's activity. Estrogens injected into the female restored near mid-cycle
levels of male grooming, but the effect was inhibited by progesterone following estrogen. In this case progesterone seems to
have an inhibitory effect on one aspect of primate social behavior.

In humans we assess the effects of progesterone on behavior
(A) by monitoring the effects of exogenous progesterone or (B) by
studying behavior which accompanies naturally occurring fluctuations of peripheral progesterone levels.

A. Behavioral effects of exogenous progesterone. Krus (68)
administered progesterone to normal males and attempted to observe
not only its effect on their behavior but also its ability to inhibit behavioral deterioration induced by LSD-25. 600 mg progesterone had little measurable effect on behavior, but it did
antagonize the effects of LSD-25. Since LSD-25 produces a state
which in some way may resemble psychosis, and since this state can
be reversed by the same pharmacological agents that are used in
treating psychosis, Krus' findings suggest a possible anti-psycho-
tic role for progesterone.

Yalom (69) administered pharmacological doses of progesterone (400 mg intramuscularly) to psychiatric female patients in mid-cycle who were prone to high levels of anxiety. There was a general tendency to report a mild decrease in anxiety and depression. Drowsiness was the most commonly encountered symptom beginning on the second or third day. This is probably related to the hypnotic effect of pharmacological doses of progesterone.

B. Naturally occurring fluctuations in the level of peripheral progesterone. The menstrual cycle and pregnancy are both characterized by dramatic changes in the plasma level of several hormones. In the normal ovulatory menstrual cycle there are two peaks of estrogen excretion (70), an ovulation peak which occurs near the end of the follicular phase and a luteal peak which occurs in the middle of the luteal phase. Progesterone is secreted by the corpus luteum beginning in the mid-cycle and reaches a peak four to seven days prior to menstruation after which it falls off quite rapidly (71).

There is a ten-fold increase in progesterone synthesis during pregnancy (72). Recent work indicates that progesterone levels in the peripheral blood rises progressively until the separation of the placenta, so that there is no reduction in circulating progesterone levels until the onset of labor at term (73). At this time there is a swift decline in plasma levels.

In Moos' study of the menstrual cycle (62) he found that women tend to report lower activation at the phase of the cycle which has the highest progesterone blood levels. The outer directed sense of well-being and alertness described by Benedek (63) is confirmed by Moos et al. His scales of self-rated pleasantness, activation and sexual arousal all increase during the follicular stage. His findings of increased tension in the premenstrual period is consistent across many studies.

The premenstrual phase is known as a period of mild discomfort for some to extreme pain and anguish for others. Frank (74) coined the term premenstrual tension to describe these disorders. The most common complaints are usually anxiety, depression, irritability, insomnia, mild confusion and headache (75). Estimates of its prevalence has ranged from 25% to 100% (76). Many studies have shown behavioral and perceptual disorders which occur with disproportionate frequency during the premenstrual phase. They include (1) accident proneness (77), (2) emergency psychiatric hospital admissions (78), (3) suicide attempts (78), (4) neurotic and psychotic depression (78) and (5) crimes of violence (79).

Pregnancy was described by Benedek as a time

when even the neurotic woman tends to lose her depression and
anxiety: a time when a woman enjoys her body. Yet the postpartum
period is a time when women tend to cry, become upset and irritable.
The "postpartum blues" syndrome was recently studied by Yalom et
al (8). Of the 39 women studied in the postpartum phase the com-
monest symptom included insomnia, restlessness and undue concern
for the welfare of the child. Confusional states, fatigue and
irritability have been reported by other authors (81). Estimates
of the incidence of postpartum blues vary from 5% to 80% (80).

The postpartum period is also a period of high risk for serious psychiatric illness. Pugh (82) reports a four-fold rise in
the probability of serious psychiatric illness in the three months
following delivery. Melges, in his study of 100 postpartum psychiatric patients, found that many of these women had had severe "post-
partum blues" following previous pregnancies.

The relationship between rapidly changing hormone levels and
increased probability of psychopathology has led Hamburg (1) to
stress that individual differences in progesterone metabolism
deserve investigation as one of the possible variables in differential susceptibility at these periods. He states, "It is an interesting possibility, but one that has not as yet been investigated,
that genetically-determined abnormalities in progesterone metabolism may predispose to some premenstrual or postpartum difficulties.
Partial enzymatic defects, such as would be found in a single-gene,
heterozygous situation, might make little if any difference under
most circumstances, yet might become clinically significant under
extreme conditions such as those at the end of pregnancy. Individual differences in progesterone metabolism on a genetic basis
might lead, for instance, to the accumulation in some individuals
of a metabolite whose effects on the brain are particularly potent.
In this connection, it is worth noting that the progesterone metabolite, pregnane-3, 20-dione has quite potent anesthetic properties (83), but there is so far no information as to whether this
metabolite ever occurs in brain."

It would also be of value to explore individual differences
in the blood-brain barrier for progesterone and its metabolites.
Recent work has shown (73) that there is a one to ten differential
in the progesterone concentration between the cerebrospinal fluid
and plasma. In the four patients reported on the level at term in
the cerebrospinal fluid varied between undetectable to .55 µg/
100 ml. It is evident that there is a pressing need not only to
study behavioral modification accompanying changes in peripheral
progesterone levels, but also to systematically examine the interactions between behavior, and both peripheral levels and cerebrospinal levels of progesterone.

REFERENCES

1. Hamburg, D.A.: Effects of Progesterone on Behavior. In Endocrines and the Central Nervous System. Edited by the Association for Research in Nervous and Mental Diseases. The Williams and Wilkins Co. 43:251-265 (1966).

2. Rothchild, I.: Interrelations between progesterone and the ovary, pituitary, and central nervous system and the control of ovulation and the regulation of progesterone secretion. Vitamins and Hormones 23:209-327 (1965).

3. Flerko, B.: Control of gonadotropin secretion in the female. In Neuroendocrinology. Ed. L. Martini and W.F. Ganong. Academic Press, New York, 613-688 (1966).

4. Woodbury, L.A. and Swinyard, C.A.: Stimulus parameters for electroshock seizures in rats. Am. J. Physiol. 170:661-667 (1950).

5. Woodbury, D.M. and Vernadakis, A.: Influence of hormones on brain activity. In Neuroendocrinology. Ed. Martini and Ganong. Academic Press, New York, 335-375 (1967).

6. Spiegel, E.A. and Wycis, H.: Anticonvulsant effects of steroids. J. Lab. Clin. Med. 30:947-953 (1945).

7. Woolley, D.E. and Timiras, P.S.: The gonad-brain relationship: effects of female sex hormones on electroshock convulsions in the rat. Endocrinology 70:196-209 (1962).

8. Stitt, S.L. and Kinnard, W.J.: The effect of certain progestins on the threshold of electrically-induced seizure patterns. Neurology 18:213-216 (1968).

9. Laidlaw, J.: Catamenial epilepsy. Lancet ii:1235-1237 (1956).

10. Logothetis, J., Harner, R., Morel, F. and Torres, F.: The role of estrogens and catamenial exacerbations of epilepsy. Neurology 9:352-360 (1959).

11. Cashin, M.F. and Moravek, V.: Physiological action of cholesterol. Am. J. Physiol. 82:294 (1927).

12. Selye, H.: Anesthetic effect of steroid hormones. Proc. Soc. Exp. Biol. Med. 46:116 (1941).

13. Merryman, W.: Progesterone anesthesia in human subjects. J. Clin Endocrin. 14:1567 (1954).

14. Gyermek, L.: Pregnanolone: a highly potent naturally occurring hypnotic anesthetic agent. Soc. Exp. Biol. Med. Proc. 125:1058-1062 (1967).

15. Gyermek, L., Genther, G. and Fliming, N.: Some effects of progesterone and related steroids on the central nervous system. Int. J. Neuropharmacol. 6:191-198 (1967).

16. Meyerson, B.J.: Relationship between the anesthetic and gestagenic action and estrous behavior inducing activity of different progestins. Endocrinology 81:369-374 (1967).

17. Heuser, G., Ling, G.M. and Cluver, M.: Sleep induction by progesterone in the pre-optic area of cats. Electroenceph. Clin. Neurophysiol. 22:122--127 (1967).

18. Lindsley, D. and Rubenstein, B.B.: Relationship between brain potentials and some other physiological variables. Proc. Soc. Exp. Biol. Med. 35:558 (1937).

19. Dusser de Barrenne, D. and Gibbs, F.A.: Variations in electroencephalogram during the menstrual cycle. Am. J. Obstet. Gynecol. 44:687-690 (1942).

20. Gibbs, F.A. and Reid, D.E.: Electroencephalogram in pregnancy. Am. J. Obstet. Gynecol. 44:672-675 (1942).

21. Cress, C.H. and Greenblatt, M.: Absence of alteration in the EEG with stilbesterol and progesterone. Proc. Soc. Exp. Biol. Med. 60:139 (1945).

22. Arai, Y., Horoi, M., Mitra, J. and Gorski, R.A.: Influence of intravenous progesterone administration on the cortical electroencephalogram of the female rat. Neuroendocrinology 2:275-282 (1967).

23. Bayer, C., Ramirez, V.D., Whitmoyer, D.I. and Sawyer, C.H.: Effects of hormones on electrical activity of the brain in the rat and rabbit. Experimental Neurology 18:313-326 (1967).

24. Matsumoto, S., Sato, I., Ito, T. and Matsuoka, A.: Electroencephalographic changes during long term treatment with oral contraceptives. International Journal of Fertility 11:195-204 (1966).

25. Sawyer, C.H. and Kawakami, M.: Characteristics of behavioral and electroencephalographic after-reactions to copulation and vaginal stimulation in the female rabbit. Endocrinology 65:622-630 (1959).

26. Porter, R.W., Cavanaugh, E.B., Critchlow, B.V. and Sawyer, C.H.: Localized changes in electrical activity of the hypothalamus in estrous cats following vaginal stimulation. Am. J. Physiol. 189:145-151 (1957).

27. Barraclough, C.A.: Hypothalamic activation associated with stimulation of the vaginal cervix in proestrous rats. Anat. Record   136:159 (1960).

28. Kawakami, M. and Sawyer, C.H.: Conditioned induction of paradoxical sleep in the rabbit. Experimental Neurology 9:470 (1964).

29. Kawakami, M. and Sawyer, C.H.: Induction of behavioral and electroencephalographic changes in the rabbit by hormone administration or brain stimulation. Endocrinology 65:631 (1959).

30. Magoun, H.W.: The Waking Brain, Charles C. Thomas, Springfield, Ill., 1958.

31. Kawakami, M. and Sawyer, C.H.: Neuroendocrine correlates of changes in brain activity thresholds by sex steroids and pituitary hormones. Endocrinology 65:652-668 (1959).

32. Kawakami, M. and Sawyer, C.H.: Effects of sex hormones and anti-fertility steroids on brain thresholds in the rabbit. Endocrinology 80:857-871 (1967).

33. Penfield, W. and Jasper, H: Epilepsy and the Functional Anatomy of the Human Brain. Little, Brown, Boston, 1954.

34. Barraclough, C.A. and Cross, B.A.: Unit activity in the hypothalamus of the cyclic female rat: effect of genital stimuli and progesterone J. Endocrin. 26:339-359 (1963).

35. Cross, B.A. and Silver, I.A.: Effect of luteal hormone on the behavior of hypothalamic neurons in pseudopregnant rats. J. Endocrin. 31:251-263 (1965).

36. Ramirez, V.D., Komisaruk, B.R., Whitmoyer, D.I. and Sawyer, C.H.: Effects of hormones and vaginal stimulation on the EEG and hypothalamic units in rats. Am. J. Physiol. 212:1376-1384 (1967).

37. Komisaruk, B.R., McDonald, P.G., Whitmoyer, D.I. and Sawyer, C.H.: Effects of progesterone and sensory stimulation on EEG and neuronal activity in the rat. Experimental Neurology 19:494-507 (1967).

38. Papez, J.W.: A proposed mechanism of emotions. A.M.A. Arch. Neurol. Psychiat. 38:725 (1937).

39. MacLean, P.D.: Studies on the limbic system (visceral brain) and their bearing on psychosomatic problems. In Recent Developments in Psychosomatic Medicine. Ed. Wittkower, E.D. and Cleghorn, R., Lippincott, Philadelphia. 1954.

40. Kawakami, M. and Terasawa, E.: Differential control of sex hormone and oxytocin upon evoked potentials in the hypothalamus and mid-brain reticular formation. Japanese Journal of Physiology 17:65-93 (1967).

41. Goy, R.W. and Young, W.C.: Strain differences in the behavioral responses of female guinea pigs to alpha-oestradiol benzoate and progesterone Behavior 10:340-354 (1957).

42. Ring, J.R.: The estrogen-progesterone induction of sexual receptivity in the spayed female mouse. Endocrinology 34:269-275 (1944).

43. Boling, J.L. and Blandau, R.J.: The estrogen-progesterone induction of mating responses in the spayed female rat. Endocrinology 25:359-371 (1939).

44. Dempsey, E.W., Hertz, R. and Young, W.C.: The experimental induction of oestrus (sexual receptivity) in the normal and ovariectomized guinea pig. Am. J. Physiol. 16:201-209 (1936).

45. Kent, G.C. and Liberman, M.J.: Induction of psychic oestrus in the hamster with progesterone administered via the lateral brain ventricle. Endocrinology 45:29-32 (1949).

46. Robinson, T.J.: Quantitative studies on the hormonal induction of oestrus in spayed ewes. J. Endocrin. 12:163-173 (1955).

47. Phoenix, C.H., Goy, R.W. and Young, W.C.: Sexual behavior: general aspects. In Neuroendocrinology Ed. Martini and Ganong. Academic Press, New York, 163-196 (1967).

48. Makepeace, A.W., Weinstein, G.L. and Friedman, M.H.: J. Physiol. 119:512-516 (1937).

49. Marshall, F.H.A. and Hammond, J.: Experimental control
by hormone action of the oestrus cycle in the ferret. J. Endocrin.
4:159-168 (1945).

50. Lunde, D.: Stimulation versus hormone induction of copulatory behavior in female rats. Master of Arts thesis, Department
of Psychology and Graduate Division, Stanford University, 1964.

51. Edwards, D.A., Whalen, R.E. and Nadler, R.D.: Induction
of oestrus: estrogen-progesterone interactions. Physiology and
Behavior 3:29-33 (1968).

52. Sawyer, C.H. and Everett, J.W.: Stimulatory and inhibitory effects of progesterone on the release of pituitary ovulating
hormone in the rabbit. Endocrinology 65:644-651 (1959).

53. Zarrow, M.X., Grota, L.J. and Denenberg, V.H.: Maternal
behavior in the rat: survival of new born fostered young after
hormonal treatment of the foster mother. Anat. Rec. 157:13-18.

54. Kislach and Beach: Inhibition of aggressiveness by ovarian hormones. Endocrinology 56:684-692 (1955).

55. Campbell, H.J.: Acute effects of pregnane steroids on
septal self-stimulation in the rabbit. J. Physiol. 196:134-135
(1968).

56. Overton, D.A.: Psychopharmacologia 10:6 (1966).

57. Stewart, J., Krebs, W.H. and Kaczender, E.: State-
dependent learning produced with steroids. Nature 216:1223-1224
(1967).

58. Ball, J.: Sexual responsiveness in female monkeys after
castration and subsequent estrin administration. Psychol. Bull.
33:811 (1936).

59. Michael, R.P., Herbert, J. and Welegalla, J.: Ovarian
hormones and the sexual behavior of the male rhesus monkey under
laboratory conditions J. Endocrin. 39:81-98 (1965).

60. Michael, R.P., Saayman, G.S. and Zumpe, D.: Inhibition of
sexual receptivity by progesterone in rhesus monkeys. J. Endocrin.
39:309-310 (1967).

61. McCance, R., Luff, M. and Widdowson, E.: The physical
and emotional periodicity in women. J. Hygiene 37:571 (1937).

62. Moos, R.H., Kopell, B.S., Melges, F.T., Yalom, I.D. Lunde, D.T., Clayton, R.B. and Hamburg, D.A.: Variations in symptoms and mood during the menstrual cycle. **Psychosomatic Research** (In press) (1968).

63. Benedek, T.F.: Sexual function in women and their disturbances. In American Handbook of Psychiatry Ed. Arieti. Basic Books, Inc., 1959, 727-748.

64. Yerkes, R.M. and Elder, J.H.: Concerning reproduction in the chimpanzee. Science 81:542-543 (1937).

65. Heller, C.G., Moore, D.J., Paulsen, C.A., Nelson, W.O. and Laidlaw, W.M.: Effects of progesterone and synthetic progestins on the reproductive physiology of normal men. Federation Proceedings 18:1057-1064 (1959).

66. Washburn, S.L. and DeVore, I.: The social life of baboons. Scient. Am. 204:62-71 (1961).

67. Michael, R.P., Herbert, J. and Welegalla, J.: Ovarian hormones and grooming behavior in the rhesus monkey (macca mulatta) under laboratory conditions J. Endocrin. 36:263-279 (1966).

68. Krus, D.M., Wapner, S., Bergen, J. and Freeman, H.: The influence of progesterone on behavioral changes induced by lysergic acid diethylamide (LSD-25) in normal males. Psychopharmacologia 2:177-184 (1961).

69. Yalom, I.: Unpublished observations.

70. Brown, J.B. and Matthew, G.D.: The application of urinary estrogen measurements to problems in gynecology. Rec. Prog. Horm. Res. 18:337 (1962).

71. VanderMolen, H.J., Runnebaum, B. and Nishizawa, E.E.: On the presence of progesterone in blood plasma from normal women. J. Clin. Endocrin. 25:170 (1965).

72. Zander, J.: The chemical estimation of progesterone and its metabolites in body fluids and target organs. In Progesterone ed. by A.C. Barnes, 77-90 Brook Lodge Press, Augusta, Mich. 1961.

73. Lurie, A.O. and Weiss, J.B.: Progesterone in cerebrospinal fluid during human pregnancy. Nature 215:1178 (1931).

74. Frank, R.T.: The hormonal causes of premenstrual tension. Arch. Neural. Psychiat. 26:1053 (1931).

75. Rogers, J.: _Endocrine and Metabolic Aspects of Gynecology_ W.B. Saunders, Philadelphia, 1963.

76. Moos, R.H.: The development of a menstrual distress questionnaire. Psychosomatic Medicine, in press, 1968.

77. Dalton, K.: Menstruation and accidents. Brit. Med. J. 2:1425 (1960).

78. Dalton, K.: Menstruation and acute psychiatric illness Brit. Med. J. 1:148 (1959).

79. Morton, J.H., Addison, H., Addison, R., Hunt, L. and Sullivan, J.: Clinical study of premenstrual tension. Am. J. Obstet. Gynecol. 65:1182 (1953).

80. Yalom, I., Lunde, D., Moos, R. and Hamburg, D.: The "postpartum blues" syndrome: description and related variables. Archives of General Psychiatry, in press, 1968.

81. Hamilton, J.: _Postpartum Psychiatric Problems_ Mosby, St. Louis, Missouri, 1962.

82. Pugh, T.: Rates of mental disease related to childbearing. New England Journal of Medicine 268:1224-1228 (1963).

83. Heftmann, E. and Mosettig, E.: _Biochemistry of Steroids_ Reinhold, New York, 1960.

THE PHYSIOLOGIC BASIS FOR THE TEMPERATURE RAISING EFFECT

OF PROGESTERONE

Irving Rothchild

Department of Reproductive Biology, Case Western Reserve
University School of Medicine, Cleveland, Ohio

The body temperature of regularly ovulating women tends to be
about 0.75° F higher in the interval between ovulation and the next
menstrual period than in the interval between menses and the next
ovulation (1,2). This phenomenon, which has been recognized since
before the turn of the century (3-5), has been shown to be due to
the progesterone secreted by the corpus luteum (6-8,1,2). During
pregnancy the tremendously increased duration of progesterone secretion is also associated with a prolongation of the body temperature
elevation, although the latter does not last as long as does the
secretion of progesterone (9). Other animals in which either an
elevation of body temperature occurs during the luteal phase or in
response to treatment with progesterone or both, are the cow (10-12),
African dwarf goat (13), rat (14-16) and monkey (17). No relation
between the ovulation cycle and the body temperature has been seen
in the pig (18). Several other steroids of the pregnane and androstane series also raise the body temperature of human subjects,
some to a much greater degree than progesterone does (19: See 20
for review).

The exact nature of this temperature raising* (TR) effect is
not known. It could be the result of either an increase in heat
production, a decrease in heat loss, or some combination of both
effects. The available evidences for and against these possibilities are discussed in what follows.

---

*The term "thermogenic", commonly used to describe the temper-
ature raising effect of progesterone, is misleading since it implies
that progesterone increases heat production. Until this is proved,
however, it would be more exact to use the term "temperature
raising (TR) effect."

EVIDENCE FOR AN EFFECT OF PROGESTERONE ON HEAT PRODUCTION

The major sources of heat production are: 1) increased body activity as a whole (e.g., exercise); 2) increased activity of specific groups of muscles (e.g., shivering); 3) increased general metabolic rate (e.g., hyperthyroidism); or 4) increase in metabolic activity of a relatively large viscus, such as the liver.

Body activity as a whole tends to be decreased, rather than increased, under the influence of progesterone (1,14,15), and may be related to its anesthetic effect (1). Although the depressing effect of progesterone on general body activity speaks against increased heat production as essential to the TR effect, it does not preclude a stimulating effect of progesterone on shivering. That is, the quiescent animal may still shiver and thus increase its heat production. As far as I can determine, however, this possibility has not been studied, so the question of whether progesterone has any effect on shivering must remain open.

There is no good evidence that progesterone increases the basal metabolic rate (BMR) since the slight increase in O_2 consumption of women during the luteal phase of the cycle (21) is almost certainly a reflection of its stimulating effect on respiration (22). Furthermore, even if the increase in BMR were real, the increase in body temperature itself could be its cause rather than its result, since the weight of the evidence is against any effect of progesterone on the thyroid gland. Thus, cretins show just as significant a rise in body temperature as do otherwise physiologically normal but feeble-minded subjects, and the latter show no significant change in PBI associated with the progesterone-induced rise in body temperature (21).

Although progesterone may effect the activity of some of the liver enzymes in a way which might increase heat production by the liver, there is no direct evidence that this is the case (see section on Liver and GI tract). Some indirect evidence from my own laboratory, however, suggests that this is probably not the mechanism through which progesterone acts. We have some data which shows that the prepubertal rat does not show the TR effect of progesterone under conditions in which her adult counterpart does (16). Since these rats were between 26 and 36 days of age, it it extremely unlikely that any marked difference between rats of this age and adults in the activity of such viscera as the liver could have accounted for this finding.

EVIDENCE FOR AN EFFECT OF PROGESTERONE ON HEAT LOSS

Progesterone could reduce heat loss by acting either directly on the physiologic processes through which body heat is lost, or

by acting centrally on the neural controls over these processes.
That is, progesterone could reduce heat loss by affecting directly
the activity of the sweat glands, the conductance of heat through
the skin, or the rate of loss of heat contained in the moisture of
expired air, urine or feces, or it could act on the presumed hypothalamic or other neural centers which control the activity of the
sweat glands, the circulation of blood through the skin, or the
control of respiration, excretion and defecation.

These several possibilities are not distinguished by any
wealth of conclusive evidence for or against any one of them. For
example, the literature contains very little evidence for any effect of progesterone on the skin, or on the circulation through it,
and, except possibly for the reports of MacKinnon (see below),
what there is is either non-contributory or does not account for
the TR effect. Thus, progesterone may increase the activity of the
sebaceous glands in somewhat the same way that androgens do, but to
a much smaller degree (see, for example, Strauss and Kligman (23)),
so it is doubtful that this effect could explain the TR effect.
Venous distensibility in the skin of the fingers seems to follow
the curve of progesterone secretion during the ovulation cycle,
the peak being seen one week before menstruation (24). The data of
McCausland et al, however, are not very extensive, and although the
effect, if confirmed, would tend to increase rather than decrease
heat loss, the importance of such an effect of progesterone on
temperature regulating processes could be determined only by comparison with the other possible effects of progesterone on pathways
of heat production and loss.

Only suggestive data are available for an effect of progesterone on sweating. No conclusions can be drawn form the data of
Sargent and Weinman (25) and of Kawahata (26) since they studied
only the mid-cycle and menstrual phases of the cycle, but MacKinnon
and collaborators have shown that progesterone treatment, the
luteal phase of the cycle, and pregnancy, are all associated with
a definite decrease in the number of active sweat glands in the
palmar skin (27-29). This finding would be consistent with an
effect of reducing heat loss, but the data so far available do not
allow us to distinguish between a direct effect on the sweat glands
or on the central control of sweating.

Some heat could also be lost with the water of expired air,
urine or feces. What little evidence there is, however, suggests
that the effect of progesterone on these possible routes of heat
loss would be unimportant or would tend to increase rather than decrease heat loss. For example, progesterone increases the respiratory rate, and it has been suggested that this effect is a centrally
mediated one, possibly involving a decreased threshold of the
respiratory center to the arterial partial pressure of CO_2 (see

Lyons (22)). I know of no experimental studies of the effect of
progesterone on the rate of urine flow or on the frequency of urina-
tion, but it is common knowledge that one of the symptoms of early
pregnancy is increased urinary frequency, which would, if anything,
tend to increase heat loss. One assumes that the tendency to urin-
ate more frequently in early pregnancy is an effect of progesterone,
but even if it were not, it occurs when the body temperature is
elevated and so could not account for the mechanism of the TR effect.

No data are available for an effect of progesterone on defecation, but loss of heat through the feces could be only a very
minor contribution to all heat losing processes, and it is very
unlikely that the common tendency for women to be constipated during
the luteal phase, or in early pregnancy, could account for the TR
effect of progesterone.

POSSIBLE EFFECTS OF PROGESTERONE ON THE CENTRAL
CONTROL OF TEMPERATURE REGULATION

The evidence thus far does not allow one to draw any but tentative conclusions. It looks as though progesterone does not increase heat production, but the possibility of an effect on shivering has not been ruled out. On the other hand, the effects of progesterone on pathways of heat loss, with the exception of sweating,
are to increase rather than decrease heat loss. I am inclined to
suggest that progesterone increases the body temperature by reducing heat loss, primarily through an effect on sweating (including
insensible loss of perspiration), but I must admit that there is
no really firm evidence for this as yet.

What evidence is there that progesterone acts on the central
regulation of body temperature?

That progesterone does affect certain kinds of central nervous system (CNS) activity (2) only suggests but does not prove
that it can also affect the neural control of body temperature.
At least two of the CNS effects of progesterone - the anesthetic
effect, which is certainly on the CNS, and the effect on respiration,
which is probably on the CNS - are clearly not connected with the
TR effect. Anesthesia induced by progesterone, as is true for most
anesthetics, is associated with a fall rather than with a rise in
body temperature (personal observations). The respiratory effect,
which involves a significant decrease in alveolar and arterial
partial pressure of CO_2, would also lead to a fall in body temperature, since a decrease in the arterial partial pressure of CO_2
causes an increase in hypothalamic temperature (30) which would act
as a signal to set heat losing processes in operation (31-34).
Furthermore, some of the synthetic progestogens, such as ethister-
one and norethisterone, which have a TR effect, do not have any

effect on respiration (35).

Lauritzen (9) has postulated that progesterone has a central effect on body temperature control. This is based primarily on two findings, neither of which, however, is conclusive. One is that the effect wears off with time (e.g., as in pregnancy), the other is that it can be blocked by barbiturates. Although the return of the body temperature of pregnant women, at about the fourth month, to the pre-pregnancy level resembles, in its temporary nature, several other effects of progesterone on the CNS (2), one can only take such evidence as contributory but not conclusive. The fact that more potent body temperature raising steroids, such as nor-ethisterone, raise the body temperature of pregnant women after it has returned to normal values, but again for only a limited period of time (36), strengthens this possibility but does not clearly establish it. The blocking effect of barbiturates on the TR effect of both progesterone and norethisterone (36) could mean that a central effect is being blocked, but since the doses used were in the anesthetic range and since anesthetics, in general, lower body temperature, the blocking effect could be nonspecific.

Salicylates have no effect on the normal body temperature but lower fever temperatures. There seems to be general agreement that their primary site of action is the central control of heat losing processes, so that body temperature is lowered through increased sweating and conductance of blood through the skin (37). The effect of salicylate treatment on the TR effect of progesterone in one study was not uniform although a body temperature lowering effect was seen in some of the subjects (38). Since salicylates act centrally one may tentatively conclude that progesterone does so also, but it is still possible for the central effect of salicylates to override a peripheral one of progesterone.

Another bit of indirect evidence is the failure of prepubertal rats to show the TR effect. An attractive explanation for this finding is that the changes in CNS control of pituitary gonado-trophin in the way progesterone causes a rise in body temperature. There is some evidence that the CNS control over sexual behavior, running activity, and appetite also change around the time of puberty (for review and references, particularly to the work of Kennedy, see Rothchild (39)) so this possibility is not a remote one, and the phenomenon itself, therefore, could derive from the fact that the particular neural process through which progesterone affects body temperature does not become fully active until after puberty.

CONCLUSIONS

The explanation of the TR effect of progesterone presents an

interesting challenge to workers in the field of both temperature
regualtion and endocrinology. The effect is not specific to progesterone but is seen with several other naturally occurring steroids of the pregnane and androstane series, as well as with some of
the synthetic progestogens. With the reservation that an effect on
shivering has not been ruled out, the TR effect does not seem to
depend on an increase in heat production. One promising possibility
seems to be that progesterone decreases heat loss, primarily by
reducing sweating, but the evidence for this is still meager and no
clear distinction can be made as yet between a central and a peripheral effect. If the effect should prove to be central, it is
clearly not mediated through either the respiration-increasing or
anesthetic effects of progesterone, but may be related in some way
to the neural control over gonadotrophin secretion, sexual behavior
and other processes connected with reproduction.

REFERENCES

1. Southam, A.L. and Gonzaga, F.P.: Amer. J. Obstet. and
Gynec. 91:142 (1965).

2. Rothchild, I.: Vitam. and Horm. 23:209 (1965).

3. Squire, W.: Trans. Obstetr. Soc. London 9:129 (1868).

4. Fraenkel, L.: Arch f. Gynaek. 64:438 (1903).

5. van de Velde, T.H.: Uber die Zusammenhang zwischen Ovarial-
funktion, Wellenbewegungen und Menstrualblutung Haarlem, (1904).

6. Barton, D.S.: Yale J. Biol. and Med. 12:503 (1940).

7. Nieburgs, H.E.: J. Obstet. and Gynec. Brit. Emp. 52:435
(1945).

8. Palmer, A.: Obstet Gynec. Surv. 4:1 (1949).

9. Lauritzen, D.: Arch. f. Gynaek. 191:122 (1958).

10. Wrenn, T.R., Bitman, J. and Sykes, J.F.: J. Dairy Sci.
41:1071 (1958).

11. Wrenn, T.R., Bitman, J. and Sykes, J.F.: Endocrinology
65:317 (1959).

12. Fallon, G.R.: Queensl. J. Agricult Sci. 16:439 (1959).

13. Parer, J.T.: Amer. J. Veter. Res. 24:1223 (1963).

14. Richter, C.P.: Josiah Macy, Jr. Foundation Conference on Gestation; Trans. 2nd Conference, Princeton, 1955; p. 11, (1956).

15. Brobeck, J.R., Wheatland, M. and Strominger, J.L.: Endocrinology 40:65 (1947).

16. Roller, R.J. and Rothchild, I.: Unpublished findings.

17. Balin, H. and Wan, L.S.: Fert. and Steril. 19:228 (1968).

18. Sanders, D.P., Heidenreich, C.J. and Jones, H.W.: Amer. J. Veter. Res. 25:851 (1963).

19. Epstein, J., Kupperman, H.S. and Cutler, H.: Ann. N.Y. Acad. Sci. 71:560 (1958).

20. Kappas, A. and Palmer, R.H.: Methods in Hormone Res. 4:1 (1965).

21. Rothchild, I. and Rapport, R.L.: Endocrin. 50:580 (1952).

22. Lyons, H.: (this conference, 1969).

23. Strauss, J.S. and Kligman, A.M.: J. Invest. Dermat. 36:309 (1961).

24. McCausland, A.M., Holmes, F. and Trotter, A.F.: Amer. J. Obstet. and Gynec. 86:640 (1963).

25. Sargent, F. and Weinman, K.P.: J. Appl. Physiol. 21:1685 (1966).

26. Kawahata, A.: Essential Problems in Climatic Physiology (ed. S. Itoh, H. Ogata and H. Yoshimura) Nankodo Publ., Kyoto, p. 169, (1960).

27. MacKinnon, P.C.B.: J. Obstet and Gynec. Brit. Emp. 61:390 (1954).

28. MacKinnon, P.C.B. and MacKinnon, I.L.: J. Obstet. and Gynec. Brit. Emp. 62:623 (1955).

29. MacKinnon, P.C.B. and Harrison, J.: J. Endo. 23:217 (1961).

30. Hayward, J.H. and Baker, M.A.: Am. J. Physiol. 215:389 (1968)

31. von Euler, C.: Pharm. Rev. 13:361 (1961).

32. Hardy, J.D.: Physiol. Rev. 41:521 (1961).

33. Bligh, J.: Biol. Rev. 41:317 (1966).

34. Hammel, H.T.: Ann. Rev. Physiol. 30:641 (1968).

35. Tyler, J.M.: J. Clin. Invest. 39:34 (1960).

36. Lauritzen, C.: Geburtsh. u. Frauenheilk. 9:807 (1957).

37. Woodbury, D.: In The Pharmacologic Basis of Therapeutics, 3rd
ed. (ed. L.S. Goodman and A. Gilman), McMillan, N.Y., p. 312 (1965).

38. Rothchild, I. and Barnes, A.C.: Endocrin. 50:485 (1952).

39. Rothchild, I.: In Reproduction in the Female Mammal (ed.
G.E. Lamming and E.C. Amoroso) Butterworth, London, p. 30 (1967).

ASSESSMENT OF PSYCHOLOGICAL CONCOMITANTS OF ORAL CONTRACEPTIVES

Rudolf H. Moos

Department of Psychiatry, Stanford University School of
Medicine, Stanford, California

This paper will review research on the menstrual cycle and on
oral contraceptives currently in progress in the Department of
Psychiatry at Stanford University. The psychological aspect of the
work is oriented around two major purposes. The first is an attempt
to develop a standard technique for the assessment of symptoms and
change of symptoms throughout the menstrual cycle. The second involves the comparison of women on oral contraceptives with women
not on oral contraceptives in terms of the symptom changes throughout their menstrual cycles.

The essential strategy has been to initially develop an assessment technique for the measurement of menstrual cycle symptomatology.
This technique was first utilized in a cross-sectional study, i.e.,
in a study concentrating on one menstrual cycle in a relatively
large number of women over two menstrual cycles. The comparison of
women on and not on oral contraceptives has proceeded in a similar
manner. Initially, there was a cross-sectional comparison of a
large number of women, some of whom were currently taking, and
others who were not currently taking, oral contraceptives. A follow-
up study is concerned with investigating the psychological effects
of an oral contraceptive by studying a small group of women over
four menstrual cycles in a double blind design, with each woman serving as her own control.

As has been previously pointed out, there are several reasons
why there should be special current interest in the physiological
actions and psychological effects of the oral contraceptive (1-3).

This research was supported in part by USPHS Grant MH 10976.

Never have so many people taken such potent drugs voluntarily over such a protracted period for objectives other than for the control of disease. For oral contraceptives the objectives are complete protection, or nearly complete protection, from pregnancy, increased pleasure and spontaneity in sexual expression, and the absence of undesirable side effects. Most studies suggest that there are few, if any, problems to be expected with the use of oral contraceptives, and yet sometimes up to 25% of women discontinue their use of the drug and state that they will not use it again (4). Our studies attempted to focus on the question of whether there were undesirable symptomatic and psychological side effects of the oral contraceptives which might underlie this fact.

Our initial research problem revolved around the development of a technique for the assessment of changes in menstrual cycle symptomatology.

A comprehensive review of the literature (5) on menstrual symptomatology indicated that there were many conflicts of results with regard to specific symptoms, e.g., Altman et al (6) reported both "fatigue" and "bursts of energy" as premenstrual tension symptoms, and Greene and Dalton (7) reported a 6% incidence of depression, whereas Paulson (8) reported an 82% incidence of depression. These differences appeared to be related to the lack of comparability of various authors' methods of study and selection of subjects. For example, three recent studies utilized three different questionnaires and obtained three different sets of results (8-10). No standard method for collecting data about menstrual cycle symptomatology had been developed, and each investigator had utilized a data gathering technique which was not comparable to those utilized in previous studies.

DEVELOPMENT OF MENSTRUAL DISTRESS QUESTIONNAIRE (MDQ)

A list of 47 symptoms for inclusion in the MDQ was obtained from open-ended questionnaires and interviews, previous research (5) and items from the Blatt Menopausal Index (11). These latter items, e.g., buzzing or ringing in ears, numbness or tingling in hands or feet, feelings of suffocation, were symptoms which menopausal women endorsed with relatively high frequency but which women in the age range of our sample (20-30) endorsed with very low frequency (12). These control symptoms were included in order to obtain some measure of how likely a woman was to complain of a variety of different symptoms, regardless of whether or not these symptoms were usually associated with menstrual cycle changes.

The women were asked to rate their experience of each of the 47 symptoms on the MDQ on a six point scale ranging from no experience of the symptom to an acute or partially disabling experience

TABLE 1

MENSTRUAL DISTRESS QUESTIONNAIRE (MDQ) SYMPTOM SCALES

1. PAIN

Muscle stiffness
Headache
Cramps
Backache
Fatigue
General aches and pains

2. CONCENTRATION

Insomnia
Forgetfulness
Confusion
Lowered judgment
Difficulty concentrating
Distractible
Accidents
Lowered motor coordination

3. BEHAVIORAL CHANGE

Lowered school or work
    performance
Take naps; stay in bed
Stay at home
Avoid social activities
Decreased efficiency

4. AUTONOMIC REACTIONS

Dizziness, faintness
Cold sweats
Nausea, vomiting
Hot flashes

5. WATER RETENTION

Weight gain
Skin disorders
Painful breasts
Swelling

6. NEGATIVE AFFECT

Crying
Loneliness
Anxiety
Restlessness
Irritability
Mood swings
Depression
Tension

7. AROUSAL

Affectionate
Orderliness
Excitement
Feelings of well-being
Bursts of energy, activity

8. CONTROL

Feeling of suffocation
Chest pains
Ringing in the ears
Heart pounding
Numbness, tingling
Blind spots, fuzzy vision

TABLE 2

PERCENT OF WOMEN WITH MILD, MODERATE, STRONG AND
SEVERE COMPLAINTS ON SELECTED SYMPTOMS ON MDQ

Scale Symptom	Menstrual		Premenstrual	
	mild moderate	strong severe	mild moderate	strong severe
Pain				
Cramps	35.6	11.0	12.3	1.9
Backache	31.9	8.1	20.7	3.7
Concentration				
Difficulty concentrating	12.3	1.9	12.9	1.2
Accidents	11.7	1.3	12.6	1.8
Behavior Change				
Take naps; stay in bed	22.4	3.8	10.4	2.1
Decreased efficiency	23.4	2.6	16.0	2.6
Autonomic Reaction				
Dizziness, faintness	9.7	1.5	3.8	0.9
Nausea, vomiting	5.3	1.2	3.6	0.7
Water Retention				
Weight gain	20.7	2.2	30.8	3.1
Swelling	31.4	4.0	30.4	5.1
Negative Affect				
Irritability	40.5	8.4	39.2	13.0
Depression	27.5	7.1	33.4	9.5
Arousal				
Well being	23.6	4.4	20.5	5.0
Energy, activity	19.4	4.5	20.0	6.6
Control				
Suffocation	1.1	0.5	1.2	0.1
Ringing in ears	1.8	0.7	1.6	0.4

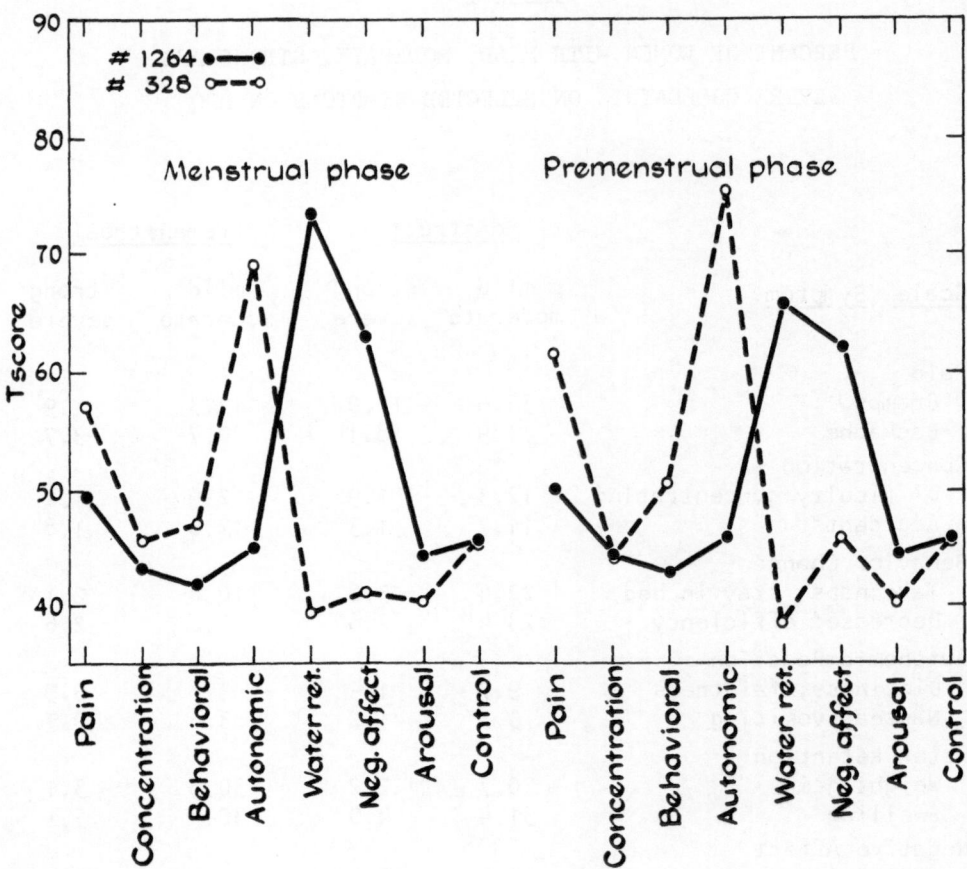

Fig. 1. Comparison of menstrual cycle symptom profiles for women numbers 1264 and 328.

of the symptom. Each woman made these ratings separately for the
menstrual, premenstrual and intermenstrual phases of her most recent
menstrual cycle and for her worst menstrual cycle. Thus women could
differentiate between their experience of different symptoms in
terms of the different phases during the cycle in which they occurred. After an initial pretest had perfected the instructions,
the MDQ was filled out by a sample of 839 young married women.

RESULTS

The 47 symptoms in the MDQ were intercorrelated and factor
analyzed (principal components solution with orthogonal rotation of
the factor matrix) for the total sample of 839 women separately for
the menstrual, premenstrual and intermenstrual phases of the most
recent cycle and for the worst menstrual cycle. The eight resulting
symptom groups shown in Table 1, reflect factors which were replicated in all four of the factor analyses. There are only 46 symptoms listed because one symptom, "change in eating habits" could
not be located consistently on any one factor. Each of these eight
groups reflect an empirically intercorrelated cluster of symptoms;
the scale labels have been chosen to reflect the major content of
the symptoms as closely as possible.

Table 2 gives the percentage of women showing mild, moderate,
strong and severe complaints on selected symptoms. Each of the
symptoms on the first six scales shows a cyclical variation with
the menstrual cycle, whereas the symptoms on the last two scales
show no such cyclical variation. The symptoms on the pain, behavior change, water retention and negative affect scales occur in
approximately 30% of the women.

In order to compare the symptom scale scores with each other
in one phase and across phases, a transformation was made that resulted in obtaining a mean of 50 and a standard deviation of 10 for
each scale. This transformation makes it possible to compare
scales with each other within one phase, to compare scales and to
draw menstrual symptom profiles for each woman which depict her
symptoms graphically.

Figure 1 contrasts a woman who complained of symptoms on the
pain and behavior change scales in both the menstrual and premenstrual phases with another woman who complained of symptoms on the
negative affect scale in both phases. Both these women had cyclical symptoms (neither scored above 50 on any of the eight scales
in the intermenstrual phase); however, they had these symptoms in
entirely different symptom areas. This example also indicates that
complaints in the area of negative affect do not necessarily decrease from the premenstrual to the menstrual phase (and thus premenstrual tension may also become menstrual tension) and that women

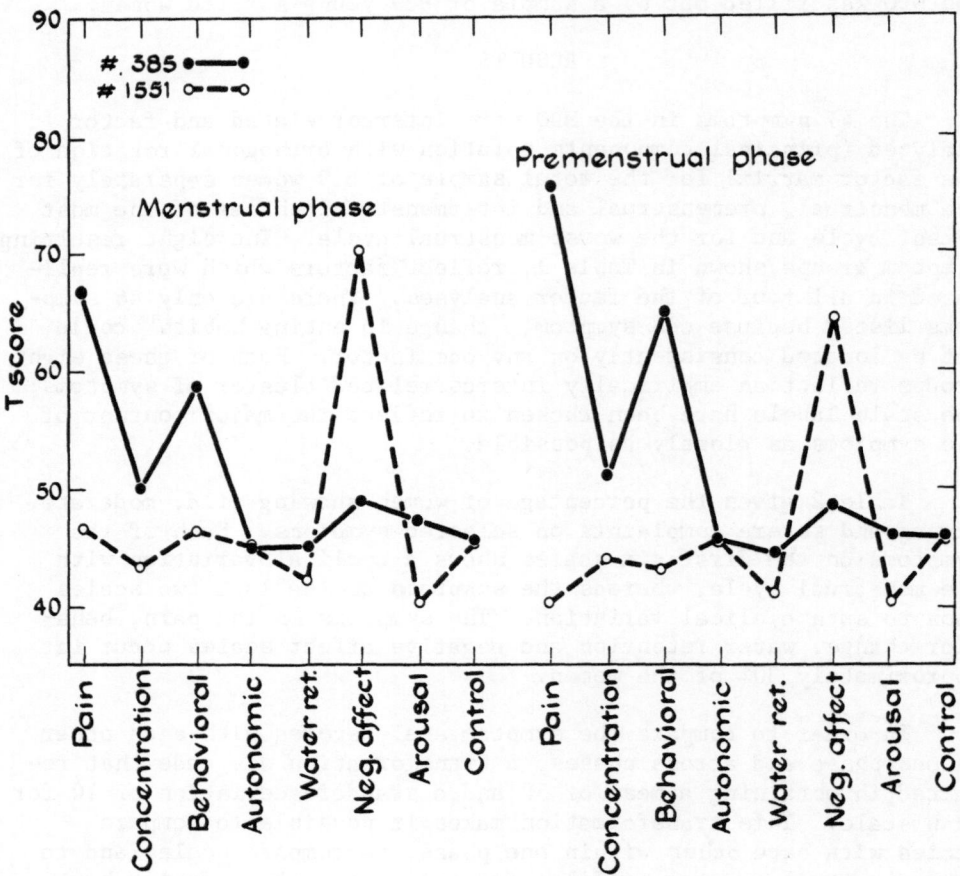

Fig. 2. Comparison of menstrual cycle symptom profiles for women numbers 385 and 1551.

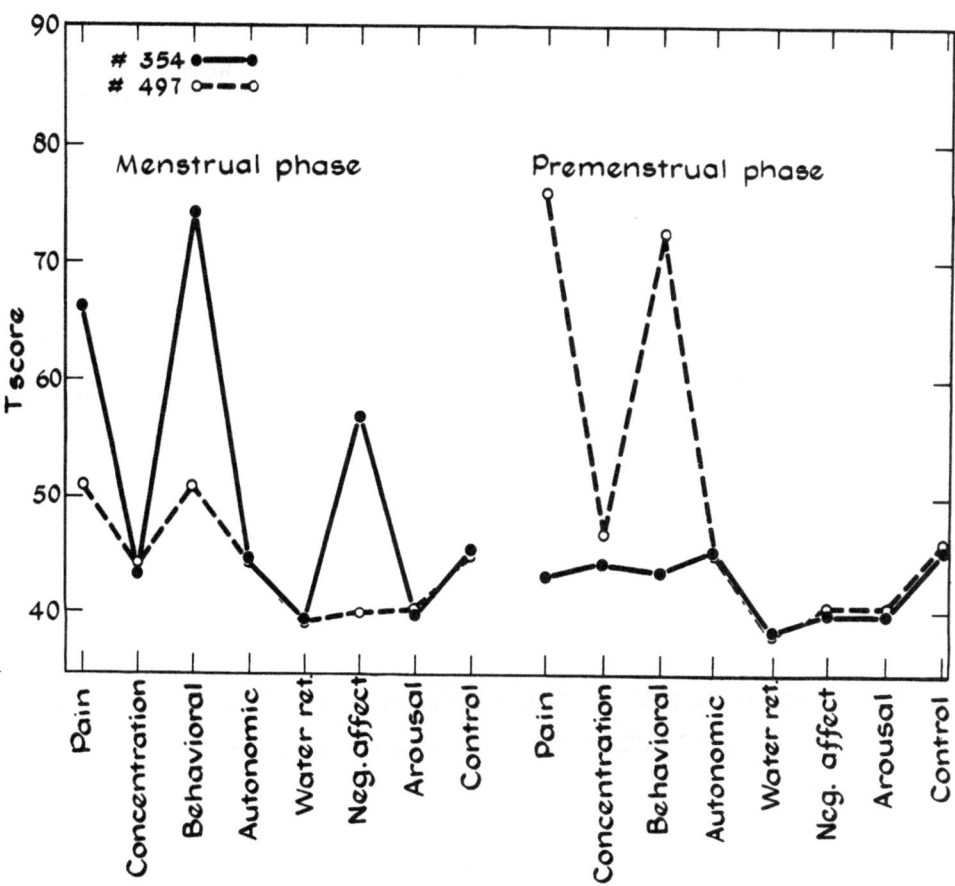

Fig. 3.   Comparison of menstrual cycle symptom profiles for women numbers 354 and 497.

TABLE 3

COMPARISON OF WOMEN ON ORAL CONTRACEPTIVES WITH
WOMEN NOT ON ORAL CONTRACEPTIVES - BACKGROUND VARIABLES

	Women on Orals (N = 420)		Women Not on Orals (N = 298)	
	Mean	SD	Mean	SD
Age (yr)	24.3	3.6	26.1	4.2
Education (yr)	15.4	1.5	15.2	1.7
Length of marriage	3.2	2.7	2.9	2.0

TABLE 4

COMPARISON OF WOMEN ON ORAL CONTRACEPTIVES WITH WOMEN NOT ON
ORAL CONTRACEPTIVES - MENSTRUAL CYCLE VARIABLES

	Women on Orals (N = 420)		Women Not on Orals (N = 298)	
	Mean	SD	Mean	SD
Length of cycle (days)	28.3	7.9	31.3	5.6
Length of flow (days)	4.9	1.0	5.9	2.1

Regularity of cycle 4-point scale %	1	2	3	4	1	2	3	4
	70.8	22.1	2.2	4.9	35.7	35.4	16.4	12.6

who have symptoms of pain in the menstrual phase may also have
similar symptoms in the premenstrual phase (and thus dysmenorrhea
may be heralded by premenstrual pain).

Figure 2 compares one woman who was high on water retention
and negative affect in both menstrual and premenstrual phases with
another woman who was high on **autonomic** reactions and moderately
elevated on pain in both menstrual and premenstrual phases. These
two women had about the same number and severity of complaints overall; however, they were in entirely different symptom areas.

Figure 3 compares a woman who complained of pain and behavior
change symptoms in the menstrual phase and of no symptoms in the
premenstrual phase with another woman who did just the reverse,
i.e., complained of pain and behavior change symptoms in the premenstrual rather than the menstrual phase. This example suggests
that the same symptoms may occur either premenstrually with significant relief at the time of menstruation, or only menstrually without having occurred premenstrually.

A typology of menstrual symptoms is of importance because of
the possibility that women who have different types of menstrual
symptoms may react differentially to oral contraceptives. Thus a
typology might help account for the large individual variability
in reactions to oral contraceptives.

Other analyses of the MDQ indicated that neither the length
of time between a woman's experience of the symptoms and her responding, had very much influence on symptom recall. Further details about the MDQ and its uses may be found elsewhere (13-15).

A CROSS-SECTIONAL COMPARISON OF
WOMEN ON AND NOT ON ORAL CONTRACEPTIVES

Of the 839 women in our initial study, one group of 420 women
was currently taking, whereas another group of 298 women was currently not taking oral contraceptives (16). The difference between these 718 women and the total sample of 839 women reflects
the number of women who were pregnant (N = 81) or who did not answer the questions about their use of oral contraceptives (N = 40).

Table 3 shows that the two groups were closely comparable on
the variables of age, education and length of marriage.

Table 4 indicates that the women on oral contraceptives reported a slightly shorter average cycle length, a slightly shorter
average length of menstrual flow, and a more regular menstrual
cycle than the women not on oral contraceptives.

TABLE 5

SYMPTOMS SIGNIFICANTLY DIFFERENTIATING* BETWEEN WOMEN IN ORAL AND NONORAL GROUPS IN MENSTRUAL AND PREMENSTRUAL PHASES[†]

Pain
Cramps	M	
Backache	M	
General aches and pains	M	PM

Concentration
Confusion		PM
Lowered judgment		PM
Difficulty concentrating	M	PM
Distractible		PM
Lowered motor coordination	M	PM

Behavioral Change
Lowered school or work performance	M	PM
Decreased efficiency	M	PM

Autonomic Reactions
No differences

Water Rentention
Weight gain		PM
Skin disorders	M	PM

Negative Affect
Restlessness		PM
Irritability		PM
Mood swings	M	PM
Depression		PM
Tension	M	PM

Arousal
No differences

Control
No differences

---

* $P < 0.01$.

[†] Women on oral contraceptives lower on all symptoms.

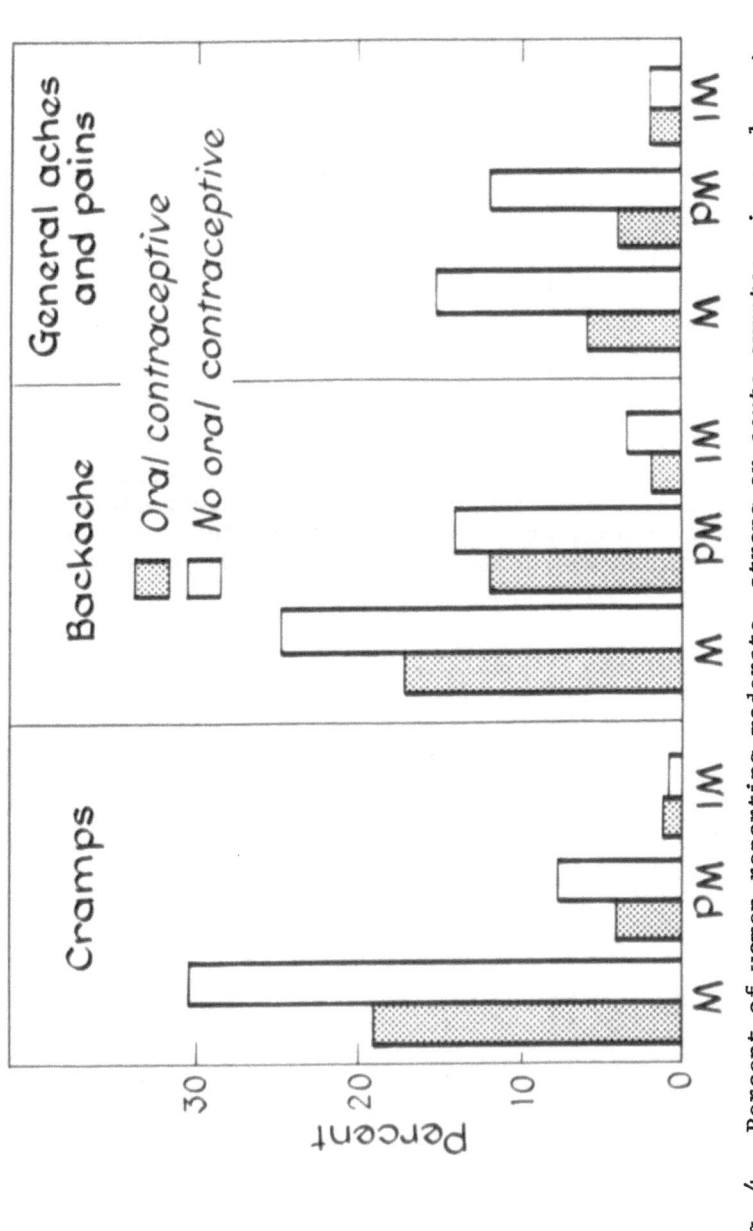

Fig. 4. Percent of women reporting moderate, strong or acute symptoms in oral contraceptive (O) and no oral contraceptive (NO) groups in menstrual (M), premenstrual (PM) and intermenstrual (IM) phases of most recent menstrual cycle - selected symptoms on pain scale.

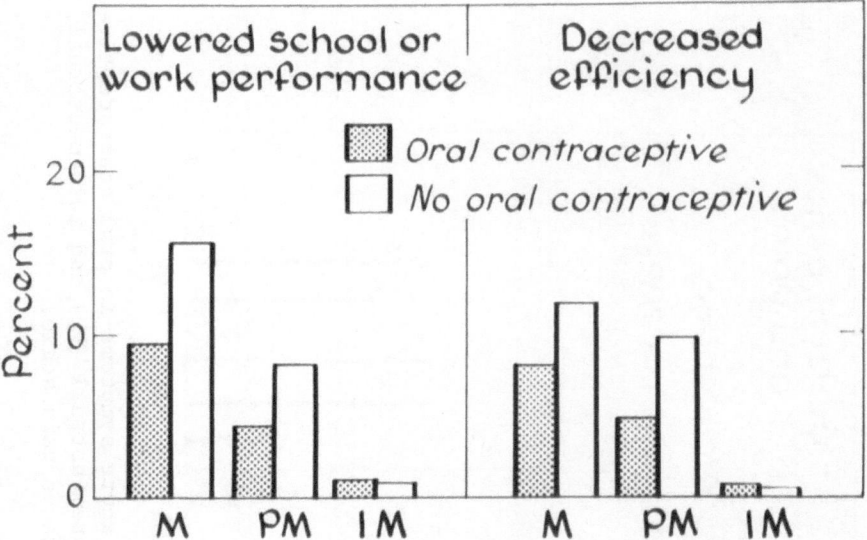

Fig. 5. Percent of women reporting moderate, strong or acute symptoms in oral contraceptive (O) and no oral contraceptive (NO) groups in menstrual (M), premenstrual (PM) and intermenstrual (IM) phases of most recent menstrual cycle - selected symptoms on behavior change scale.

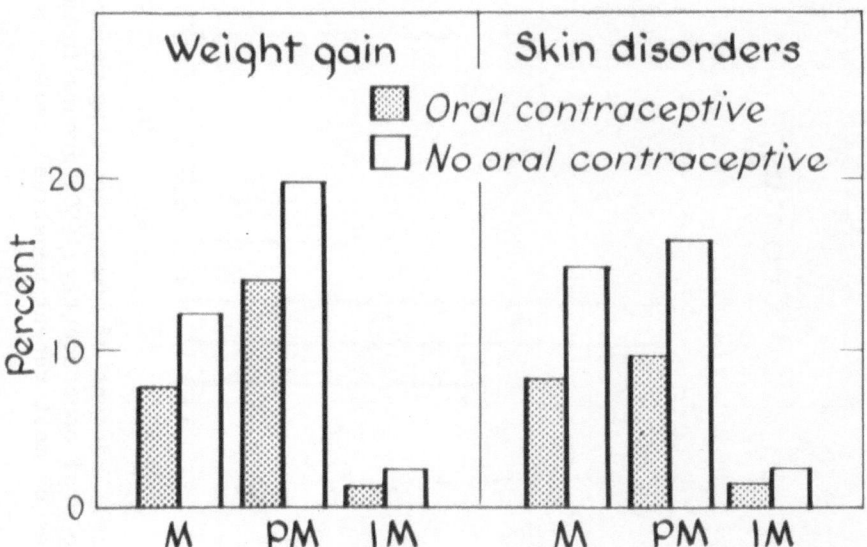

Fig. 6. Percent of women reporting moderate, strong or acute symptoms in oral contraceptive (O) and no oral contraceptive (NO) groups in menstrual (M), premenstrual (PM) and intermenstrual (IM) phases of most recent menstrual cycle - selected symptoms on water retention scale.

These differences are clearly consistent with earlier reports
on the effects of oral contraceptives. They are also consistent
with the verbal descriptions which many women gave on the questionnaires regarding the differences between their menstrual cycles
when they were on as compared to when they were not on oral contraceptives (17).

A special derivation of the Mann-Whitney U test for use with
large groups (18) was utilized in the comparison of symptom severity in the oral and nonoral groups. The women not on oral contraceptives complained of greater severity of various symptoms in both
menstrual (P < 0.01 for 10 of 47 symptoms) and premenstrual
(P < 0.01 for 15 of 47 symptoms) phases. Table 5 shows that these
symptoms were mainly in the areas of pain (cramps, general aches
and pains), concentration (lowered judgment, distractibility),
negative affect (restlessness, tension, depression, irritability),
and behavior change (lowered school or work performance, decreased
efficiency).

None of the symptoms differentiated significantly between the
two groups in the intermenstrual phase, and there were only three
symptoms which significantly differentiated the groups in the worst
menstrual cycle symptom reports.

These results show that, on the average, women who were not
currently on oral contraceptives complained more of a variety of
menstrual and premenstrual symptoms than comparable women who were
currently on oral contraceptives. The important facts that there
were no control symptoms which significantly differentiated the
groups, and that there were no differences between the two groups
in symptoms during the intermenstrual phase indicates that the
women not on oral contraceptives were not merely "high complainers".

Figures 4-7 give examples of the actual percent of women who
had moderate, strong or acute complaints of selected symptoms in
the two groups in the menstrual, premenstrual and intermenstrual
phases of the most recent menstrual cycle. It can be seen that
some of the differences between the two groups complained of moderate, strong or acute cramps in the menstrual phase whereas only
18.8% of the oral group showed similar complaints. In addition,
36.1% of the nonoral group complained of moderate, strong or acute
irritability in the premenstrual phase whereas only 23.8% of the
oral group showed similar complaints.

COMPARISONS OF WOMEN ON DIFFERENT TYPES OF PREPARATIONS

The next step in the data analysis was a comparison of symptoms
in three groups of women on different oral contraceptives. The
first group of 60 women were on Enovid, a combination preparation

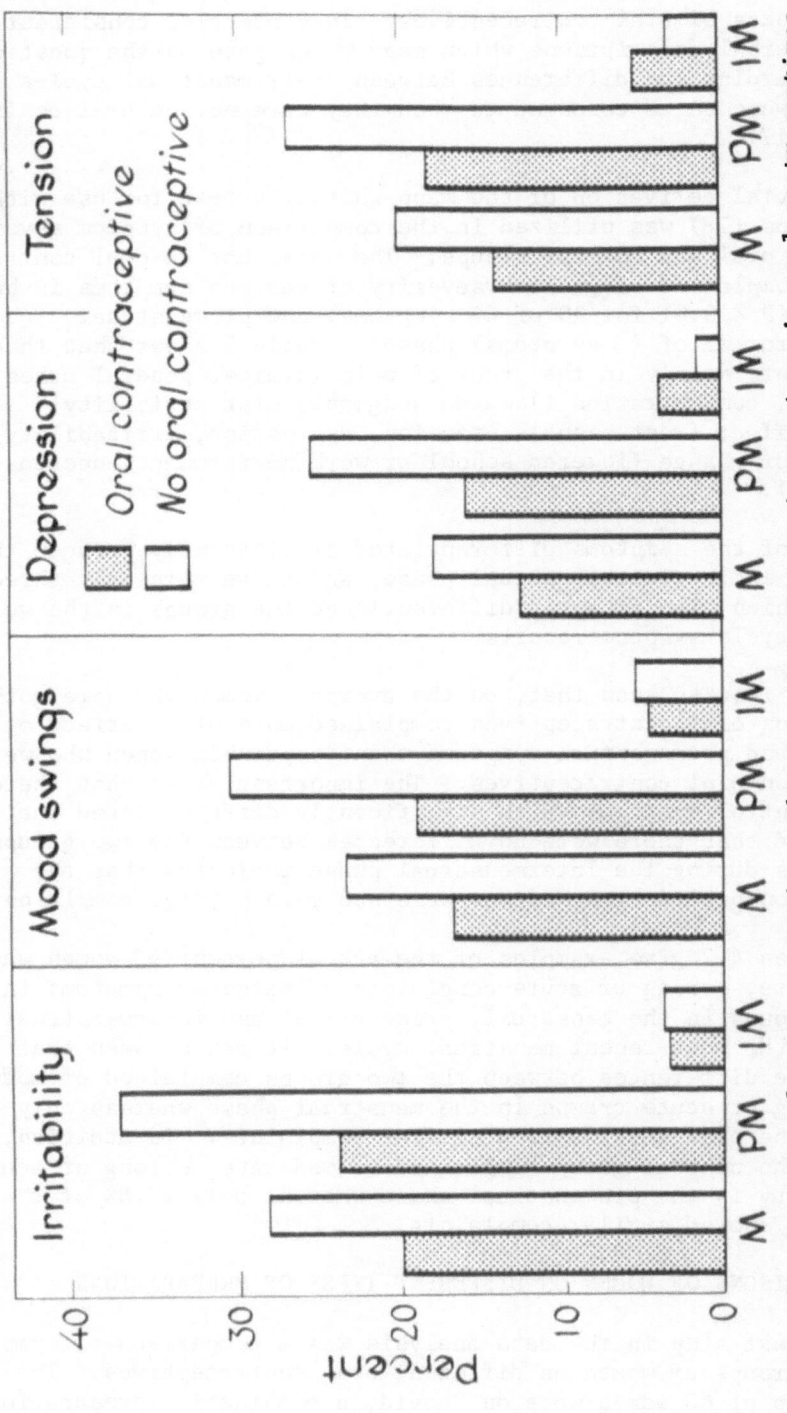

Fig. 7. Percent of women reporting moderate, strong or acute symptoms in oral contraceptives (O) and no oral contraceptive (NO) groups in menstrual (M), premenstrual (PM) and intermenstrual (IM) phases of most recent menstrual cycle - selected symptoms on negative affect scale.

TABLE 6

COMPARISON OF WOMEN ON DIFFERENT ORAL CONTRACEPTIVES – MENSTRUAL CYCLE VARIABLES

	Women on Enovid (N=60)		Women on Norinyl, Norlestrin, Orthonovum (N=56)		Women on C-Quens, Oracon (N=21)	
	Mean	S.D.	Mean	S.D.	Mean	S.D.
Length of cycle (days)	26.7	4.4	27.1	4.1	29.7	3.6
Length of flow (days)	5.6	1.3	4.8	0.9	5.7	1.4

	Women on Enovid (N=60)				Women on Norinyl, Norlestrin, Orthonovum (N=56)				Women on C-Quens, Oracon (N=21)			
	1	2	3	4	1	2	3	4	1	2	3	4
Regularity of cycle %	% 68	12	5	14	% 72	20	2	6	% 55	30	5	10

with estrogenic and progestational agents in each tablet. The
second group of 56 women were on one of three other combination
preparations, i.e., Orthonovum, Norinyl or Norlestrin. These preparations are comparable in the amount of progestin they contain,
each having between 2 to 2.5 milligrams per tablet. The third
group of 21 women were on one of two sequential preparations, i.e.,
C-Quens or Oracon. In these preparations the woman gets an estrogenic agent alone for the first 15 or 16 days and then a combination
of estrogenic and progestational agents for the last five days.

The differences between these three groups must be interpreted
with caution since they constitute a selected sample of these women
who answered the initial questionnaire and who identified which
preparation they were taking. The three groups were comparable in
the background variables of age, education and length of marriage.

Table 6 indicates that the groups on Enovid and the three
other combination preparations reported a significantly shorter menstrual cycle length than the group on the sequential preparations
(t-test, p < .05). The women on the three combination preparations
also reported a significantly shorter length of menstrual flow than
the women on the two sequential preparations (t-test, p < .05). In
addition, the women on the combination preparations were more likely to report that their menstrual cycles had been very regular
within the past year. This evidence suggests that the women currently on sequential preparations had slightly longer and less regular menstrual cycles and a slightly longer duration of menstrual
flow than the women currently on combination preparations.

The three groups were next compared on their average scores
on the eight MDQ symptom scales. There were only two significant
differences between the three groups on the scales in the menstrual
phase. In general, the women on the three combination preparations
tended to complain somewhat less of symptoms than the women in
either of the other two groups. These women complained significantly less (t-test, p < .05) of symptoms on the concentration and
control scales than did the women on Enovid.

Figure 8 compares the premenstrual phase symptoms on the eight
symptom scales in the three groups of women. The women currently
on the sequential preparations tended to complain more of symptoms
than either of the other two groups of women. Two of these differences reached statistical significance. The women on sequential
preparations showed significantly (t-test, p < .05) more complaints
on the water retention scale than did the women on the three combination preparations and significantly (t-test, p < .05) more
complaints on the negative affect scale than those women on Enovid.
The differences between the women on sequential and combination
preparations on both the concentration and autonomic reactions

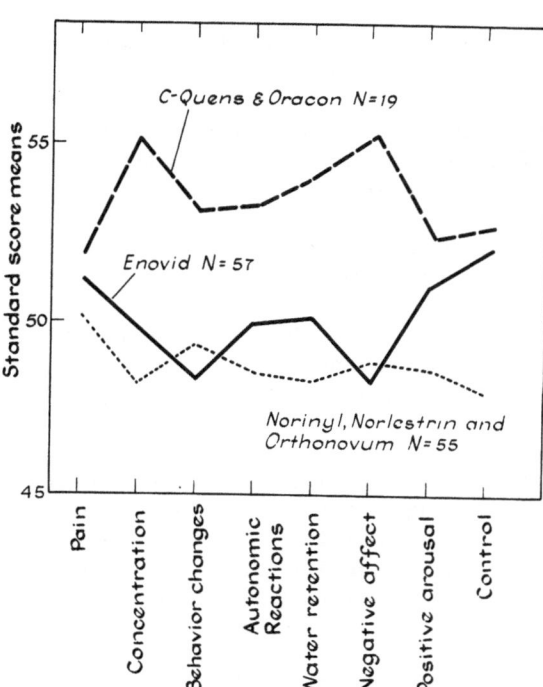

Fig. 8. Comparison of premenstrual symptoms in women on different types of oral contraceptives.

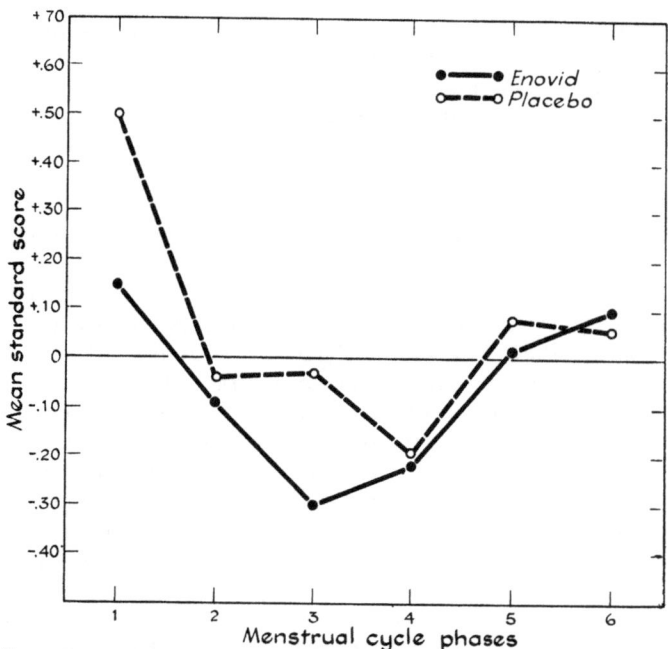

Fig. 9. Comparison of ratings of pain of eight women on Enovid (5 mg) and on placebo.

scales were in the same direction, but fell just short of statistical significance.

There were no statistically significant differences between the three groups of women on any of the symptom scales in the intermenstrual phase of the most recent cycle.

The two groups of women on combination pills were separately compared with the women on sequential pills on their reports of symptoms in their worst menstrual cycle. There was only one significant difference (t-test, $p < .05$). The women on the three combination pills reported having had significantly less symptoms on the water retention scales than the women on the sequential pills.

In contrasting the changes in symptoms shown by these three groups, it is important to note that the women on sequential preparations showed relatively greater changes throughout the cycle than did the women in the other two groups. For example, on each of the first six symptom scales the women on sequential preparations were relatively higher in their complaints in the premenstrual than in the menstrual phase, and they showed greater changes from the premenstrual to the menstrual phase on these scales than the women in either of the other two groups. These results suggest that the women on sequential preparations had a more clear-cut premenstrual rise in symptomatology than do the women on combination preparations.

Another important finding is that the women on sequential preparations showed greater variances on all symptoms scales in the premenstrual phase of the most recent cycle than did the women in the other two groups, suggesting that there may be greater individual variability of withdrawal reactions to sequential than to combination preparations.

A further analysis of the written comments on the questionnaires indicated that approximately 10% of the women who either were currently on or who previously had taken oral contraceptives stated that they had far less menstrual symptomatology while they were on the pills. However, approximately another 10% stated that they had a great deal more menstrual symptomatology when they were on the pills. Most of these latter women stated that they had discontinued the pills for this reason. This suggests that about 20% of women may experience either a significant increase or a significant decrease of menstrual symptomatology when they take oral contraceptives. These overall data and individual comments clearly show that there are significant individual differences in reactions to oral contraceptives (19).

In this connection it is important to note the extent of change and experimentation which occurs in the use of different

types of contraceptives. Almost 40% of women in the sample stated
that they had changed contraceptive methods in the past, and over
20% stated that they were contemplating a future change in contraceptive methods. In this population of young married women, then,
there is clearly a great deal of dissatisfaction and change from
one method to another, a large part of which appears to be related
to the experience of undesirable concomitant reactions.

LONGITUDINAL COMPARISON OF WOMEN ON AND NOT ON ENOVID

In a further investigation in our laboratories Silbergeld,
Brast and Noble studied eight healthy unmarried female students who
served as paid volunteers. They ranged in age from 19-31 years,
had never used oral contraceptives, and were not on any drugs
during the experiment. Their personal histories showed no endocrine, gynecological or psychiatric disorders.

The eight subjects were randomly assigned to two groups of
four each and were studied over four consecutive menstrual cycles
(approximately four months). Those in Group A received five mgm
Enovid, for the first two cycles and placebo for the last two. For
Group B the situation was reversed: the first two cycles were on
placebo and the last two on Enovid. This cross-over design permitted each girl to serve as her own control.

The experiment was conducted on a double-blind basis. The
subjects were instructed to take one tablet at bedtime for twenty
days beginning on the fifth day of the cycle counting from the
first day of bleeding. They were told that in any given cycle the
drug would be either Enovid or a placebo.

Each volunteer measured her daily A.M. basal body temperature
prior to arising with a basal temperature thermometer calibrated
from 96-100°F. Every night the subjects filled out a supplemented
Green-Nowlis Mood Adjective Check List (MACL) (20) as well as the
Menstrual Distress Questionnaire (MDQ).

In order to analyze the data for cyclic variations despite the
wide variation in the lengths of the subjects' cycles, each cycle
was divided into six phases on the basis of two detectable events
in each cycle, namely, the onset of menses (as determined by a
marked drop in basal body temperature). In anovulatory cycles, a
fixed point corresponding to ovulation was established by counting
back fourteen days from the onset of the next menses. The cycle
was partitioned into four phases of fixed length and two of variable length. For each variable, data obtained in the same phase
of the same cycle were averaged to yield a single score for the
phase and thus six scores for each cycle.

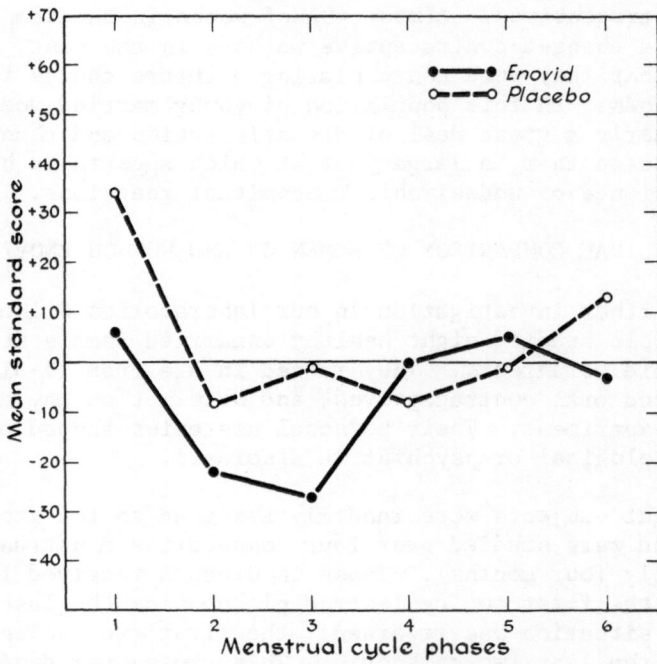

Fig. 10. Comparison of ratings of behavior change of eight
women on Enovid (5 mg) and on placebo.

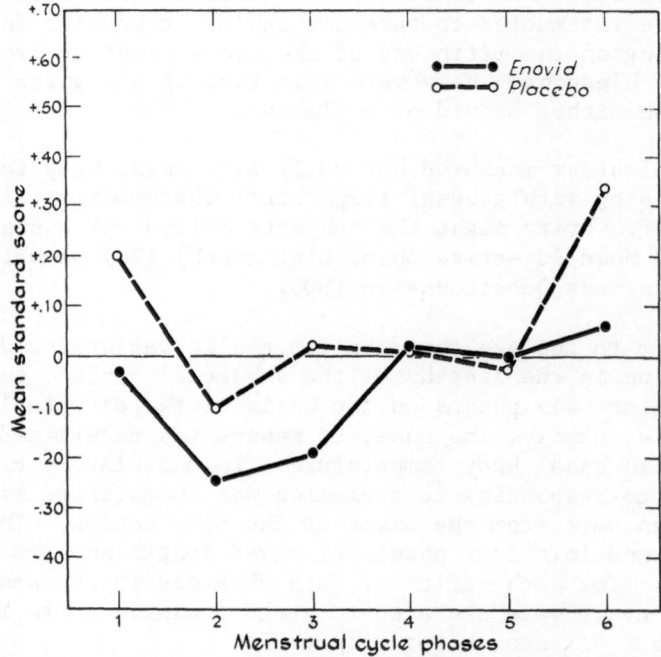

Fig. 11. Comparison of ratings of negative affect on eight
women on Enovid (5 mg) and on placebo.

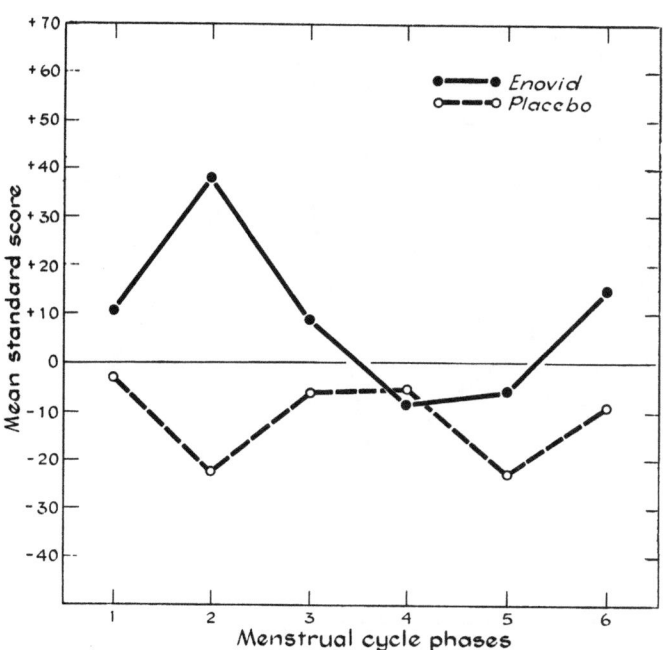

Fig. 12. Comparison of ratings of autonomic reactions of eight women on Enovid and on placebo.

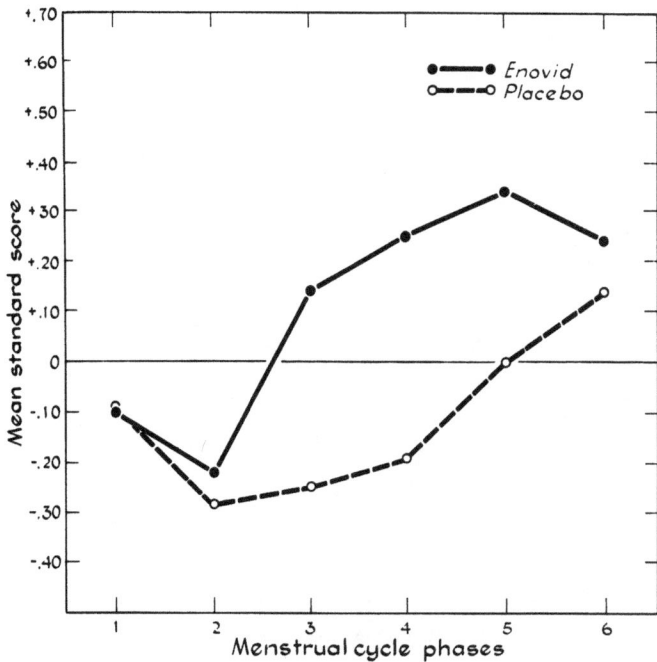

Fig. 13. Comparison of ratings of water retention of eight women on Enovid (5 mg) and on placebo.

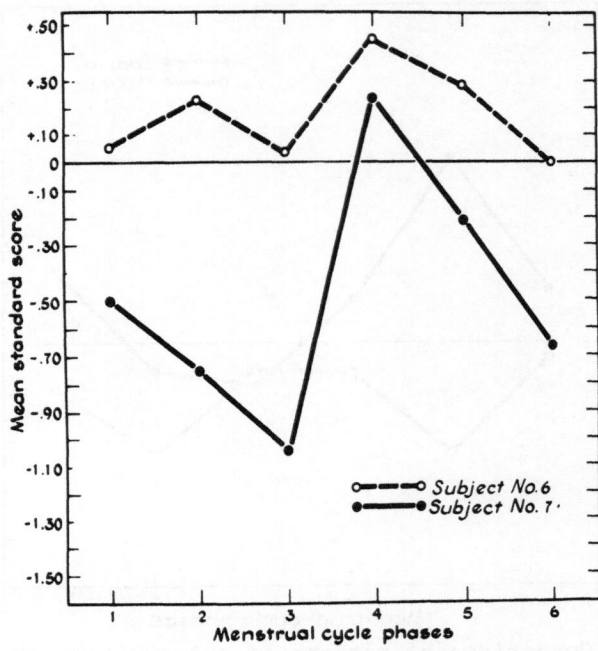

Fig. 14. Example of Enovid-placebo differences for ratings of pain for two women.

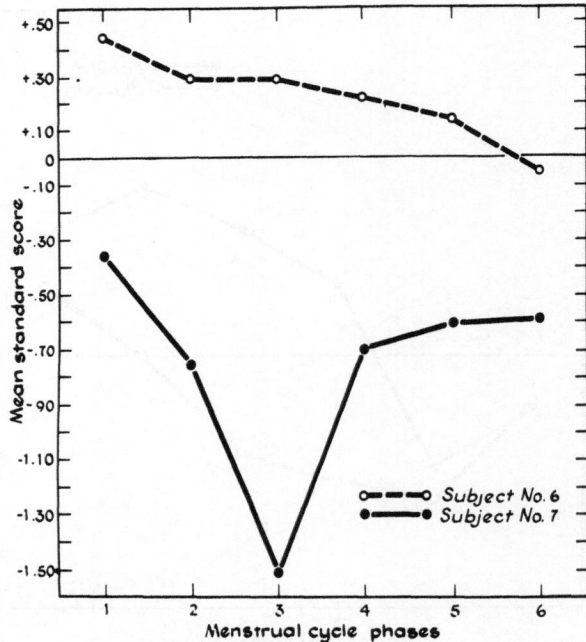

Fig. 15. Example of Enovid-placebo differences for ratings of negative affect for two women.

Most of the data obtained in this study is still being
analyzed; however, some preliminary results have emerged from the
MDQ. Cluster analyses using the Holzinger-Harman F-coefficient (21)
were done for the MDQ variables with averaged normal deviates serving as the measures of association between variables. The resulting eight MDQ clusters obtained were essentially the same as those
previously constructed.

There were a few variables which significantly differentiated
between the Enovid and the placebo cycles. Women complained of more
water retention symptoms, particularly painful and tender breasts,
and more nausea and vomiting in the Enovid than in the placebo
cycles. On the other hand, they complained of more pain, particularly muscle stiffness and backache, of more behavioral change,
particularly taking naps or staying in bed, and of more irritability in the placebo than in the Enovid cycles.

Figures 9-13 graphically show some of these results. Figures
9-11 show that the placebo cycles are higher on pain, negative affect and behavior change, especially during the first part of the
cycle, and, for the latter two variables, during the premenstrual
phase. Figures 12 and 13, on the other hand, show that the Enovid
cycles are generally higher on water retention and autonomic
reactions.

Figures 14 and 15 illustrate the large individual variability
masked by the mean differences. These figures plot the average
Enovid minus placebo scores for the six cycle phases. Subject 6
shows more complaints of pain and negative affect in the Enovid
cycles whereas subject 7 complains more of these symptoms in the
placebo cycles.

DISCUSSION

These results are both consistent with and serve to amplify
those of previous studies. For example, there seems to be little
doubt that progestin-estrogen combinations relieve a number of
symptoms associated with premenstrual tension (22-26). There have
also been many reports that these medications relieve dysmenorrhea.
For example, Andrews and Andrews (27) observed that norethynodrel
with mestranol (Enovid) prevented or significantly relieved dysmenorrhea in 87.5% of patients. Rice-Wray et al (28) reported that
with ten mg of norethindrone with mestranol (Orthonovum) there was
decreased dysmenorrhea in 15% of women but increased pain in 6%.
Similar results have been reported with other medications (29,30).

On the other hand, associated side effects do appear to be consistently prevalent from study to study. For example, Dickinson
and Smith (31) studied 117 private patients over a total of 998

menstrual cycles on five mg of norethindrone with mestranol. They
found that 11 patients (9%) had side effects which caused them to
discontinue use of the medication. Also, 14% of the total sample
reported nausea as a side effect and 13% reported fatigue, irritability, or increased premenstrual tension as side effects.

Wearing (32) studied 62 patients who were also on norethindrone with mestranol over a total of 312 cycles. Of these, 28% of
the women complained of headache, fatigue or tension, 20% complained
of nausea and 16% complained of depression. Wearing concluded that
depression was the most distressing side effect encountered, and
that it seemed that depression, when it occurred, became more prominent the longer the patient remained on medication. Others have
also reported depression as a distressing side effect, especially
in patients with previous history of depressive episodes (33,34),
and Daly et al (35) have reported two cases of psychosis associated with the use of a sequential oral contraceptive.

Nillson and Almgren (36) compared 54 women who were prescribed
oral contraceptives during the postpartum period with 104 women who
used other contraceptive methods. There were no differences between the two groups in respect to psychiatric symptoms and psychological or social factors before medication, i.e., before and
during pregnancy. During the postpartum period a significantly
higher frequency of psychiatric symptoms was found in the oral contraceptive group as regards both the total number of psychiatric
symptoms and individual symptoms of a neurasthenic and depressive
nature.

Nillson et al (37) studied all women who were prescribed an
oral contraceptive during 1964 in a Department of Obstetrics and
Gynecology. Results suggest that psychiatric side effects were almost as common as purely somatic symptoms, and that in many cases
their intensity was sufficiently great to motivate earlier cessation of the oral contraceptive treatment. Individual symptoms of
a neurasthenic or depressive character were the most common encountered. Frequency of psychiatric side effects was not related
to age, parity, marital state or social class. Women with a previous history of psychiatric symptoms and women who had experienced
emotional problems or severe nausea and vomiting during an earlier
pregnancy reported more symptoms.

Nillson and Solvell(38), in a double-blind design, studied
126 women for 12 periods each. Each received four preparations
randomly distributed throughout four cycles and then in the same
order of distribution during eight more cycles. Volidan showed a
very high incidence of spotting and breakthrough bleeding. Ovulen
gave less spotting and breakthrough bleeding than Volidan but significantly more than Anovlar mite and Lyndiol mite. Ovulen caused

more nausea than the other preparations.   The weight increase was
significantly higher for Anovlar mite.

Pincus, after conducting several studies (2,39), has concluded
that only a very small proportion of the side effects actually involve the physiological effects of transition from a woman's characteristic ovarian hormone controlled cyclic events to those insti-
tuted by exogenous hormone control.

However, various physiological effects related to oral contraceptive medication which themselves show individual variability have
been demonstrated.   For example, there is some evidence of increases
in protein-bound iodine (PBI) (40) and decreases in excretion of
17-hydroxycorticosteroids in norethynodrel with mestranol users (41).
There is also evidence of increase in plasma cortisol due at least
in part to increased binding of cortisol to transcortin in subjects
taking estrogen or progestin-estrogen combinations (42).   A recent
study has reported a slow spindle as seen in patients with amenorrhea and anovulatory cycles in the natural sleeping electroencephalogram of patients using oral contraceptives, indicating that
these drugs may alter hypothalamic function (43).   In this connection, there is evidence that the progestins alter arousal thresholds
for stimuli in the hypothalamus of various animals (44).

There certainly are individual differences in these and other
physiological effects of oral contraceptive medication, and these
differences may underlie, at least in part, the large individual
variability in reactions to these medications.   It should be expected that some women will experience endocrine-associated effects
when oral contraceptives are taken clinically.   For example, when
relatively fixed doses of estrogen-progestin preparations are taken
by large numbers of women, the response-distribution curve must be
such that for a certain percentage of women the dose administered
will be either too high or too low.

In this connection it should be pointed out that there is no
à priori evidence to support that curious asymmetrical hypothesis
that increases in menstrual symptomatology are due to psychogenic
factors whereas decreases in menstrual symptomatology are due to
the physiological actions of drugs.

Also, complaints of side effects tend to be most evident
early during the use of drugs and tend to be reported as a rather
low, fairly constant, level thereafter.   It has therefore been suspected that apprehension or other psychogenic causes occasioned by
the use of a new drug might underlie many of the reported side
effects.   However, the length of time an effect exists is not necessarily a good index of whether or not that effect is psychogenic.
There may be increased tolerance in some women in the various

physiological effects of the medication. In addition, the figures
on the percentage of women who report side effects are always based
on the number of women still taking the medication at the time the
evidence for side effects is assessed. Since this number often
declines drastically over several months, partially because the
women who do have disturbing side effects discontinue taking the
medication, these percentage figures may be misleadingly low.

It is of some interest to note that the rejection rate for the
intrauterine contraceptive device (IUCD) appears to be in the same
range as that for the oral contraceptives (45,46). However, there
were enough women who stated, on our questionnaire, that they were
dissatisfied with oral contraceptives but satisfied with the IUCD,
or vice versa, that the hypothesis that women who reject one method
will also redject another must itself be rejected.

The possible psychological ramifications of fertility control
have had most inadequate study. Some relevant questions which need
to be investigated inclued the following: Do oral contraceptives
exert the same effect on emotions as does naturally produced progesterone? Does the continued use of a predominately progestational cycle have the same effect as the naturally produced sequential estrogen-progesterone cycle? Are there interactions between
oral contraceptives and other medications taken concurrently, e.g.,
tranquilizers, which may affect a woman's reaction? To what extent
are some of the observed effects dose-related? Finally, might not
some women who show either particularly marked alleviation or ex-
acerbation of menstrual symptomatology concurrently with oral contraceptive medication have genetically determined differences in
the pathways utilized for steroid medications? The large individual variability in reactions to oral contraceptive medication
would seem to make these questions crucial for further study.

REFERENCES

1. Food and Drug Administration Report on Oral Contraceptives
by the Advisory Committee on Obstetrics and Gynecology, F.D.A.,
Aug. 1, 1966.

2. Pincus, G.: Control of conception by hormonal steroids
Science 153:493-500 (1966).

3. Ryder, N.B. and Westoff, C.F.: Use of oral contraception
in the United States, 1965. Science 153:1199-1205 (1966).

4. Ratner, H.: Oral contraception drop-out rate. Science
155:951 (1967).

5. Moos, R.H. and Baker, K.: Literature review and summary of the premenstrual tension syndrome. Unpublished research report, Stanford University, 1965.

6. Altman, M., Knowles, E. and Bull, H.: A psychometric study of the sex cycle in women. Psychosom. Med. 3:199 (1941).

7. Greene, R. and Dalton, K.: The premenstrual syndrome. Brit. Med. J. 1:1007 (1953).

8. Paulson, M.: Psychological concomitants of premenstrual tension. Doctoral dissertation, University of Kansas, 1956.

9. Coppen, A. and Kessel, N.: Menstruation and personality. Brit. J. Psychiat. 109:711 (1963).

10. Sutherland, H. and Steward, I.: A critical analysis of the premenstrual syndrome. Lancet i:1180 (1965).

11. Blatt, M., Wiesbader, H. and Kupperman, H.: Vitamin E and climacteric syndrome. A.M.A. Arch. Int. Med. 91:792 (1953).

12. Neugarten, B. and Kraines, R.: Menopausal symptoms in women of various ages. Psychosom. Med. 27:266 (1965).

13. Moos, R.H.: The development of a menstrual distress questionnaire. Psychosom. Med., In Press.

14. Moos, R.H.: A typology of menstrual cycle symptoms. Amer. J. Obstet. Gynecol. In Press.

15. Moos, R.H., Kopell, B.S., Melges, F.T., Yalom, I.D., Lunde, D.T., Clayton, R.B. and Hamburg, D.A.: Variations in symptoms and mood during the menstrual cycle. J. Psychosom. Res. In Press.

16. Moos, R.H.: Psychological aspects of oral contraceptives. Archives of General Psychiatry 19:87-94 (1968).

17. Drill, V.A.: Oral Contraceptives. New York: McGraw-Hill Book Co., Inc., 1966.

18. Goldstein, A.: Biostatistics: An Introductory Text. New York, Macmillan Co., Publishers, 1964.

19. Glick, I.D.: Mood and behavioral changes associated with the use of the oral contraceptive agents--A review of the literature. Psychopharmacologia 10:363-374 (1967).

20. Newlis, V.: Research with the mood adjective check list.
In Affect, Cognition and Personality, Tomkins, S. and Izard, C.
(eds.), New York, Springer, pp. 353-389 (1965).

21. Harmon, H.H.: Modern Factor Analysis. University of
Chicago Press, Chicago, 1960.

22. Binks, R., Cambourn, P. and Papworth, R.A.: Preliminary
report of a clinical trial of oral norethynodrel for fertility
control. Med. J. Aust. 49(1):716-717 (1962).

23. Pullen, D.: "Conovid-E" as an oral contraceptive. Brit.
Med. J. 2:1016-1019 (1962).

24. Goldzieher, J.W., Moses, L.E. and Ellis, L.T.: Study of
norethindrone in contraception. JAMA 180:359-361 (1962).

25. Mears, E. and Grant, E.C.G.: "Anovlar" as an oral contraceptive. Brit. Med. J. 2:75-79 (1962).

26. Gould, J.: Control of ovulation with Provest. Int. J.
Fertil. 8:737-741 (1963).

27. Andrews, W.C. and Andrews, M.C.: The use of progestins
for oral contraception. Southern Med. J. 55:454-456 (1962).

28. Rice-Wray, E., Schultz-Contreras, M., Guerrero, I. and
Aranda-Rosell, A.: Long-term administration of norethindrone in
fertility control. JAMA 180:355-358 (1962).

29. Andrews, W.C. and Andrews, M.C.: Reduction of side-effects
from ovulation suppression by the use of newer-progestin conbina-
tions. Fertil. Steril. 15:75-83 (1964).

30. Jungck, E.C.: Sequential estrogen-progestogen therapy in
gynecology. Amer. J. Obstet. Gynec. 94:165-169 (1966).

31. Dickinson, J.H. and Smith, G.G.: A new and practical
oral contraceptive agent: norethindrone with mestranol. Canad.
Med. Assoc. J. 89:242-245 (1963).

32. Wearing, M.P.: The use of norethindrone (two mg) with
mestranol (one mg) in fertility control. Canad. Med. Assoc. J.
89:239-241 (1963).

33. Kaye, B.M.: Oral contraceptives and depression. JAMA
186:522 (1963).

34. Kane, F., Daly, R., Ewing, J. and Keeler, M.: Mood and
behavioral changes with progestational agents. Brit. J. Psychiat.
113:265-268 (1967).

35. Daly, R.J., Kane, F.J. and Ewing, J.A.: Psychosis associated with the use of a sequential oral contraceptive. Lancet
ii:444-445 (1967).

36. Nillson, A. and Almgren, P.E.: Psychiatric symptoms
during the postpartum period as related to use of oral contraceptives. Brit. Med. J. 2:453-455 (1968).

37. Nillson, A., Jacobson, L. and Ingemanson, C.A.: Side-
effects of an oral contraceptive with particular attention to mental symptoms and sexual adaptation. Acta. Obst. et Gynec. Scand.
46:537-556 (1967).

38. Nillson, L. and Solvell, L.: Clinical studies on oral
contraceptives - a randomized doubleblind crossover study of four
different preparations (Anovlar mite, Lyndiol mite, Ovulen and
Volidan). Acta Obst. et Gynec. Scand. 46:537-556 (1967).

39. Pincus, G.: Frontiers in methods of fertility control.
In Human Fertility and Population Problems, Greep, R.O. (ed.),
Schenkman Publishing Co., Inc., Cambridge, Mass., pp. 177-203 (1963).

40. Pincus, G.: The Control of Fertility. Academic Press,
Inc., New York, 1965.

41. Pincus, G.: Long term administration of Enovid to human
subjects. In Proceedings of Symposium on 19-Norprogestational
Steroids, G.D. Searle and Co., Chicago, p. 105 (1957).

42. Carter, A.C., Feldman, E.B. and Wallace, E.Z.: The
effects of steroids on the levels of the plasma 17-hydroxycortico-
steroids and the serum protein-bound iodine. In Biological
Activities of Steroids in Relation to Cancer, Pincus, G. and
Vollmer, E.P. (eds.), Academic Press, Inc., New York, p. 77 (1960).

43. Matsumoto, S., Sato, I., Ito, T. and Matsuoka, A.: Electroencephalographic changes during long term treatment with oral
contraceptives. Int, J. Fertil. 11:195-204 (1966).

44. Sawyer, C.H.: Neuroendocrine Blocking Agents: Discussion
In Advances in Neuroendocrinology, University of Illinois Press,
Urbana, Ill., pp. 451-459 (1963).

45. King, A.G.: Selection of patients for the intrauterine
contraceptive device. Obstet. Gynec. 29:139-141 (1967).

46. Silbar, E.L. and Solomon, E.M.; Intrauterine contraception and the private patient. Clin. Med. 74:25-27 (1967).

BEHAVIORAL EFFECTS OF GONADAL HORMONES AND CONTRACEPTIVE STEROIDS IN PRIMATES

Richard P. Michael

Primate Research Center (Institute of Psychiatry),
Bethlem Royal Hospital, Beckenham, Kent, England

Although there is no doubt that ovarian steroids are essential for the expression of sexual receptivity in those female mammals which show well-defined periods of oestrus or heat, the extent to which this holds true for the higher primates, including man, remains controversial. Although the basic observations on primate sexual behavior must be made in the field, significant contributions to our understanding of the hormonal factors controlling sexual activity have been made by controlled studies under laboratory conditions (1). Nevertheless, a systematic approach to these questions is only just beginning.

The catarrhine monkeys and apes alone among infra-human mammals have true menstruation and, in the case of the rhesus monkey, the cycle is about 28 days. From the many field studies that have been made, certain generalizations may be drawn concerning the sexual interactions between adults of opposite sex: the females of several species of anthropoid primates appear to have periods of heightened receptivity, usually near mid-cycle, when they are more ready to permit the male to copulate (Alouatta palliata, (2); on vaginal plug evidence in Ateles geoffroyi Kuhl, (3); Presbytes entellus, (4); Macaca mulatta, (5-8); M. fuscata, (9); Papio ursinus and P. anubis, (10-12); P. hamadryas, (13); Pan troglodytes schweinfurthii, (14,15)). The conclusions drawn from these field studies receive added support

---
The original work reported here with contraceptive steroids was supported by grants from the Medical Research Council and the Population Council which are gratefully acknowledged. Mr. T.M. Plant was supported by a Research Studentship from the Science Research Council.

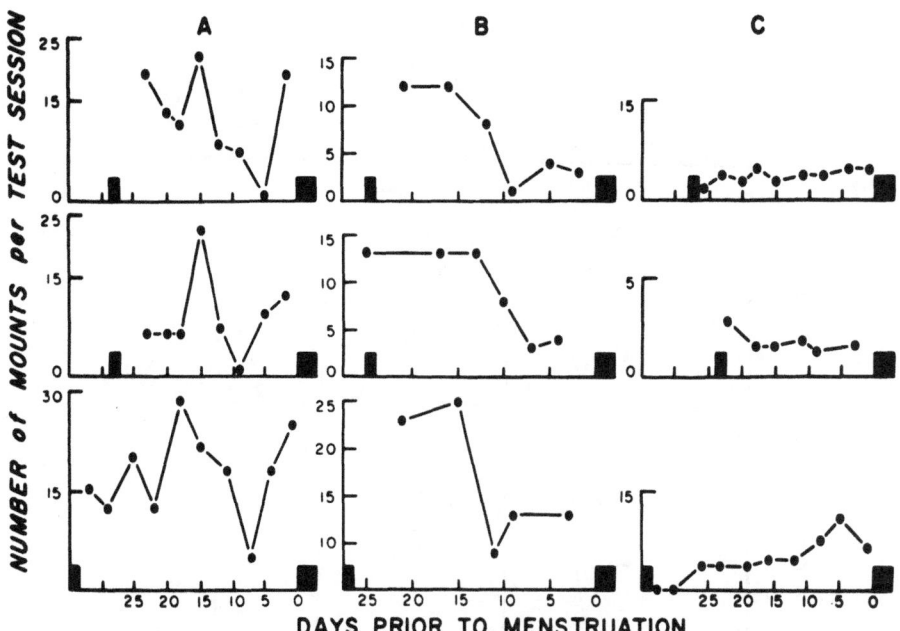

A Maxima at mid-cycle and secondary pre-menstrual rise

B High activity in follicular phase and low activity in luteal phase

C No rhythmic changes

Fig. 1.   Rhythmic changes in the mounting activity of male
rhesus monkeys during the menstrual cycles of their female partners.
Examples from nine pairs of animals illustrating the three main
types of changes that are observed.   Solid rectangles indicate
vaginal bleeding.

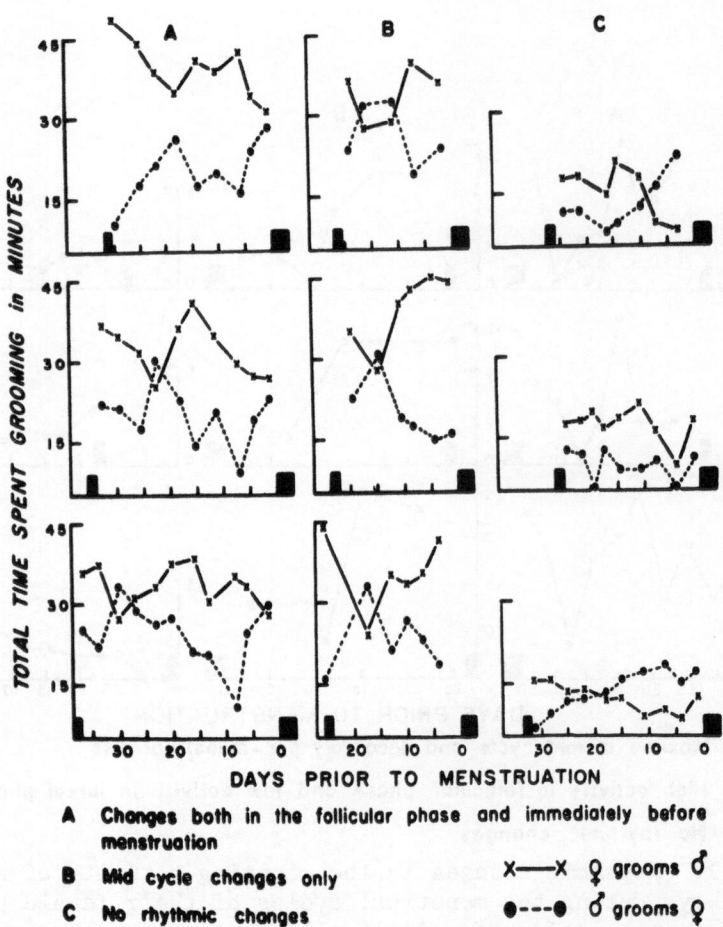

Fig. 2. Rhythmic changes in the grooming activity of pairs of adult rhesus monkeys of opposite sex during the menstrual cycle of the female of the pair. Examples from nine pairs of animals illustrating the three main types of changes that are observed. Grooming times in mins. per one hour test session. Solid rectangles indicate vaginal bleeding.

from more recent experiments conducted in the laboratory. Copulation in the rhesus monkey is particularly suitable for quantitative study as it consists of a series of separate mounts, each with an intromission and thrusting, the series being terminated in the final, ejaculatory mount. When a female rhesus monkey is introduced into a spacious cage with an active male, some aspects of the copulatory sequence already referred to are usually observed together with grooming behavior. In the laboratory, rhythmic changes in both these aspects of primate behavior have been noted to occur in relation to the menstrual cycle of the female of the pair (16-21).

HORMONAL INFLUENCES ON MOUNTING AND GROOMING BEHAVIOR

Considering, first, the rhythmic fluctuations in the mounting activity of the pair: if a count is made of the sexual mounts by the male on the female during 60-minute test sessions conducted on successive days of the menstrual cycle, depending on the identity of the pair, the numbers tend to increase towards mid-cycle, when ejaculation times also become shorter, and then decline in number during the luteal phase of the cycle. Figure 1 shows examples of the three main patterns of mounting that are observed: A) those with well-defined maxima near mid-cycle, sharp declines early in the luteal phase and secondary increases immediately before menstruation; B) those with sustained high levels of mounting activity throughout the follicular phase, again sharp declines early in the luteal phase and with these low levels persisting until the next menstruation; C) those pairs not showing any evidence of rhythmic changes in mounting activity, which may be at high or low levels during the cycle, although low levels are the ones illustrated. Very striking individual variations and partner preferences exist which are not encountered to anything like the same extent in lower mammals, but which will be familiar to those working in the clinical field. Nevertheless, clear-cut rhythms in sexual activity have been observed in some 50% of the pairs studied by us, and these now number several dozen. Grooming is also a conspicuous feature of primate behavior. Although originally regarded as subserving the needs of hygiene, it is now apparent that this activity has wider significance. Not only is it related to the establishment of hierarchies of dominance and submission between animals, but it also serves to define the position of an individual within the highly organized primate society (5,6,11,22,23). Changes in mutual grooming behavior also form part of the changing interaction between males and females that occur in relation to the menstrual cycle of the female (17,31); thus, it provides a subtle indication of the state of the socio-sexual integration existing between partners (Fig. 2). Both mounting rhythms and grooming rhythms are abolished by bilateral ovariectomy of the female of the pair, and the behavior can be restored by administration of oestrogens to the ovariectomized female (Figs. 3,4). There can be no doubt then, that

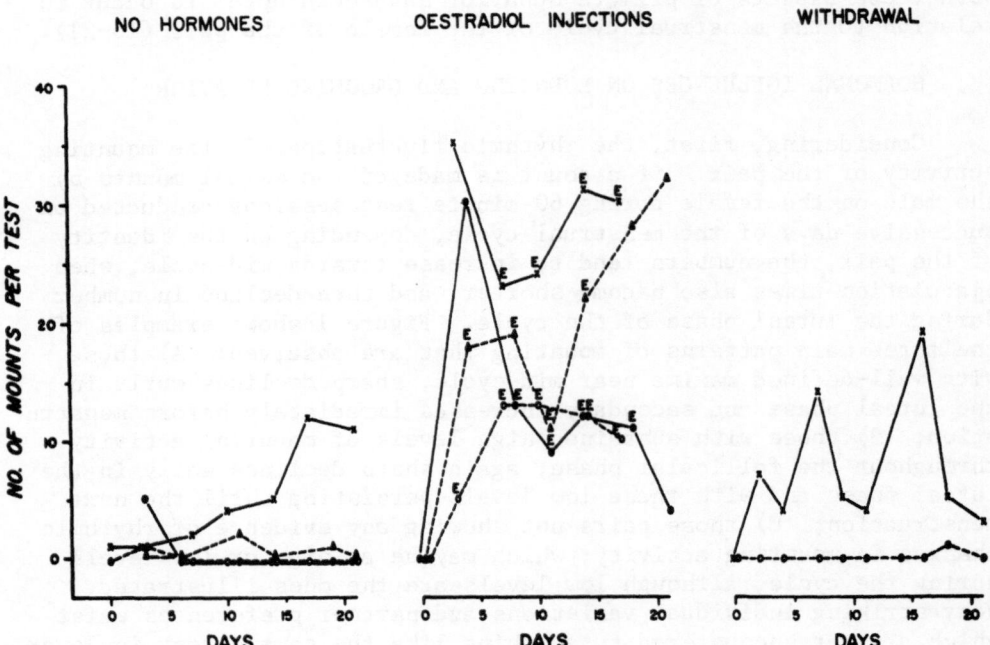

Fig. 3. Ovariectomy results in a depression of mounting activity and a loss of mounting rhythms. Male mounting and ejaculations are restored when their ovariectomized partners receive oestradiol (25 µg/day, s.c.). When the hormone is withdrawn, behavior may return rapidly to base-line or remain unstable for prolonged periods. E = tests with ejaculations.

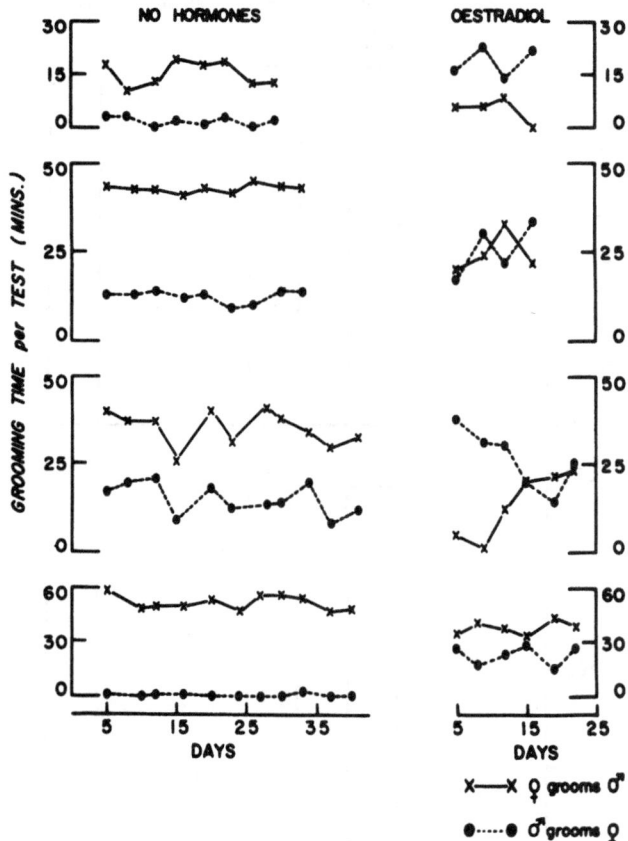

Fig. 4. The effect of ovariectomy and of the administration
of oestradiol on grooming times in four pairs of rhesus monkeys.
Ovariectomy abolishes all grooming rhythms and the stability of the
grooming times is noteworthy. Oestradiol administration to the female results in increased grooming by males and decreased grooming
by females, thus reproducing the pattern observed near mid-cycle.

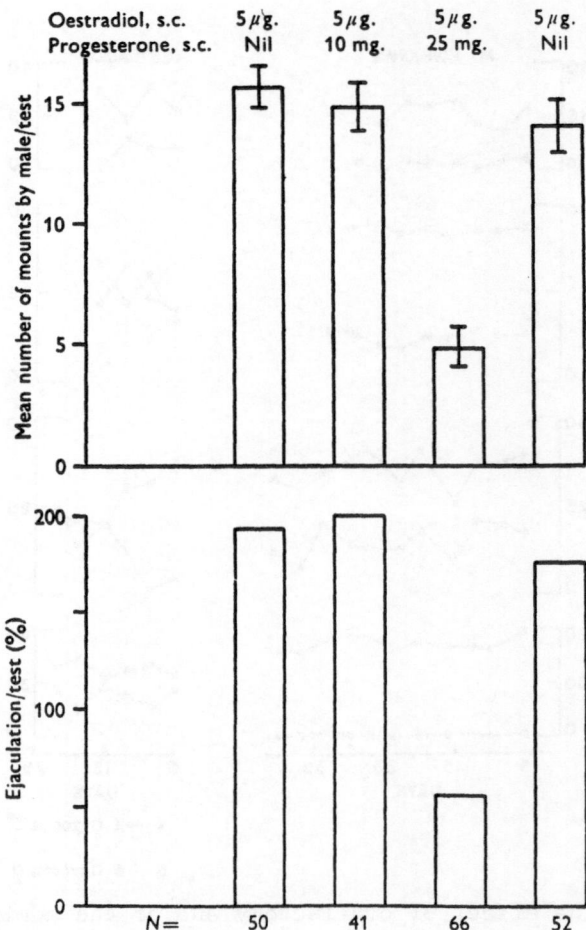

Fig. 5. The suppression of mounting activity and of ejaculation in male rhesus monkeys by the administration of progesterone
to their ovariectomized, oestrogen-treated female partners. N =
number of one-hour tests (six pairs). Vertical lines show the
standard errors of the means. (Where values exceed 100%, more than
one ejaculation occurred per test.)

that these behaviors are influenced by endocrine mechanisms and
that gonadal hormones play a significant role in determining both
the social and the sexual activity of these higher primates.

EFFECTS OF PROGESTERONE

The role of progestational agents in controlling primate sexual behavior has not been systematically investigated to date but
has a fresh importance now that oral progestins are taken by large
numbers of women for contraception. Progesterone facilitates sexual receptivity in the ovariectomized, oestrogen-primed mouse (24),
rat (25), guinea pig (26) and hamster (27); in these forms, progesterone induces psychic oestrus, usually with a latency of a few
hours and acts synergistically with oestrogen. In contrast, rabbits
in postpartum oestrus are thrown out of heat by progesterone treatment (28) and implants of progesterone inhibit stilbestrol-induced
oestrus in the spayed ferret (29); in these latter cases there is
clear antagonism. These striking species differences made it necessary to approach this problem afresh in the primate (30-32). The
changes in the mean number of mounts by males per test in six pairs
(209 tests) are shown in Figure 5 (upper part). When ovariectomized
females receiving constant daily doses of oestradiol (5 μg per day
subcutaneously (s.c.)) were given in addition 25 mg progesterone
s.c. daily, the number of mounts per test was reduced significantly
(P < 0.001) as compared with all other treatment conditions. When
progesterone was withdrawn, mounting returned to levels that did
not differ significantly from those before its administration.
During the administration of oestradiol to the females, there was a
high incidence of ejaculation by male partners, with two ejaculations occurring in the majority of tests. Treatment of these females with progesterone in addition to the oestrogen resulted in a
marked decrease in the incidence of ejaculation in five of the six
pairs: in three pairs, it was abolished; in two pairs, reduced to
less than half; and, in the remaining pair, it was relatively unchanged. Comparison of the group results for different treatments
showed that the incidence of ejaculation decreased significantly
with 25 mg progesterone (χ^2 = 62.5, P < 0.001), and was restored
when progesterone was withdrawn (Fig. 5, lower part). Without entering here into a discussion of the behavioral mechanisms underlying these changes, it is evident that the administration of progesterone to the female results in a marked suppression of the
mounting activity of the male partner and in a dramatic decline in
the ejaculatory performance of these males.

BEHAVIORAL EFFECTS OF SOME CONTRACEPTIVE STEROIDS

In view of these findings it was considered of interest to investigate the sexual activity of male rhesus monkeys during the
treatment of their female partners with combinations of an oestrogen

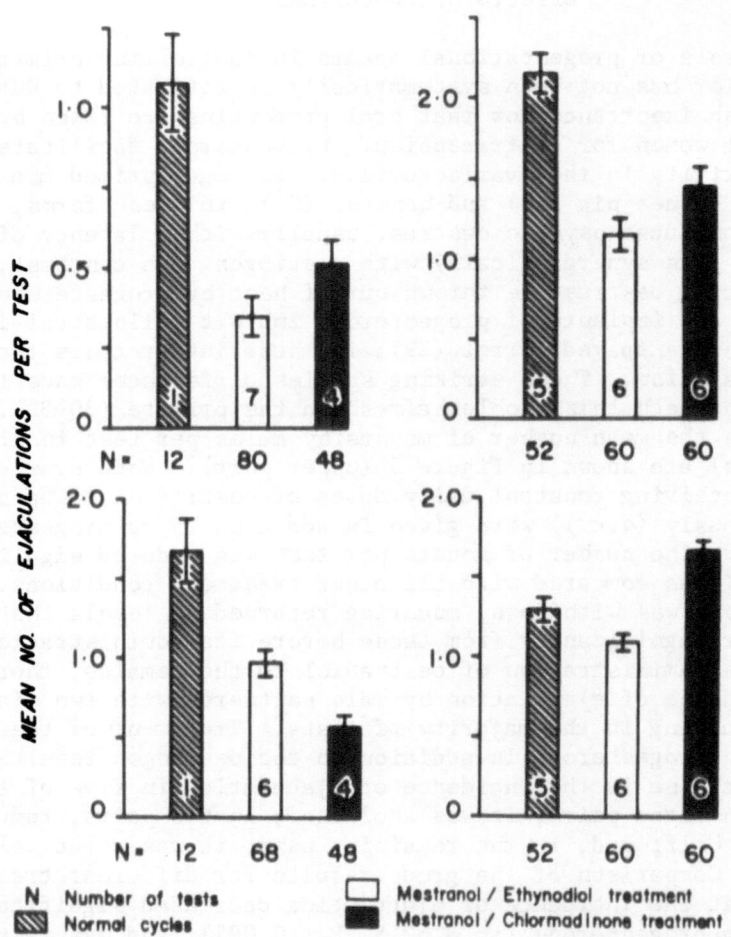

Fig. 6. Effect on the ejaculatory performance of male rhesus monkeys of treating their partners with contraceptive steroids. In three of the four pairs, a marked depression of ejaculation resulted. Vertical bars give standard error of means. Numbers within columns give the number of menstrual cycles or of treatment cycles. (612 tests of one-hour). Michael and Plant - unpublished observations.

and different progestins that are currently used by women for oral
contraceptive purposes. The studies reported here were conducted
in collaboration with Mr. T.M. Plant of this laboratory. Two mature
female and four adult, sexually active, male rhesus monkeys, all
jungle-bred have been investigated for periods of 14-17 months.
Each female was paired with two different males making a total of
four paired combination. The females were introduced regularly, by
means of a wheeled transfer cage, into large testing compartments
occupied by a male for tests of 60-minute duration. Each pair was
tested two to three times/week, and, between tests, animals were
housed together in the same room in individual cages without access
to each other. Observers scored the behavior during tests from be-
hind one-way vision mirrors, using techniques described previously
(33). In order to prevent pregnancies during the pre-treatment period, the Fallopian tubes of the females were ligated. After one to
five months observation without treatment, each female received daily
0.05 mg mestranol and 1.0 mg ethynodiol diacetate for 21 days, followed by seven days without treatment, when the cycle of treatment
was repeated. This routine was maintained for six to seven months
and was then changed to a sequential regimen consisting of 0.05 mg
mestranol for 11 days, then 0.05 mg mestranol with 0.75 mg chlormadinone acetate for the next ten days, followed by seven days without treatment; this latter routine was maintained for four to six
months. Thus, the schedules of treatment were similar to those recommended for human contraception. All compounds were given subcutaneously because the oral route of administration proved unreliable in these primates. Since the testing routing remained unchanged
throughout with the same pairs of animals, a direct comparison of
the effects of the two types of treatment was possible.

Although changes in several behavioral measures were observed
and scored, we are only describing here effects on male ejaculatory
capacity and thrusting performance. The latter is known to be a
sensitive indicator of male sexual activity and increases at times
when female receptivity is low, for example, after ovariectomy.
Figure 6 shows a marked decrease in the mean number of ejaculations
per test in three of the four pairs studied when both the combined
and the sequential treatments were compared with normal menstrual
cycles. In three pairs, also, the depression of ejaculation was
somewhat less marked during the sequential regime than during the
combined treatment regime. As was mentioned above, the total number
of intromitted thrusts occurring prior to ejaculation provided an
additional measure of male sexual performance in those tests in
which ejaculation was not abolished (34). When ejaculation times
are short, for instance near mid-cycle, and stimulation of the penis
by the vagina is optimal, the male works less hard and the number of
thrusts required for ejaculation is lower. Figure 7 shows an increase in the mean number of thrusts to ejaculation in all four
pairs while the females were receiving contraceptive agents. This

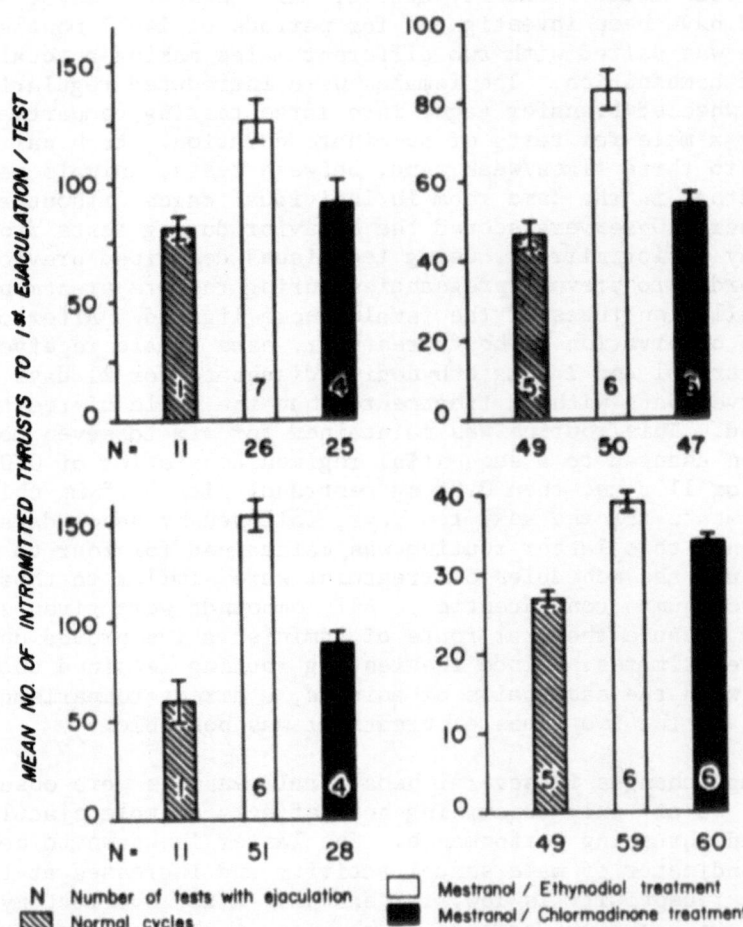

Fig. 7. Effect on the thrusting performance of male rhesus
monkeys of treating their partners with contraceptive steroids. In
all four pairs, more thrusts were required to achieve ejaculation
during treatment, and this effect was more marked with the combined
than with the sequential regime. The same pairs and cycles as in
Figure 6. Michael and Plant - unpublished observations.

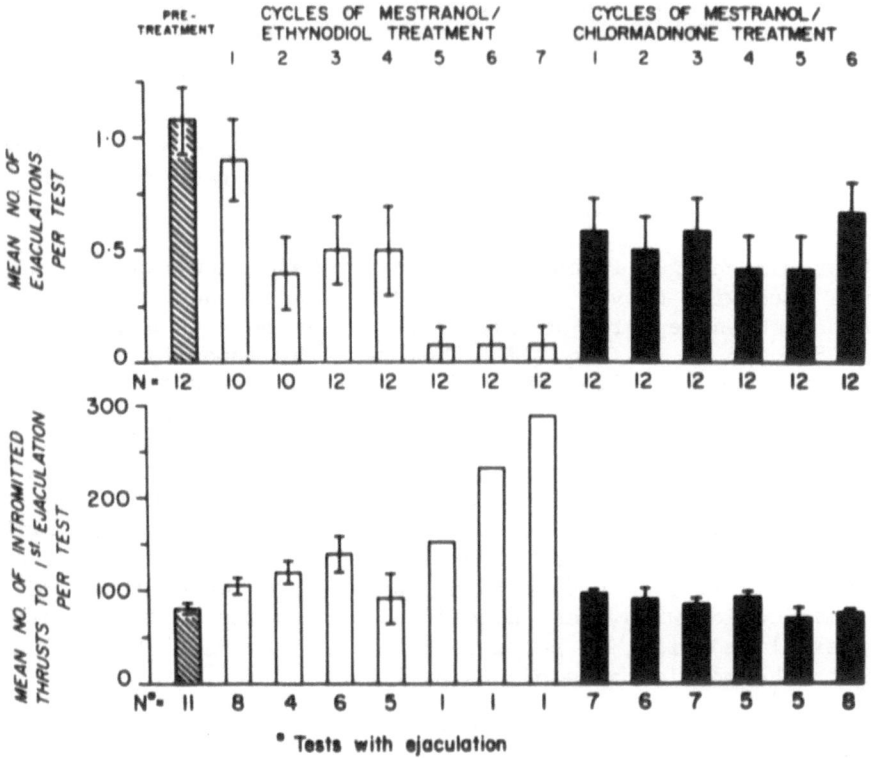

Fig. 8. Effect on the sexual behavior of a male rhesus
monkey of successive cycles of treatment of the female partner with
contraceptive steroids. With a mestranol-ethynodiol regime, the
depression of ejaculation and increase in thrusting was progressive.
With a mestranol-chlormadinone regime, the impairment of ejaculation was not progressive and thrusting was not changed. (164 tests).
Michael and Plant - unpublished observations.

effect was more marked during the combined than during the sequential treatment since, over all, the number of thrusts made by males
to achieve ejaculation nearly doubled.

When the effects of successive cycles of treatment on the behavior of individual pairs were examined in more detail, clear differences between the two treatment regimes emerged that were not so
obvious in the group data. With mestranol-ethynodiol both the depression of ejaculation and the increase in thrusting changed progressively with successive cycles of treatment, and in one pair
during the seventh month of treatment, ejaculation occurred only
once in twelve tests while the number of thrusts required to achieve
it had trebled (Fig. 8). With mestranol-chlormadinone, in contrast,
the impairment of ejaculation was not obviously progressive and
thrusting remained virtually unchanged.

Profound changes in mood and behavior have been reported in
patients receiving Enovid (35,36), and depression and loss of
libido have been reported in 30% of 136 women on Anovlar, and in
34% of 85 women on Volidan (37). However, the majority of reports
refer to increased desire for, and greater satisfaction from, coitus because of removal of the fear of pregnancy. Data from infra-
human primates cannot substitute for adequate clinical evaluation
and it is never wise to extrapolate across species boundaries:
this is especially the case for human sexual behavior which is influenced by so many subtle, social and cultural factors. Nevertheless, the data on contraceptive agents reported here are clear-cut,
and the possibility should certainly not be overlooked that prolonged medication with these powerful steroids may in time modify
human sexual behavior, in particular that of the male, by influencing the hormonal status of his partner.

REFERENCES

1. Michael, R.P.: Gonadal hormones and the control of primate
behavior, in Endocrinology and Human Behavior. ed. Michael, R.P.
Oxford University Press, London, p. 69-93 (1968).

2. Carpenter, C.R.: A field study of the behavior and social
relations of howling monkeys (Alouatta palliata). Comp. Psychol.
Monogr. 10:1-168 (1934).

3. Carpenter, C.R.: Behavior of red spider monkeys in Panama
J. Mammal. 16:171-180 (1935).

4. Jay, P.: The common langur of North India. In Primate
Behavior ed. deVore, I., Holt, Rinehart and Winston, New York,
pp. 197-249 (1965).

5. Carpenter, C.R.: Sexual behavior of free-ranging rhesus monkey (Macaca mulatta). I. Specimens, procedures and behavioral characteristics of estrus. J. Comp. Psychol. 33:113-142 (1942).

6. Carpenter, C.R.: Sexual behavior of free-ranging rhesus monkeys (Macaca mulatta). II. Periodicity of estrus, homosexual, autoerotic and non-conformist behavior. J. Comp. Psychol. 33:143-162 (1942).

7. Altmann, S.A.: A field study of the sociobiology of rhesus monkeys (Macaca mulatta). Ann. N.Y. Acad. Sci. 102:338-435 (1962).

8. Southwick, G.B., Beg, M.A. and Siddiqi, M.R.: Rhesus monkeys in North India. In Primate Behavior ed. deVore, I. Holt, Rinehart and Winston, New York, p. 111-159 (1965).

9. Imanishi, E.: Social behavior in Japanese monkeys, (Macaca fuscata) In Primate Social Behavior ed. Southwick, C.H. London, p. 68-81 (1963).

10. Bolwig, N.: A study of the behavior of the chacma baboon (Papio ursinus) Behavior 14:136-163 (1959).

11. Washburn, S.L. and deVore, I.: The social life of baboons Sci. Amer. 204:62-71 (1961).

12. Hall, K.R.L. and deVore, I.: Baboon social behavior. In Primate Behavior. ed. deVore, I. Holt, Rinehart and Winston, New York, p. 53-110 (1965).

13. Kummer, H. and Kurt, F.: Social units of a free-living population of hamadryas baboons. Folia primat. 1:4-19 (1963).

14. Young, W.C. and Orbison, W.D.: Changes in selected features of behavior in pairs of oppositely-sexed chimpanzees during the sexual cycle and after ovariectomy. J. Comp. Psychol. 37:107-143 (1944).

15. Goodall, J.: Chimpanzees of the Gombe Stream Reserve. In Primate Behavior. ed. deVore, I. Holt, Rinehart and Winston, New York, p. 425-473 (1965).

16. Ball, J. and Hartman, C.G.: Sexual excitability as related to the menstrual cycle in the monkey. Amer. J. Obstet. Gynec. 39:117-119 (1935).

17. Michael, R.P. and Herbert, J.: Menstrual cycle influences grooming behavior and sexual activity in the rhesus monkey. Science 140:500-501 (1963).

18. Michael, R.P.: Some aspects of the endocrine control of sexual activity in primates. Proc. Roy. Soc. Med. 58:595-598 (1965).

19. Michael, R.P., Herbert, J. and Welegalla, J.: Ovarian hormones and grooming behavior in the rhesus monkey (Macaca mulatta) under laboratory conditions. J. Endocr. 36:263-279 (1966).

20. Michael, R.P., Herbert, J. and Welegalla, J.: Ovarian hormones and the sexual behavior of the male rhesus monkey (Macaca mulatta) under laboratory conditions. J. Endocr. 39:81-98 (1967).'

21. Michael, R. P. and Welegalla, J.: Ovarian hormones and the sexual behavior of the female rhesus monkey (Macaca mulatta) under laboratory conditions. J. Endocr. 41: 407-420 (1968).

22. Zuckerman, S.: The Social Life of Monkeys and Apes. Kegan Paul, London (1932).

23. Maslow, A.H. and Flanzbaum, S.: Role of dominance in the social and sexual behavior of infra-human primates. II. An experimental determination of the behavior syndrome of dominance. J. Genet. Psychol. 48:278-309 (1936).

24. Ring, J.R.: The estrogen-progesterone induction of sexual receptivity in the spayed female mouse. Endocr. 34:269-275 (1944).

25. Boling, J.L. and Blandau, R.J.: The oestrogen-progesterone induction of mating responses in the spayed female rat. Endocr. 25:259-364 (1939).

26. Dempsey, E.W., Hertz, R. and Young, W.C.: The experimental induction of oestrus (sexual receptivity) in the normal and ovariectomized guinea pig. Am. J. Physiol. 116:201-209 (1936).

27. Kent, G.C. and Liberman, M.J.: Induction of psychic estrus in the hamster with progesterone administered via the lateral brain ventricle. Endocr. 45:29-32 (1949).

28. Makepeace, A.W., Weinstein, G.L. and Friedman, M.H.: The effect of progestin and progesterone on ovulation in the rabbit. J. Physiol. Lond. 119:512-516 (1937).

29. Marshall, F.H.A. and Hammond, J.: Experimental control by hormone action of the oestrus cycle in the ferret. J. Endocr. 4:159-168 (1945).

30. Michael, R.P., Herbert, J. and Saayman, G.: Loss of ejaculation in male rhesus monkeys after administration of progesterone to their female partners. Lancet ii:1015-1016 (1966).

31. Michael, R.P., Saayman, G. and Zumpe, D.: Sexual attractiveness and receptivity in rhesus monkeys. Nature 215:554-556 (1967).

32. Michael, R.P., Saayman, G. and Zumpe, D.: Inhibition of sexual receptivity by progesterone in rhesus monkeys (Macaca mulatta), J. Endocr. 39:309-310 (1967).

33. Michael, R.P. and Saayman, G.: Individual differences in the sexual behavior of male rhesus monkeys (Macaca mulatta) under laboratory conditions. Anim. Behav. 15:460-466 (1967).

34. Michael, R.P. and Saayman, G.: Sexual performance and the timing of ejaculation in male rhesus monkeys (Macaca mulatta). J. Comp. Physiol. Psychol 64:213-218 (1967).

35. Keeler, M., Kane, F. and Daly, R.: An acute schizophrenic episode following abrupt withdrawal of Enovid in a patient with previous postpartum psychiatric disorder. Am. J. Psychiat. 120:1123-1124 (1964).

36. Kane, F., Daly, R., Ewing, J. and Keeler, M.: Mood and behavioral changes with progestational agents. Brit. J. Psychiat. 113:265-268 (1967).

37. Grant, E.C.G. and Mears, E.: Mental effects of oral contraceptives. Lancet i: 945-946 (1967).

ROLE OF THE CENTRAL NERVOUS SYSTEM IN THE CONTROL OF

REPRODUCTIVE MECHANISMS BY GONADAL STEROIDS

Julian M. Davidson

Department of Physiology, Stanford University Medical
School, Stanford, California

Modification of gonadotropin secretion is the principal means whereby the oral contraceptive agents control fertility, and their natural counterparts - the ovarian hormones - regulate the reproductive cycle. Estrogenic steroids have inhibitory or "negative feedback" effects on the secretion of FSH and LH; progestins have a similar relationship to LH. Under certain circumstances both types of steroid can have stimulatory ("positive feedback") effects on LH secretion. Synergistic relationships have been demonstrated between the inhibitory effects of the two ovarian steroids (1).

In the physiological control of ovulation it is probable that both stimulatory and inhibitory effects of estrogen play a role, and that progesterone is important in the inhibition of gonadotropin secretion in pregnancy, pseudopregnancy, and the normal cycle. The stimulatory role of estrogen has been best substantiated in the rat (2). Progesterone apparently does not have this type of triggering function in ovulation since its level does not rise until after the ovulatory release of gonadotropin in rats and humans (3-5). In rabbits, however, it has been suggested that ovarian progestin exerts positive feedback action after the initial release of LH to maintain high LH levels during the preovulatory period (6).

A clear-cut negative feedback relationship exists between testosterone and gonadotropin secretion in the male, and this could be the basis for a future male antifertility "pill". Another possibility for future utilization of the feedback action of gonadal

Supported by USPHS Grant #HD-00778.

steroids in fertility control is the inhibition, perhaps by an anti-estrogen, of the stimulation by estrogen of the ovulatory surge of LH secretion.

In view of the practical and theoretical importance of these feedback systems, it is regrettable that so little is known of the mechanisms involved. It fact, we are woefully lacking even in much of the basic information on the dynamic interactions between gonadal steroids and gonadotropic hormones. How long does it take for changes in gonadal steroid concentration to "turn on" or "turn off" secretion of FSH and LH? How do different steroids interact in their feedback functions under physiological conditions? Indeed, what are the precise dose-response relationships between administered steroid and secreted gonadotropin? Not least, in view of the important controlling action of the CNS on gonadotropin secretion, is the question of whether the gonadal steroids act directly on the pituitary or indirectly on those CNS regions which exert that control.

Localization of the sites of the feedback actions of the various steroid hormones is important for an understanding of neuro-endocrine control mechanisms, as a basis for future work on the biochemical mechanisms of feedback action, and as a matter of practical importance in the provision of new agents for fertility control. The most direct experimental approach to this problem is by the intracranial implantation of small amounts of crystalline steroids, although various less direct methods have also proved useful (7). Some of the available information resulting from implantation experiments will be briefly reported here; more complete discussions may be found in recent review articles (7,8).

The method of chronic intracranial implantation of crystalline steroids was introduced by Harris, Michael and Scott (9) in order to localize the effect of estrogen on sex behavior in cats, and was later applied by Lisk to the study of gonadotropin feedback mechanisms in rats (10). Comparison of the feedback effects of intra-hypothalamic and intrapituitary estrogen was first made on rabbits (11). Implants in the median eminence region inhibited copulation-induced ovulation and eventually led to ovarian atrophy, while similar implants in the anterior pituitary and adjacent hypothalamic areas were ineffective. Subsequent work confirmed and extended these findings (12), and similar results have been obtained in rats by others (13). It appears, however, that implants in the pituitary of rats may also have some inhibitory action (14,15), and it is possible that part of the effects of estrogen implants in the median eminence may result from transport of the implanted steroid through the portal vessel system to the pituitary (16). Investigations using a variety of other methods have generally supported the view that the primary site of negative feedback action of estrogen is

at the hypothalamic level (17-19), even though secondary effects on
the pituitary cannot be ruled out.

The site of the stimulatory action of estrogen on gonadotropin
secretion has been studied in reference to the phenomenon that small
amounts of estrogen administered to immature female rats will advance the onset of puberty (20-22). When various hypothalamic sites
of implantation were compared, it was found that placement of crystalline estradiol benzoate in the anterior hypothalamic-preoptic
region was effective in inducing precocious vaginal opening and estrous cycles, while similar implants in the median eminence region
had no significant effect (21). This suggests a separation of the
stimulatory and inhibitory effects of estrogen on gonadotropin secretion, in that their actions are exerted on different regions of
the hypothalamus. These findings were incorporated into a tentative hypothesis on the mechanism controlling the onset of puberty
in the female rat. The possibility that another site of the stimulatory action of estrogen in the prepuberal animal is the pituitary could not, however, be eliminated in the study of Smith and
Davidson (21), and is strongly suggested by the work of Docke and
Dorner (20).

We have recently applied the method of intracranial implantation to the investigation of the site of inhibitory feedback action
of progesterone (Smith, Weick and Davidson, unpublished). Ovulation and estrous cycles were suppressed by implantation of progesterone in the median eminence region of rats, but not in neighboring hypothalamic regions or the anterior pituitary itself. Follicular development was generally unimpaired, suggesting that the
predominant effect is not on FSH but on LH secretion. While the
evidence is against a direct pituitary action for LH inhibition by
progesterone, the possibility of a pituitary site of its stimulatory action in the advancement of ovulation in adult rats is raised
by recent findings in this laboratory (Weick and Davidson, unpublished). Other investigators have provided evidence for a hypothalamic site of action of the orally active progestational anti-
fertility agents (23-25).

The evidence relating to testosterone is less equivocal than
for the ovarian steroids. Crystalline testosterone implants in
the median eminence region, but not in the neighboring hypothalamus
or in the pituitary resulted in testicular atrophy in dogs (26) and
rats (27-29). This result cannot be explained by spread of implanted androgen to the pituitary, since hypothalamic implants of
testosterone also inhibit gonadotropin secretion from ectopic pituitary transplants in hypophysectomized male rats (30). The converse
aspect of negative feedback regulation - stimulation of gonadotropin secretion by decreased testosterone concentrations - has also
been localized to the median eminence region. Implants of a

specific anti-androgen, cyproterone (1,2 α-methylene 6-chloropregn-4, 6-diene-17-α-ol-3, 20-dione), in this area but not in other neighboring regions or in the pituitary itself, resulted in stimulation of gonadotropin secretion in male rats (31,8). Evidence has been supplied that a change in hypothalamic sensitivity to the negative feedback effect of testosterone may account for the onset of puberty in the male rat (29,8).

Another effect of testosterone which has been localized to the hypothalamus is the activation of sexual behavior responses. The complete pattern of mating may be restored in long-term castrate male rats by single intrahypothalamic implants of testosterone, the effective area being more widespread than is the case for the negative feedback-sensitive region (32).

An attempt to compare some of the functional characteristics of these two actions of testosterone on the hypothalamus has been made (8). Among differences noted were the fact that considerably more testosterone is required to activate negative feedback inhibition of LH secretion than to maintain sexual behavior in male rats; the opposite relationship applies to the differential sensitivity of these systems to estrogen. Of particular interest in this regard, however, are recent findings on the effects of anti-androgen implantation (8).

When a relatively large quantity of crystalline cyproterone (4-600μg) was implanted via double stainless steel tubes in the anterior and posterior hypothalamus of normal male rats, no effects on patterns of sexual behavior could be found. When these animals were castrated, however, it was noted that the decline in this behavior was retarded in animals implanted with cyproterone. Furthermore, the recovery of behavioral responses in castrated rats injected with testosterone was significantly facilitated by the presence of intrahypothalamic cyproterone (8). In addition, subcutaneous injections of cyproterone acetate significantly slowed the decline in sexual behavior following castration of male rats (Bloch and Davidson, unpublished).

Interestingly enough, we have now observed that cyproterone acetate, which was previously thought to be devoid of androgenic activity (33), will, on systemic administration, maintain the androgen-dependent cornified papillae on the glans penis of castrated male rats (Bloch and Davidson, unpublished). These results suggest, therefore, both a difference between the hypothalamic receptors for the feedback and behavioral actions of testosterone, as well as a similarity between hypothalamic androgen receptors subserving the sex behavioral function and the receptors located in the penile epithelium.

An alternate interpretation is that cyproterone has inherent though very weak androgenicity, and that these two types of receptor are extremely sensitive to androgen in the conditions of these experiments. This possibility is currently under investigation. In either case, the resemblance between the two androgen substrates is a matter which merits future study because of its possible relevance to the investigation of the cellular and molecular actions of androgen.

REFERENCES

1. McCann, S.M.: Effect of progesterone on plasma luteinizing hormone activity. Amer. J. Physiol. 202:601-604 (1962).

2. Schwartz, N.B.: New concepts of gonadotropin and steroid feedback control mechanisms. In Textbook of Gynecologic Endocrinology (J.J. Gold, ed) pp. 33-50 (1968).

3. Feder, H.H., Brown-Grant, K., Corker, C.S. and Exley, D.: Systemic plasma progesterone levels during the pro-oestrous critical period in rats. J. Endocrin. (In press) (1969).

4. Miyake, T.: Interrelationship between the release of pituitary luteinizing hormone and secretions of ovarian estrogen and progestin during estrous cycle of the rat. Integrative Mechanism of Neuroendocrine System. (S. Itoh, ed.) Hokkaido University Medical Library Series No. 1, pp. 139-149 (1968).

5. Neill, J.D., Johansson, E.D.B., Datta, J.K. and Knobil, E.: Relationship between plasma levels of luteinizing hormone and progesterone during the normal menstrual cycle. J. Clin. Endocrin. 27:1167-1173 (1967).

6. Hilliard, J. Penardi, R. and Sawyer, C.: A functional role for 20 α hydroxypregn-4-en-3-one in the rabbit. Endocrinology 80:901-909 (1967).

7. Davidson, J.M.: Feedback regulation of gonadotropin secretion. In Frontiers in Neuroendocrinology (In press) Oxford, New York, (1969).

8. Davidson, J.M. and Bloch, G.J.: Neuroendocrine control of male reproduction. Biology of Reproduction (In press) (1969).

9. Harris, G.W., Michael, R.P. and Scott, P.P.: Neurological site of action of stilbestrol in eliciting sexual behavior. Ciba Foundation Symposium on the Neurological Basis of Behavior, p.236-254 (1958).

10. Lisk, R.D.: Estrogen-sensitive centers in the hypothalamus of the rat. J. Exp. Zool. 145:197-208 (1960).

11. Davidson, J.M. and Sawyer, C.H.: Effects of localized intracerebral implantation of oestrogen on reproductive function of the female rabbit. Acta Endocrin. 37:385-393 (1961).

12. Kanematsu, S. and Sawyer, C.H.: Effects of hypothalamic and hypophysial estrogen implants on pituitary and plasma LH in ovariectomized rabbits. Endocrinology 75:579-585 (1964).

13. Lisk, R.D.: Maintenance of normal pituitary weight and cytology in the spayed rat following estradiol implanted in the arcuate nucleus. Anat. Rec. 146:281-292 (1963).

14. Ramirez, V.D., Abrams, R.M. and McCann, S.M.: Effect of estradiol implants in the hypothalamo-hypophysial region of the rat on the secretion of luteinizing hormone. Endocrinology 75:243-248 (1964).

15. Chowers, I. and McCann, S.M.: Comparison of the effect of hypothalamic and pituitary implants of estrogen and testosterone on reproductive system and adrenal of female rats. Proc. Soc. Exp. Biol. Med. 124:260-266 (1967).

16. Bogdanove, E.M.: Direct gonad-pituitary feedback: an analysis of effects of intracranial estrogenic depots on gonadotrophin secretion. Endocrinology 73:696-712 (1963).

17. Flerko, B. and Szenthgothai, J.: Oestrogen sensitive nervous structures in the hypothalamus. Acta Endocrinol. (Kbh.) 26:121-127 (1957).

18. McCann, S.M.: A hypothalamic luteinizing hormone releasing factor. Amer. J. Physiol. 202:395-400 (1962).

19. Meites, J., Piacsek and Mittler, J.C.: Effects of castration and gonadal steroids on hypothalamic content of FSH-RF and LH-RF. Proc. 2nd Inter. Congr. Hormonal Steroids. Excerpta Med. Intern. Congr. Series No. 132. pp. 958-965 (1966).

20. Docke, F. and Dorner, G.: The mechanism of the induction of ovulation by oestrogens. Journal of Endocrinology 33:491-499 (1965).

21. Smith, E.R. and Davidson, J.M.: Role of estrogen in the cerebral control of puberty in female rats. Endocrinology 82:100-108 (1968).

22. Motta, M., Fraschini, F., Giuliani, G. and Martini, L.: The central nervous system, estrogen and puberty. Endocrinology 83:1101-1107 (1968).

23. Kanematsu, S. and Sawyer, C.H.: Blockade of ovulation in rabbits by hypothalamic implants of norethindrone. Endocrinology 76:691-699 (1965).

24. Dorner, G. and Docke, F.: The influence of intrahypothalamic and intrahypophysial implantation of estrogen or progestogen on gonadotrophin release. Endocrinol. exp. 2:65-71 (1967).

25. Ectors, F. and Pasteels, J.L.: Action antiovulatoire de la medroxyprogesterone, implantee en quantites minimes dans l'hypothalamus anterieur de la ratte. C. R. Acad. Sc., Paris 265:758-760 (1967).

26. Davidson, J.M. and Sawyer, C.H.: Evidence for a hypothalamic focus of inhibition of gonadotropin by androgen in the male. Proc. Soc. Exp. Bio. Med. 107:4-7 (1961).

27. Lisk, R.D.: Testosterone-sensitive centers in the hypothalamus of the rat. Acta Endocrin. (Kbh.) 41:195-204 (1962).

28. Chowers, I. and McCann, S.M.: The effects on ACTH and gonadotropin secretion of implants of gonadal steroids in the hypothalamo-hypophysial region. Israel Med. J. 22:420-432 (1963).

29. Smith, E.R. and Davidson, J.M.: Differential responses to hypothalamic testosterone in relation to male puberty. Amer. J. Physiol. 212:1385-1390 (1967).

30. Smith, E.R. and Davidson, J.M.: Anti-androgen implanted in brain stimulates male reproductive system. Science 155:593-595 (1967).

32. Davidson, J.M.: Activation of the male rat's sexual behavior by intracerebral implantation of androgen. Endocrinology 79:783-794 (1966).

33. Junkmann, K. and Neumann, F.: Zum wirkumgsmechanismus von an fetan antimaskulin wirksamen gestagenen. Acta. Endoc. Suppl. 90:139-154 (1964).

DISCUSSION AND APPENDIX

DISCUSSION

Over fifteen tapes of discussion were monitored in this conference, and while much of the discussion was pertinent, interesting, and even exciting, it was impossible to properly edit it and still achieve our goals - early publication date, a single volume rather than two and as moderate cost as possible. Consequently, the editors have extracted some of the discussion pertinent to the contraceptive agents with emphasis on those comments which give supplementary data or touch upon key interpretations. Most of the comments printed here have been reviewed by the authors and, while edited for brevity and levity, remain intact.

The Editors

EFFECTS ON LIVER AND GASTROINTESTINAL TRACT

E.L. Bierman: Do you have any information on the relative increase of porphyrin precursors or metabolites in the urine of normal females taking various oral contraceptive preparations?

C.S. Song: There are a few studies on a limited number of patients. Burton et al (Lancet ii:1326, 1967) have shown that as many as 26% of normal women taking an oral contraceptive had significant increases in coproporphyrins 1 and 3. Porphyrin precursors such as PBG or ALA were not determined. In porphyric patients, the urinary excretion of these compounds is also increased. The predominant effect in normal subjects appears to be on the excretion of porphyrins rather than the precursors and such effect is not quite as specific as the precursor excretion in determining the derangement of porphyrin metabolism specifically related to ALA synthetase activity.

W.R. Hazzard: Can you confirm and explain the effects of oral contraceptives upon acute intermittent porphyria?

C.S. Song: The sex steroid influence on acute intermittent porphyria is confusing. I can only cite the published records. Oral contraceptives have been implicated as precipitating agents for acute intermittent porphyria. On the other hand, there have been reports that certain sex steroids had ameliorating effects in some individuals. There is no ready biochemical explanation for these effects although it is possible that they might be the result of different dosages or influences on the endogenous production of other porphyrin-inducing substances.

EFFECTS ON CARBOHYDRATE METABOLISM

D.M. Kipnis: Dr. Spellacy, would you comment on your short- and
long-term glucose tolerance tests?

W.N. Spellacy: We have been using the intravenous glucose tolerance
test in our prospective studies. There are no abnormal tests up
through one year of drug ingestion. After two years, four percent
of the tests were abnormal, and after three years, which is as far
as we have gone in that series, there are 12.5% abnormal tests. In
the cross-sectional studies, where we have no prior information on
the subjects and where we used an oral glucose tolerance test, approximately 20% to 30% of the tests are abnormal after five to six
years of drug usage and by ten years approximately 75% of the results are abnormal. These data may be reflecting a number of factors including the type of drug used, the test used, and also the
duration of treatment.

E.M. Gold: I am interested in Dr. Kalkhoff's data because our
findings concur with his in the overt diabetic patient. I would
like to comment on the terms used, i.e., "suppressive effect" because I suspect that some of our difficulties in understanding these
changes are semantic ones. In describing the hyperglycemic effects
seen with oral contraceptives, such terms imply that carbohydrate
utilization has undergone an unfavorable "deterioration" due to
insulin "suppression." However, an elevation in blood glucose
during the estrogen-treated state may not, for all we know, be harmful to the individual. While this may be heresy, particularly here
in the city of Boston, the point merits consideration in view of
considerable evidence which currently questions the long-term
implications of hyperglycemia -- even in established diabetes mellitus.

R.K. Kalkhoff: I called it a suppressed response because the normal, carefully selected, control subject shows a brisk elevation of
plasma insulin during steroid glucose tolerance test, whereas the
same individual treated with an oral contraceptive agent does not
in association with deterioration of the steroid glucose tolerance
test.

E.M. Gold: Does that not assume that the glucose-sensing mechanism
is unchanged? If it were simply reset, i.e., no longer responsive
to the same threshold level of blood glucose, might not similar
changes occur?

R.K. Kalkhoff: I agree. This could be functional rather than an
absolute disturbance and not deleterious. It might be completely
reversible. Nevertheless, there are a few patients in whom subclinical diabetes continues despite the withdrawal of the contraceptive
agent. Then, the question is raised if all cases are reversible.

EFFECTS ON LIPID METABOLISM

R.H. Furman: Dr. Wynn, it seems to me that your data on the young woman with familial hypercholesterolemia are consistent with the view that the oral contraceptive may produce qualitatively, if not quantitatively, changes similar to those occurring in pregnancy. This may reflect the enormous quantities of estrogen produced during the third trimester.

V. Wynn: It's hard to know what the oral contraceptives are doing in relation to metabolism and what pregnancy is doing in relation to metabolism. One cannot compare an alkylated oestrogen combined with an alkylated testosterone derivative or 17-hydroxyprogesterone derivative with the hormones which are produced in pregnancy. This is a fallacy which is so widespread that it really astonishes me that serious individuals can continue to call the oral contraceptive substances "hormones". I doubt if the changes in lipid pattern induced by pregnancy could be explained by hormonal effects on a quantitative basis. First, the serum lipid values start to change at about the sixth month of pregnancy or sooner before there is an obvious increase in cortisol-binding globulin, if one uses this as a quantitative index of oestrogen secretion. Second, in pregnancy, there is a pronounced elevation of the serum cholesterol as well as triglyceride and an increase in high density lipoproteins. Such changes are unlike that found in patients taking as much as four times the usual contraceptive dose.

P. Beck: We have studied fasting serum triglyceride and cholesterol concentrations in women taking three different oral contraceptive agents (Fig. 1). Mean serum triglyceride and cholesterol levels were elevated during pregnancy. Five weeks postpartum, the serum concentrations of these two lipids had declined, but were still higher than normal. Treatment with mestranol-containing oral contraceptive agents (Ovulen or C-Quens) for periods of two weeks to six months produced no further increase in triglyceride or cholesterol levels. Not until six weeks after stopping these agents did fasting serum triglyceride and cholesterol concentrations return to normal. It's worth emphasizing that the triglyceride levels five weeks postpartum were still above normal range even though the carbohydrate tolerance had returned to normal. Moreover, we found no correlation between the basal-insulin levels and the fasting triglyceride concentrations. Subsequently, 20 of these patients were treated with chlormadinone alone (0.5 mg daily) for contraceptive purposes. In these patients fasting serum concentrations of cholesterol and triglycerides have remained normal for intervals ranging from two weeks to six months on chlormadinone. These findings lend support to the thesis that the estrogenic component of oral contraceptive agents increases circulating triglycerides, but I feel it would be wise to examine the nortestosterone derivatives for lipemic activity.

E.L. Bierman: I would like to pose several general questions to the panel of speakers on the lipid effects. First, what might be the role of the lipid alterations produced by oral contraceptives in the production of disease such as atherosclerosis? Are you concerned with such changes in normal young women?

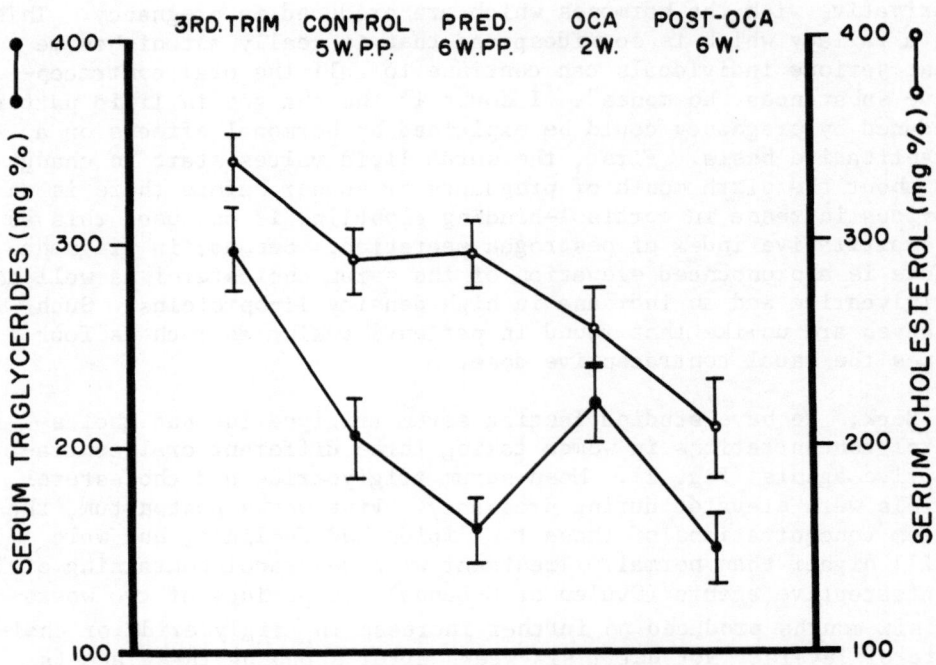

Fig. 1. Mean ± SEM fasting serum triglyceride and cholesterol concentrations in 27 women before, during and after treatment with mestranol 0.08 mg daily or with mestranol 0.1 mg plus ethynodiol diacetate 1 mg daily for 2 weeks. Triglyceride and cholesterol levels in these same women during gestation and following acute challenge with prednisolone (10 mg 2 and 12 hours before testing) 6 weeks postpartum are shown for comparison. (Beck and Wells, in press.)

R.H. Furman: If you consider the normal young woman without any
steroid treatment, she has a serum triglyceride level probably between 50-75 mg per cent; a high proportion of her serum cholesterol
is in the form of high density lipoprotein which is protein and
phospholipid-rich (and, therefore, a very stable particle), and, at
this time of her life, she has the least amount of cholesterol circulating as a beta-lipoprotein. If we now consider the increased
vulnerability to atherosclerosis and coronary artery disease generally extant in the various hyperlipidemic syndromes, one cannot
escape the conclusion that any steroid or environmental change that
increases the amount of cholesterol circulating as lower density
lipoprotein must increase the predisposition to atherogenesis. On
what is a quantitatively important magnitude of change, however, I
am not prepared to draw the line. In some of the epidemiologic
data reported by Oliver and Boyd and by Winkleman, there is evidence
that atherosclerotic complications (specifically manifestations of
coronary heart disease) parallel parity in women, suggesting that
if the gravid state is repeated often enough, it does predispose to
an accelerated atherogenesis.

E.L. Bierman: What is the possibility that a combination of
steroids can be found whose effects on altering lipid transport
would be minimized?

A. Svanborg: I think that we should not discuss the contraceptive
steroids as a group. It may be possible that some are less danger-
ous than others.

R.H. Furman: When we studied, by analytical ultracentrifugation,
the serum lipid effects of combinations of estrogens and androgens,
in what we might regard as physiologically equivalent doses, androgen completely wiped out the estrogen effect. So it is conceivable
that a weak androgenic-anabolic agent in an oral contraceptive
combination could eliminate the triglyceride effect of the estrogen
without eliminating the ovulatory suppressive effect.

U.S. Seal: It would be worthwhile to consider that these compounds
have different activities on a molar basis. The direct comparison
of two substances is suggestive but dose-response curves should be
done. In dose-response studies which we have done with a number of
estrogens, we found as much as hundred-fold differences between
several of the substances on a molar basis. Premarin, for example,
has about 1/100 of the activity and diethylstilbestrol about one-
tenth of the activity of ethinyl estradiol on a weight basis in
seven systems which we examined.

DISCUSSION

TABLE I

EFFECT OF ORAL CONTRACEPTIVES ON BLOOD PRESSURE

Subject	Age	Oral Agent	Average B.P. mm Hg Before O.C.P.	During O.C.P.	After O.C.P.	Months on OCP before known BP>150/100	Months off OCP before BP<145/95	Comments
J.P.+	22	Enovid	128/80	170/120	140/95	12	8	
J.P.*+	24	Enovid	140/95	170/110		1		Still under observation
J.G.	30	Enovid Provest	132/92	185/95	130/80	6	7	
J.G.*	31	C-Quens	130/70	180/90	132/80	7	4	
L.T.	39	C-Quens	110/70	192/106	116/76	24	1	Normal aortogram
S.L.	52	Norlestrin	126/80	200/120	140/60	22	.5	Mild recurrent hypertension
P.E.	48	Norlestrin	124/75	200/100	140/80	11	6	Diabetic GTT
C.B.	31	Norinyl	110/80	170/110	120/88	8	¼	
P.M.	20	three kinds	130/70	210/110	130/70	24	1.5	Severe headaches
J.Si.	24	Orthonovum	126/68	162/100	142/82	52	1	
S.M.	42	Orthonovum	122/75	200/115	134/84	72	3	Mild recurrent hypertension
C.H.	27	Orthonovum	130/70	180/110	130/88	8	1	Severe headaches
P.C.	43	Provest Norlestrin	125/72	190/98	124/80	2	5	Diabetic GTT - Severe headaches
B.A.	32	Enovid	130/80	238/130	120/80	60	5	Normal aortogram
C.M.	48	Premarin (not OCP)	135/70	180/110	134/84	5	3	
Average 35.2			125/76	191/110	131/81	23.5	3.6	

*Repeat course not included in average.

+B.P. could be brought to normal with Aldactone while taking O.C.P.

HYPERTENSION

M.G. Crane: I would like to present some data on a group of
patients who developed hypertension while on oral contraceptives.
We have been able to document that their blood pressures were normal before starting the pills. The first table (Table 1) shows
the length of time that the patients were treated before hypertension was discovered. Quite likely, the hypertension had been present for several months before it was recognized. In some instances
the patients were followed well enough to know that they had been
normotensive for as long as four years (one patient) on the medication before they developed hypertension.

The second table (Table 2) presents the data on six other
patients who developed hypertension after starting on oral contraceptives and who have not yet had a return of blood pressure to
normal since discontinuing the pills. Perhaps, after further time
will have elapsed, their blood pressures will return to normal.

TABLE 2

EFFECT OF ORAL CONTRACEPTIVES ON BLOOD PRESSURE

Subject	Age	Oral Con- traceptive	Average B.P. mm Hg Before O.C.P.	During O.C.P.	After O.C.P.	Mos. on OCP before known B.P. >150/100	Months follow- up off O.C.P.
S.H.	26	Ovulen	130/80	165/115	140/98	6	6
N.S.[2]	32	Orthonovum	120/62	170/120	146/100	48	2
B.S.[2,4]	30	Orthonovum	120/60	185/120	130/94*	48	6
J.S.[-2]	34	Orthonovum	108/84	170/110	150/100	48	1
H.P.[1]	31	Norlutin Provest	120/80	150/110	112/94*	12	6
L.H.[3]	25	Enovid	114/76	214/140		24	1
Average	30		120/75	185/121		35.1	

*Value while on Aldactone
1. B.P. could be brought to normal with Aldactone while taking O.C.P.
2. Normal Aortogram
3. Fibromuscular hyperplasia. Deceased postoperatively.
4. We thank Dr. Fred Havens, Jr. for permission to use the results
   of patient B.S.

The third table (Table 3) shows preliminary results of plasma renin activity (PRA) and aldosterone excretion rates on certain of the patients cited above. First, the PRA values were significantly lower three to six weeks after the contraceptive agent was discontinued than during its administration, and in the few patients studied, the PRA values tended to increase slightly in the third set of observations. Second, four of seven patients had suppressed PRA values at the three-six week period.

TABLE 3

EFFECT OF ORAL CONTRACEPTIVES ON PLASMA RENIN ACTIVITY
AND ALDOSTERONE EXCRETION

Subject	PRA: Normal Na$^+$ Supine			PRA: Low Na$^+$ Upright			Urinary Aldosterone	
	On OCP	Off OCP 3-6 wk	Off OCP 5-8 mo	On OCP	Off OCP 3-6 wk	Off OCP 5-8 mo	On OCP	Off OCP 3-6 wk
S.L.	66	69	150	363	263	180	4.1	4.7
P.E.	260	110	150	520	110	280	15.3	4.2
C.B.	500	90	260	1000	270	560	15.4	10.3
C.H.	170	100		720	790		12.7	3.8
N.S.	270	71		750	213		11.2	3.7
C.M.*	6	72	150	220	272	820	7.8	6.1
J.Si.	90	99		895	520		9.0	
S.H.	380	250	260	905	553	200	17.0	15.0
L.T.	530		230	2188		360	22.7	
L.H.	1700			7380			38.7	
B.S.	15			3000			27.0	

*C.M. took Premarin.
Note: PRA units = ng of Angiotensin II/100 ml plasma.
       Urinary aldosterone - µg/24 hours.

I do not know how to predict which patients are likely to develop hypertension on the medication. Perhaps, those patients have a predisposition to hypertension.

EFFECTS ON THE VASCULAR SYSTEM

E.L. Bierman: Dr. Doll, the striking difference observed in cerebral as compared to coronary thrombosis in the British studies suggests that atherosclerosis may not be an underlying factor in the pathogenesis of the observed thrombosis. My first question is: do the autopsy findings in the deaths from cerebral thrombosis confirm the idea that atherosclerosis was not an underlying problem in women below age forty? The second question relates to the lipid session. In view of the striking alterations in lipid transport and in the concentration of circulating lipoproteins, atherosclerosis might eventually become a problem. Do you plan on extending your studies in such a way as to detect this phenomenon in older age women, namely forty to fifty?

R. Doll: We do not plan to extend our studies to cover older age groups. I am afraid I cannot give any direct answer to the first question as no detailed examination was made of the state of the cerebral arteries in women who developed cerebral thrombosis. I would say, however, that the fact that an agent is related to thrombosis in one set of arteries but not in another is not necessarily surprising. There is ample epidemiological evidence that the environmental factors that predispose to cerebral thrombosis are different from those that predispose to coronary thrombosis. Cigarette smoking, for example, is related to coronary thrombosis but not to cerebral thrombosis and one condition occurs commonly in some populations (for example, the United States and Finland) while the other occurs commonly in others (for example, in Japan and in the African populations of South Africa).

M. Novy: Dr. Doll, frequently in making judgments about the use of oral contraceptives, one is asked what the relative risk of embolism in pregnancy is. Would you comment on this?

R. Doll: I hate having to compare the risks of using oral contraceptives with the risk of pregnancy because oral contraceptives may be taken daily for years and, in the absence of oral contraceptives, even the best women are not pregnant all of the time. A direct comparison is, therefore, extremely difficult. The sort of question you might ask is: what is the balance of risk between taking oral contraceptives for say, ten years, and the effect of the number of pregnancies a woman might expect to have over the same period using other methods of contraception? As a first approximation, the risk of thrombo-embolism from one year's use of oral contraceptives is about the same as the risk associated with one pregnancy.

DRUGS CITED IN TEXT

Many drugs are cited in the text by trade name or various
trivial names. For convenience, a summary of most of these drugs
is tabulated below. The Roman numerals in parentheses refer to the
chemical structures on the following pages. This list is not complete and dosages and treatment regimens have been omitted although
the "sequential drugs" are marked with asterisks. Additional information should be sought in the original references or in the pharm-
aceutical literature.

Drug	Manufacturer	Composition (Structure Number)
Anovlar	Schering	Norethindrone Acetate (XIII) Ethinyl Estradiol (III)
C-Quens*	Lilly	Chlormadinone Acetate (XX) Mestranol (IV)
Delalutin	Squibb	Hydroxyprogesterone Caproate (XVII)
Delpregnin	Nova Industri A/S	Megestrol Acetate (XIX) Mestranol (IV)
Duphaston	Philips Roxane	Dydrogesterone (XXI)
Enovid	Searle	Norethynodrel (VIII) Mestranol (IV)
Lormin	Lilly	Chlormadinone Acetate (XX) Mestranol (IV)
Lyndiol	Organon	Lynestrenol (XII) Mestranol (IV)
Norinyl	Syntex	Norethindrone (XI) Mestranol (IV)
Norlestrin	Parke-Davis	Norethindrone (XI) Ethinyl Estradiol (III)
Norlutate	Parke-Davis	Norethindrone (XI)
Oracon*	Mead Johnson	Dimethisterone (XIV) Ethinyl Estradiol (III)
Ortho-Novum	Ortho	Norethindrone (XI) Mestranol (IV)

Ovral	Wyeth	Norgestrel (d-norgestrel) (XV)
		Ethinyl Estradiol (III)
Ovulen	Searle	Ethynodiol Diacetate (VII)
		Mestranol (IV)
Premarin	Ayerst	Equilin Sulfate (20-30%) (VI)
		Estrone Sulfate (50-60%) (V)
Provera	Upjohn	Medroxyprogesterone Acetate (XVIII)
Provest	Upjohn	Medroxyprogesterone Acetate (XVIII)
		Ethinyl Estradiol (III)

STRUCTURES

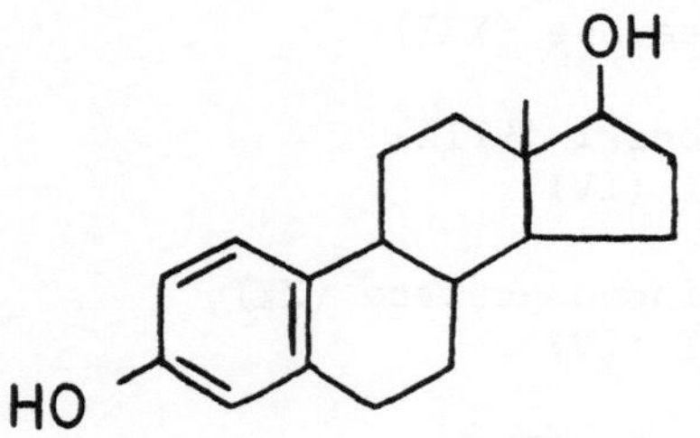

Estradiol
I

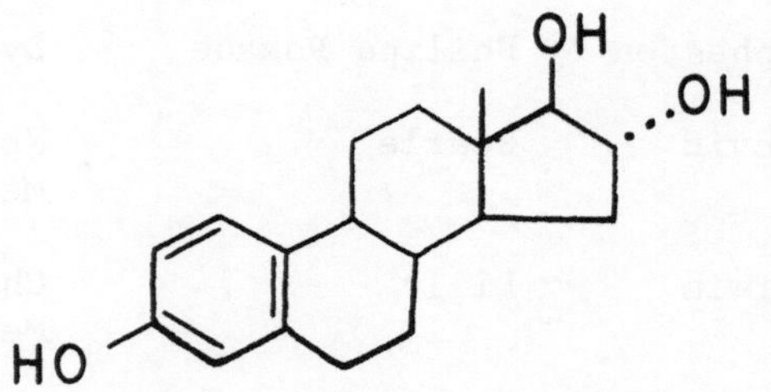

Estriol
II

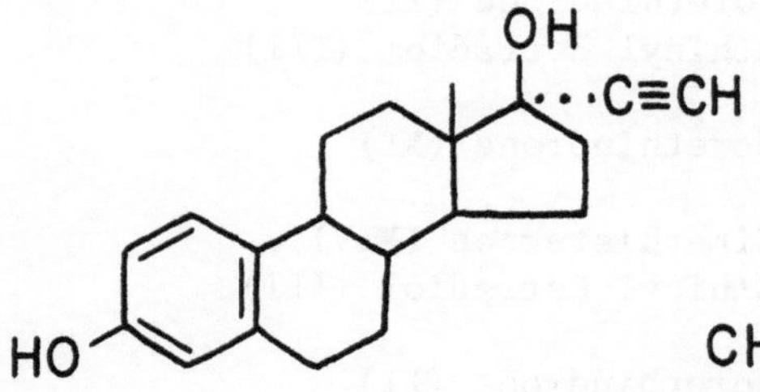

Ethinyl Estradiol
III

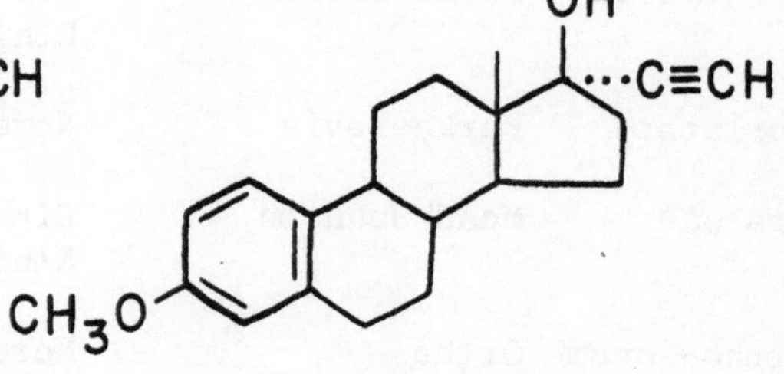

Mestranol
IV

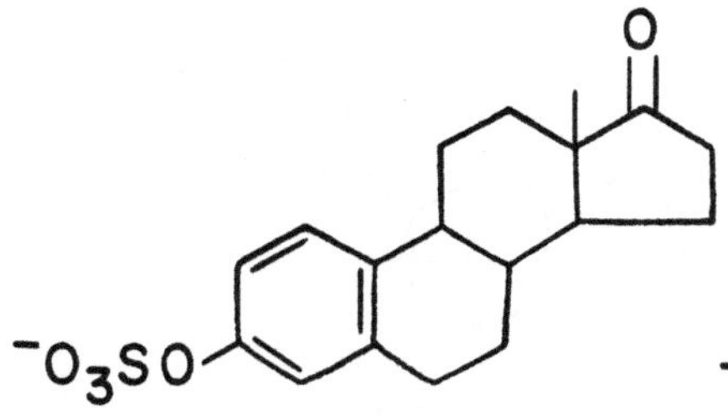

Estrone Sulfate
V

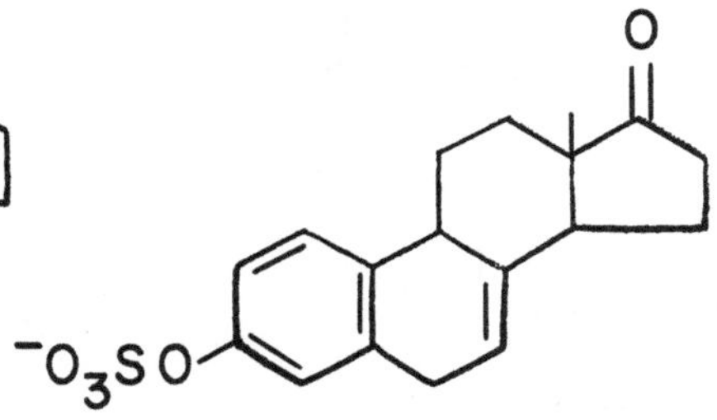

Equilin Sulfate
VI

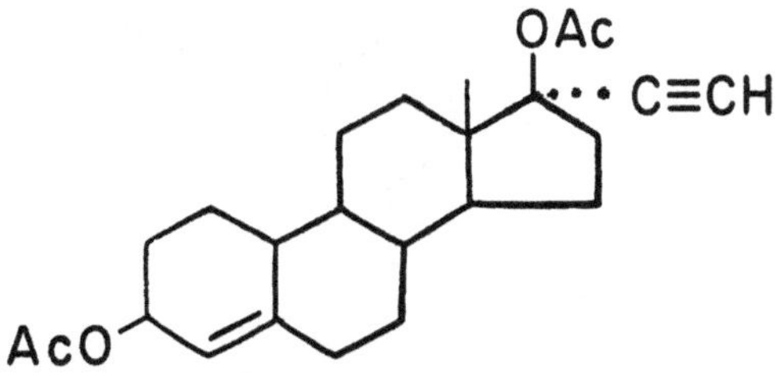

Ethynodiol Diacetate
VII

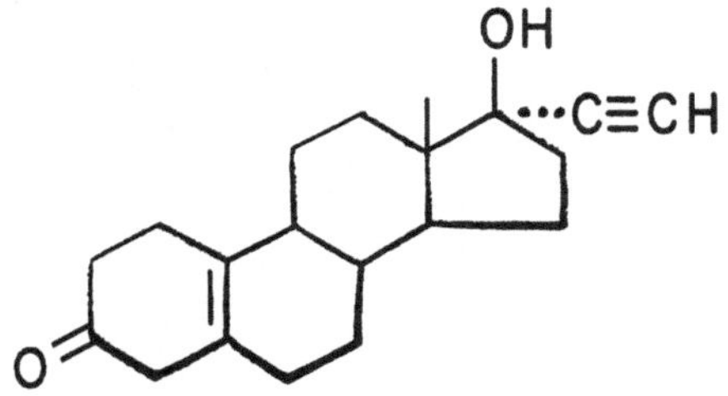

Norethynodrel
VIII

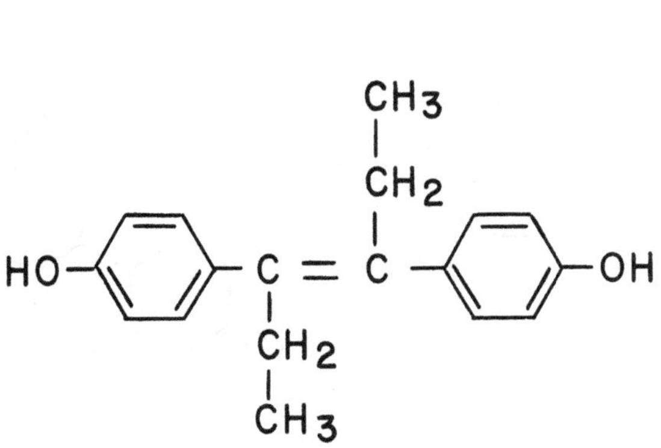

Diethylstilbestrol
IX

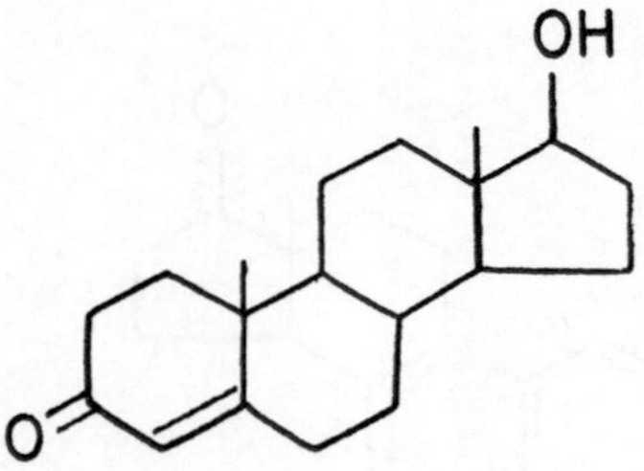

Testosterone
X

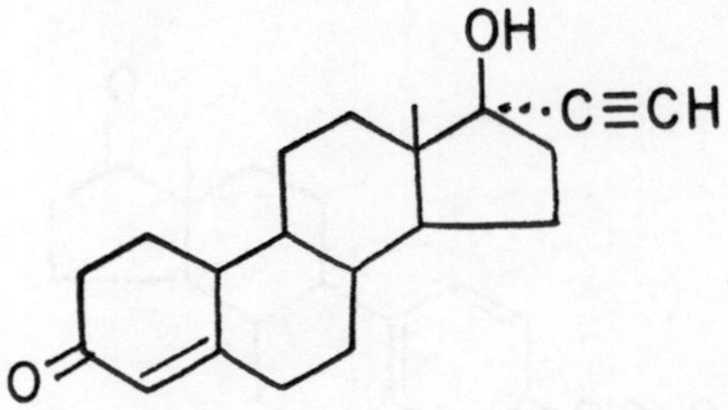

Norethindrone
XI

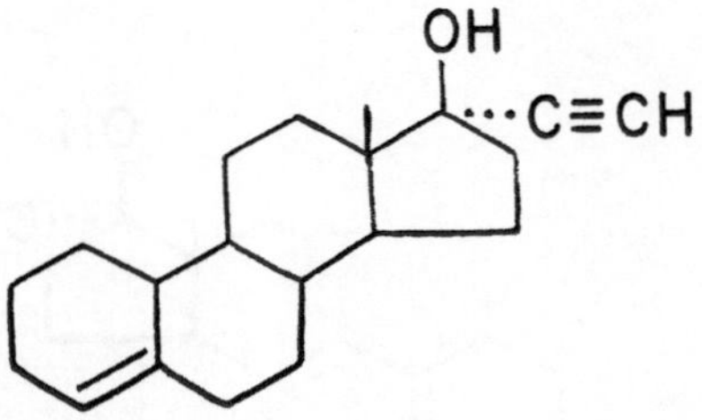

Lynestrenol
XII

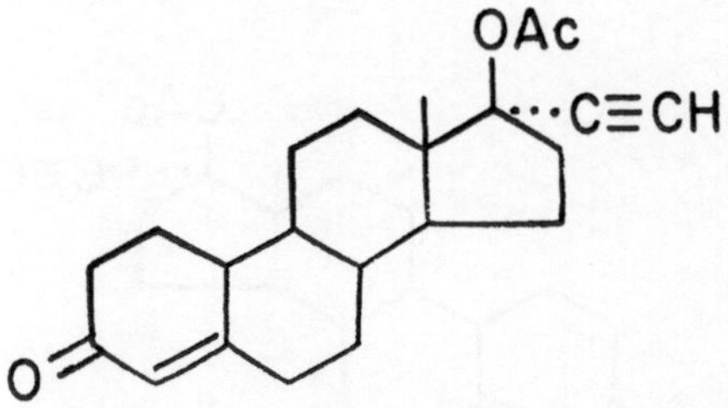

Norethindrone Acetate
XIII

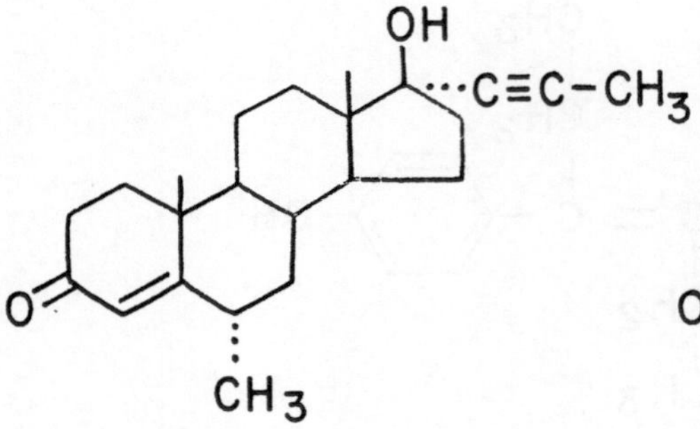

Dimethisterone
XIV

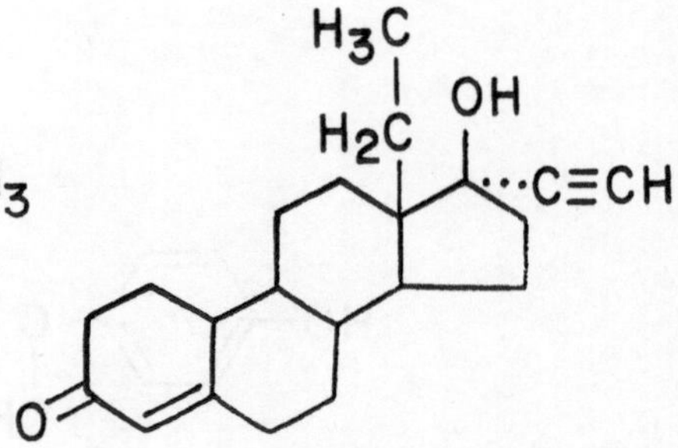

Norgestrel
(d-norgestrel)
XV

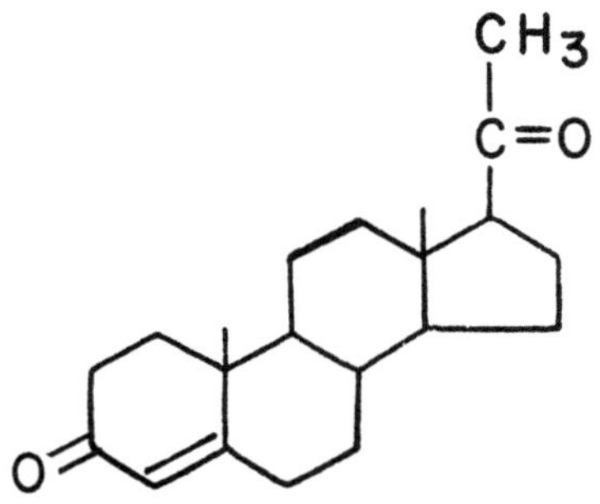

Progesterone
XVI

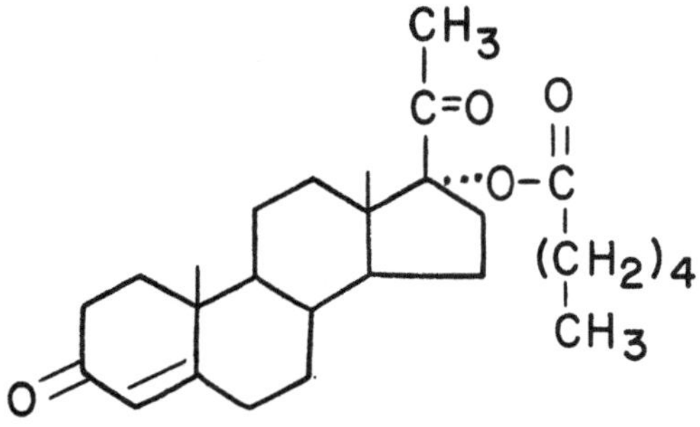

Hydroxyprogesterone Caproate
XVII

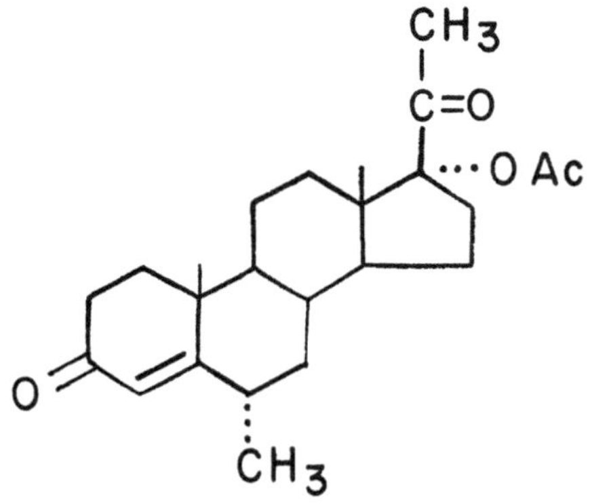

Medroxyprogesterone Acetate
XVIII

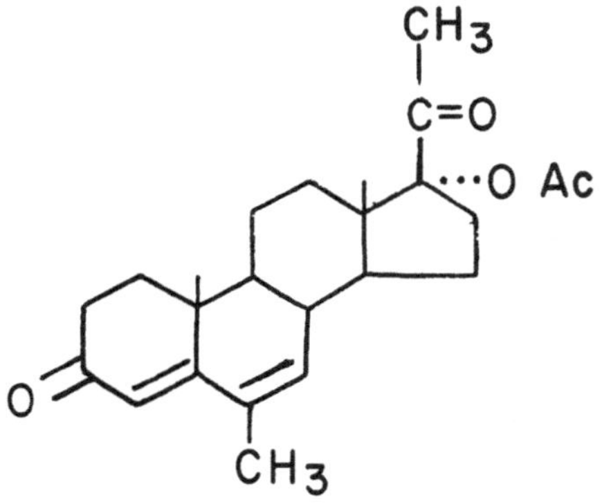

Megestrol Acetate
XIX

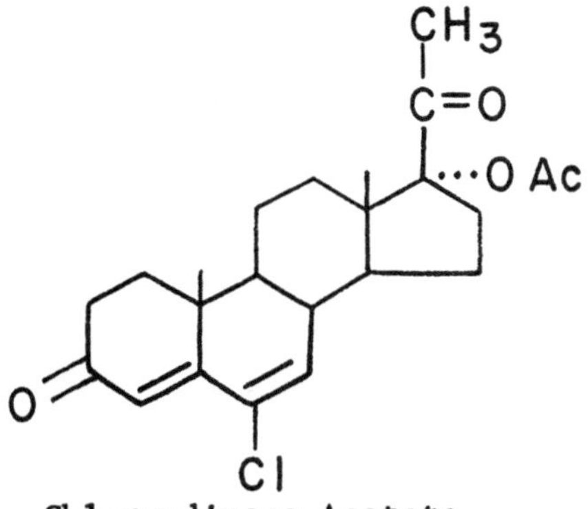

Chlormadinone Acetate
XX

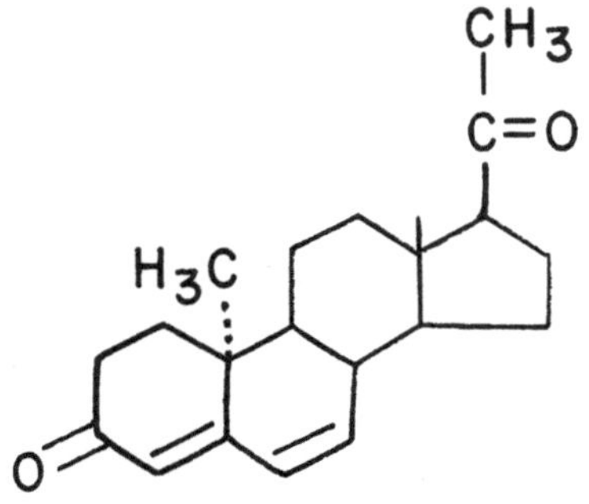

Dydrogesterone
XXI

Hydroxyprogesterone caproate
XVI

Progesterone
XV

Megestrol Acetate
XIX

Medroxyprogesterone acetate
XVIII

Hydrogesterone
XXI

Chlormadinone Acetate
XX

INDEX